PROGRESS IN HEMODIALYSIS – FROM EMERGENT BIOTECHNOLOGY TO CLINICAL PRACTICE

Edited by **Angelo Carpi, Carlo Donadio**
and **Gianfranco Tramonti**

Progress in Hemodialysis – From Emergent Biotechnology to Clinical Practice
Edited by Angelo Carpi, Carlo Donadio and Gianfranco Tramonti

Published by InTech

Janeza Trdine 9, 51000 Rijeka, Croatia

Publishing Process Manager Masa Vidovic

Technical Editor Teodora Smiljanic

Cover Designer InTech Design Team

Additional hard copies can be obtained from orders@intechopen.com

Progress in Hemodialysis – From Emergent Biotechnology to Clinical Practice,
Edited by Angelo Carpi, Carlo Donadio and Gianfranco Tramonti
p. cm.
ISBN 978-953-307-377-4

For EU product safety concerns:
IN TECH d.o.o., Prolaz Marije Krucifikse Kozulić 3, 51000 Rijeka, Croatia,
info@intechopen.com or visit our website at intechopen.com.

Meet the editors

Dr. Angelo Carpi is a clinical professor of medicine and Director of the Division of Male Infertility of the Department of Reproduction and Aging in the Pisa University Medical School, Pisa, Italy. He earned his M.D. and postgraduate degrees in internal medicine and nuclear medicine from the University of Pisa, as well as a diploma of qualification on peptide hormones from the Collegio Medico Giuridico-Scuola Normale Superiore and the Scuola Superiore Sant'Anna, Pisa, Italy. He is the author of about 300 publications, member of editorial boards of the international journals Biomedicine & Pharmacotherapy and Frontiers in Bioscience and organizer of 52 scientific meetings and editor of 20 books often including nephrologic aspects. Additional information at www.carpimed.it.

Professor Carlo Donadio is the clinical professor of nephrology and Director of the Laboratory of Renal Functional Evaluation and of the hemodialysis unit at Pisa University. He is also Director of the Master Course of Dialytic Treatment of Renal Failure held at the Department of Internal Medicine of Pisa University. Professor Donadio graduated as M.D. and post-graduated in internal medicine, nephrology, and nuclear medicine at Pisa University. His major research interests and clinical activities are in different nephrological topics, from the patho-physiology of renal diseases, through the validation of methods to measure renal function in man, the assessment of new serum and urinary markers of glomerular and tubular impairment, the evaluation and prevention of nephrotoxicity due to drugs and contrast media. Studies in chronic kidney disease (CKD) patients addressed the evaluation of bone turnover and parathyroid hormone, the inflammatory status, the global approach to the cardiovascular risk, the analysis of body composition and nutritional status in CKD, renal transplant recipients and maintenance hemodialysis patients. Recently, Prof. Donadio applied proteomic techniques to the study of patho-physiology of uremic syndrome and to the evaluation of depurative and inflammatory characteristics of resins, high and low-flux membranes for hemodialysis.

Professor Gianfranco Tramonti is the clinical professor of nephrology at the Department of Internal Medicine at the Pisa University Medical School, Pisa, Italy. He earned his M.D. and postgraduate degrees in internal medicine, nuclear medicine and nephrology from the University of Pisa. He also attended as visiting professor at Northwestern University of Chicago Medical School from November 1999 through October 2000, from July 2003 through November 2003 and from December 2010 through March 2011. Field of research: renal function and new markers to detect renal function, renal metabolism of low molecular weight proteins, nephrotoxicity, activity and expression of tubular cell transporters in vivo and in renal tubular cell line cultures. His research activities have produced more than 50 publications, most of which on nephrology.

Contents

Preface

Hemodialysis (HD) represents the first successful long term substitutive therapy with an artificial organ for severe failure of a vital organ. Because HD was started many decades ago, a book on HD may not appear up-to-date.

Indeed, HD covers many basic and clinical aspects and this book reflects the rapid expansion of new and controversial aspects either in the biotechnological or in the clinical field.

The related topics are multiple because HD includes either biotechnology or multi-organ involvement as well as different pathogenetic factors. Many efforts to reduce dialysis complications and their treatment are made. This book revises new technologies and therapeutic options to improve dialysis treatment of uremic patients.

This book consists of three parts:

- modeling, methods and technique
- prognosis
- complications

The first part includes twelve chapters, five on modeling, water and electrolyte preparation or regulation, four face membranes and biocompatibility, the remaining three deal with procedures or controversies.

Besides important progress in biotechnology, a common and principal aim crossing most of these chapters is the attempt to reduce morbidity by the use of more compatible devices.

Prediction of morbidity or mortality by progress in the laboratory is a principal general topic or aim of the second group of four chapters. These chapters underline the relevance of the residual renal function and of the main laboratory biomarkers to predict cardiovascular complications.

The third part includes seven chapters on clinical complications. The principal topic crossing two chapters is the importance of metabolic disorders for the origin and the development of the most important clinical complications (cardiovascular and bone).

The remaining five chapters deal with lifestyle aspects (sleep or physical activity) and local (vascular access) or systemic (infections) complications.

Therefore, this book reflects either emergent biotechnological or updated clinical aspects concerning HD. These two topics include suggestions to improve prognosis and therapy of the patients on HD.

The book will help not only general physicians, nephrologists, internists, cardiologists, endocrinologists but also basic researchers, including bioengineers, to approach, understand and manage the principal problems related to HD.

Finally, we consider that we were medical students in the same university hospital in the sixties and successively we worked in the same university hospital department. Our original department of internal medicine specialized in nephrology, under the leadership of the late Prof. Gabriele Monasterio, who first proposed and validated the low protein diet and included teachers who were pioneers in projecting and using the artificial kidney.

Thanks to them, the authors of these book chapters and the publisher, we once more have the pleasure to work together in this project including colleagues from multiple continents.

Prof. Angelo Carpi, M.D.,
Department of Reproduction and Aging, University of Pisa,
Italy

Prof. Carlo Donadio, M.D.,
Department of Internal Medicine, University of Pisa,
Italy

Prof. Gianfranco Tramonti, M.D.,
Department of Internal Medicine, University of Pisa,
Italy

Part 1

Modeling, Methods and Technique

1

Kinetic Modeling and Adequacy of Dialysis

Malgorzata Debowska[1], Bengt Lindholm[2] and Jacek Waniewski[1]
[1]*Institute of Biocybernetics and Biomedical Engineering, Polish Academy of Sciences, Warsaw,*
[2]*Divisions of Baxter Novum and Renal Medicine, Karolinska Institutet, Stockholm,*
[1]*Poland*
[2]*Sweden*

1. Introduction

The mathematical description of hemodialysis (HD) includes two parts: 1) explanation of the exchange between patient's blood and dialysate fluid across a semipermeable membrane of the dialyzer, and 2) characterization of the solute removal from the patient. The solute transport across the dialyzer membrane depends on the difference in hydrostatic pressure and solute concentration gradients between both sides of the membrane and also on the permeability of the membrane to the solute. The local equations for solute and fluid transport through the membrane are based on a phenomenological (thermodynamic) description according to the Staverman-Kedem-Katchalsky-Spiegler approach (Staverman, 1951; Kedem & Katchalsky, 1958; Katchalsky & Curran, 1965; Spiegler & Kedem, 1966). The two compartment model describes the functioning of the patient – dialyzer system, assuming that body fluid is divided into two parts: one directly (extracellular compartment) and one indirectly (intracellular compartment) accessible for dialysis (Schneditz & Daugirdas, 2001). The one compartment model of the solute distribution volume assumes that the solute is distributed in a single, homogenous pool. Solute kinetic modeling is based on a set of ordinary differential equations describing the changes of solute mass, concentration and distribution volume in body compartments and in the dialyzer. Using solute kinetic modeling one is able to evaluate dialysis efficiency.
The question concerning dialysis dosing has been debated and remains controversial since the beginning of the dialysis treatment era. Between 1976 and 1981, the National Cooperative Dialysis Study (NCDS) was performed in the United States to establish objective, quantitative criteria for the adequate dose of dialysis (Gotch & Sargent, 1985; Sargent & Gotch, 1989; Locatelli et al., 2005). The primary analysis showed that morbidity was less at lower levels of time average urea concentration. The secondary 'mechanistic' analysis of the NCDS data done by Gotch and Sargent launched the issue of urea KT/V (Gotch & Sargent, 1985).
Single-pool KT/V overestimates the removed amount of urea because of the postdialysis urea rebound, i.e., a fast postdialysis increase in urea concentration in plasma, which is a compartmental effect; therefore, the equilibrated KT/V (eqKT/V), estimated by the Daugirdas formula, was introduced to clinical practice (Daugirdas et al., 2001). Equilibrated KT/V values can be also calculated using an alternative equation by Daugirdas and

Schneditz (Daugirdas & Schneditz, 1995), or the formula derived from observations during the HEMO Study (Depner et al., 1999; Eknoyan et al., 2002; Daugirdas et al., 2004), or that introduced by Tattersall et al. (Tattersall et al., 1996).

The usage of the KT/V index as a sole and optimal measure of dialysis dose is questioned by many authors. Fractional solute removal (FSR) and equivalent continuous clearance (ECC) are two such alternative options, which can be used instead of KT/V. FSR was suggested by Verrina et al. (Verrina et al., 1998) and Henderson (Henderson, 1999) for comparative studies of various dialysis modalities and schedules. By definition FSR is the removed mass over the reference solute mass in the body. The concept of FSR is closely related to the concept of the solute removal index (SRI) proposed by Keshaviah (Keshaviah, 1995). Standard KT/V (stdKT/V), introduced by Gotch, is another variant of FSR (Gotch, 1998). The time-average solute concentration (C_{ta}) has been introduced to define 'equivalent renal clearance' (EKR), as a solute removal rate over C_{ta} (Casino & Lopez, 1996). Using other reference concentrations in the definition of EKR instead of C_{ta}, the general idea of equivalent continuous clearance, ECC, can be formulated (Waniewski et al., 2006; Waniewski et al., 2010). There are at least four different reference methods: 1) peak, p, 2) peak average, pa, 3) time average, ta, and 4) treatment time average, trta, reference values of volume, mass, and concentration applied in KT/V, FSR and ECC (Waniewski et al., 2006; Waniewski et al., 2010). KT/V, FSR and ECC are mathematically related for the same reference method. However, the choice of an adequacy index and the respective reference method is not obvious. It is not possible to decide whether this or the other definition is better although some authors have declared their preferences (Keshaviah, 1995; Casino & Lopez, 1996; Verrina et al., 1998; Henderson, 1999). The difference between different hypotheses and the indices based on them may be investigated theoretically, but the choice, if any, may be done only on the basis of a large set of clinical data. Future research should hopefully provide more information about the relationship between various definitions and the probability of clinical outcome in dialyzed patients.

Recent studies report some advantages of low-efficiency, frequent schedule over short, high-efficiency HD (Depner, 1998; Charra et al., 2004). The two compartment variable volume urea kinetic model can be applied to examine the whole set of dialysis adequacy indices in different dialysis treatments, e.g. 1) conventional HD with 3 sessions per week, 2) daily HD with 6 sessions per week and 3) nocturnal HD with 6 long sessions using typical patient and treatment parameters. The peak average reference method used in FSR and ECC calculations seem to be a more sensitive to the frequency and time of dialysis than the method based on time average reference (Waniewski et al., 2006; Waniewski et al., 2010).

The unified approach to the definition of dialysis adequacy indices proposed by Waniewski et al. is valid for all modalities of dialysis performed in end-stage renal disease and acute renal failure patients and for the assessment of residual renal function (Waniewski et al., 2006; Debowska et al., 2010; Waniewski et al., 2010). The integrated system of dialysis adequacy indices takes into account all currently applied indices and allows to explain their relationships and specificities.

The theory and practical application of this system of adequacy indices are here presented on the basis of our previous publications and a (unpublished) PhD thesis (Waniewski & Lindholm, 2004; Debowska & Waniewski, 2005; Debowska et al., 2005; Waniewski et al., 2006; Debowska et al., 2007a; Debowska et al., 2007b; Debowska et al., 2010; Waniewski et al., 2010).

2. Theory of fluid and solute transport in hemodialysis

The mathematical description of hemodialysis includes two parts: 1) one part that explains the fluid and solute transport across a semi-permeable membrane of the dialyzer, and 2) one part that characterizes the global solute transport between removal device and patient.

2.1 Solute and fluid transport in dialyzer

The fluid and solute transport in dialyzer consists of two processes: transport through a permselective membrane between blood and dialysate and transport in blood and dialysate channels.

The theoretical description of transport through a permselective membrane is based on phenomenological (thermodynamic) descriptions according to the Staverman-Kedem-Katchalsky-Spiegler approach (Staverman, 1951; Kedem & Katchalsky, 1958; Katchalsky & Curran, 1965; Spiegler & Kedem, 1966; Weryński & Nowosielcew, 1983; Werynski & Waniewski, 1995; Waniewski, 2006). Diffusion is the dominant factor for small solute transport in hemodialyzer. The transport due to convection prevails in hemofilters, plasma separators, etc. In hemodialyzer with highly permeable membrane used in hemodiafiltration, the convective transport component plays a leading role in the removal of middle molecules and small proteins (Werynski & Waniewski, 1995).

Considering the dialyzer as shown in Fig. 1, the system will soon after the start of dialysis be at the quasi-steady state with the mass balance:

$$Q_{b,i}C_{b,i} + Q_{d,i}C_{d,i} = \left(Q_{b,i} - Q_v\right)C_{b,o} + \left(Q_{d,i} + Q_v\right)C_{d,o} \tag{1}$$

where $Q_{b,o} = Q_{b,i} - Q_v$ and $Q_{d,o} = Q_{d,i} + Q_v$ are the rates of blood and dialysate flows at the outlet of hemodialyzer, respectively, Q_v is ultrafiltration rate, $C_{b,i}$ and $C_{d,i}$ are the inlet blood and dialysate concentrations and $C_{b,o}$ and $C_{d,o}$ are the outlet blood and dialysate concentrations, respectively.

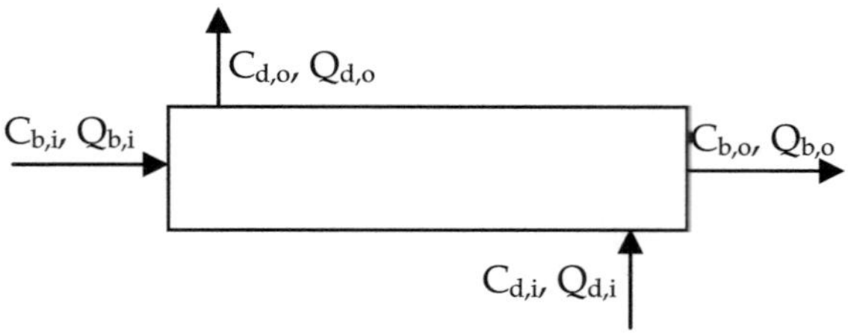

Fig. 1. Schematic description of concentration and flows in dialyzer.

After rearrangement of equation (1):

$$Q_{b,i}\left(C_{b,i} - C_{b,o}\right) + Q_v C_{b,o} = Q_{d,i}\left(C_{d,o} - C_{d,i}\right) + Q_v C_{d,o} \tag{2}$$

The left side of equation (2) represents the solute leaving the blood; the right side is the solute appearing in dialysate. The first term on each side of equation (2) is the diffusive component of flux and the second term represents the convective contribution.

At any specific blood and dialysis fluid flow rates, the diffusive dialysance D is the change in solute amount of incoming blood over concentration driving force ($C_{b,i} - C_{d,i}$):

$$D = \frac{Q_{b,i}\left(C_{b,i} - C_{b,o}\right)}{C_{b,i} - C_{d,i}} = \frac{Q_{d,i}\left(C_{d,o} - C_{d,i}\right)}{C_{b,i} - C_{d,i}} \tag{3}$$

Assuming that solute concentration in the inflowing dialysate is zero ($C_{d,i} = 0$) equation (3) yields the definition of diffusive clearance K:

$$K = \frac{Q_{b,i}\left(C_{b,i} - C_{b,o}\right)}{C_{b,i}} \tag{4}$$

Dialyzer clearance is a parameter that describes the efficiency of membrane devices, i.e. the solute removal rate from the blood related to blood solute concentration at the inlet to the hemodialyzer (Darowski et al., 2000; Waniewski, 2006).

Ultrafiltration Q_v from blood to dialysate increases diffusive solute transport from blood to dialysate and therefore the clearance of the hemodialyzer or hemofilter may be described as:

$$K = K_0 + T_r \cdot Q_v \tag{5}$$

where K_0 is the diffusive clearance for $Q_v = 0$ and T_r is the transmittance coefficient (Werynski & Waniewski, 1995; Darowski et al., 2000; Waniewski, 2006). Although the dependence of K on Q_v in the one-dimensional theory is slightly nonlinear, one may assume the linear description used in equation (5) that was confirmed experimentally with high accuracy (Waniewski et al., 1991). T_r may be estimated from the experimental data using the equation:

$$T_r = \frac{K - K_0}{Q_v} \tag{6}$$

The measurements of K_0 and K for a few different values of Q_v allow determining T_r using equation (6) and linear regression.

2.2 One and two compartment models for the distribution of fluid and solutes in the body

Compartment models consider the patient body as a single compartment (thick line in Fig. 2) or as two compartments: intracellular and extracellular (dashed line in Fig. 2).

The one compartment model of the solute distribution volume assumes that solute mass, M_b, is distributed in the body in a single, homogenous pool of volume V_b with concentration C_b. The two compartment model assumes that body fluid is divided into two parts: one directly (extracellular compartment, described by solute mass M_e, concentration C_e and fluid volume V_e) and one indirectly (intracellular compartment, with solute mass M_i, concentration C_i and fluid volume V_i) accessible for dialysis (Schneditz & Daugirdas, 2001). It is assumed that solute generation, at the rate G, and water intake, at the rate G_w, occur only in the extracellular space. In the two compartment model, solute and water removal by the kidneys, with clearances K_r and K_{rw}, respectively, are also related only to the extracellular compartment.

Some authors use more general terminology for the two compartment model with perfused and non-perfused compartments, without deciding a priori about their physiological interpretation. This terminology may be used for the description of the distribution of small

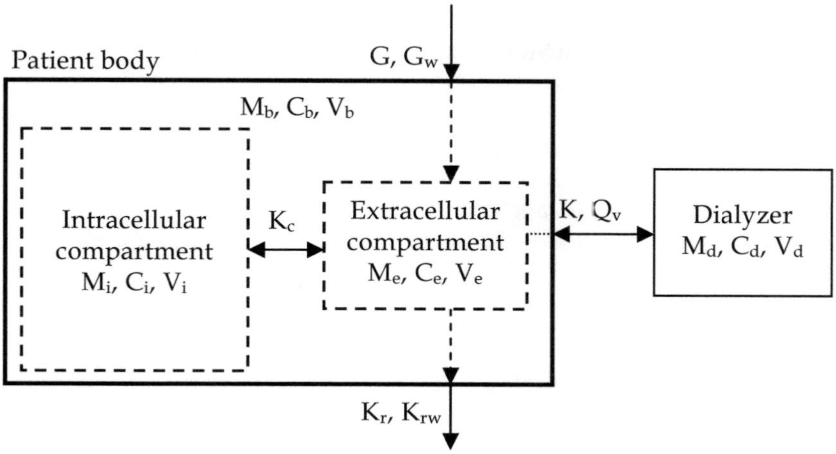

Fig. 2. One and two compartment models for the distribution of water and solutes in the body.

solutes (as urea and creatinine) and proteins (as β_2-microglobulin). In some papers, extracellular and intracellular water were called perfused and non-perfused compartments, respectively (Clark et al., 1999; Leypoldt et al., 2003; Leypoldt et al., 2004).

In one compartment model the rate of the change of solute mass in the body, $dM_b/dt = d(C_bV_b)/dt$, and in dialysate, $dM_d/dt = d(C_dV_d)/dt$, during hemodialysis, are described by the following ordinary differential equations:

$$\begin{cases} \dfrac{d(C_bV_b)}{dt} = G - K(C_b - C_d) - K_rC_b \\ \dfrac{d(C_dV_d)}{dt} = K(C_b - C_d) \end{cases} \tag{7}$$

In the two compartment model, the removal of solute by the dialyzer with clearance K and by the kidneys with residual clearance K_r, is a function of the solute concentration in the extracellular compartment, C_e, but indirectly depends also on the intercompartmental mass transport coefficient K_c:

$$\begin{cases} \dfrac{d(V_eC_e)}{dt} = K_c(C_i - C_e) - K(C_e - C_d) + G - K_rC_e \\ \dfrac{d(V_iC_i)}{dt} = -K_c(C_i - C_e) \\ \dfrac{d(V_dC_d)}{dt} = K(C_e - C_d) \end{cases} \tag{8}$$

For urea and creatinine, $C_d = 0$ in standard hemodialysis and hemofiltration treatments, because fresh dialysis fluid without these solutes is continuously provided. The rate of total solute mass removal from the body, dM_R/dt, during hemodialysis is:

$$\frac{dM_R}{dt} = K(C_e - C_d) + K_rC_e \tag{9}$$

The total solute amount removed from the body ΔM_R is the mass removed by dialyzer with clearance K and by the kidneys with residual clearance K_r. The solute removal by dialyzer is proportional to the solute concentration gradient between dialysate and extracellular compartment (C_e - C_d) when using the two compartment model. In the one compartment model, the body solute concentration C_b is used in equation (9) instead of C_e.
In the two compartment model, the changes of fluid volume in extracellular and intracellular compartments, $V_e(t)$ and $V_i(t)$, respectively, are assumed to be proportional to the volumes of these compartments (Canaud et al., 1995; Clark et al., 1998; Ziolko et al., 2000):

$$V_e(t) = \alpha \cdot V_b(t),\ V_i(t) = (1-\alpha) \cdot V_b(t) \tag{10}$$

where α is usually about 1/3, V_b for urea and creatinine is assumed to be equal to total body water (TBW) and V_b as well as V_e can be measured by bioimpedance (Zaluska et al., 2002).
During HD the change of solute distribution volume is described by a linear relationship:

$$V_b(t) = V_b(t_0) + \beta \cdot t \tag{11}$$

where $V_b(t_0)$ is the initial volume of solute distribution and the rate of volume change:

$$\beta = G_w - K_{rw} - Q_v \tag{12}$$

consists of water intake with rate G_w, residual water clearance K_{rw} and ultrafiltration with rate Q_v.

3. Hemodialysis efficiency: history and definitions of dialysis adequacy indices

The questions concerning how to quantify dialysis dose and how much dialysis should be provided, are controversial and have been debated since the beginning of the dialysis treatment era. Between 1976 and 1981, the National Cooperative Dialysis Study (NCDS) was performed in the United States to establish objective, quantitative criteria for the adequate dose of dialysis (Gotch & Sargent, 1985; Sargent & Gotch, 1989; Locatelli et al., 2005). It included 165 patients and had a 2 x 2 factorial design: the patients were randomized to two different midweek pre-dialysis blood urea nitrogen (BUN) levels (70 vs. 120 mg/dL) and two different treatment times (2.5 - 3.5 vs. 4.5 – 5.0 h).
Concentration targeting in this study used a time average BUN concentration (C_{ta}) of 50 mg/dL (groups I and III) and 100 mg/dL (groups II and IV). Dialysis time was fixed for the protocol; hence, dialyzer clearance was the main treatment parameter that was adjusted. A one compartment variable volume model was used to prescribe and control the treatment. Urea kinetic modeling was applied to determine protein catabolic rate (pcr) and the parameters of dialysis necessary to achieve a specified BUN level with thrice weekly treatments. BUN changes in an individual patient were quantified as the product of dialyzer urea clearance (K, mL/min) and the treatment time (T, min), normalized to the urea distribution volume (V, mL). KT/V exponentially determines the total decrease in BUN during a dialysis treatment:

$$C_{post} = C_{pre} e^{-\frac{KT}{V}} \tag{13}$$

C_{post} and C_{pre} are postdialysis and predialysis blood urea concentration. KT/V was prescribed in the NCDS as a function of pcr and C_{pre}:

$$-\frac{KT}{V} = \ln\left(1 - \frac{0.49pcr - 0.16)}{C_{pre}}\right) \tag{14}$$

The primary analysis showed that morbidity was less at lower levels of urea C_{ta} and the number of deaths in patients assigned to groups II and IV was very high (Parker et al., 1983). No significant effect of treatment time was found, although there was a clear trend towards a benefit from longer dialysis ($p = 0.06$).

The 'mechanistic' analysis of the NCDS data done by Gotch and Sargent launched the issue of urea KT/V (Gotch & Sargent, 1985). The patient groups II and IV, with high BUN, had low KT/V values at all levels of pcr and the groups I and III, with low pcr, had low levels of BUN and KT/V. For Kt/V > 0.8 the data base was comprised almost entirely of patient groups I and III with pcr > 0.8. KT/V < 0.8 provided inadequate dialysis with high probability of failure irrespective of pcr.

The factor KT/V was described as the "fractional clearance of urea" (Gotch & Sargent, 1985). If K is the urea clearance and T is time, the term KT is a volume. The ratio of KT to V expresses the fraction of the urea distribution volume that is totally cleared from urea.

3.1 Fast hemodialysis: two compartment effects, single-pool and equilibrated KT/V

The human body has a large number of physical compartments. The mathematical description of body is usually simplified by considering it as single pool (one compartment) or as a few interconnected pools. In a multicompartment model, the solute and fluid transport between body spaces should be described.

The one compartment model assumes that the body acts as a single, well mixed space and is characterized by: 1) high permeability of cells to the solute being modeled, 2) rapidly flowing blood that transports the solute throughout a totally perfused body. The assumptions of one compartment model for urea or creatinine during dialysis are valid as long as the flux of solute into and out of cells is faster than the flux of solute from the extracellular space accessible to dialysis. When the intercompartment flow between body compartments is too slow and constrained in comparison with the solute removal rate from the perfused compartment, then the solute behavior increasingly deviates from that of one compartment kinetics.

With the available high efficiency dialyzers and the tendency to short-time, rapid dialysis at least the two compartment modeling appears to be necessary. The two compartment model assumes solute generation to and removal from the perfused space, which is for urea and creatinine typically the extracellular compartment. This assumption is considered reasonable because urea is produced in the liver and enters body water from the systemic circulation (Sargent & Gotch, 1989). Regarding creatinine, in most studies the previously determined urea distribution volumes for each patient were successfully used as an approximation for creatinine distribution space (Canaud et al., 1995; Clark et al., 1998; Waikar & Bonventre, 2009).

The perfused (extracellular) compartment communicates with the non-perfused compartment (intracellular) according to the concentration gradient with an intercompartmental mass transport coefficient (K_c, mL/min). For a low value of K_c, the

discrepancy between one and two compartment modeling is larger because the immediate intercompartmental flow is precluded (Debowska et al., 2007b).
Assuming one compartment model, a fixed distribution volume (no ultrafiltration) and no generation during the dialysis, as during a short HD session, the concentration of any solute can be described by the equation (Sargent & Gotch, 1989; Daugirdas et al., 2001):

$$C_t = C_{pre} \cdot e^{-K \cdot t / V} \tag{15}$$

where C_t is the blood concentration of the solute at any time t during dialysis, C_{pre} is the blood concentration at the beginning of HD, K is the clearance of applied dialyzer, and V is the solute distribution volume.
The single pool KT/V (spKT/V) for urea is determined from equation (15) as the natural logarithm (ln) of the ratio of postdialysis (C_{post}) to predialysis (C_{pre}) plasma urea concentrations (Gotch & Sargent, 1985; Daugirdas et al., 2001):

$$spKT / V = -\ln\left(\frac{C_{post}}{C_{pre}}\right) \tag{16}$$

The expression 1 - C_{post}/C_{pre}, is called urea reduction ratio (URR):

$$URR = 1 - R \tag{17}$$

where

$$R = \frac{C_{post}}{C_{pre}} \tag{18}$$

A solute like urea or creatinine is however removed during hemodialysis more efficiently from the extracellular than from the intracellular compartment and its concentration in plasma falls faster than expected when assessed by one compartment modeling; this effect is called urea inbound (Daugirdas et al., 2001), Fig. 3. When dialysis is completed, the flow from intracellular to extracellular compartment causes a fast increase of postdialysis urea concentration in plasma, i.e., urea rebound (Daugirdas et al., 2001; Daugirdas et al., 2004), Fig. 3. Even if solute removal from a compartment directly accessible to dialyzer is relatively efficient during an intermittent therapy, the overall solute removal may be limited by slow intercompartmental mass transfer. Urea concentration measured in plasma represents the extracellular urea concentration.
The effects of urea generation and urea removal due to solute convective transport that are not included in the basic relation between spKT/V and URR can be corrected by Daugirdas formula (Daugirdas, 1993):

$$spKT / V = -\ln(R - 0.008 \cdot T) + (4 - 3.5 \cdot R) \cdot UF / W \tag{19}$$

where T is treatment time in hour, UF is ultrafiltration volume and W is the postdialysis weight (in kilograms). Single-pool kinetics overestimates however the removed amount of urea because of the postdialysis urea rebound, which is an compartmental effect, and therefore the equilibrated KT/V (eqKT/V) was introduced to clinical practice to be estimated by the following formula (Daugirdas et al., 2001):

$$eqKT / V = -\ln(R_{eq} - 0.008 \cdot T) + (4 - 3.5 \cdot R_{eq}) \cdot UF / W \tag{20}$$

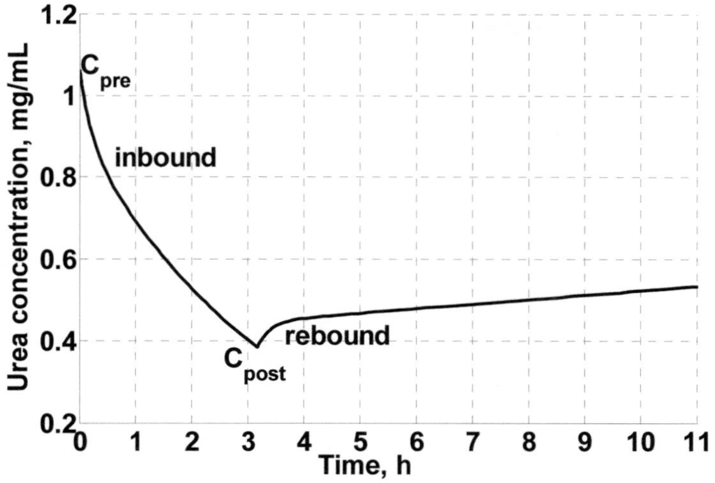

Fig. 3. The phenomena of the intradialytic drop in urea concentration in plasma (inbound), and the postdialysis increase in urea concentration in plasma (rebound).

where

$$R_{eq} = \frac{C(T_{eq})}{C_0} \tag{21}$$

$C(T_{eq})$ is the urea concentration 30 to 60 minutes after the dialysis session. The eqKT/V is typically about 0.2 KT/V unit lower than the spKt/V, but this difference depends on the efficiency, or rate of dialysis (Daugirdas et al., 2001). Equilibrated KT/V values can be also calculated using an alternative equation, as described by Daugirdas and Schneditz (Daugirdas & Schneditz, 1995):

$$eqKT/V = spKT/V - 0.6 \cdot \frac{spKT/V}{T} + 0.03 \tag{22}$$

or the formula derived from observations during the HEMO Study (Depner et al., 1999; Eknoyan et al., 2002; Daugirdas et al., 2004):

$$eqKT/V = spKT/V - 0.39 \cdot \frac{spKT/V}{T} \tag{23}$$

or that introduced by Tattersall et al. (Tattersall et al., 1996):

$$eqKT/V = spKT/V \cdot \frac{T}{T+36} \tag{24}$$

where T indicates treatment time in minutes. Equations (22) and (23), were derived from regression using the rebounded BUN measured 30 or 60 minutes after dialysis. The Tattersall equation was derived from theoretical considerations of disequilibrium and rebound, but the coefficient was derived from fitting to clinical data.

3.2 Urea KT/V and creatinine clearance for the kidneys

To assess the residual renal function (RRF) urine is usually collected for 24 hours and analyzed for urea as well as creatinine (Daugirdas et al., 2001). Residual renal clearance for a particular substance can be calculated as follows:

$$K_r = \frac{\text{excretion rate}}{C_e} = \frac{C_{urine} V_{urine}}{T_{urine}} \frac{1}{C_e} = \frac{\Delta M_r}{T_{urine}} \frac{1}{C_e} \tag{25}$$

where V_{urine} is urine volume, C_{urine} is solute concentration in urine, T_{urine} is time of urine collection, C_e is plasma solute concentration and ΔM_r is solute mass removed by the kidneys. Weekly KT/V for the kidney for 1 week time is expressed as follows:

$$\text{weekly } (KT/V)_{RRF} = \frac{7 \cdot C_{urine} V_{urine}}{C_e V_b} = \frac{7 \cdot \Delta M_r}{M_b} \tag{26}$$

where M_b is solute mass in the body, V_b is TBW and other symbols have the same meaning as in equation (25).

In clinical practice, the most popular methods used for evaluation RRF is creatinine clearance (Cl_{Cr}), calculated as follows:

$$\text{weekly } Cl_{Cr,\,RRF} = \frac{7 \cdot \Delta M_{R,Cr}}{1\text{week} \cdot C_{e,Cr}} \frac{1.73}{BSA} \tag{27}$$

where $\Delta M_{R,Cr}$ is creatinine total mass removed during one day due to therapy and by residual renal function, $C_{e,Cr}$ is serum creatinine concentration, BSA is body surface area and 1.73 is the average BSA for a typical human. Weekly creatinine clearance is the most often expressed in L for 1 week.

3.3 Equivalent renal clearance (EKR)

In a steady state, during continuous dialytic treatment or/and with renal function, the solute generation rate G is balanced by the solute removal rate K_{ss} determining in this way the constant concentration C_{ss} within the patient body (Gotch, 2001):

$$C_{ss} = G/K_{ss} \tag{28}$$

The K_{ss} is defined by rearrangement of equation (28):

$$K_{ss} = G/C_{ss} \tag{29}$$

Calculation of a continuous clearance K_{ss}, equivalent to the amount of dialysis provided by any intermittent dialysis schedule, K_{eq}, requires calculation of G and the concentration profile, and selection of a point on this profile, which may be considered to be equivalent to, e.g. weekly, the oscillating concentration (C_{eq}) according to: $K_{eq} = G/C_{eq}$. This approach to the clearance calculation has been reported using different definitions of C_{eq}. The peak concentration hypothesis defined C_{eq} as the maximum solute concentration, within e.g. one week duration. The mean predialysis (peak average) solute concentration was used to define standard K (stdK) (Gotch, 1998). The time-average solute concentration (C_{ta}) has been introduced to define 'equivalent renal clearance' (EKR) (Casino & Lopez, 1996):

$$\mathrm{EKR} = \frac{G}{C_{ta}} \tag{30}$$

The equation (30) may be used in metabolically stable patients, whereas in acute renal failure patients the definition for EKR requires a more unifying form (Casino & Marshall, 2004):

$$\mathrm{EKR} = \frac{\Delta M_R / T}{C_{ta}} \tag{31}$$

where ΔM_R is total solute amount removed by replacement therapy and the kidneys, and T is arbitrary assumed time. EKR, in the form of equation (31), is determined as solute removal rate over time average solute concentration.

3.4 Standardized KT/V

Taking into account the average predialysis urea concentration, Gotch introduced the standard KT/V (stdKT/V) concept to measure the relative efficiency of the whole spectrum of dialytic therapies whether intermittent, continuous or mixed (Gotch, 1998). The stdKT/V was defined with a relation between urea generation, expressed by its equivalent normalized protein catabolic rate (nPCR) and the peak average urea concentration (C_{pa}) of all the weekly values (Gotch, 1998; Diaz-Buxo & Loredo, 2006):

$$\mathrm{stdKT/V} = \frac{0.184(\mathrm{nPCR} - 0.17) \cdot V \cdot 0.001}{C_{pa}} \cdot \frac{7 \cdot 1440}{V} \tag{32}$$

where 0.184(nPCR - 0.17) V·0.001 is equal to urea generation rate G (mg/min), V is body water in mL and 7·1440 is number of minutes in one week´s time. Predialysis urea concentration (C_{pa}) - for any combination of frequency of intermittent HD (IHD), automated peritoneal dialysis (APD) and continuous dialysis between IHD or APD sessions - was defined as follows (Gotch, 1998):

$$C_{pa} = \frac{\dfrac{G}{(\mathrm{spKT/V}) \cdot V / T}\left(1 - e^{-\mathrm{eqKT/V}}\right) e^{-\frac{(K_p + K_r)((7/N)1440 - T)}{V}} + \dfrac{G}{K_p + K_r}\left(1 - e^{-\frac{(K_p + K_r)((7/N)1440 - T)}{V}}\right)}{\left(1 - e^{-\mathrm{eqKT/V}}\right) e^{-\frac{(K_p + K_r)((7/N)1440 - T)}{V}}} \tag{33}$$

where K, K_p and K_r are dialyzer, peritoneal and renal urea clearances, respectively, T is duration of treatment sessions, N is the frequency of IHD or APD per week and eqKT/V is the equilibrated KT/V calculated according to equation (22).

Assuming a symmetric weekly schedule of dialysis sessions, no residual renal function, and a fixed solute distribution volume V, Leypoldt et al. obtained an analytical relationship between stdKT/V, spKT/V and eqKT/V (Leypoldt et al., 2004):

$$\mathrm{stdKT/V} = \frac{10080 \dfrac{1 - e^{-\mathrm{eqKT/V}}}{T}}{\dfrac{1 - e^{-\mathrm{eqKT/V}}}{\mathrm{spKT/V}} + \dfrac{10080}{N \cdot T} - 1} \tag{34}$$

where N is number of treatments per week and eqKT/V is derived from spKT/V by using one of the equations (20), (22), (23) or (24). stdKT/V calculated using equation (34) differs slightly from stdKT/V using the exact method, equation (32), that takes into account among other things asymmetry of weekly schedule and K_r (Leypoldt et al., 2004). The stdKT/V is a method to measure the efficiency of HD of variable frequency, continuous peritoneal dialysis (PD), intermittent PD, continuous renal replacement therapies and residual renal function (Diaz-Buxo & Loredo, 2006).

3.5 Solute removal index (SRI) and fractional solute removal (FSR)

An alternative for KT/V is fractional solute removal (FSR), which was suggested by Verrina et al. (Verrina et al., 1998) and Henderson (Henderson, 1999) for comparative studies of different dialysis modalities and schedules. The concept of FSR is closely related to the concept of the solute removal index (SRI) proposed by Keshaviah (Keshaviah, 1995).
SRI was defined for HD as the ratio of net solute removed during a dialysis session (i.e., the solute amount removed minus the solute amount generated in the same time period) over the initial solute amount in the body. This parameter is however useless for comparative analysis of different dialysis modalities and schedules. Its numerical value for the kidneys and continuous therapies, such as continuous ambulatory peritoneal dialysis (CAPD), is by definition equal to zero (Waniewski & Lindholm, 2004). Therefore, Keshaviah (Keshaviah, 1995) used for CAPD and automated peritoneal dialysis the definition of SRI as the ratio of solute removed during a dialysis session over its initial amount in the body, i.e., the definition of FSR.

3.6 International guidelines on HD dose

According to the Kidney Disease Outcomes Quality Initiative (KDOQI) guidelines the minimally adequate dose of thrice-weekly HD in patients with residual renal clearance (K_r) less than 2 mL/min/1.73 m^2 should be urea single pool KT/V (excluding residual renal function) of 1.2 per dialysis (i.e., an average urea reduction ratio of 65%), (Work Group, 2001). KDOQI Work Group emphasizes that the literature clearly supports the delivery of a minimum hemodialysis dose of at least urea spKt/V = 1.2, but does not suggest an optimal dose. Identification of an optimal dose of hemodialysis would require evaluation of patient status and clinical outcomes including survival analyses and assessment of quality of life as well as the cost-effectiveness of different hemodialysis regimens. Until such data are available, the Work Group states that the hemodialysis dose recommended is to be regarded as a minimum value only (Work Group, 2001; Work Group, 2006).
The European Best Practice Guidelines recommend higher values: the minimum prescribed HD dose per session for thrice-weekly schedule as equilibrated KT/V for urea is set at 1.2; this corresponds to a value of spKT/V equal to 1.4 (Work Group, 2002).

4. Integrated system of dialysis adequacy indices

The integrated system of dialysis adequacy indices aims to include currently applied indices, systemize their definitions and explain relationships between them. The unified approach to the dialysis adequacy proposed by Waniewski et al. is valid for all modalities of dialysis performed in end-stage renal disease and acute renal failure patients, and for the assessment of residual renal function (Waniewski et al., 2006; Debowska et al., 2010; Waniewski et al., 2010).

4.1 Different definition variants of KT/V, equivalent continuous clearance (ECC) and fractional solute removal (FSR)

For the assessment of dialysis efficacy, a few different adequacy indices can be used: a) KT/V (K - dialyzer clearance, T - treatment time, V - solute distribution volume), b) equivalent continuous clearance, ECC and c) fractional solute removal, FSR.

There are at least four different reference methods: 1) peak, *p*, 2) peak average, *pa*, 3) time average, *ta*, and 4) treatment time average, *trta*, reference values of concentration, mass and volume, applied in ECC, FSR and KT/V definitions, respectively (ref = p, ref = pa, ref = ta and ref = trta), (Waniewski et al., 2006). For certain applications also minimal average or minimal reference methods are used, e.g. in equation (19) post-dialysis minimal weight is included in calculation of spKT/V. The peak value is the maximal value of solute concentration or mass, the peak average value is calculated as the average of pretreatment values (before each HD session), the time average value is the average calculated over the whole cycle of dialysis, T_c, and the treatment time average value is calculated as the average for the time T when dialysis was performed, Fig. 4.

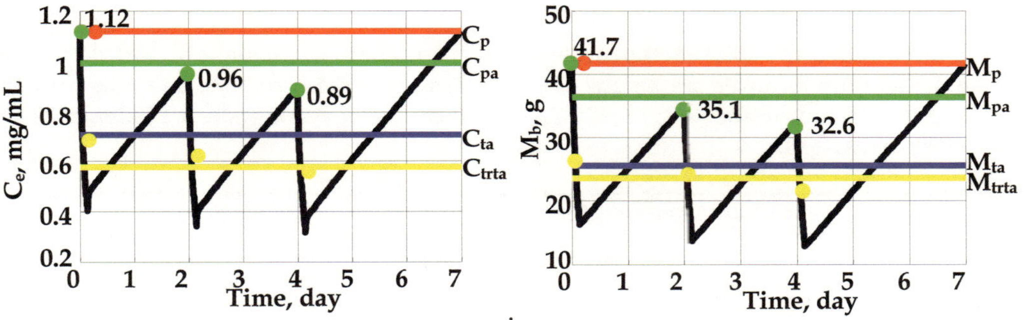

Fig. 4. Examples showing urea concentration in extracellular compartment (left side) and urea mass in patient body (right side) during a cycle of three hemodialysis sessions.

The reference solute distribution volume is calculated as the reference mass over the reference concentration:

$$V_{ref} = M_{b,ref} / C_{ref} \tag{35}$$

Note, that V_{ref} defined in this way may be different from the volume calculated in analogy to C_{ref} or $M_{b,ref}$; for example, V_{ta} is in general different from the average volume over the treatment time.

For HD, dialyzer clearance K is equal to the average effective dialyzer clearance K_T defined as solute mass removed from the body during dialysis M_{Rd}, per the treatment time, T, and per the average solute concentration in extracellular compartment during treatment time, C_{trta} ($K = K_T = \Delta M_{Rd}/T/C_{trta}$), (Waniewski & Lindholm, 2004; Waniewski et al., 2006).

Another concept of clearance, equivalent renal clearance, EKR (mL/min), was proposed by Casino & Lopez for metabolically stable patients, equation (30), but for metabolically unstable patients equation (31) should be used (Casino & Lopez, 1996; Casino & Marshall, 2004), c.f. section 3.3. Using a different concentration in EKR instead of C_{ta}, a general definition of equivalent continuous clearance, ECC, may be formulated (Waniewski et al., 2006; Waniewski et al., 2010), Table 1:

$$ECC_{ref} = \frac{\Delta M_R}{t \cdot C_{ref}} \tag{36}$$

where index "ref" denotes a reference concentration, e.g. ref = ta or ref = p, etc. If the patient is in a steady metabolic state, i.e. after a cycle time (T_c) the solute concentration and solute mass in the body return to their initial values, then the total amount of solute removed during T_c is equal to the solute amount generated during T_c. Thus, for the metabolic steady state and $t = T_c$:

$$\Delta M_R = G \cdot T_c \tag{37}$$

If one scales the total removed solute mass to some reference mass ($M_{b,ref}$) then a nondimensional parameter - fractional solute removal, FSR - may be defined as follows (Gotch, 1998; Waniewski & Lindholm, 2004; Waniewski et al., 2006), Table 1:

$$FSR_{ref} = \frac{\Delta M_R}{M_{b,ref}} \tag{38}$$

FSR is often called the solute removal index (SRI), although originally SRI was defined as the solute amount removed minus the solute amount generated in the same time over the initial solute amount in the body, Table 1, (Keshaviah, 1995; Waniewski & Lindholm, 2004, Waniewski et al., 2010).

Reference method	*Equivalent Continuous Clearance ECC*	*Fractional Solute Removal FSR*
peak, p	$ECC_p = \frac{\Delta M_R / T_c}{C_p}$	$FSR_p = \frac{\Delta M_R}{M_{b,p}}$ (Henderson, 1999), SRI, (Keshaviah, 1995)
peak average, pa	$ECC_{pa} = \frac{\Delta M_R / T_c}{C_{pa}}$ stdK, (Gotch, 1998)	$FSR_{pa} = \frac{\Delta M_R}{M_{b,pa}}$ stdKT/V (Gotch, 1998)
time average, ta	$ECC_{ta} = \frac{\Delta M_R / T_c}{C_{ta}}$ EKR, (Casino & Lopez, 1996; Casino & Marshall, 2004)	$FSR_{ta} = \frac{\Delta M_R}{M_{b,ta}}$
treatment time average, trta	$ECC_{trta} = \frac{\Delta M_R / T_c}{C_{trta}}$ $K \cdot T/T_c$ (Lowrie et al., 1999; Waniewski et al., 2006)	$FSR_{trta} = \frac{\Delta M_R}{M_{b,trta}}$ $K \cdot T/V_{trta}$ (Waniewski et al., 2006)

Table 1. Summary of dialysis adequacy indices.

In particular, EKR is equal to a particular version of ECC (ECC_{ta}), equation (36), that was used in many clinical and theoretical studies, Table 1 (Casino & Lopez, 1996; Verrina et al., 1998; Clark et al., 1999; Leypoldt et al., 2003; Casino & Marshall, 2004; Waniewski et al., 2006). If ref = pa (where pa denotes the average predialysis concentration) then ECC_{pa} is equal to stdK defined by Gotch and used in some clinical and theoretical studies, Table 1 (Gotch, 1998; Gotch et al., 2000; Leypoldt et al., 2003; Leypoldt et al., 2004; Waniewski et al., 2006). Both these clearances were defined initially for the metabolic steady state using formula (30), (Casino & Lopez, 1996; Gotch, 1998; Gotch et al., 2000), and were later generalized to the general case using formula (36), (Casino & Marshall, 2004; Debowska et al., 2010).

ECC and FSR are not independent indices but they are correlated (Debowska et al., 2005; Waniewski et al., 2006):

$$ECC_{ref} = \frac{V_{ref}}{t} FSR_{ref} \tag{39}$$

where ECC_{ref} and FSR_{ref} may be calculated for the same time interval t; a practically important case is $t = T_c$. The coefficient of proportionality, V_{ref}/t, depends on the choice of reference method, because V_{ref} is defined as $V_{ref} = M_{b,ref}/C_{ref}$, equation (35). Furthermore, if $t = T_c$ and the residual renal clearance is K_r, then FSR is related to KT/V (Waniewski et al., 2006):

$$FSR_{ref} = \frac{C_{trta}}{C_{ref}} \frac{KT}{V_{ref}} + \frac{C_{ta}}{C_{ref}} \frac{K_r T_c}{V_{ref}} \tag{40}$$

because

$$\Delta M_R = \Delta M_{Rd} + \Delta M_r , \; \Delta M_{Rd} = K \cdot T \cdot C_{trta} , \; \Delta M_r = K_r \cdot T_c \cdot C_{ta} \tag{41}$$

where ΔM_{Rd} and ΔM_r are the removed solute mass by replacement therapy and the kidneys, respectively. Another correlation can be found between ECC and K for $t = T_c$ (Waniewski et al., 2006):

$$ECC_{ref} = \frac{C_{trta}}{C_{ref}} \frac{T}{T_c} K + \frac{C_{ta}}{C_{ref}} K_r \tag{42}$$

The relationships between ECC and FSR, FSR and KT/V and between ECC and K, equations (39), (40) and (42), respectively, follow directly from their definitions and are valid for all reference methods and any patient and treatment modality (Waniewski et al., 2006). They do not depend on the assumption of the metabolic steady state. However, the coefficients in these relationships, which involve the ratios of different reference concentrations, must be calculated for each patient and treatment schedule separately.

4.2 Typical modalities and schedules for hemodialysis

Different dialysis modalities and schedules are applied in clinics to treat patients with end-stage renal diseases. Although solute removal indices are normalized by the solute amount in the body (with the body size included), many other parameters and conditions may differ as the patients are treated by different forms of dialysis (continuous or automated PD, HD, or combination of PD and HD), different number of sessions per week, different duration of each session, and therefore the values of dialysis adequacy indices depend on the details of dialysis. Numerical simulations of different HD regimes were performed using solute kinetic modeling and the obtained solute mass, concentration and distribution volume profiles in body compartments and solute concentration, mass and volume of dialysate were used to calculate dialysis adequacy indices. The two compartment variable volume model, equation (8), was implemented in the computer program Matlab and solved by numerical integration (Runge-Kutta method) to describe the solute and fluid transport between patient and removal device during dialysis.

4.3 Comparison of adequacy indices for different HD regimes based on computer simulations

The objective of the analysis presented here was to compare different adequacy parameters and their different definitions for different schedules of HD, Table 2:

1. Conventional, daily hemodialysis with three 219-minute sessions (*HD3x*)
2. Daily hemodialysis with six 147-minute sessions (*HD6xd*)
3. Nocturnal hemodialysis with six 401-minute sessions (*HD6xn*)

Values of HD duration and dialyzer clearance were taken to be the average for patients groups enrolled in the Frequent Hemodialysis Network Daily and Nocturnal clinical trails (Daugirdas et al., 2010). Computer simulations were carried out for several weeks of the treatment to achieve the metabolic steady state of the patient.

Label	*Time schedule*	*K, mL/min*
HD3x	3 x 219 min	272
HD6xd	6 x 147 min	277
HD6xn	6 x 401 min	170

Table 2. Time schedule and dialyzer clearance K for: conventional hemodialysis provided three times a week (HD3x), daily hemodialysis carried out six times a week (HD6xd) and long, nocturnal hemodialysis (HD6xn).

Other parameters were: urea generation rate, $G = 7$ mg/min, residual urea clearance $K_r = 0.6$ mL/min. The convective transport of the solute was characterized by transmittance coefficient, $T_r = 0.3$, equation (5), for hemodialyzer. For the two compartment model, it was assumed that the intercompartmental clearance $K_c = 600$ mL/min and volumes of extracellular and intracellular compartments were changed according to equation (10) with $\alpha = 1/3$. The postdialysis water distribution volume was $V_b = 40$ L; water was generated with constant rate ($G_w = 1.04$ mL/min); weekly 10.5 L of water was removed by means of residual water clearance ($K_{rw} = 0.1$ mL/min) and as a result of ultrafiltration Q_v.

The changes of urea concentration in the extracellular compartment of the body and the values of FSR, as obtained by computer simulations using parameters from Table 2, were shown in Fig. 5 and Fig. 6. The time average concentration, C_{ta}, was 0.5 mg/mL in conventional HD performed three times per week and 0.36 mg/mL and 0.22 mg/mL for daily and nocturnal HD carried out six times per week, respectively, Fig. 5 and Table 3. The amplitude of urea concentration changes had the highest values for HD3x and the lowest for HD6xn, Fig. 5 and Table 3.

The weekly values of ECC and FSR, according to all methods for the definition of reference values, equations (36) and (38), and the respective values of urea concentrations in blood, C_{ref}, are shown in Table 3. The adequacy indices were different, with the indices ECC and FSR for HD3x being lower than for HD6xd and HD6xn, Table 3.

The adequacy indices, ECC and FSR, had the highest values for the definitions based on treatment time (trta) reference method and the lowest values for the definitions based on the peak reference method (Table 3), and were between weekly $ECC_{ta} = 14.03$ mL/min and

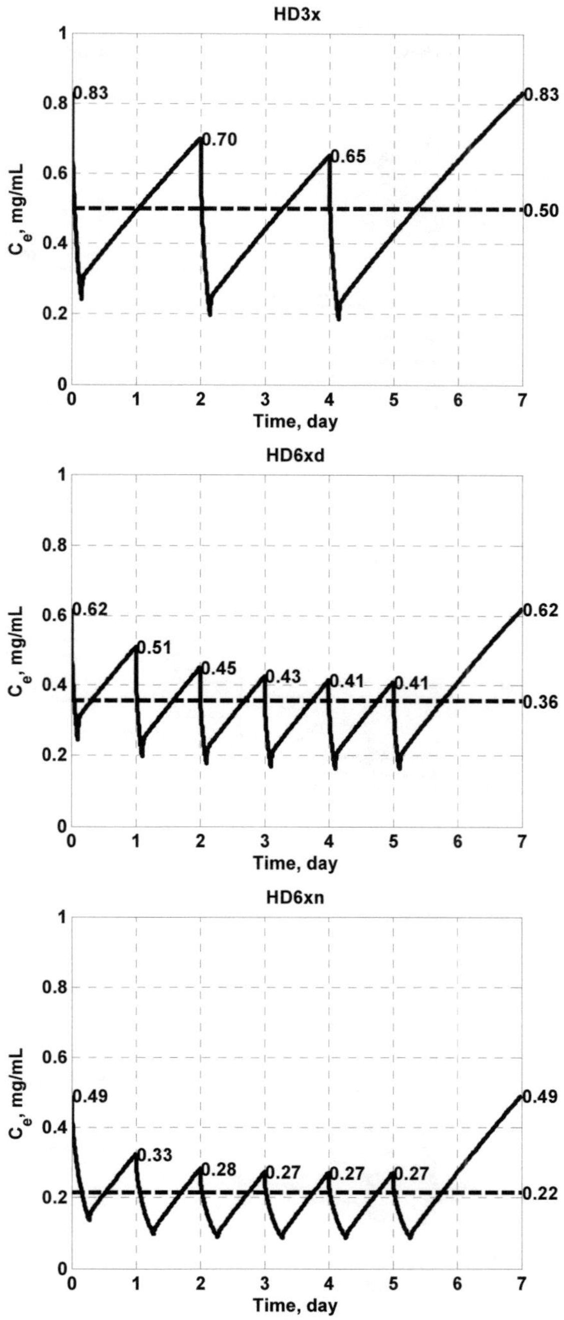

Fig. 5. Urea concentration, C_e, in the extracellular compartment during conventional hemodialysis provided three times a week (HD3x), daily hemodialysis carried out six times a week (HD6xd) and long, nocturnal hemodialysis (HD6xn). Average urea concentration was plotted with dashed line.

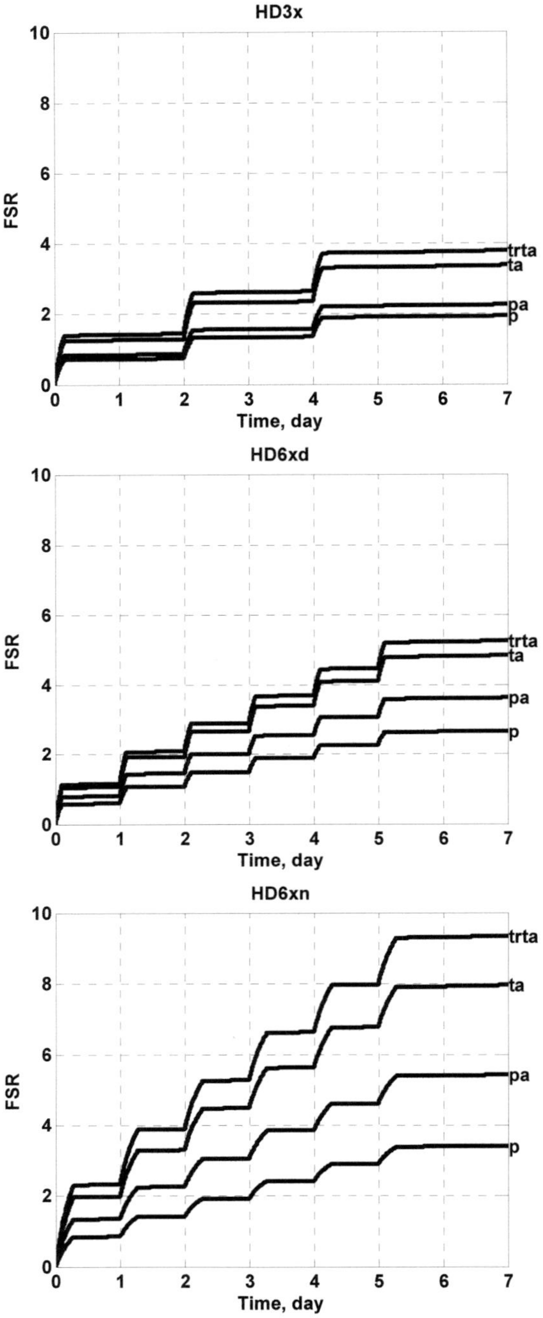

Fig. 6. FSR, normalized by peak, p, peak average, pa, time average, ta, and treatment time average, trta, urea mass in the body during conventional hemodialysis provided three times a week (HD3x), daily hemodialysis carried out six times a week (HD6xd) and long, nocturnal hemodialysis (HD6xn).

FSR_{pa} = 2.26 for HD3x and weekly ECC_{ta} = 32.3 mL/min and FSR_{pa} = 5.44 for HD6xn, indicating more efficient solute removal with HD6xn. The difference between the values of the indices calculated according to different definitions (treatment time average, time average, peak average, peak) was high (up to 192%).
The ratio of ECC and FSR differed slightly between the modalities and definitions (range, 4.04 - 4.96 mL/min) and correlated with the fluctuations of water volume and urea concentration in the body, as shown by V_{ref}, Table 3. Nevertheless, equation (39) is valid for all investigated applications. Because the cycle time was the same for all simulated dialysis modalities, T_c = 1 week, thus the correlation between the ratio of ECC to FSR and water volume confirmed the relationship described by equation (39).

		ECC	*FSR*	$\frac{ECC}{FSR}$	V_{ref}	C_{ref}
HD3x	p	8.42	1.94	4.34	43.76	0.83
	pa	9.62	2.26	4.25	42.85	0.73
	ta	14.03	3.38	4.16	41.90	0.50
	trta	18.83	3.80	4.96	50.01	0.37
HD6xd	p	11.28 (34%)	2.69 (39%)	4.20	42.32	0.62
	pa	14.84 (54%)	3.64 (61%)	4.08	41.11	0.47
	ta	19.71 (40%)	4.85 (43%)	4.07	40.99	0.36
	trta	25.31 (34%)	5.26 (38%)	4.81	48.46	0.28
HD6xn	p	14.25 (69%)	3.42 (76%)	4.17	41.99	0.49
	pa	21.94 (128%)	5.44 (141%)	4.04	40.69	0.32
	ta	32.3 (130%)	7.95 (135%)	4.06	40.93	0.22
	trta	41.66 (121%)	9.35 (146%)	4.45	44.90	0.17

Table 3. Weekly ECC, FSR, the ratio of ECC to FSR, the solute distribution volume, V_{ref}, and urea concentration in extracellular compartment, C_{ref}, calculated according to four different definitions: peak (p), peak average (pa), time average (ta) and treatment time average (trta) for conventional hemodialysis provided three times a week (HD3x), daily hemodialysis carried out six times a week (HD6xd) and long, nocturnal hemodialysis (HD6xn). Values in brackets present the difference in relation to conventional HD (in percent).

The formula for the relationship between FSR and KT/V, equation (40), shows that FSR may be represented as a weighted sum of KT/V and K_rT_c/V, with the first term representing the urea removal by dialysis and the second one, the urea removal by residual clearance. The weighing coefficients are the ratios of the average urea concentration in blood during dialysis treatment over the reference urea concentration and the average urea concentration in blood during the whole treatment cycle over the reference concentration, respectively, Table 4. These coefficients depend on the reference method as well as the treatment modality and schedule.
ECC may be related to K and K_r using equation (42). For that purpose K must be recalculated by the factor T/T_c, and then the recalculated value of K and the value of K_r are summed up with the same weighing coefficients that appear in formula (40) for the relationship of FSR and KT/V. The weighing coefficients show how much the average concentrations, during effective treatment time T, and during the whole cycle time T_c, respectively, differ from the reference concentration, Table 4.

		$\frac{KT}{V_{ref}}$	$\frac{K_rT_c}{V_{ref}}$	$\frac{C_{trta}}{C_{ref}}$	$\frac{C_{ta}}{C_{ref}}$	FSR
HD3x	p	4.15	0.14	0.45	0.60	1.94
	pa	4.24	0.14	0.51	0.69	2.26
	ta	4.34	0.14	0.75	1.00	3.38
	trta	3.63	0.12	1.00	1.34	3.80
HD6xd	p	5.85	0.14	0.45	0.57	2.69
	pa	6.02	0.15	0.59	0.75	3.64
	ta	6.04	0.15	0.78	1.00	4.85
	trta	5.10	0.12	1.00	1.28	5.26
HD6xn	p	9.82	0.14	0.34	0.44	3.42
	pa	10.13	0.15	0.53	0.68	5.44
	ta	10.07	0.15	0.78	1.00	7.95
	trta	9.18	0.13	1.00	1.29	9.35

Table 4. Nondimensional parameters KT/V_{ref}, residual K_rT_c/V_{ref}, the ratio of treatment time average to reference urea concentration C_{trta}/C_{ref}, the ratio of time average to reference urea concentration C_{ta}/C_{ref} and fractional solute removal, FSR, equation (40), for conventional hemodialysis provided three times a week (HD3x), daily hemodialysis carried out six times a week (HD6xd) and long, nocturnal hemodialysis (HD6xn).

ECC and FSR were found to be equivalent descriptions of dialysis, if the same reference method (peak, peak average, time average, treatment time average) was used, as suggested by equation (39). The ratio of ECC and FSR was similar for all definitions, in contrast to much different values of the indices themselves.

5. Adequacy indices for steady and non-steady metabolic state

The change of solute mass in the body during dialysis is due to the generation minus removal, but, in general, one can not assume that the solute removal is equal to the generation during the cycle time (i.e. intra- plus inter-dialysis time), especially in acute renal failure, ARF, patients; thus, even the measurement of removed solute in spent dialysate or filtrate does not necessarily accurately reflect the generated mass. In such cases, the real solute generation rate needs to be estimated using computer simulations for specific patients and dialysis parameters by fitting the theoretical predictions to the solute concentration profile using equation (8) for simulation. The calculation of FSR and ECC should then be based on equations (38) and (36) as it was shown by Debowska et al. (Debowska et al., 2010).

6. Conclusions

A unified scheme was proposed for the definitions of the adequacy indices on the basis of the reference values for: 1) normalization of removed solute mass to body solute mass (FSR), 2) cleared water volume to urea distribution volume (KT/V), and 3) solute generation rate to solute concentration in blood (ECC). The selection of the reference method can be done using respectively: peak (p), peak average (pa), time average (over the whole treatment cycle, ta) and treatment time average (over time of all dialysis sessions during the treatment cycle, trta) values of solute mass or concentration. It is not clear a priori which reference method should be used (ref = p, ref = pa, ref = ta or ref = trta) for the assessment of the treatment adequacy. To get a consistent scheme of definitions and relationships, the reference solute distribution volume was defined as $V_{ref} = M_{b,ref} / C_{ref}$. For each reference method, three adequacy indices, FSR, KT/V and ECC, can be defined. The computer simulations demonstrated that these indices are related, and that the relationships follow their definitions.

In general, ECC is equivalent to FSR, equation (39), if the same type of reference method is applied for both parameters (Debowska et al., 2005; Waniewski et al., 2006). The coefficient of proportionality, V_{ref}/T_c, depends only slightly on the details of the procedure, especially on the schedule of water removal and the degree of total body water variation during the treatment cycle as well as the difference between urea concentrations in intracellular and extracellular compartments that may develop during dialysis sessions. Nevertheless, the variations of V_{ref} between different definitions and procedures for the same patient are small. If a reference method (p, pa, ta, trta) of FSR and ECC definitions is fixed, then the changes in FSR are reflected by the changes in ECC and vice versa for the same patient. However, this relationship is different for patients with different total body water, which may also differ between patient populations.

One advantage of using equivalent continuous clearance, ECC, or fractional solute removal, FSR, is that these indices permit comparison of hemodialysis and peritoneal dialysis doses, and allow the addition of the contributions from HD, PD and residual renal function into the whole index for solute removal efficiency, and thus these indices could provide a basis for setting one standard target dose for all patients regardless of dialysis modality, frequency and duration (Depner, 2005; Debowska et al., 2007a). Note that ECC and FSR may also be successfully applied in continuous and semi-continuous therapies (e.g. continuous veno-venous hemofiltration, CVVH, slow low-efficiency daily dialysis, SLEDD) in patients with acute renal failure (Clark et al., 1999; Leypoldt et al., 2003; Debowska et al., 2010).

From the beginning of the era of dialysis treatment, there has been a quest for the optimal dialysis index. The history reflects the complexity of this matter, and attempts to simplify the meander way of this process that has not yet been finished because different versions of existing dialysis modalities are applied, new therapies are being introduced into clinical practices as new techniques become available. Compartmental models and solute kinetic analysis, presented here, used for the mathematical and computer-based description of delivered dose of dialysis are important tools for the evaluation of dialysis adequacy.

7. References

Canaud, B., Garred, L. J., Argiles, A., Flavier, J. L., Bouloux, C. & Mion, C. (1995). Creatinine kinetic modelling: a simple and reliable tool for the assessment of protein nutritional status in haemodialysis patients. *Nephrol Dial Transplant*, Vol. 10, No. 8, pp. (1405-10)

Casino, F. G. & Lopez, T. (1996). The equivalent renal urea clearance: a new parameter to assess dialysis dose. *Nephrol Dial Transplant*, Vol. 11, No. 8, pp. (1574-81)

Casino, F. G. & Marshall, M. R. (2004). Simple and accurate quantification of dialysis in acute renal failure patients during either urea non-steady state or treatment with irregular or continuous schedules. *Nephrol Dial Transplant*, Vol. 19, No. 6, pp. (1454-66)

Charra, B., Terrat, J. C., Vanel, T., Chazot, C., Jean, G., Hurot, J. M. & Lorriaux, C. (2004). Long thrice weekly hemodialysis: the Tassin experience. *Int J Artif Organs*, Vol. 27, No. 4, pp. (265-83)

Clark, W. R., Leypoldt, J. K., Henderson, L. W., Mueller, B. A., Scott, M. K. & Vonesh, E. F. (1999). Quantifying the effect of changes in the hemodialysis prescription on effective solute removal with a mathematical model. *J Am Soc Nephrol*, Vol. 10, No. 3, pp. (601-9)

Clark, W. R., Mueller, B. A., Kraus, M. A. & Macias, W. L. (1998). Quantification of creatinine kinetic parameters in patients with acute renal failure. *Kidney Int*, Vol. 54, No. 2, pp. (554-60)

Darowski, M., Orłowski, T., Weryński, A. & Wójcicki, J. M. (2000). *Biocybernetyka i Inżynieria Biomedyczna* Akademicka Oficyna Wydawnicza Exit, 83-87674-25-7, Warszawa

Daugirdas, J. T. (1993). Second generation logarithmic estimates of single-pool variable volume Kt/V: an analysis of error. *J Am Soc Nephrol*, Vol. 4, No. 5, pp. (1205-13)

Daugirdas, J. T., Blake, G. & Ing, T. S. (2001). *Handbook of Dialysis* (3rd ed.), Lippincott Williams & Wilkins, 0-316-17381-9, Philadelphia

Daugirdas, J. T., Depner, T. A., Greene, T., Levin, N. W., Chertow, G. M. & Rocco, M. V. (2010). Standard Kt/Vurea: a method of calculation that includes effects of fluid removal and residual kidney clearance. *Kidney Int*, Vol. 77, No. 7, pp. (637-44)

Daugirdas, J. T., Greene, T., Depner, T. A., Leypoldt, J., Gotch, F., Schulman, G. & Star, R. (2004). Factors that affect postdialysis rebound in serum urea concentration, including the rate of dialysis: results from the HEMO Study. *J Am Soc Nephrol*, Vol. 15, No. 1, pp. (194-203)

Daugirdas, J. T. & Schneditz, D. (1995). Overestimation of hemodialysis dose depends on dialysis efficiency by regional blood flow but not by conventional two pool urea kinetic analysis. *Asaio J*, Vol. 41, No. 3, pp. (M719-24)

Debowska, M. & Waniewski, J. (2005). Comparison of dialysis adequacy indices calculated according to one and two compartment model. *Bio-Algorithms And Med-Systems*, Vol. 1, No. 1, pp. (205-208)

Debowska, M., Waniewski, J. & Lindholm, B. (2005). Dialysis adequacy indices for peritoneal dialysis and hemodialysis. *Adv Perit Dial*, Vol. 21, pp. (94-7)

Debowska, M., Waniewski, J. & Lindholm, B. (2007a). Bimodal dialysis: theoretical and computational investigations of adequacy indices for combined use of peritoneal dialysis and hemodialysis. *Asaio J*, Vol. 53, No. 5, pp. (566-75)

Debowska, M., Waniewski, J. & Lindholm, B. (2007b). An integrative description of dialysis adequacy indices for different treatment modalities and schedules of dialysis. *Artif Organs*, Vol. 31, No. 1, pp. (61-9)

Debowska, M., Waniewski, J. & Lindholm, B. (2010). Adequacy indices for dialysis in acute renal failure: kinetic modeling. *Artif Organs*, Vol. 34, No. 5, pp. (412-419)

Depner, T., Beck, G., Daugirdas, J., Kusek, J. & Eknoyan, G. (1999). Lessons from the Hemodialysis (HEMO) Study: an improved measure of the actual hemodialysis dose. *Am J Kidney Dis*, Vol. 33, No. 1, pp. (142-9)

Depner, T. A. (1998). Benefits of more frequent dialysis: lower TAC at the same Kt/V. *Nephrol Dial Transplant*, Vol. 13 Suppl 6, pp. (20-4)

Depner, T. A. (2005). Hemodialysis adequacy: basic essentials and practical points for the nephrologist in training. *Hemodial Int*, Vol. 9, No. 3, pp. (241-54)

Diaz-Buxo, J. A. & Loredo, J. P. (2006). Standard Kt/V: comparison of calculation methods. *Artif Organs*, Vol. 30, No. 3, pp. (178-85)

Eknoyan, G., Beck, G. J., Cheung, A. K., Daugirdas, J. T., Greene, T., Kusek, J. W., Allon, M., Bailey, J., Delmez, J. A., Depner, T. A., Dwyer, J. T., Levey, A. S., Levin, N. W., Milford, E., Ornt, D. B., Rocco, M. V., Schulman, G., Schwab, S. J., Teehan, B. P. & Toto, R. (2002). Effect of dialysis dose and membrane flux in maintenance hemodialysis. *N Engl J Med*, Vol. 347, No. 25, pp. (2010-9)

Gotch, F. A. (1998). The current place of urea kinetic modelling with respect to different dialysis modalities. *Nephrol Dial Transplant*, Vol. 13 Suppl 6, pp. (10-4)

Gotch, F. A. (2001). Is Kt/V Urea a Satisfactory Measure for Dosing the Newer Dialysis Regimens? *Semin Dial*, Vol. 14, No. 1, pp. (15-17)

Gotch, F. A. & Sargent, J. A. (1985). A mechanistic analysis of the National Cooperative Dialysis Study (NCDS). *Kidney Int*, Vol. 28, No. 3, pp. (526-34)

Gotch, F. A., Sargent, J. A. & Keen, M. L. (2000). Whither goest Kt/V? *Kidney Int Suppl*, Vol. 76, pp. (3-18)

Henderson, L. W. (1999). Critical interpretation of adequacy parameters in peritoneal dialysis and hemodialysis. *Perit Dial Int*, Vol. 19 Suppl 2, pp. (S38-44)

Katchalsky, A. & Curran, P. (1965). *Nonequilibrium thermodynamics in biophysics* Harvard University Press, Cambridge

Kedem, O. & Katchalsky, A. (1958). Thermodynamic analysis of the permeability of biological membranes to non-electrolytes. *Biochim Biophysic Acta*, Vol. 27, pp. (229-246)

Keshaviah, P. (1995). The solute removal index--a unified basis for comparing disparate therapies. *Perit Dial Int*, Vol. 15, No. 2, pp. (101-4)

Leypoldt, J. K., Jaber, B. L., Lysaght, M. J., McCarthy, J. T. & Moran, J. (2003). Kinetics and dosing predictions for daily haemofiltration. *Nephrol Dial Transplant*, Vol. 18, No. 4, pp. (769-76)

Leypoldt, J. K., Jaber, B. L. & Zimmerman, D. L. (2004). Predicting treatment dose for novel therapies using urea standard Kt/V. *Semin Dial*, Vol. 17, No. 2, pp. (142-5)

Locatelli, F., Buoncristiani, U., Canaud, B., Kohler, H., Petitclerc, T. & Zucchelli, P. (2005). Dialysis dose and frequency. *Nephrol Dial Transplant*, Vol. 20, No. 2, pp. (285-96)

Lowrie, E. G., Chertow, G. M., Lew, N. L., Lazarus, J. M. & Owen, W. F. (1999). The urea [clearance x dialysis time] product (Kt) as an outcome-based measure of hemodialysis dose. *Kidney Int*, Vol. 56, No. 2, pp. (729-37)

Parker, T. F., Laird, N. M. & Lowrie, E. G. (1983). Comparison of the study groups in the National Cooperative Dialysis Study and a description of morbidity, mortality, and patient withdrawal. *Kidney Int Suppl*, No. 13, pp. (S42-9)

Sargent, J. A. & Gotch, F. A. (1989). *Replacement of renal function by dialysis* Kluwer Academic Publishers,

Schneditz, D. & Daugirdas, J. T. (2001). Compartment effects in hemodialysis. *Semin Dial*, Vol. 14, No. 4, pp. (271-7)

Spiegler, K. & Kedem, O. (1966). Thermodynamics of hyperfiltration (reverse osmosis): criteria for efficient membranes. *Desalination*, Vol. 1, pp. (311-326)

Staverman, A. (1951). The theory of measurement of osmotic pressure. *Rac trav chim*, Vol. 70, pp. (344-352)

Tattersall, J. E., DeTakats, D., Chamney, P., Greenwood, R. N. & Farrington, K. (1996). The post-hemodialysis rebound: predicting and quantifying its effect on Kt/V. *Kidney Int*, Vol. 50, No. 6, pp. (2094-102)

Verrina, E., Brendolan, A., Gusmano, R. & Ronco, C. (1998). Chronic renal replacement therapy in children: which index is best for adequacy? *Kidney Int*, Vol. 54, No. 5, pp. (1690-6)

Waikar, S. S. & Bonventre, J. V. (2009). Creatinine kinetics and the definition of acute kidney injury. *J Am Soc Nephrol*, Vol. 20, No. 3, pp. (672-9)

Waniewski, J. (2006). Mathematical modeling of fluid and solute transport in hemodialysis and peritoneal dialysis. *J. Membr. Sci.*, Vol. 274, pp. (24-37)

Waniewski, J., Debowska, M. & Lindholm, B. (2006). Theoretical and numerical analysis of different adequacy indices for hemodialysis and peritoneal dialysis. *Blood Purif*, Vol. 24, No. 4, pp. (355-66)

Waniewski, J., Debowska, M. & Lindholm, B. (2010). Can the diverse family of dialysis adequacy indices be understood as one integrated system? *Blood Purif*, Vol. 30, No. 4, pp. (257-65)

Waniewski, J. & Lindholm, B. (2004). Fractional solute removal and KT/V in different modalities of renal replacement therapy. *Blood Purif*, Vol. 22, No. 4, pp. (367-76)

Waniewski, J., Werynski, A., Ahrenholz, P., Lucjanek, P., Judycki, W. & Esther, G. (1991). Theoretical basis and experimental verification of the impact of ultrafiltration on dialyzer clearance. *Artif Organs*, Vol. 15, No. 2, pp. (70-7)

Werynski, A. & Waniewski, J. (1995). Theoretical description of mass transport in medical membrane devices. *Artif Organs*, Vol. 19, No. 5, pp. (420-7)

Weryński, A. & Nowosielcew, W. (1983). *Kompartmentowe modelowanie procesów sterowania w systemach fizjologicznych* Wydawnictwo Komunikacji i Łączności, 83-206-0284-X, Warszawa

Work Group (2001). I. NKF-K/DOQI Clinical Practice Guidelines for Hemodialysis Adequacy: update 2000. *Am J Kidney Dis*, Vol. 37, No. 1 Suppl 1, pp. (S7-S64)

Work Group (2002). Section II. Haemodialysis adequacy. *Nephrol Dial Transplant*, Vol. 17 Suppl 7, pp. (16-31)

Work Group (2006). Clinical practice guidelines for hemodialysis adequacy, update 2006. *Am J Kidney Dis*, Vol. 48 Suppl 1, pp. (S2-90)

Zaluska, W. T., Malecka, T., Swatowski, A. & Ksiazek, A. (2002). Changes of extracellular volumes measured by whole and segmental bioimpedance analysis during hemodialysis in end-stage renal disease (ESRD) patients. *Ann Univ Mariae Curie Sklodowska Med*, Vol. 57, No. 2, pp. (337-41)

Ziolko, M., Pietrzyk, J. A. & Grabska-Chrzastowska, J. (2000). Accuracy of hemodialysis modeling. *Kidney Int*, Vol. 57, No. 3, pp. (1152-63)

2

Automated Blood Volume Regulation During Hemodialysis

Isabelle Chapdelaine, Clément Déziel and François Madore
Hôpital du Sacré-Coeur de Montréal, Montréal
Canada

1. Introduction

Intradialytic hypotension (IDH) is the most common complication of hemodialysis (HD), occurring in up to 20 to 33% of sessions (Daugirdas, 2001). IDH is responsible for various minor symptoms (nausea, vomiting, muscle cramps, dizziness, and fatigue) during dialysis, but is also associated with more severe adverse events such as myocardial infarction (Burton et al., 2009) and cerebral ischemia (Mizumasa et al., 2004). Moreover, as a result of frequent interruption of sessions and repetitive administration of intravenous fluids, underdialysis and inability to reach dry weight, with subsequent chronic overhydration, can follow.

Traditionally, HD prescriptions are based on clinical evaluation and laboratory measurements, and are re-evaluated periodically or when an adverse event, such as hypotension, commands it. The drawback of this prescription is that it relies on previous observations, with the assumption that the same will hold true for the next sessions. Hence, it implies discomfort for the patients, as the actions to remediate to IDH, for example, by stopping ultrafiltration (UF) or adjusting dry weight, are taken on an *a posteriori* basis (Locatelli et al., 2005).

In an attempt to prevent IDH, technological advances have made possible the detection of subclinical predictors of hemodynamic instability, for example relative blood volume variations. With repetitive measurement of such specific parameters during HD (Mercadal & Petitclerc, 2009), actions can be implemented to correct the monitored parameter toward a desired target, with the aim of preventing overt IDH. When this action is automatic and regulated by a closed feedback loop, it is called biofeedback.

In this chapter, we will review some of the physiological basis of IDH and blood volume reduction during HD, and we will examine the technical aspects of the various devices used to adjust blood volume during dialysis, with special emphasis on biofeedback systems. Finally, we will study the literature published on the effects of automated blood volume regulation devices on the occurrence of hypotensive episodes, volume overload control, hypertension management and quality of life in chronic HD patients.

2. Intradialytic hypotension

The causes of IDH are multifactorial. On one side, a number of patient-related conditions can promote blood pressure (BP) fall during HD: age, comorbidities such as diabetes and cardiomyopathy, anemia, large interdialytic weight gain (IDWG), use of anti-hypertensive medication, etc. On the other hand, factors associated with the dialysis prescription itself can also contribute to hemodynamic instability: short HD sessions, high ultrafiltration rate, high dialysate temperature, low dialysate sodium concentration, inflammation caused by membrane activation, etc. As a consequence, various interventions aimed at modulating these parameters have been proposed to ameliorate the vascular tolerance to ultrafiltration (UF), but with variable efficacy and limited benefits.

On a physiological basis, IDH can be viewed as the inability of the cardio-vascular system to respond adequately to the reduction of blood volume. Cardio-vascular reactivity involves reflex activation of the sympathetic system, with appropriate tachycardia and arterial and venous vasoconstriction in response to cardiac underfilling and hypovolemia. These compensatory mechanisms are altered in some patients, which put them at risk of developing IDH. However, these are difficult to assess and to modify. Comprehensive study of blood volume regulation during HD can help understand IDH susceptibility of individual patients.

3. Blood volume regulation

3.1 Concept of plasma refilling

Blood volume is dependent on two main factors: plasma refilling capacity and UF rate. During HD, fluid is removed directly from the intravascular compartment. Total body water (TBW), which is about 60% of body weight (BW), is distributed in part in the intracellular (40% BW) and in part in the extracellular (20% BW) compartments. The latter is further subdivided in the interstitial (15% BW) and the intravascular (5% BW) spaces. Thus, only 8% of the TBW is readily available for UF. Therefore, in order to remove a substantial amount of fluid during a short period of time, the vascular compartment needs to be continuously refilled from the interstitial space.

Plasma refill is mostly driven by hydrostatic and oncotic forces. During the first part of a HD session, the vascular oncotic pressure raises and the hydrostatic pressure lessens as a result of progressive UF. Pressure gradients thus created drive the water back into the vascular space until a new equilibrium is reached. As UF and water withdrawal from the intravascular space continue, the new disequilibrium thereby generated has to be once again balanced, and so on until the end of the session (Santoro et al., 1996). Several factors can influence rate of plasma refilling by acting on these forces: hydration status, plasma osmolality, and plasma protein concentration. Patient's proper refilling capacity, which is not measurable as a parameter, also has an effect on the rate at which water moves back in the blood vessels. Overall, IDH is generated when the imbalance between UF rate and plasma refilling capacity cannot be surpassed by cardio-vascular compensatory reflexes.

3.2 Relative blood volume measurement

Cardio-vascular reactivity and plasma refilling capacity of each patient, albeit central in the pathogenesis of IDH development, are difficult to assess and therefore are not convenient as monitoring tools. Direct measurement of blood volume is feasible, classically using dilution of radioactively labelled blood elements (such as ^{131}I albumin or ^{51}Cr red blood cells), but it implies serial blood tests and radiation, and so is clearly impractical for the repetitive assessment of blood volume. One way to circumvent this problem is to measure blood volume change during HD which, as a surrogate marker of vascular refilling, can be estimated using bedside devices.

Relative blood volume (RBV) is the term used to describe « the blood volume at any time as a percentage of the blood volume at the commencement of treatment » (Nesrallah et al., 2008). Most of the non-invasive devices extrapolate the RBV change from the variation of the hemoconcentration of a blood element. The basic premise of this calculation is that if the blood component remains constant throughout the HD session (i.e., the numerator), the variation of its concentration is necessarily due to the change in the blood volume (i.e., the denominator). The various devices available vary in the blood element they measure (i.e., red blood cells, hematocrit, total protein concentration) and in the method used to measure it (i.e., optical absorbance, ultrasound, etc.).

One caveat of these techniques is that they are based on the assumption that uniform mixing of the measured blood element and plasma occurs throughout the whole circulation (Dasselaar et al., 2007a). Venous (or systemic) hematocrit (Hct_{sys}) is usually higher than whole-body hematocrit (Hct_{w}), due to the dynamic reduction of hematocrit in the microcirculation during blood flow through capillaries and venules. This is expressed as the F-cell ratio, Hct_{w}/Hct_{sys}. However, during UF, it was shown that the F-cell ratio rises as a result of the compliance of the microcirculation and fluid transfer to the macrocirculation. Therefore, the equations on which the inference of the blood volume change during HD is based may not be always valid (Mitra et al., 2004).

In a study from Dasselaar et al. (2007a), the blood volume reduction estimated by three commonly used devices (Crit-line®, Hemoscan® and BVM®, see below) was compared to a standard laboratory-derived Hb relative blood volume measurement during two HD sessions. It was shown that all three devices systematically overestimate the RBV reduction at modest RBV change, and underestimate the real fall in blood volume at higher RBV decline.

In addition, RBV monitoring also assumes that red blood cell mass or plasma protein density remains constant throughout the length of the session, which may not be true if hemolysis or blood leak happens, or when a blood transfusion is given.

3.3 Relation between relative blood volume and intradialytic hypotension

While hypovolemia is clearly a major determinant in the pathogenesis of IDH, the link between blood volume reduction and appearance of arterial hypotension is still a matter of debate. Recent studies have been unable to find a linear relationship between RBV and blood pressure, and a specific threshold to which hypotension will certainly occur does not seem to exist, even in an individual patient. This is probably because of variations, for each treatment, in the patient's ability to activate cardio-vascular compensatory mechanisms, in order to offset BP reductions induced by a wide range of hypovolemic states.

In fact, in many trials where blood volume (BV) biofeedback was effective in reducing the occurrence of IDH, there was no difference in the final RBV reached by either the standard treatment or the BV-controlled treatment. According to some authors, it is possible that RBV reduction *per se* is not the main risk factor for development of IDH. Rather, the excessive fluctuations of BV and the form of the RBV slope during HD may contribute more to hemodynamic instability (Andrulli et al., 2002). Indeed, the slope of the RBV curve with BV regulation device is different from that produced by standard HD (Franssen et al, 2006). The initial phase is usually steeper (meaning higher UF rate), which is rendered possible and tolerable because of higher initial interstitial pressures and better plasma refilling rate. The second phase is characterized by a reduced UF rate, which in turn make the RBV more stable and the patient less prone to IDH in this vulnerable period.

4. Biofeedback system

While monitoring may help to understand how BV is regulated during UF in an individual patient, the HD prescription often remains empirical. The hemodynamic stability during the previous HD sessions dictates the delivered parameters of the next HD treatments. Dialytic parameters such as UF rate and dialysate sodium concentration are usually set at the start of the HD session, and remain fixed throughout the treatment, with the assumption that they continue to be adequate for the whole treatment duration. However, this is not taking into account that patients may undergo physiologic variations during HD, and that fixed parameters, creating labile gradients, may not always be appropriate and may promote IDH. In fact, the standard HD prescription lacks a rapid retroactive response in case of variation of the monitored parameter, as the action to bring it back towards the desired value are taken manually (by the operator, a nurse or physician) or semi-automatically (authorized by the operator) (Locatelli et al., 2005), thus implying a certain lag of time that may be deleterious if IDH is to be prevented.

The method used to traditionally prescribe HD parameters is far from how the kidneys really behave to maintain internal homeostasis, keeping biologic variables in very tight ranges through instantaneous adjustments in response to precise negative or positive feedback loops. To try to get closer to what would be called « physiological dialysis », technological advances of the last decades have conducted to the development of sophisticated softwares that allow automated biofeedback. The concept of biofeedback is based on repetitive on-line measurements of the patient's biochemical parameters with biosensors, which are then constantly analysed by an automatic controller as being within the target values pre-set by the operator, or not. If the measured parameter is within the desired values considered safe, the treatment continues unchanged. If not, an action to bring it back towards the aimed values is immediately and automatically undertaken through the effectors, in a closed-loop that insures the stability of the monitored parameter.

The theoretical advantage of such devices is that they not only rapidly detect physiological abnormalities which may predict hemodynamic instability (blood volume reduction for example), but they automatically adjust one or more dialytic parameters to correct the situation. This obviates the need to perform manual changes by the operator and, at the same time, avoids the time lag before the action is undertaken. By modulating on-line some of the delivered dialysis parameter, these devices also address the physiological variations occurring during HD (and the variability of the patient's parameters from session to session), and thus provide more physiological dialysis, which may be more suited to prevent IDH.

At the present time, biofeedback systems are available for different parameters: relative blood volume, thermal energy balance, plasmatic conductivity, to which arterial pressure feedback using fuzzy logic control can be added. These devices are described here, with emphasis on blood volume biofeedback.

5. Blood volume biofeedback

Currently, only two commercially blood volume biofeedback devices are available: the Hemocontrol® (Gambro) and the BVM® (Fresenius) systems. Although both monitor change in relative blood volume during HD, they use different technologies and different integration systems. They are reviewed here.

5.1 Hemocontrol® system

The Hemocontrol® blood volume management system was first designed by Santoro and colleagues (Santoro et al., 1994) and afterwards modified in collaboration with the Hospal-Gambro research group. It is available on the Integra® and Artis® machines (with a few updates on the latter).

This biofeedback system is based on an automatic multi-input multi-output controller (MIMO) capable of integrating a multitude of signals and to modulate controlled variables to force the blood volume reduction along a pre-defined trajectory towards a pre-defined target of blood volume reduction (Locatelli et al., 2005). This results in a smoother and more gradual decline of relative blood volume, limiting the irregularity of BV variation that was shown to be predictive of IDH (Andrulli et al., 2002).

Basically, the monitored parameters are the actual UF (or weight loss), the actual dialysate sodium (or conductivity) and the actual blood volume change. The differences between the target values of the same three parameters (that is: desired UF, desired dialysate sodium (or equivalent conductivity) and desired final blood volume change) and the actual parameters serve as inputs to the MIMO controller. At any moment, the actual BV curve is plotted against the pre-determined BV trajectory and, should it deviate the least, automatic modulation of the UF rate and dialysate sodium (or conductivity) allows smooth redirection to the « ideal » curve (figures 1 and 2).

The blood volume change during dialysis is monitored using an optical sensor located in the arterial line that measures on-line hemoglobin (Hb) concentration by optical absorbance, according to Lambert-Beer law. The law states that Hb is a function of monochromatic light absorbance. Provided that the amount of Hb does not change, the blood volume variation from the start of the session can be inferred from the change in Hb concentration.

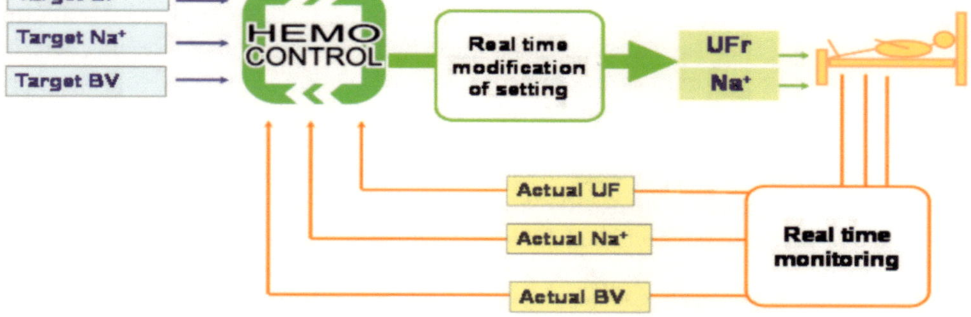

Fig. 1. Hemocontrol® biofeedback system (from Gambro).

The three targets prescribed by the physician (total UF, final dialysate sodium, and final BV reduction) are computed in the Hemocontrol® software and are compared to the actual same parameters (UF, dialysate sodium, and RBV) on a continuous basis during HD. The controller can modulate the UF rate and dialysate sodium in order to bring the actual parameters back on the pre-determined trajectory of the RBV curve.

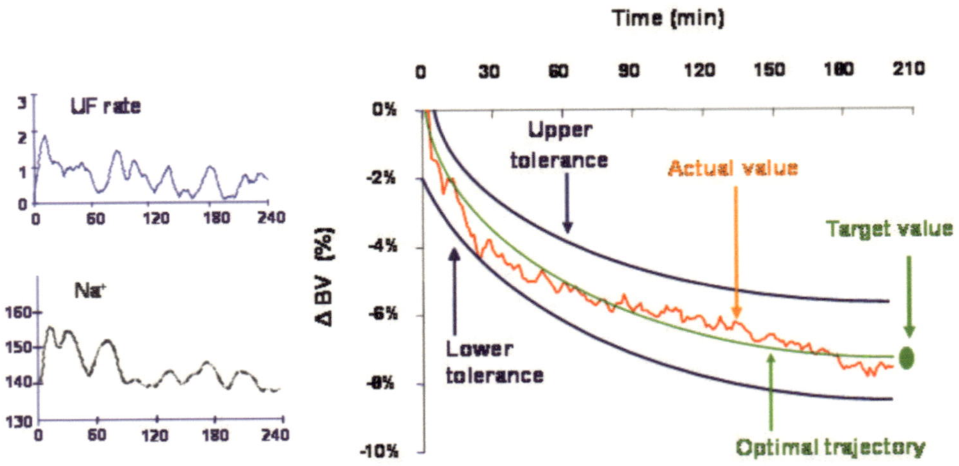

Fig. 2. Optimal trajectory of Relative blood volume (RBV) reduction during HD with Hemocontrol® (from Gambro).
The Hemocontrol® software designs the ideal RBV reduction curve, for each patient at each session, based on both initial and target parameters. Upper and lower tolerance limits are set to ensure safety. UF rate and dialysate sodium vary continuously during HD to keep the actual curve parallel to the optimal trajectory.

In practical terms, several parameters need to be set. Before the first use, data on the patient's sex, age, height and weight are needed to calculate total body water with any of the proposed formula. Treatment duration is also determined before the beginning of the treatment. Then, the three main targets need to be specified:

1. Total body weight loss or total UF (for water balance), based on clinical evaluation of dry weight;
2. Final sodium or equivalent dialysate conductivity. Conductivity refers to the electrical conducting property of the dialysis solution given by the dissociation of inorganic salts into charged ions. Since sodium is the principal ion in solution, conductivity is used as a surrogate for sodium concentration. For simplification purpose, conductivity was replaced by sodium concentration in the recent devices. Equivalent conductivity represents the dialysate conductivity that produces the same sodium balance at the end of a BV regulated session as a HD session with constant dialysate conductivity (Franssen et al., 2005);
3. Relative BV change to be reached at the end of HD which is individually determined for each patient on the basis of anterior sessions. A short observation period (approximately two weeks) is usually required to analyse each patient's BV curve morphology and to determine their respective BV/UF ratio. This ratio represents the %BV per each kilogram of UF fluid, and indirectly reflects the individual patient refilling plasma capacity. Depending on this ratio, and on the total UF prescribed for each dialysis, the final %BV can be adjusted.

Of note, these three targets may sometimes be in conflict with each other, for example when large UF is prescribed for a patient with low plasma refilling rate (i.e. a high BV/UF ratio). The closed feedback loop system has then to reach the best compromise between the various targets and produce the most appropriate BV curve for this patient during that specific session.

Because of safety concerns, limits (or tolerance range) concerning maximum UF rate and sodium/conductivity range are also pre-specified (figure 2). Of note, there is no specific probe for plasmatic sodium with Hemocontrol®, as it is the case for Diacontrol® (see below). The dialysate conductivity is modulated toward a mean final value, but not in an automatic feedback response to patient's plasmatic sodium.

Overall, the goal of the Hemocontrol® system is to reach the same sodium and water balance as would a traditional approach, while the hemodynamic tolerability is enhanced by the profiling of the UF rate and the dialysate conductivity. Indeed, when the blood volume approaches the lower acceptable value for a given patient, UF is diminished or ceased while the dialysate conductivity is raised. Conversely, UF rate can be increased and/or dialysate conductivity decreased when blood volume is higher than expected on the pre-defined BV trajectory.

5.2 BVM® Fresenius

The Blood Volume Management (BVM®) module designed by Fresenius is available on the 4008 and 5008 HD machines. This system also has relative blood volume as the core feature of the feedback loop, but rather deals with the « critical relative blood volume (cRBV) » concept instead of tracking an optimal curve to reach a final BV.

The BV monitor is based on the measurement of total protein concentration (which includes plasma protein and Hb) by on-line ultrasound technology. Initially described by Schneditz (Schneditz et al., 1990), this method uses a probe in the arterial line that continuously measures the speed at which the ultrasounds travel through a specially designed cuvette. Since the sound speed is positively correlated to blood density, and, once again, assuming that the total content of blood does not change during UF, blood volume variations can be calculated from the changes in sound transmission velocity.

The critical relative blood volume (cRBV) is individually determined for each patient. It is the threshold at which a particular patient would be at risk of IDH, based on the anterior sessions. The monitored parameter is the blood volume reduction, and a defined algorithm modulates the UF rate according to the relation of the actual BV to the cRBV. The algorithm is designed to allow the maximal UF rate at the beginning of the session, where the plasma refilling capacity is generally at its best, with a gradual decrease afterwards to avoid reaching the cRBV:

$$\text{Actual UF rate} = \text{initial UF rate x factor} \quad (1)$$

$$\text{Initial UF rate} = 2 \text{ x (remaining UF/remaining time)} \quad (2)$$

The actual UF rate is the delivered UF rate and the initial UF rate is two times the ratio between the remaining UF and the remaining time (remaining UF/remaining time). The factor is a coefficient between 0 and 1 determined according to the current RBV. When the cRBV is reached, the factor is 0 and so the UF is transitorily suspended until the RBV rises again. When the relative blood volume is more than halfway the distance between the cRBV and 100%, the factor is 1 and maximal UF is allowed. Finally, when the RBV is more than halfway towards the cRBV, the factor is between 0 and 1 and decreases in a linear fashion (figure 3). This automatic feedback loop thus constantly adjust the UF rate to ensure, on one hand, that RBV stays over the predefined threshold and, on the other hand, that the UF rate is maximal at the beginning of the session and minimal at the end, where hypovolemia is

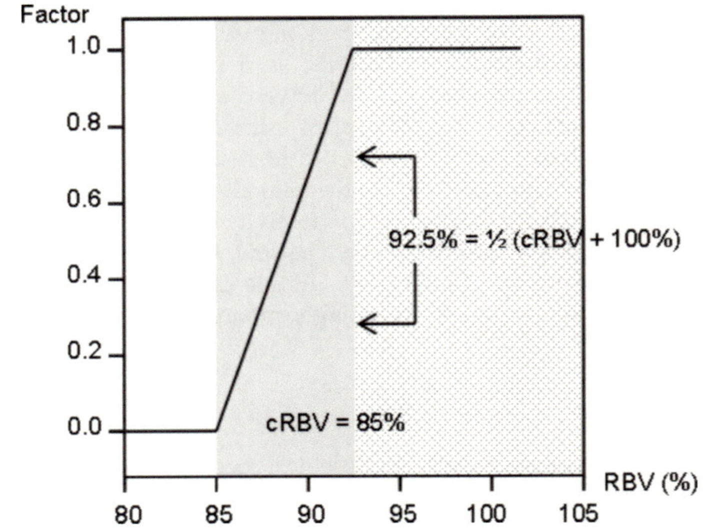

Fig. 3. BVM® algorithm (from Fresenius).
This figure illustrates an example where the cRBV is set at 85%. When the actual RBV is 85% or less (white area), factor is 0 and UF stops. When RBV is greater than halfway between cRBV and 100% (here, halfway between 85% and 100% is 92,5%), the factor is 1,0 and UF is maximal (shaded area). In between (gray area), factor is between 0 and 1, and UF is not maximal.

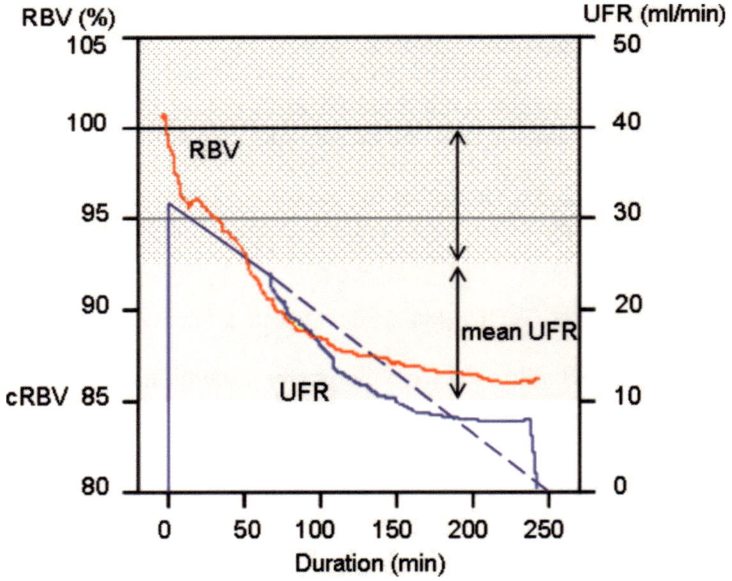

Fig. 4. UF rate in relation to RBV with the use of BVM® algorithm (from Fresenius).
This figure illustrates the changes in UF rate (UFR) and RBV during HD given a cRBV set at 85% (same as Figure 3). The UFR is initially higher and progressively declines following reduction of RBV.

more likely to happen (figure 4). Of note, the dialysate conductivity is not an effector in this system and, unless a specific sodium profile is prescribed, remains unchanged.

5.3 Impact of blood volume biofeedback systems

The two biofeedback systems described above are designed differently but share the same goal: stabilizing blood volume reduction to avoid IDH and, ideally, its related complications. Many studies have been published on the ability of these devices to reduce vascular instability, mostly with the Hemocontrol® system, but few studies assessed other outcomes. Table 1 summarizes published trials that evaluated the impact of blood volume biofeedback systems.

5.3.1 Reduction of intradialytic hypotension and nursing interventions

Definition of IDH in the literature is not standardized and so differs between studies. Some authors use a strict definition based on an absolute or relative reduction of arterial pressure, while others report IDH as a drop in BP accompanied by symptoms and/or requiring nursing intervention (such as stopping or slowing UF, saline infusion or Trendelenburg's position). Regardless of the definition used, the great majority of published trials, conclude that blood volume biofeedback systems are valuable in reducing IDH compared to standard hemodialysis (cf. table 1). Reduction of the proportion of HD sessions with at least one IDH episode ranges from 10 to 60%. However, it must be emphasized that most of these studies recruited patients who were already prone to hemodynamic instability, at varying degrees. As a general rule, the more severe and/or frequent the hemodynamic instability, the greater the benefits are from the automatic volume regulation.
The largest randomized controlled trial assessing the impact of biofeedback regulation on IDH occurrence was published by Santoro in 2002. Thirty-two hypotension-prone patients recruited in ten Italian nephrology centers were analysed in a cross-over, parallel group study of 4 months duration, comparing conventional HD to automatic BV-controlled HD. Although UF rate, pre and post-dialysis BP, and end-dialysis BV were the same with both treatments, a 30% reduction in dialysis sessions complicated by acute hypotension (systolic blood pressure ≤ 90 mm Hg or a ≥ 25 mm Hg decrease with symptoms) was observed with the use of automatic biofeedback. An additional aim of this trial was to identify which patient's parameters influence individual response to biofeedback. Clinical characteristics, dialysis prescriptions and plasma sodium values did not differ between the two treatment arms. However, two parameters appeared to be linked to responsiveness to BV-regulated feedback. First, good responders had higher final BV reduction and higher BV/UF ratio, suggesting a certain plasma refilling impairment. Second, poor responders had lower mean arterial pressure at the start of the HD sessions, and smaller increase in heart rate when standing from the lying position. Overall, these results indicate that IDH secondary to decreased plasma refilling capacity responds better to BV regulation than IDH due to impaired cardio-vascular reactivity. Of note, most studies that reported beneficial effects of biofeedback systems found similar results with regard to RBV changes during HD suggesting that reduction of IDH might not be exclusively explained by RBV preservation. As postulated by several authors, it is possible that treatment with BV automatic feedback exerts its favourable hemodynamic effect by preventing rapid RBV fluctuations (Santoro et al., 1994).
To evaluate whether BP stabilisation obtained per-dialysis with Hemocontrol® in IDH-prone patients was also sustained in the post-HD period, Franssen et al. (2005) used 24h BP

monitoring in a small prospective study. Following Hemocontrol®-driven HD, systolic blood pressure was significantly higher in the first 16 hours following HD, but this difference disappeared on the next morning. There was no difference in diastolic blood pressure. The authors concluded that the higher post HD systolic BP may explain the improvement of inter-HD symptoms observed in other studies (see below), although their study did not specifically evaluate interdialytic symptoms.

Only one randomized controlled trial did not restrict patient selection on the basis of previous hemodynamic instability or fluid overload (Déziel et al. 2007). This study included 57 patients (55% of them hypotension-prone) who were randomized to either standard HD or Hemocontrol®-driven HD. At 6 months, there was a 43% reduction in the number of sessions that required nursing interventions for IDH in the Hemocontrol® group (35% to 19%), compared with a 36% increase in nursing interventions in the control group (23% to 32%, p=0,04 for changes between groups). These results are in accordance with those reported by Ronco et al. (2000), who also demonstrated a significant decrease in the number of nursing interventions in a population prone to IDH when treated with BV biofeedback.

Finally, two non-randomized, short-term prospective studies specifically assessed the value of BV-regulated HD among non hypotensive-prone patients (Wolkotte et al., 2002 and McIntyre et al., 2003). Both found a statistically significant improvement in dialysis tolerance in terms of reduction of IDH.

Randomized trials

Author	Study design	Patients	Intervention (control)	Duration	Main endpoint(s)	Results (treatment vs. control)	
Ronco (2000)	RCT Cross-over	12 patients IDH-prone	AFB + HC vs. AFB	4 weeks	Sessions with IDH (%)	33 vs. 82	p<0,001
					Equilibrated Kt/V	1,13 vs. 1,03	p<0,001
Santoro (2002)	RCT Cross-over Multicenter	32 patients IDH-prone	Std HD+HC vs. Std HD	4 months	Sessions with IDH (%)	24 vs. 34	p=0,004
					Mean no. of interdialytic symptoms	2,7 vs. 3,1	p<0,001
Moret (2006)	RCT Cross-over	10 patients IDH-prone	Std HD+HC vs. Std HD	4 months	Post-HD plasm. conduct.	14,11 vs. 14,11	NS
					Ionic mass removal (mmol)	432 vs. 383	NS
					IDH (%)	16 vs. 8	NS
Selby (2006)	RCT Cross-over	8 patients IDH-prone LVH	Std HD+HC vs. Std HD	4 weeks	No. of regional wall motion abnormalities	23 vs. 42	OR 1,8; 95%CI, 1,1-3,0
					No. of IDH	12 vs. 24	OR 2,0; 95%CI, 1,0-4,4

Randomized trials							
Déziel (2007)	RCT	57 patients Unselected	Std HD+HC vs. Std HD	6 months	Home SBP change (mm Hg)	142 to 135 vs. 148 to 140	NS between groups
					Nursing interventions (% change)	-16 vs. +9	p=0,04
					Kidney burden score (change in score)	-6 vs. +5	p=0,004
Dasselaar (2007)	RCT	28 patients with hypertension and volume overload	Std HD+HC vs. Std HD	16 weeks	Pre-HD weight reduction (kg)	0,2 vs. 0,1	NS
					Pre-HD SBP reduction (mm Hg)	-23 vs. +3	p<0,01
					Pre-HD DBP reduction (mm Hg)	-8 vs. +1	p<0,05
Garzoni (2007)	RCT Cross-over Multi-center	56 patients IDH-prone	Std HD+BVM vs. Std HD	6 weeks	Sessions with IME requiring intervention (%)	43 vs. 46	NS
					Subgroup of high IDH incidence	57 vs. 65	p=0,016
Nesrallah (2008)	RCT	60 patients with volume overload	Std HD+BVM vs. Std HD	6 months	Change in ECFV (%)	1,8 vs. 0,87	NS
					Frequency of IDH	0,11 vs. 0,19	p<0,01
Gabrielli (2009)	RCT Cross-over Multi-center	26 patients IDH-prone	Std HD+BVM vs. Std HD	12 weeks	Sessions with IME requiring intervention (%)	32 vs. 40	p=0,02
					Mean no. of IME/session	0,42 vs. 0,53	p=0,04
					Equilibrated Kt/V	1,17 vs. 1,12	NS
Non-randomized trials							
Santoro (1998)	Prospective Cross-over	8 patients IDH-prone	Std HD + HC vs. Std HD	3 months	% of IDH	26 vs. 44 (A_1) and 27(A_2)	NS
					% of severe IDH	3 vs. 27 (A_1) vs. 17(A_2)	p<0,01

Non-randomized trials							
Basile (2001)	Prospective Cross-over	19 patients IDH-prone	Std HD + HC vs. Std HD	20 – 36 months	% sessions with IDH Post-HD asthenia score	21 vs. 32 6,2 vs. 4,3	p<0,0001 p<0,0001
Bégin (2002)	Prospective Cross-over	7 patients IDH-prone	Std HD + HC vs. Std HD	12 weeks	% of event-free sessions (sessions without intervention for IDH)	51 vs. 29	p<0,01
Wolkotte (2002)	Prospective Cross-over	16 patients Non IDH-prone	Std HD + HC vs. Std HD	9 weeks	% of IDH % of minor symptoms	6 vs. 16 11 vs. 18	p<0,05 p<0,05
McIntyre (2003)	Prospective Cross-over	15 patients Non IDH-prone	Std HD + HC vs. Std HD	8 weeks	% sessions with IDH	3,5 vs. 7	p<0,001
Franssen (2005)	Prospective	12 patients IDH-prone	Std HD + HC vs. Std HD	12 weeks	% sessions with IDH Post-HD SBP o 24h recording (mm Hg) Dry weight reduction (kg)	28 vs. 64 Same at 24h 2,1 vs. 2,0	p<0,01 NS NS
Winkler (2008)	Observational Cohort	18 patients IDH-prone with diabetes	Std HD + HC vs. baseline	48 weeks	No. of IDH per session Dry weight reduction (kg) % Cardiac ejection fraction	1 vs. 9 -1,7 vs. 0 53 vs. 43	p<0,01 NS NS

Trials are subdivided in randomized or non-randomized studies and listed by year of publication. AFB: acetate-free biofiltration, BVM: blood volume monitor (Fresenius), DBP: diastolic blood pressure, ECVF: extracellular fluid volume, IDH: intradialytic, hypotension, IME: intradialytic morbid events, HC: Hemocontrol® (Gambro), HD: hemodialysis, LVH: left ventricular hypertrophy, NS: non-significant, RCT: randomized controlled trial, SBP: systolic blood pressure, Std HD: standard bicarbonate-based hemodialysis

Table 1. Trials on the use of blood volume biofeedback control system in chronic hemodialysis

5.3.2 Reduction of intra- and inter- dialytic symptoms and improvement in quality of life

Regarding improvement of patient's symptoms during HD, some data are available in the literature but they are mostly based on secondary outcome analysis and show only limited evidence of benefit. Basile et al. (2001) prospectively followed patients for up to 36 months with BV-regulated HD during which period nurses and patients had to fill a symptoms questionnaire for each HD session. A reduction of muscle cramps during HD and an improvement in the post-HD asthenia score were found to be significantly associated with biofeedback system. However, self-evaluation of other intra- and inter- HD symptoms (notably, thirst) was not significantly different between the two treatment arms.

Ronco et al. (2000) found a significant reduction of the proportion of sessions with self-reported intradialytic symptoms following treatment with BV-controlled UF (21% vs. 76%, $p<0{,}001$). In addition, Santoro et al. (2002) also showed a 10% decrease of interdialytic symptoms following treatment with BV-controlled HD.

In a study by Déziel et al. (2007), the Kidney Disease and Quality of Life questionnaire (KDQOL) was used to evaluate quality of life at baseline and after 6 months of treatment with either Hemocontrol® or standard HD. Among the 20 items related to physical and mental health, only one parameter, burden of kidney disease, was significantly improved in the Hemocontrol® group versus the control group. Finally, in a randomized controlled trial of 60 patients, Nesrallah et al. (2008) did not find any significant difference with regard to dialysis-related symptoms and quality of life between the two treatment groups (Hemocontrol® versus standard HD) despite the fact that a reduction of IDH could be observed.

5.3.3 Hypertension and volume control

Three RCT specifically assessed the utility of BV regulation devices in improving fluid status and/or BP control in chronic hemodialysis patients. First, Dasselaar et al. (2007b) studied 12 hypertensive and mild volume-overloaded patients managed with either standard HD or BV tracking, where dry weight reduction was gradually undertaken by nephrologists according to clinical judgement. At 12 weeks, patients treated with BV regulation had a significantly lower pre- and post- HD systolic and diastolic blood pressure. Patients achieved larger UF volume without any change in RBV and showed reduction in extracellular water (determined by bioimpedance analysis). Despite these improvements in surrogate markers of volume status, no difference in mean weight from baseline could be observed. Authors concluded that this observation could result from increase in lean body mass; however, other specific nutritional parameters were not measured.

Second, in a trial published by Nesrallah et al. in 2008, volume-overloaded patients were included if bioimpedance displayed an extracellular fluid volume (ECFV) of at least 45%. In the treatment group, dry weight was adjusted by an algorithm guided by the Hemocontrol® biofeedback software based on plasma-refilling characteristics. At 6 months, there was no statistically significant difference between the two groups in the primary endpoint (change in ECFV) nor were there any significant differences in systolic blood pressure, total UF and interdialytic weight gain.

Finally, in a trial by Déziel et al. (2007), change in home blood pressure was evaluated following treatment with BV device versus standard HD. Patients were not selected on the basis of prior hypertension or volume overload history. While the use of Hemocontrol® effectively reduced home systolic BP, the clinical-based decision algorithm to manage BP in the standard group was as effective, and the overall difference between the groups was not significant.

In summary, no randomized trial has clearly demonstrated that the use of biofeedback devices is superior to standard HD and clinical judgement in reducing dry weight in volume expanded patients. Biofeedback devices may be of value in reducing blood pressure in hypertensive patients, although a systematic and clinical treatment algorithm may be as useful.

5.3.4 Reduction of left ventricular dysfunction

Cardiovascular morbidity and mortality are extremely high among chronic HD patients. Aside from the conventional risk factors for atherosclerosis, it was proposed that recurrent subclinical myocardial ischemia occurring during HD, as a result of silent decrease in myocardial perfusion, may contribute to the excessive cardio-vascular burden. In support of this hypothesis, Selby et al. (2006) demonstrated that reversible regional wall motion abnormalities which develop in a majority of hypotension-prone patients during HD, were substantially reduced with biofeedback dialysis. However, the observation period in this study was only 4 weeks, and it is unknown at the present time whether biofeedback HD provides any benefit on long-term cardiac dysfunction.

5.3.5 Improvement of dialysis delivery

Hemodialysis and UF may cause vasoconstriction of peripheral vascular beds, thus reducing peripheral tissue perfusion. This phenomenon may cause sequestration of urea, as only a central vascular loop of blood remains to be dialyzed. When hypotension occurs, this phenomenon may be aggravated leading to enhanced urea compartmentalization and reduced HD efficiency. Hence, it was proposed that improved hemodynamic stability during dialysis may improve urea removal and increase Kt/V.

Ronco et al. (2000) conducted a multi-center, cross-over randomized trial of 12 IDH-prone patients treated for two weeks with acetate-free biofiltration (AFB, schedule A) and for two weeks with AFB plus Hemocontrol® (schedule B). Parameters of urea kinetics were significantly improved when patients were on schedule B, with higher equilibrated Kt/V (1,12 vs. 1,03, $p<0,001$), and lower urea rebound at 30 minutes post-HD (6,4 vs. 14,2 g, $p<0,001$), despite similar predialysis urea concentration, HD prescriptions and treatment time.

However, a larger randomized trial of 26 patients followed for 12 weeks and treated with standard HD or BVM-controlled HD in a cross-over fashion did not find any significant improvement of equilibrated Kt/V in the treatment group (1,17 vs. 1,12, $p=0,156$) in spite of a slightly but significant higher treatment time and a 20% reduction of intradialytic morbid events (Gabrielli et al., 2009).

5.3.6 Morbidity and mortality

With improved hemodynamic tolerance, reduction of left ventricular wall dysfunction, and superior dialysis delivery, it would be reasonable to assume that the use of biofeedback systems would improve morbidity and mortality in chronic dialysis patients. Unfortunately, no trial to date has examined this issue and the question remains open.

Nevertheless, one large trial published in 2005 assessed the effect on morbidity of a BV-monitor based algorithm of UF control versus conventional management of volemia. The CLIMB (Crit-Line® Intradialytic Monitoring Benefit) study (Reddan et al., 2005) was a multi-centered, randomized, controlled trial of 443 chronic HD patients followed for 6 months during which ultrafiltration was either managed according to Crit-Line® values of RBV reduction, or by usual clinical strategies. Patients were not selected on a basis of prior IDH history, and the algorithm of the treatment group was only proposed and not mandatory. During the follow-up period, there were no statistically significant differences between the two groups regarding the number of IDH, the occurrence of intradialytic symptoms and the control of BP. Surprisingly, the risk ratios for both non-access and access-related hospitalizations were higher in the Crit-Line® group (adjusted RR 1,61 and 1,52; p-value 0,01 and 0.04, respectively). Mortality was 8.7% in the treatment group and 3.3% in the control group (p=0.021). The authors concluded that the availability of Crit-Line® may alter clinicians' behaviour and may cause a risk for patients, although these results have to be interpreted cautiously since the control group had an atypically low hospitalization and mortality rate.

5.4 Blood volume biofeedback and sodium overload

One of the potential risks of automated BV regulation using sodium (Na) or conductivity modulation is alteration in sodium removal, with consequent Na overload and increased thirst, which can theoretically lead to increased interdialytic weight gain and worsening hypertension. Most of the studies described above did not find a significant change in pre and post HD sodium concentration (Santoro et al., 2002; Wolkotte et al., 2002; Dasselaar et al., 2007b, etc.), although plasma Na is a poor surrogate of real sodium balance.

Moret et al. (2006) assessed the effect of such devices on sodium transfer during hemodialysis. In a cross-over randomized trial of 10 patients with frequent hypotension, plasma conductivity (PC) and ionic mass balance (IMB) were compared in four different HD modalities: standard HD with fixed Na concentration (140 mmol/L), linear Na profiling (150 to 140 mmol/L), BV-controlled feedback with Hemocontrol® (mean dialysate conductivity (DC) 14,0 mS/cm) and plasma-conductivity (PC)-controlled feedback with Diacontrol® (see below) (post-dialytic PC target of 14,0 mS/cm). Mean pre- and post-dialytic PC were statistically higher during Na-profiled HD, and post-dialytic PC was lower in PC-controlled feedback, compared to the other three modalities. The effects of BV-regulated HD on PC and IMB did not differ from those of standard HD, and thus it seems that BV-regulated HD can be prescribed without any safety concern regarding sodium loading.

6. Other biofeedback systems

Three other biofeedback systems were designed to reduce the occurrence of hypotensive episodes during HD. Rather than focusing on BV changes during HD, these devices use other targets (e.g. arterial BP) or other means of action (e.g. thermal balance, plasma conductivity). They are reviewed here briefly.

6.1 Arterial pressure biofeedback

Arterial pressure biofeedback aimed at stabilizing BP during HD uses repetitive measurement of arterial blood pressure as the monitored parameter and a fuzzy-logic system as the controller of fluid removal. Created by B. Braun and implemented on the Dialog Advanced machines, the APBS® (Automatic Blood Pressure Stabilization system) puts blood pressure itself as the main input to the automatic fuzzy controller rather than a surrogate marker (e.g. blood volume). Fuzzy logic is a problem-solving system, rather than a mathematical model, and is reported to be better suited to analyse and compute non-linear data systems. It mimics how a person would make a decision, based on judgments such as: « if X, then Y», according to the rules pre-set by the operator. In a practical manner, the operator has to set two parameters for each patient: the BP set point and the maximal UF rate. The set-point is the critical BP level at which the patient experiences symptomatic hypotension, or simply the BP threshold at which the nurse or the physician would consider stopping the UF in that particular patient. The maximal UF rate is defined as the maximal rate of fluid removal that can be applied at any time, since this system is designed to maximise UF rate at the start of the HD session and to minimize it towards the end. With a specialized arm cuff that takes BP measurements every five minutes, three variables are calculated (Mancini et al., 2007): 1) Relative difference between actual systolic BP and the pre-adjusted set point; 2) Short-term pressure trend (15 min); 3) Long-term pressure trend (25 min). These input data are then computed by the fuzzy controller through several steps that involve probabilistic reasoning according to specific rule bases, and ultimately result in modulation of the UF rate, in a closed feedback loop (figure 5). This system allows gradual and continuous variations of the UF rate, as it varies proportionally to the changes of the BP trends.

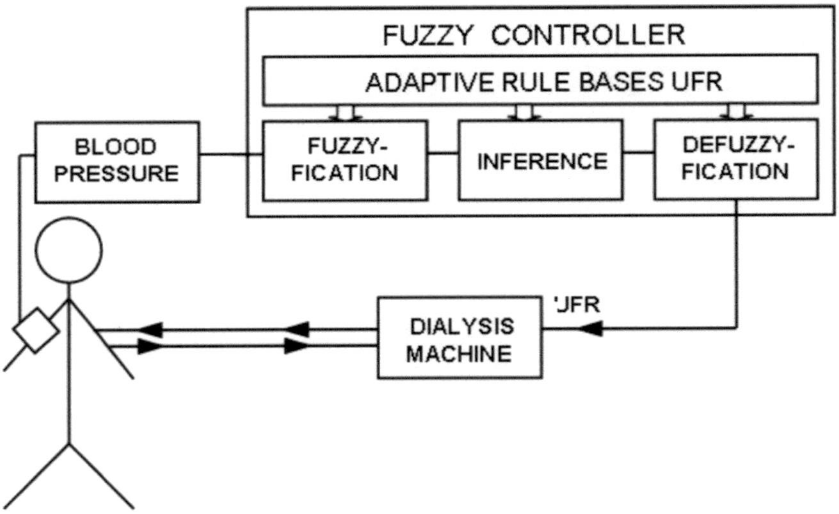

Fig. 5. Fuzzy control of the UF rate.
Technical scheme of the closed-loop system for the fuzzy control of the UF rate. (Adapted from Mancini et al., 2007)

Literature on the use of fuzzy logic control in preventing IDH is still scarce, but a prospective multi-center study published in 2007 (Mancini et al., 2007) showed a significant decrease of 25% in IDH incidence in 55 hypotension-prone patients. The authors emphasized the need to introduce correct critical BP for each patient for the fuzzy controller to perform adequately (Mancini et al., 2007).

6.2 Thermal balance system

During HD, body temperature usually rises due in part to an increased production of heat secondary to inflammatory reactions induced by imperfect dialysate water and biocompatibility of membranes, and in part by decreased blood flow to the skin, with subsequent heat retention. This phenomenon can contribute to hemodynamic instability. Cooler dialysate, by inducing vasoconstriction, is known to enhance vascular stability, but poor tolerance due to chills and discomfort is a major drawback to its use.

Blood temperature control (BTC®, Fresenius) is a biofeedback system aimed at keeping body temperature stable throughout the session, with progressive decline of dialysate temperature in response to progressive increased in heat production, resulting in « isothermic dialysis » (Mercadal & Petitclerc, 2009). Designed by Fresenius, the blood temperature monitor (BTM) is composed of sensors in the arterial and venous lines and monitors blood temperature change by a thermodilution technique. Thermal balance can be maintained through the automatic modulation of the dialysate temperature (the output) by the BTC® software (the controller) in response to BTM measurements compared to the set target temperature (the input).

A systematic review, published in 2006, reviewed the most pertinent publications on the clinical effects of cool dialysate (Selby & McIntyre, 2006). Six of them, which were all cross-over studies of relatively short duration, evaluated the use of BTM compared to various control groups. Overall, there was a significant decrease in IDH frequency with reduction in dialysate temperature using BTM, with a rate of IDH 2.0 (95% CI, 1.9-2.1) times less than control group.

6.3 Plasma conductivity biofeedback system

This biofeedback system was designed to allow variation in the dialysate sodium (Na) concentration to better suit the patient's initial plasmatic value and parallel the changes in plasma Na concentration occurring during dialysis. Instead of a fixed dialysate Na concentration, a target final plasma conductivity (as a surrogate for Na) is rather prescribed, and thus the patient's post-dialysis sodium concentration is independent of the initial status. The goal of this system is to maximise sodium removal individually for each session, but avoiding large gap between plasmatic and dialysate sodium, which can produce patient's discomfort, hypotension and cramps (if dialysate Na is lower) or sodium loading, thirst and worsening hypertension (if dialysate Na is higher).

The Diascan® (Gambro) module monitors the patient's plasma conductivity every 15 minutes through conductivity probes located at the dialysate inlet and outlet. The software Diacontrol® (Gambro) computes this information and softly and gradually modulates the dialysate conductivity in order to reach the prespecified target plasmatic conductivity at the end of the session. The curve of the conductivity trajectory is pre-defined and minimizes large variations to avoid rapid shift of plasmatic osmolality and disequilibrium syndrome.

Again, large randomized trials are lacking to evaluate the utility of this feedback system, and results of two small prospective studies published recently are conflicting. Both compared Diacontrol® to standard dialysis in stable patients to assess whether gradual decrease in target conductivity, and consequent increased ionic mass balance (meaning increased sodium removal) could be achieved. Manlucu and colleagues (2010) found a significant reduction in end plasmatic conductivity and in ionic mass balance, with consequent reduction in IDWG and BP. On the contrary, Selby and al. (2007) found a lower final conductivity with fixed dialysate conductivity, and no difference in BP, IDH frequency or dialysis tolerability. Hence, demonstration of a Diacontrol® beneficial effect remains to be proven.

7. Conclusions

IDH is the most frequent complication of dialysis, and is associated with significant patient morbidity. Although pathogenesis is multifactorial, blood volume reduction appears to be central in the development of such events, especially when cardio-vascular compensatory mechanisms are impaired. In an attempt to reduce hypotensive episodes, blood volume biofeedback devices have been developed. The underlying premise of such devices is to automatically adjust dialysis parameters such as UF rate and dialysate conductivity, in response to variations of monitored patient's characteristics, in order to make dialysis sessions more physiological and to prevent IDH by acting on subclinical signs of hemodynamic instability. Evidence supports BV biofeedback in hypotensive prone patients to reduce occurrence of IDH, nursing interventions, and probably intra- and inter- dialytic symptoms, although no large scale randomized trial has been published to date. BV biofeedback may also be helpful to enhance vascular tolerance in stable patients, but literature is limited. Data concerning improvement of hypertension and volume overload, as well as improvement of dialysis delivery, is conflicting. Finally, there is no large randomized trial that assessed the impact of automatic BV control on morbidity and mortality. Data suggesting that Crit-line® based algorithm of hypertension management is associated with higher hospitalisation and mortality rates are of concern. Larger and long-term randomized trials comparing BV biofeedback devices to standard HD are needed to better define the impact of these novel technologies on patient outcomes.

8. References

Andrulli, S., Colzani, S., Mascia, F., Lucchi, L., Stipo, L., Bigi, MC., Crepaldi, M., Redaelli, B., Albertazzi, A. & Locatelli, F. (2002). The role of blood volume reduction in the genesis of intradialytic hypotension. *Am J Kidney Dis.* Vol.40, No.6, pp. 1244-54

Basile, C., Giordano, R., Vernaglione, L., Montanaro, A., De Maio, P., De Padova, F., Marangi, AL., Di Marco, L., Santese, D., Semeraro, A. & Liogorio, VA. (2001). Efficacy and safety of haemodialysis treatment with the Hemocontrol biofeedback system: a prospective medium-term study. *Nephrol Dial Transplant.* Vol.16, No.2, pp. 328-334

Bégin, V., Déziel, C. & Madore, F. (2002). Biofeedback regulation of ultrafiltration and dialysate conductivity for the prevention of hypotension during hemodialysis. *ASAIO J.* Vol.48, No.3, pp. 312-315

Burton, JO., Jefferies, HJ., Selby, NM. & McIntyre CW. (2009). Hemodialysis-induced cardiac injury: determinants and associated outcomes. *Clin J Am Soc Nephrol.* Vol.4, No.5, pp. 914-20

Dasselaar, JJ., Huisman, RM., De Jong, PE. & Franssen, CFM. (2007a). Relative blood volume measurements during hemodialysis: Comparisons between three noninvasive devices. *Hemodialysis International.* Vol.11, No.4, pp. 448-455

Dasselaar, JJ., Huisman, RM., De Jong, PE., Burgerhof, JGM. & Franssen, CFM. (2007b). Effects of relative blood volume-controlled hemodialysis on blood pressure and volume status in hypertensive patients. *ASAIO J.* Vol.53, No.3, pp. 357-364

Daugirdas, JT. (2001). Pathophysiology of dialysis hypotension: an update. (2001). *Am J Kidney Dis.* Vol.38, No.4, suppl 4, pp. S11-S17

Déziel, C., Bouchard, J., Zellweger, M. & Madore, F. (2007). Impact of Hemocontrol on hypertension, nursing interventions, and quality of life: A randomized, controlled trial. *Clin J Am Soc Nephrol*. Vol.2, No.4, pp. 661-668

Franssen, CFM., Dasselaar, JJ., Sytsma, P., Burgerhof, JGM., De Jong, PE. & Huisman, RM. (2005). Automatic feedback control of relative blood volume changes during hemodialysis improves blood pressure stability during and after dialysis. *Hemodialysis International*. Vol.9, No.4, pp. 383-392

Gabrielli, D., Kristal, B., Katzarski, K., Youssef, M., Hachache, T., Lopot, F., Lasseur, C., Gunne, T., Draganov, B., Wojke, R. & Gauly, A. (2009). Improved intradialytic stability during haemodialysis with blood volume-controlled ultrafiltration. *J Nephrol*. Vol.22, No.2, pp. 232-240

Garzoni, D., Keusch, G., Kleinoeder, T., Martin, H., Dhondt, A., Cremaschi, L., Tatsis, E., Ibrahim, N., Boer, W., Kuehne, S., Claus, M., Zahn, M., Schuemann, E., Engelmann, J., Hickstein, H., Wojke, R., Gauly, A. & Passlick-Deetjen, J. (2007). Reduced complications during hemodialysis by automatic blood volume controlled ultrafiltration. *Int J Artif Organs*. Vol.30, No.1, pp. 16-24

Locatelli, F., Buoncristiani, U., Canaud, B., Köhler, H., Petitclerc, T. & Zucchelli, P. (2005). Haemodialysis with on-line monitoring equipment: tool or toys? *Nephrol Dial Transplant*. Vol.20, No.1, pp. 22-33

Mancini, E., Mambelli, E., Irpinia, M., Gabrielli, D., Cascone, C., Conte, F., Meneghel, G., Cavatorta, F., Antonelli, A., Villa, G., Dal Canton, A., Cagnoli, L., Aucella, F., Fiorini, F., Gaggiotti, E., Triolo, G., Nuzzo, V. & Santoro, A. (2007). Prevention of dialysis hypotension episodes using fuzzy logic control system. *Nephrol Dial Transplant*.Vol.22, No.5, pp. 1420-1427

Manlucu, J.,Gallo, K., Heidenheim, PA. & Lindsay, RM. (2010). Lowering postdialysis plasma sodium (conductivity) to increase sodium removal in volume-expanded hemodialysis patients: A pilot study using a biofeedback software system. *Am J Kidney Dis*. Vol.56, No.1, pp. 69-76

McIntyre, CW., Lambie, SH. & Fluck, RJ. (2003). Biofeedback controlled hemodialysis reduces symptoms and increases both hemodynamic tolerability and dialysis adequacy in non-hypotension prone stable patients. *Clin Nephrol*. Vol.60, No.2, pp. 105-112

Mercadal, L. & Petitclerc, T. (2009). Technical advances in haemodialysis. *Néphrologie & Thérapeutique*. Vol.5, No.2, pp. 109-113

Mitra, S., Chamney, P., Greenwood, R. & Farrington, K. (2004). The relationship between systemic and whole-body hematocrit is not constant during ultrafiltration on hemodialysis. *J Am Soc Nephrol*.Vol.15, No.2, pp. 463-469

Mizumasa, T., Hirakata, H., Yoshimitsu, T., Kubo, M., Kashiwagi, M., Tanaka, H., Kanai, H., Fujimi, S. & Iida, M. (2004). Dialysis-related hypotension as a cause of progressive frontal lobe atrophy in chronic hemodialysis patients: a 3-year prospective study. *Nephron Clin Pract*. Vol.97, No.1, pp. 23–30

Moret, K., Aalten, J., van den Wall Bake, W., Gerlag, P., Beerenhout, C., van der Sande, F., Leunissen, K. & Kooman, J. (2006). The effect of sodium profiling and feedback technologies on plasma conductivity and ionic mass balance: a study in hypotension-prone dialysis patients. *Nephrol Dial Transplant*. Vol.21, No.1, pp. 138-144

Nesrallah, GE., Suri, RS., Thiessen-Philbrook, H., Heidenheim, P. & Lindsay, RM. (2008). Can extra-cellular fluid volume expansion in hemodialysis patients be safely reduced using the Hemocontrol biofeedback algorithm? A randomized trial. *ASAIO J.* Vol.54, No.3, pp. 270-274

Reddan, DN., Szczech, LA., Hasselblad, V., Lowrie, EG., Lindsay, RM., Himmelfarb, J., Toto, RD., Stivelman, J., Winchester, JF., Zillman, LA., Califf, RM. & Owen Jr, WF. (2005). Intradialytic blood volume monitoring in ambulatory hemodialysis patients: A randomized trial. *J Am Soc Nephrol.* Vol.16, No.7, pp. 2162-2169

Ronco, C., Brendolan, A., Milan, M., Rodeghiero, MP., Zanella, M. & La Greca, G. (2000). Impact of biofeedback-induced cardiovascular stability on hemodialysis tolerance and efficiency. *Kidney Int.* Vol.58, No.2, pp. 800-808.

Santoro, A., Mancini, E., Paolini, F., Spongano, M. & Zuchelli, P. (1994). Automatic control of blood volume trends during hemodialysis. *ASAIO J.* Vol.40, No.3, pp. M419-422

Santoro, A., Mancini, E., Paolini, F. & Zucchelli, P. (1996). Blood volume monitoring and control. *Nephrol Dial Transplant.* Vol.11, Suppl. 2, pp. 42-47

Santoro, A., Mancini, E., Paolini, F., Cavicchioli, G., Bosetto, A. & Zucchelli, P. (1998). Blood volume regulation during hemodialysis. *Am J Kidney Dis.* Vol.32, No.5, pp. 739-748

Santoro, A., Mancini, E., Basile, C., Amoroso, L., Di Giulio, S., Usberti, M., Colasanti, G., Verzetti, G., Rocco, A., Imbasciati, E., Panzetta, G., Bolzani, R., Grandi, F. & Polacchini, M. (2002). Blood volume controlled hemodialysis in hypotension-prone patients: A randomized, multicenter controlled trial. *Kidney Int.* Vol.62, No.3, pp. 1034-1045

Schneditz, D., Pogglitsch, H., Horina, J. & Binswanger, U. (1990). A blood protein monitor for the continuous measurement of blood volume changes during hemodialysis. *Kidney Int.* Vol.38, No.2, pp. 342-346

Selby, NM., Lambie, SH., Camici, PG., Baker, CS. & McIntyre CW. (2006). Occurrence of regional left ventricular dysfunction in patients undergoing standard and biofeedback dialysis. *Am J Kidney Dis.* Vol.47, No.5, pp. 830-841

Selby, NM. & McIntyre, CW. (2006). A systematic review of the clinical effects of reducing dialysate fluid temperature. *Nephrol Dial Transplant.* Vol.21, No.7, pp. 1883-1898

Selby, NM., Taal, MW. & McIntyre, CW. (2007). Comparison of progressive conductivity reduction with diacontrol and standard dialysis. *ASAIO J.* Vol.53, No.2, pp. 194-200

Winkler, RE., Pätow, W. & Ahrenholz, P. (2008). Blood volume monitoring. *Contrib Nephrol.* Vol.161, pp. 119-124

Wolkotte, C., Hassell, D., Moret, K., Gerlag, PG., van den Wall Bake, AW., van der Sande, FM. & Kooman, JP. (2002). Blood volume control by biofeedback and dialysis-induced symptomatology. A short-term clinical study. *Nephron.* Vol.92, No.3, pp. 605-609.

3

Sodium and Hemodialysis

Matthew Gembala and Satish Kumar
University of Oklahoma
USA

1. Introduction

The original dialysate sodium prescription was 126.5 mEq/L (Kolff, 1947). Before volumetric controlled ultrafiltration, sodium was removed primarily, slowly and most predictably by diffusion. With the development of high flux dialysis membranes, dialysate osmolality asserted a faster and more dramatic effect on serum osmolality. Hypotonic dialysate rapidly drops serum osmolality that leads to net fluid shift out of the vascular space, causing significant intradialytic symptoms (Stewart et al., 1972). Further, the duration of dialysis sessions was shortened as clearance of urea was improved, requiring an accelerated rate of ultrafiltration.

To counter symptoms of hypo-osmolarity and rapid ultrafiltration, dialysate sodium concentration was increased. In the early 1970s, Stewart demonstrated less cramping with sodium of 145 mEq/L than with 132 mEq/L (Stewart et al., 1972). In the early 1980s, Locatelli showed improved cardiovascular stability when sodium concentration was raised to 148 mEq/L from 142 mEq/L (Locatelli et al., 1982). As the sodium prescription increased, concerns about sodium overloading arose. In 1985, Cybulsky demonstrated worsening of hypertension in already hypertensive patients (Cybulsky et al., 1985); and Daugirdas showed increasing thirst and interdialytic weight gain (IDWG), in both level and modelled high sodium techniques (Daugirdas et al., 1985). Nevertheless, intradialytic hemodynamic stability remained a valid concern and the data were not always clear. For example, Barré showed no worsening of hypertension and pulmonary edema at [Na^+] 145, 150 and 155 mEq/L (Barré, 1988). The technique of sodium modelling offered a theoretical means to attenuate the risk of sodium loading. By the early 1990s, Acchiardo advocated, "[s]odium modelling [149mEq/L dropping to 140 mEq/L] should always be used in patients being maintained on high flux dialysis" (Acchiardo & Hayden, 1991). This approach was widely practiced throughout the 1990s. After more than a decade of high sodium and sodium profiling dialysis, trends toward exacerbation of hypertension and interdialytic weight gain were becoming evident (Song, 2002).

Despite a growing body of literature on the effects of dialysis sodium, the sodium prescription is frequently overlooked or ineffectually utilized. Further, despite the increasing sophistication of dialysis delivery systems, the sodium prescription is often not adjusted to suit individual patient needs. First, we will erect a conceptual framework for understanding the dialysate sodium prescription. Second, we will review the primary literature regarding dialysate sodium and outcomes. Third, we will formulate recommendations on prescribing dialysate sodium. Finally, we will explore the technical and systems challenges to adjusting the actual sodium delivered to an individual patient.

2. Theoretical framework for consideration of dialysate sodium

2.1 The relationship of sodium to volume

Traditionally, sodium content of the body and extracellular volume are equivalent concepts. Sodium concentration is a function of osmotic regulation while total sodium content is a function volume regulation. In renal, hepatic, or cardiac impairment, excess sodium cannot be adequately offloaded, leading to extracellular fluid accumulation in the form of peripheral and pulmonary edema, and ascites. Dialysis offers a means of volume regulation in the form of ultrafiltration. Hydrostatic gradients generated across the dialysis membrane are used to remove (relatively) isotonic fluid from the vascular space. Intradialytic weight gain (IDWG) is a function of the salt and water intake between dialysis sessions. Increased IDWG is attributed to dietary non-compliance; conversely, decreased IDWG reflects excellent dietary compliance or can be a harbinger of poor nutritional status as low salt intake can parallel inadequate protein-calorie intake (Sarkar et al., 2006). These mutually confounding factors must always be recognized when designing or evaluating outcomes research evaluating IDWG. An occult source of sodium can offset even the most compliant diet: hypertonic dialysate. While the programmed hydrostatic gradient moves sodium (volume) out of the patient in the form of ultrafiltrate, osmotic gradients can move sodium in or out of the patient by diffusion.

2.2 Defining the sodium space

When dialyzing against hypertonic sodium, patient's sodium rises - but not so much that causes adverse osmotic sequelae. Problems arise by utilizing the osmotic utility of elevated interdialytic serum sodium without weighing the volume implications. When using profiling techniques, serum sodium concentration only increased from a predialysis average of 138.6 +/- 0.2 to 141.0 +/- 0.1 when dialyzing against an average dialysate sodium of 147mEq/L (Song et al., 2002). This change is an increase in of 2.4mEq/L; multiplying by the volume of distribution of sodium in a 70kg male patient results in 33meq of sodium transferred by diffusion. Once the set-point serum osmolality is restored by oral fluid intake, this represents just a little more than 200cc of normal saline (NS). As an osmotic agent, however, sodium's effects are distributed beyond the extracellular fluid. A change in serum sodium reflects a change in total body osmolality, or "total body cation" (Charra & Chazot, 2003; Gotch et al., 1980). When the extracellular sodium concentration rises, intracellular water will diffuse into the extracellular space reaching a new equilibrium: the predominant intracellular cation, potassium, would rise similarly to the extracellular sodium. Using the data presented by Song et al. (2002), an increase in serum sodium of 2.4mEq/L could be multiplied across the total body water; in a 70kg person this would result in a net diffusion of 100mEq of sodium, equivalent to 650cc of NS. Based on these calculations, the increase in IDWG should be between 0.20kg ($\Delta Na^{+} \approx \Delta$extracellular volume) and 0.65kg (Δsodium $\approx$ Δtotal body cation). The measured increase in IDWG, however, was greater than either calculated value. IDWG increased by 1.20kg. It is clear that the "osmolar space" is greater than the total body water. The body must be able to store sodium/osmoles outside the osmolar pool.

2.3 Non-Osmotic sodium

Increasing serum osmolality causes increased thirst leading to rapid re-accumulation of volume. As demonstrated above, this cannot account for all the sodium/volume transfer of hypertonic dialysate. Hypertonic dialysate causes sodium to accumulate in the extracellular matrix in a concentration dependent, non-osmotic fashion. In a now classic experiment, Saul Farber, Maxwell Schubert, and Nancy Schuster demonstrated how sodium behaves in connective tissue (Farber et al., 1957). Completely ionized chondroitin sulfate can complex with "countercations" at a ratio of 1:100. Every mol of chondroitin can associate with 100 mols of sodium- thereby reducing soluble (osmotically active) sodium. The proportion of sodium complexed with chondroitin is positively correlated to the concentration of sodium in the surrounding solution. In addition to chondroitin sulfate, hyaluronic acid and other mucopolysaccharides can interact with multiple sodium ions (Dunstone, 1959; Schubert, 1964). Given relative equal binding capacity of chondroitin sulfate for most cations (Na^+, K^+, Mg^{2+}, Ca^{2+}, Sr^{2+}, Ba^{2+}), the relative concentration will determine the quantity of ion bound to the polyanion (Woodbury, 1956). Therefore, when the serum sodium concentration is increased (such as when dialyzing against a high sodium dialysate), it follows that the sodium content of the mucopolysaccharides will also increase. As each ion of sodium complexes with a polyanion, it leaves the osmotic pool, leaving a lower serum sodium concentration - restoring the dialysate:serum sodium gradient. Sodium will continue to diffuse into the patient until the polyanions are saturated while the patient osmolality will not rise appreciably. Thus, the net transfer of sodium into the patient will be much more than simply the difference between the predialysis and postdialysis serum sodium as demonstrated by the calculations in paragraph 2.2. When dialysis is complete, water intake will eventually restore serum sodium to the set-point determined by the hypothalamic osmostat. The mucopolysaccharide sodium reservoir will release sodium into the osmotic pool, stimulating thirst and driving extracellular volume expansion.

Polyanions are ubiquitously distributed: bone (Woodbury, 1956), cartilage (Dunstone, 1959), blood vessels (Tobain et al., 1961), liver, intestine, brain, kidney (Law, 1984), lung and skin (Titze et al., 2003). Given this distribution, it should not be surprising that extracellular, soluble sodium makes up approximately 75% of total body sodium (Bergstrom, 1955). Therefore, 25% of total body sodium is sequestered out of the extracellular osmotic pool. The amplitude of the effect of non-osmotic sodium reservoirs should be significant.

The typical acid/base cycle in hemodialysis patients amplify pathologic sodium binding & release of polyanions, especially those of bone. Approximately 25% of total body sodium is sequestered in the bone and cartilage (Harrison, 1936). Thirty to forty percent of skeletal sodium is exchangeable with circulating sodium every 24hrs (Kaltreider, 1941; Forbes & Perley, 1951; Forbes & Lewis, 1956). During acidosis, sodium is freed from the bone, the hydrogen ion displacing the sodium ion (Levitt, 1955; Bergstrom, 1955). This model approximates the interdialytic period. The inverse process occurs during dialysis; as pH rapidly corrects, H^+ ions disassociate from bone easily leaving room for sodium – a process amplified by high dialysate sodium. After dialysis, pH begins to fall; hydrogen ions reaccumulate, displacing bound sodium back into the osmotically active sodium pool, driving volume expansion.

Polyanions are not a static quantity. A high sodium environment leads to increased glycosaminoglycans synthesis: the expression mRNA of various enzymes for the synthesis of glycosaminoglycans increases 120% to 210% during high sodium intake (Heer, 2009). Increased polyanion synthesis leads to an expansion of the non-osmotic sodium pool. Further, there is increasing evidence that hypertonic stress and sodium overload stimulate mononuclear phagocyte system cells to release vascular endothelial growth factor C (VEGF-C) promoting lymphangiogenesis (Titze & Machnik, 2010). Thus, hypertonic dialysate may stimulate the creation of reservoirs for further sodium storage.

3. Review of the primary literature: dialysate sodium and outcomes

At least fourteen studies can be identified that examine the relationship between variation in the dialysate sodium prescription and various clinical measures. Four retrospective, case-control studies and ten prospective, cohort studies were identified. Three additional studies examine variation of dialysate conductivity in a similar manner.

3.1 Retrospective studies

As seen in Table 1, we identified four retrospective studies evaluating the relationship between dialysate sodium and interdialytic weight gain and blood pressure control. In these chart-review approaches, patients were compared in a case-control manner. In two studies, 58 patients dialyzed against the same sodium bath of 143mEq/L (Keen & Gotch, 2007; Levin et al., 2001). Patient's pre-dialysis serum sodium 'set point' was compared to the dialysate sodium resulting in a positive or negative "sodium gradient." Patients with a negative gradient had a serum sodium concentration greater than the dialysate sodium concentration; these patients had better interdialytic weight gain and improved blood pressure control than those with a positive gradient, without any change in intradialytic hypotension. Therefore, the lower the dialysate (compared to the patient's sodium) the better the IDWG and BP control.

In the two audits, patients dialyzing against a relatively lower sodium concentration had less IDWG (Davenport 2006, 2008). In the initial study, lower dialysate sodium was correlated with an improvement in BP control (defined as decrease in pre-dialysis blood pressure or number of antihypertensives prescribed). However, in the larger follow-up study, this relationship did not hold. It must be remembered that this retrospective design cannot account for the prescribing physicians reasons for the choice of dialysate sodium. It is likely that hypotension prone patients would be prescribed a higher sodium bath and less antihypertensives.

Author (year)	n	Dialysate [Na+] (mEq/L)	Effect of Lower Dialysate [Na+] on		
			IDWG	BP Control	Intradialytic hypotension
Keen, Gotch (2007)	58	143 c/w patient's set point[a]	improved	improved	no change
Levin, Keen (2001)	58	143 c/w patient's set point[a]	improved	improved	N/A
Davenport (2006)	469	136-139, 140, >140	improved	improved	no change
Davenport (2008)	2187	136-139, 140, >140	improved	no change	improved

Table 1. Four retrospective studies examining the relationship of dialysate sodium prescription on interdialytic weight gain (IDWG), Blood Pressure (BP) Control, and Intradialytic hypotension. BP control is defined as improved pre-dialysis blood pressure measures and/or reduction in number of antihypertensives prescribed. n = number of patients in the study. c/w = 'compared with'. N/A = data not available. [a]"Set Point" was defined as mean monthly predialysis plasma sodium concentration.

3.2 Prospective studies

As seen in Table 2, we identified ten (10) prospective involving 165 patients evaluating the relationship between the dialysate sodium prescription and IDWG, BP control, intradialytic hypotension and thirst.

3.2.1 IDWG

Of the nine (9) prospective studies reporting data on IDWG, eight (8) showed statistically significant improvement in IDWG during dialysis on the lower sodium dialysate. The one study that did not show any change in IDWG compared the narrowest sodium difference (141mEq/L vs. 138 mEq/L), making it the most susceptible to beta error (Thein et al., 2007). This 8 month study did show a blunting of the expected seasonal increase in IDWG and BP (Argiles, 2004), perhaps due to the lower sodium dialysate used during the four months of winter typically associated with higher IDWG.

3.2.2 Blood pressure control

Six prospective studies demonstrate improvement in blood pressure control after switching patients to lower dialysate sodium. Blood pressure control is defined as reduction in predialysis blood pressure measures or reduction in number of prescribed antihypertensives. Three studies showed no change in blood pressure control. No study, however, showed worsening blood pressure on lower dialysate sodium. It seems certain that a modest reduction in dialysate sodium can have beneficial influence on blood pressure management.

3.2.3 Interdialytic hypotension

Of the five studies reporting interdialytic hypotensive events, two demonstrated more frequent hypotension on the lower sodium dialysate. The first found, 9% fewer dialysis sessions complicated by hypotension using higher dialysate sodium (Cybulsky et al., 1985). Of note, the dialysate sodium used in the "low sodium" cohort was 133mEq/L, the second lowest in all of the studies reviewed. However, given the yearlong duration of this study, the results cannot be dismissed lightly. The other study showing worsening BP stability during dialysis had an increased incident rate of approxamately 10% as well (Song, 2002). These studies highlight the limitations of reducing sodium indefinitely. There is a lower limit on decreasing serum osmolality before fluid shifts into the interstitium enough to cause hypotension. Two studies showed no change in intradialytic hypotension. One had the narrowest range of dialysate sodium (Thein et al., 2007) while the other had nearly the largest (see table 2 and Daugirdas et al., 1985). One study actually demonstrated better hemodyanamic stability on lower sodium dialysate highlighting the sometimes paradoxical effects of high sodium (de Paula et al., 2004): As hypertonic dialysate drives higher IDWG, ultrafiltration must increase in order to maintain steady dry weight. If IDWG becomes great enough, removing this excess fluid will put the patient at risk for intradialytic hypotension.

3.2.4 Thirst

Effect of dialysate sodium on thirst was quite variable. Thirst is probably most dependent on subjective patient factors than any other factor.

Author (Year)	n	t (weeks)	Dialysate [Na+] (mEq/L)	Effect of Lower Dialysate [Na+] on			
				IDWG	BP Control	Intradialytic Hypotension	Thirst
Cybulsky (1985)	16	52	133, 144	improved[c]	improved[f]	worsened	no change
Daugirdas (1985)	7	12	135, 143, 160/133 model	improved	no change	no change	improved
Barré (1988)	5	24	145, 150, 155	improved	no change	N/A	variable
Krautzig (1998)	8	24-30	135, 140	improved[d]	improved	N/A	N/A
Kooman (2000)	6	6	136, 140	N/A	no change	N/A[h]	N/A
Song (2002)	11	24	138, 140, 147[a]	improved	improved[g]	worsened	N/A
de Paula (2004)	27	6	138, serum [Na+] x 0.95	improved	improved[f]	improved	improved
Oliver (2004)	15	8	132, 137	improved[e]	N/A	N/A	worsened
Thein (2007)	52	32	138, 141	no change	improved	no change	N/A
Sayarlioglu (2007)	18	8	'higher' to 137 or 135[b]	improved	improved	N/A	N/A

Table 2. Ten prospective studies examining the relationship of dialysate sodium prescription on interdialytic weight gain (IDWG), Blood Pressure (BP) Control, Intradialytic Hypotension, and Thirst. BP control is defined as improved pre-dialysis blood pressure measures and/or reduction in number of antihypertensives prescribed. Estimated dry weight was not changed during these studies. n = number of patients in study. N/A = data not available. [a]Patients on Sodium Profiling with [Na+] expressed as Time Averaged Concentration (TAC). [b]Patients placed on 135 if serum was below 137, and on 137 if serum was above 137 (not explained what they did if it WAS 137). No record of baseline Na+ Rx prior to the change. [c]Improvement was seen in the normotensive subset. [d]Half of the participants had an unquantified improvement. [e]Improvement seen in patients with baseline IDWG greater than 1kg/day. [f]Improvement was seen in the 'previously hypertensive' subset. [g]138 & 140 groups were improved when compared to 147 group. [h]There was a 'tendency' toward worsened intradialytic hypotension, data not reported.

3.3 Conductivity studies

Electrical conductivity of solutions reflects the concentration of solute in solution. Substituting conductivity measurements for concentration measurements allows real-time estimations of solute concentrations. Modeling solute clearance, sodium mass transfer, and access recirculation by differences in pre/post dialyzer conductivity represent powerful applications of this technology (Polaschegg, 1993; Locatelli et al., 1995; Petitclerc, 1999). In its most straightforward application, dialysate conductivity can be used as a surrogate for dialysate sodium concentration with one mS/cm conductivity equivalent to 10meq/L sodium. Three short, prospective studies involving 36 patients were identified which examined the effect of lowering dialysate conductivity on blood pressure. One study showed improved control in blood pressure as conductivity was decreased (Farmer et al. 2000). Another study found improvement in blood pressure control and IDWG but worsening intradialytic hypotension with decreasing dialysate conductivity (Lambie et al., 2005). The study with the narrowest range of comparison did not show changes in any parameters (Selby et al., 2007).

Author (Year)	n	t (weeks)	Approximate [Na+] (mEq/L)[b]	Effect of Lower Dialysate Conductivity on			
				IDWG	BP Control	Intradialytic Hypotension	Thirst
Farmer (2000)	10	4	132.7, 137.7	no change	improved	N/A	N/A
Lambie (2005)	16	8[a]	130,132,134,136	improved	improved	worsened	N/A
Selby (2007)	10	6	132, 134, 136	no change	no change	no change	no change

Table 3. Three prospective studies showing the effect of lowering dialysate conductivity on interdialytic weight gain (IDWG), Blood Pressure (BP) Control, Intradialytic Hypotension, and Thirst. Estimated dry weight was not changed during these studies. n = number of patients in study. N/A = data not available. [a]Exact duration not reported, but estimated from number of stepwise changes in conductivity and duration of dialysis for each step. [b]Calculated from dialysate conductivity.

4. Recommendations for the dialysate sodium prescription

4.1 Facility-wide approach

As demonstrated above, higher dialysate sodium provides questionable and inconsistent benefit for intradialytic hemodynamic stability at the cost of proven exacerbation of hypertension and interdialytic weight gain. "Lower" dialysate sodium should therefore be preferred, however, the exact definition of "lower" concentration is variable between studies. In the prospective studies, "lower" was defined from below 132 mEq/L to 145mEq/L while "higher" was defined from 137 to 155 or higher. Of the 165 patients in these studies, we could identify 131 patients where the exact high and low settings could be identified. The weighted average for the lower sodium was 137mEq/L and 143mEq/L for the higher sodium settings.

Given the number of potential barriers to crafting an individualized approach the sodium prescription for each patient, implementing a facility-wide change to 137mEq/L may be safely recommended. Typically, each dialysis unit sets a 'usual' dialysate sodium concentration based on the decision of the medical director. The 'standard' sodium can serve as the default with each provider making individualized changes based on individual patient's needs. Therefore, the initial step is encouraging dialysis directors to choose a default dialysate sodium concentration at, or close to, 137mEq/L.

4.2 Individualized approach

Several questions must be answered when formulating an individualized dialysate sodium. Will changing dialysate sodium cause long-term changes in serum osmolality? Are serum and dialysate sodium estimations equivalent concepts? As will be demonstrated below, predialysis serum sodium tends to be relatively constant over time, eliminating the need to measure the sodium every treatment. Further, conventions in laboratory reporting and the Gibbs-Donnan effect influence the direction of diffusive mass transfer between serum and dialysate.

4.2.1 Sodium setpoint

Pre-dialysis serum sodium remains rather constant over time. The sodium setpoint in dialysis patients is the mean monthly pre-dialysis sodium concentration. In 58 patients over 9 to 16 months, dialyzing against constant dialysate sodium of 143mEq/L, within-subject variability of serum sodium was only 0.62 +/- 0.42 mEq/L (Mean +/- 2 Standard Deviations). Further, the average serum sodium among the 58 patients was 137.3 +/- 2.5 mEq/L (mean +/- SD). Therefore, 98% of this population was dialyzing against relatively hypertonic dialysate even at the rather 'physiological' sodium of 143meq/L (Keen & Gotch, 2007).
Over the short term, the sodium set point remains constant even when dialysate sodium is manipulated. During a brief evaluation, 27 patients maintained constant pre-dialysis serum sodium despite reduction of dialysate sodium to 95% of serum sodium. The average serum sodium was 134.0 +/- 1.4 during the first 3 weeks dialyzing against 138 mEq/L and remained 134.0 +/- 1.5 (mean +/- SD) after the decrease (de Paula et al., 2004).
During longer studies it appears that the sodium set point can be influenced slightly by changes of dialysate sodium. Over an 18-week period, 11 patients had a small but statistically significant increase in pre-dialysis sodium when the time-averaged concentration (TAC) of Na+ was raised from 140 to 147 mEq/L (138.1+/-0.1 to 138.6+/-0.2) (Song et al., 2002). Similar findings were seen in subgroup analysis of 52 patients over 8 months. Patients in the upper tertile of pre-dialysis serum sodium at study entry had a small but statically significant decrease in pre-dialysis serum sodium from 141 to 140 mEq/L (p=0.003) after the dialysate sodium was dropped from 141 to 138 mEq/L (Thein et al, 2007).
Several other studies show that the sodium set point may be somewhat more mutable; however, each significant change seems to be related to sub- or super-physiologic dialysate sodium concentrations (Wilkinson et al., 1977; Fischbach et al., 1988; Acchiardo & Hayden, 1991). When dialyzing across a *physiologic* range of dialysate sodium, however, the concept of a set point remains valid, as variation of predialysis serum sodium is less than 1% (Song et al., 2002; de Paula et al., 2004; Keen & Gotch, 2007; Thein et al, 2007).

4.2.2 Sodium measurements and Gibbs-Donnan considerations

By convention, ionometric serum sodium measurements are corrected to reflect sodium concentration in the total serum volume thereby giving results to historicalresults equivalent to historical flame photometry (Burnett et al., 2000). Given that sodium is distributed only in the water phase, laboratory measures will underestimate the sodium available for dialytic exchange. Actual values should be raised by 7% given usual levels of proteins and lipids. The Gibbs-Donnan effect demonstrates, however, that not all this sodium is available for dialytic exchange. Negatively charged plasma proteins interact with a portion of ionized sodium essentially removing it from the ionic pool. This effect lowers the "plasma diffusible sodium by 4-5%" (Santos, 2008), essentially cancelling out the overestimation of the lab value (Lindley, 2009). More correctly, the accounting for plasma proteins is unnecessary as lab convention and Gibbs-Donnan cancel each other out; however, lipids are uncharged and therefore do not participate in Gibbs-Donnan. Thus diffusible serum sodium is higher than expected in proportion to the lipid content of serum. In patients with relatively normal lipids, however, this difference is small enough to be ignored. In summary, dialysate sodium set to serum sodium can be considered functionally isonatric.

4.2.3 Final individualized guidelines

The default sodium prescription should be equal the serum sodium. Dialysate with identical sodium concentration to serum keeps sodium diffusion neutral; this approach relies exclusively on ultrafiltration for mass transfer of sodium/volume. If attempting to minimize variables, an isotonic dialysate is preferred; in this way ultrafiltration is responsible for the net sodium transfer while not being silently counteracted by dialysate sodium diffusing into the patient.

Dialysate with higher sodium concentration than the patient's serum sodium will provide a net sodium transfer into the patient. Hypertonic dialysate is only indicated chronically for non-hypertensive patients with significant, recurrent intradialytic hypotension or acutely for prevention of disequilibrium syndrome.

Dialysate with lower sodium concentration than the patient's serum sodium will accept a net sodium transfer out of the patient. If attempting to maximize methods for BP control and IDWG management, the utilization of hypotonic dialysate is preferred, insofar as is tolerated by interdialytic symptoms.

5. Technical & systems requirements for adjustment of dialysate sodium

As with any prescription, benefits are never greater than the level of compliance. In the case of dialysate sodium, several technical and systems issues must be understood in order to modify a dialysate sodium level. Given the many daily problems that dialysis unit staff must face, awareness of the prescribed sodium can easily be overlooked. Further, both doctors and staff may not be aware of the mechanisms required to change dialysate sodium. Depending on each unit's equipment and dialysate formulation, changing dialysate sodium may cause changes in the other electrolytes; this can cause consternation or confusion.

Staff awareness of the importance and compliance and Medical director interventions: In our experience, despite excellent and capable dialysis staff, modifications to the sodium prescription can easily be overlooked. In our unit, dialysate is delivered from a central system. The sodium concentration "out of the wall" is determined by the concentrate formula ordered by the unit - or even determined by a corporate purchasing office. There are several points of intervention. First, medical directors, need to be aware of the level of sodium in their concentrates. There are several manufactures of dialysate concentrate each with its unique formulation. Further, some manufacturers offer a variety of sodium levels within their own product lines. One intervention could be for the medical director to select the formulation that delivers the desired default sodium - based on our recommendation this would be 137mEq/L (see Paragraph 4.1). Changing the base solution is not the only method to vary the sodium in a unit and may not be economical or practical. Even if the central supply of dialysate does not match the "Facility-Wide" prescription, the staff can change to sodium concentration at each individual dialysis machine. Dialysis unit staff should be educated regarding the importance and technique of making changes to match the prescription. This education should be done even if the central supply of dialysate has the 'ideal' sodium level as eventually an "Individualized" approach should be introduced. Staff awareness, training and 'buy in' are the only way to deliver individualized sodium.

5.1 Review of dialysate generation

Modern dialysate contains bicarbonate; it also contains variable amounts of calcium and magnesium. If such a solution were stored for any length of time, calcium and magnesium would combine with bicarbonate and precipitate out of solution. Dialysate must also be at physiologic pH which is, unfortunately, ideal for bacterial growth. In order to avoid these untoward consequences, bicarbonate is kept separate from calcium and magnesium in separate solutions or powders. The nomenclatures for these concentrates are "Acid" and "Bicarbonate". The Acid typically consists of sodium, chloride, potassium, magnesium, calcium, dextrose, acetate, and sometimes citrate. The Bicarbonate concentrate consists of sodium bicarbonate with some brands containing some additional sodium chloride. Creation of dialysate is requires mixing the Acid and Bicarbonate solutions in exact proportions. This is performed in 'real time' in the dialysis machine based on the pre-mixed concentrates of Acid and Bicarbonate and the software programmed for each concentrate.

5.2 Concentrate formulations

All the liquid and dry concentrates in the Fresenius NaturaLyte® - 4000 Series of Acid and Bicarbonate will result in a final sodium concentration of 137mEq/L once mixed. Fresenius Citrasate® Series results in a base sodium of 137.3 mEq/L once mixed with the NaturaLyte® Bicarbonate (Fresenius, 2010). Rockwell Medical produces three series of formulations available in dry and liquid. The Rockwell Medical R-Series results in final sodium concentrations of 138, 139, 140, 143 mEq/L. The C-Series results in 137mEq/L. The F-Series results in 135 or 138 mEq/L (Rockwell Medical, 2009). Minntech's Centrisol® results in a final sodium concentration of 137 mEq/L and their Renasol® results in 139,140,142,or 143 mEq/L (Minntech, 2010).

Company/ Product	Final Na^+ (mEq/L)	Na^+ from Acid (mEq/L)
Fresenius		
NaturaLyte®	137	100
Citrasate®	137.3	100.3
Minntech		
Centrisol®	137	unlisted
Renasol®	139,140,142,143	unlisted
Rockwell Medical		
R-Series*	138, 139, 140, 143	79, 80, 81, 84
C-Series*	137	100
F-Series*	135, 138	100, 103

Table 4. The default sodium concentration of several available dialysate concentrates and the sodium contribution from the acid portion (Fresenius, 2010; Minntech, 2010; Rockwell Medical 2009). *RenalPure® Liquid Acid with SteriLyte® Liquid Bicarbonate or Dri-Sate® Dry Acid with RenalPure® Powder Bicarbonate.

5.3 Dialysate proportioning systems

Given that both the Acid and Bicarbonate concentrates contain significant sodium (sodium chloride in Acid and sodium bicarbonate in the Bicarbonate). The sodium can therefore varied by adjusting the dilution of the Acid, Bicarbonate or both. The mechanism of this variation is determined by the design and software of the dialysis machine. Each manufacturer may have slightly different approach. All models of the Fresenius 2008® series (2008H, 2008K, 2008K², 2008T) have an explicit mechanism behind sodium variation: the amount of Acid concentrate is varied to change the sodium concentration to the target value. The other electrolytes in the Acid component will vary in proportion to the sodium change, while the electrolytes in the Bicarbonate solution will remain unchanged (Fresenius Medical Care, 2001, 2009a, 2009b, 2010). Other manufactures advertise the ability to vary sodium across a wide range. The Gambro Artis® System can vary sodium concentration from 130-160mEq/L - much wider than the Bicarbonate variability (24-38mEq/L). Therefore the majority, if not all, of the variation in sodium is produced from variation in the Acid concentrate (Gambro, 2008). Similar ranges apply to the Gambro AK96 Advance® and Bio® models: Sodium varies 130-160mEq/L and Bicarbonate 20-40mEq/L (Gambro, 2009). B.Braun's Dialog+® has a conductivity range from 12-17mS/cm, indicating a wide range of sodium variation, however, the relative contribution of Acid and Bicarbonate portions are not readily accessible (B.Braun Medical Inc., 2009). The capability and mechanism of sodium variation for the Baxter TINA® and ARENA® systems are not easily obtainable in an "open access" format. However, given the wide use if sodium modeling over the past two decades, any modern dialysis machine probably has the capability to generate individualized sodium concentrations.

Systems like the Fresenius 2008® Series, which hold the Bicarbonate constant and vary the Acid in order to alter the sodium, will show the greatest variation in the other electrolytes in the acid component. As will be demonstrated below, however, these changes are minute and clinically irrelevant. If any of the other systems utilize a combination of Acid and Bicarbonate variations to alter sodium concentration, the changes in Acid electrolytes will be even less effected (the bicarbonate concentration would vary somewhat, however, the change would also be minimal).

5.4 Electrolyte variability during sodium individualization

The question arises, will there be a change in other electrolyte components during the sodium variation? Clinically these variations are insignificant and should not hinder the use of tailored sodium. Dialysis staff needs to be reassured of this, as many of the newer generation dialysis machines will display the changes to all electrolytes when one is changed. Some staff may see a small change in the potassium and undo the change because the potassium level does not match the prescription. Dialysis unit policy and dialysis orders should be written to accept small variation in other electrolytes during adjustment of sodium. Of note, during sodium profiling, all the acid electrolytes in the same way, resulting in wider, yet still clinically insignificant, fluctuations in the other components.

Here is an example of the nature of electrolyte variation with individualized sodium. A clinician determines that a particular patient's individualized dialysate sodium should be 133mEq/L. Some adjustment of the dialysis machine is required as none of the available base solutions result in this a sodium of 133mEq/L. A Fresenius 2008T®, for example, manipulates the final dialysate sodium by varying concentration of the Acid component

(Fresenius Medical Care, 2010a). If the available dialysate has a base sodium of 137mEq/L and the Acid concentrate contributes 100mEq/L (such as Fresenius NaturaLyte®, Citrasate® or Rockwell Medical C-Series), it is possible to predict the changes on the other electrolytes. Reducing the final sodium from 137 to 133 mEq/L requires reducing the Acid component from 100meq/L to 96mEq/L (a change of 4%). Reducing each Acid component by 4% will give the final concentration of that component. Using a standard Acid solution, such as Fresenius NaturaLyte® Product Number 08-2201-5, contributes 100mEq/L of sodium,

Electrolyte	Product Number / Acid Concentration	New Concentration After 5meq/L Sodium Decrease
	Fresenius, 08-2201-5	
Na^+ (mEq/L)	100	95 (5% reduction)
K^+ (mEq/L)	2.0	1.9
Ca^{++} (mEq/L)	2.00	1.90
Mg^{++} (mEq/L)	1.00	0.95
Cl^- (mEq/L)	105.0	99.8
Acetate (mEq/L)	4.0	3.5
Dextrose (mg/dL)	100	95
	Rockwell Medical, R-205	
Na^+ (mEq/L)	79	74 (6.33% reduction)
K^+ (mEq/L)	3	2.8
Ca^{++} (mEq/L)	3.5	3.2
Mg^{++} (mEq/L)	1.5	1.4
Cl^- (mEq/L)	86	80.6
Acetate (mEq/L)	4	3.7
Dextrose (mg/dL)	200	187
	Rockwell Medical, F-215	
Na^+ (mEq/L)	103	98 (4.85% reduction)
K^+ (mEq/L)	1	0.95
Ca^{++} (mEq/L)	2.5	2.37
Mg^{++} (mEq/L)	1	0.95
Cl^- (mEq/L)	107.5	102.3
Acetate (mEq/L)	3	2.85
Dextrose (mg/dL)	200	190

Table 5. Change in electrolyte concentrations resulting from an individualized sodium prescription. This example shows what happens to the other electrolytes after a 5mEq/L reduction in dialysate sodium. The breakdown of the Acid portion of several common concentrates is shown in the center column (Rockwell Medical, 2009; Fresenius Medical Care, 2010b). Based on the percent change of Acid sodium, the resulting values for potassium, calcium, magnesium, chloride, acetate and dextrose are listed in the left column.

2.00mEq/L of potassium and 100mg/dL of dextrose (Fresenius Medical Care, 2010b). Diluting this Acid by 4% results in Na^+ 96mEq/L, K^+ 1.92mEq/L, and dextrose 96mg/dL. None of these changes carry a significant clinical effect. The smaller the sodium contribution of the Acid, the other electrolytes will show a larger variation. Table 5 shows the final electrolyte changes of several standard dialysate solutions when using the proportioning system to decrease the base sodium by 5mEq/L.

6. Conclusions

Dialysate sodium concentration must be prescribed for each dialysis session. Dialysate sodium standards vary from 126.5mEq/L to greater than 155mEq/L through out the history of dialysis. While higher concentrations can be used to promote greater hemodynamic stability during dialysis, their cost is worsening hypertension and greater interdialytic weight gain. Glycosaminoglycans and other polyanions sequester sodium out of the osmotic pool and amplify the sodium gain during hypertonic dialysis causing greater effects than the traditional 'sodium space' model would predict. We reviewed 17 prospective and retrospective studies that quantify the effects of dialysate sodium on hypertension, interdialytic weight gain and intradialytic hypotension. In order to minimize undesired effects of high or low sodium for the most patients, "facility-wide" dialysate sodium setting of 137mEq/L should be implemented. An individualized sodium prescription can be calculated by setting dialysate sodium equal the patient's serum sodium. This calculation can be done without adjustments since laboratory conventions and the Gibbs-Donnan effect essentially negate each other. In order to deliver a facility-wide or individualized sodium prescription, changing dialysate concentrates could be undertaken but not necessary: modern proportioning systems can adjust the dilution of dialysate Acid or Bicarbonate components. Usually the dilution of the Acid is adjusted while Bicarbonate remains constant. The other Acid electrolytes will vary by the same percentage as the sodium variation: a clinically inconsequential change.

7. Acknowledgments

MG thanks Camelia, Natalie & Kaitlyn. You are the light of my world.

8. References

Acchiardo, S. & Hayden, A. (1991). Is Na+ modeling necessary in high flux dialysis? *American Society for Artificial Internal Organs Transactions*. Vol. 37, No.3, (July 1991), pp. M135-7. ISSN 0889-7190

Adair, G. (1923). On the Donnan Equilibrium and the Equation of Gibbs. *Science*. Vol.6, No.58, (July 1923), pp.13, ISSN 0036-8075

Argiles, A., Lorho, R., Servel M., Chong G., Kerr P. & Mourad, G. Seasonal modifications in blood pressure are mainly related to interdialytic body weight gain in dialysis patients. *Kidney International*. Vol.65, No.5, (May 2004), pp. 1795-1801. ISSN 0085-2538

B.Braun Medical Inc. (2009). Dialog+® Hemodialysis System, Your Clinical Assistant for Hemodialysis Therapy. April 17,2011, Available from: <http://www.bbraunusa.com/images/bbraun_usa/DIALOG_PLUS_Brochure3-09.pdf>

Barré, P., Brunelle, G. & Gascon-Barré, M. (1988). A randomized double blind trial of dialysate sodiums of 145 mEq/L, 150 mEq/L, and 155 mEq/L. *American Society for Artificial Internal Organs Transactions*. Vol.34, No.3, (July 1988), pp. 338-41, ISSN 0889-7190

Bergstrom, W. (1955). The participation of bone in total body sodium metabolism in the rat. *The Journal of Clinical Investigation*. Vol.34, No.7, (July 1955), pp. 997-1004, ISSN 0021-9738

Burnett, R., Covington, A., Fogh-Andersen, N., Kulpmann, W., Lewenstam, A., Maas, A., Muller-Plathe, O., Sachs, C., Siggaard-Andersen, O., VanKessel, A. & Zijlstra, W. (2000) *Clinical Chemistry and Laboratory Medicine*. Vol.38, No.10, (October 2000), pp.1065-1071, ISSN 1434-6621

Charra, B., Bergstrom, J. & Scribner, B. (1998). Blood pressure control in dialysis patients: importance of the lag phenomenon. *American Journal of Kidney Diseases*. Vol.32, No.5, (November 1998), pp.720-724, ISSN 1523-6838

Charra, B. & Chazot, C. (2003). Volume Control, Blood Pressure and Cardiovascular Function: Lessons from Hemodialysis Treatment. *Nephron Physiology*. Vol.93, No.4, (May 2003), pp. 94–101, ISSN 1660-2137

Cybulsky A., Matni A. & Hollomby D. (1985). Effects of high sodium dialysate during maintenance hemodialysis. *Nephron*. Vol.41, No.1, (1985), pp. 57-61, ISSN 0028-2766

Daugirdas, J., Al-Kudsi, R., Ing, T. & Norusis, M. (1985). A double-blind evaluation of sodium gradient hemodialysis. *American Journal of Nephrology*. Vol.5, No.5, (July 1985), pp. 163-8, ISSN 0250-8095

Davenport, A. (2006). Audit of the effect of dialysate sodium concentration on inter-dialytic weight gains and blood pressure control in chronic haemodialysis patients. *Nephron. Clinical practice*. Vol.104, No.3, (Epub July 2006), pp. c120-c125, ISSN 1660-2110

Davenport A., Cox C. & Thuraisingham R; PanThames Renal Audit Group. (2008). The importance of dialysate sodium concentration in determining interdialytic weight gains in chronic hemodialysis patients: the PanThames Renal Audit. *The International Journal of Artificial Organs*. Vol. 31, No.5, (May 2008), pp. 411-417, ISSN 0391-3988

de Paula, F., Peixoto, A., Pinto, L., Dorigo, D., Patricio P. & Santos, S. (2004). Clinical consequences of an individualized dialysate sodium prescription in hemodialysis patients. *Kidney International*. Vol.66, No.3, (September 2004), pp. 1232-1238, ISSN 0085-2538

Dunstone, J. (1959). Some Cation-binding Properties of Cartilage. *The Biochemical Journal*. Vol.72, (July 1959), pp. 465-473, ISSN 0264-6021

Farber, S., Schubert, M. & Schuster, N. (1957). The binding of cations by chondroitin sulphate. *Journal of Clinical Investigation*. Vol.36, No.12, (December 1957), pp.1715-1722, ISSN 0021-9738

Farmer, C., Donohoe, P., Dallyn, P., Cox, J., Kingswood, J. & Goldsmith, D. (2000). Low-sodium haemodialysis without fluid removal improves blood pressure control in chronic haemodialysis patients. *Nephrology*. Vol.5, No.4, (December 2000), pp.237-241, ISSN 1440-1797

Fischbach, M., Tarral, E. & Geisert, J. (1988). Sequential hypertonic haemodialysis in children. *Pediatric Nephrology*. Vol.2, No.4, (October 1988), pp. 442-446, ISSN 0931-041X

Forbes, G. & Perley, A. (1952). Estimation of total body sodium by isotopic dilution. I. Studies on young adults. *The Journal of Clinical Investigation*. Vol. 30, No.6, (June 1951), pp. 558-65, ISSN 0021-9738

Forbes, G. & Lewis, A. (1956). Total sodium, potassium and chloride in adult man. *The Journal of Clinical Investigation*. Vol.35, No.6, (June 1956), pp. 596-600, ISSN 0021-9738

Fresenius Medical Care. (2001). *Operator's Manual, Fresenius 2008H Hemodialysis Machine*. (Revision H), Fresenius USA, Inc. Retrieved from: <http://www.fmcna.com/fmcna/OperatorsManuals/operators-manuals.html>

Fresenius Medical Care. (2009). *2008K Hemodialysis Machine Operator's Manual*. (Rev. K). Fresenius USA, Inc. Retrieved from: <http://www.fmcna.com/fmcna/OperatorsManuals/operators-manuals.html>

Fresenius Medical Care. (2009). *2008K² Hemodialysis Machine Operator's Manual*. (Rev. E) Fresenius USA, Inc. Retrieved from: <http://www.fmcna.com/fmcna/OperatorsManuals/operators-manuals.html>

Fresenius Medical Care. (2010). *2008T Hemodialysis Machine Operator's Manual* (Rev E). Fresenius USA, Inc. Retrieved from: <http://www.fmcna.com/fmcna/OperatorsManuals/operators-manuals.html>

Fresenius Medical Care. (2010). Dialysis Product Catalog. April 17, 2011, Available from: <http://www.fmcna.com/fmcna/DialysisProducts/dialysis-products.html>

Gambro. (2008). Artis dialysis system, Advanced Simplicity. April 17,2011, Available from: <http://www.gambro.com/PageFiles/5982/Artis,%20Produktdatablad.pdf?epslanguage=en>

Gambro. (2009). The AK 96 machine, Advance version. April 17, 2011, Available from: <http://www.gambro.com/Global/Globalweb/Products/HD/Monitors/Ak_96/Documents/HCEN4966_2_AK96_advance_Low.pdf?epslanguage=en>

Gotch, F., Lam, M., Prowit, M. & Keen, M. (1980). Preliminary Clinical results with Sodium-Volume Modeling of Hemodialysis Therapy. *Proceedings of the Clinical Dialysis and Transplant Forum*. Vol.10, (1980), pp. 12-17, ISSN 0094-6044

Harrison, H., Darrow, D. & Yannet, H. (1936). The total electrolyte content of animals and its probable relation to the distribution of body water. *The Journal of Biological Chemistry*. Vol.113, (March 1936), pp. 515-529, ISSN 0021-9258

Heer, M., Frings-Meuthen, P., Titze, J., Boschmann, M., Frisch, S., Baecker, N. & Beck, L. (2009). Increasing sodium intake from a previous low or high intake affects water, electrolyte and acid-base balance differently. *The British Journal of Nutrition*. Vol.101, No.9, (May 2009), pp. 1286-1294, ISSN 1475-2662

Kaltreider N., Meneely, G., Allen, J. & Bale, W. (1941). Determination of the volume of the extracellular fluid of the body with radioactive sodium. *Journal of Expimental Medidine*. Vol.74, (December 1941), pp. 569-590

Keen, M. & Gotch, F. (2007). The association of the sodium "setpoint" to interdialytic weight gain and blood pressure in hemodialysis patients. *The International Journal of Artificial Organs*. Vol.30, No.11, (November 2007), pp. 971-979, ISSN 0391-3988

Kolff, W. (1947). *New Ways of Treating Uraemia: The Artificial Kidney, Peritoneal Lavage, Intestinal Lavage*. J & A Churchill, Ltd. London

Kooman J., Hendriks E., van Den Sande F. & Leumissen K. (2000). Dialysate sodium concentration and blood pressure control in hemodialysis patients. *Nephrology, Dialysis, Transplant*. Vol.15, No.4, (April 2000), ISSN 0931-0509

Krautzig, S., Janssen, U., Koch, K., Granolleras, C. & Shaldon, S. (1998). Dietary salt restriction and reduction of dialysate sodium to control hypertension in maintenance haemodialysis patients. *Nephrology, Dialysis, Transplantation*. Vol.13, No.3, (March 1998), pp. 552-553, ISSN 0931-0509

Lambie, S., Taal, M., Fluck, R. & McIntyre, C. (2005). Online Conductivity Monitoring: Validation and Usefulness in a Clinical Trial of Reduced Dialysate Conductivity. *ASAIO Journal*. Vol. 51, No.1, (January 2005), pp. 70-76, ISSN 1058-2916

Law, R. (1984). Characteristics of ionic binding by rat renal tissue in vitro. *The Journal of Physiology*. Vol.353, (August 1984), pp.67-80, ISSN 0022-3751

Levin, N., Zhu, F. & Keen, M. (2001). Interdialytic weight gain and dry weight. *Blood Purification*. Vol.19, No.2, (2001), pp. 217-221, ISSN 0253-5068

Levitt, M., Turner, L., Sweet, A. & Pandiri, D. (1956). The response of bone, connective tissue, and muscle to acute acidosis. *The Journal of Clinical Investigation*. Vol. 35, No.1, (January 1956), pp. 98-105, ISSN 0021-9738

Locatelli, F., Pedrini, L., Ponti, R., Costanzo, R., Di Filippo, S., Marai, P., Pozzi, C. & Bonacina, G. (1982). "Physiological" and "Pharmacological" Dialysate Sodium Concentrations. *The International Journal of Artificial Organs*, Vol.5, No.1, (June 1982), pp. 17-24, ISSN 0391-3988

Locatelli, F., Di Filippo, S., Manzoni, C., Corti, M., Andrulli, S. & Pontoriero, G. (1995). Monitoring sodium removal and delivered dialysis by conductivity. *The International Journal of Artificial Organs*. Vol.18, No.11, (November 1995), pp. 716-721, ISSN 0391-3988

Minntech. (2010). Product Guide. April 17, 2011, Available from: < http://www.minntech.com/renal/products/2010-catalog.pdf>

Oliver, A., Wright, M., Matson, A., Woodrow, G., King, N. & Dye, L. (2004) Low sodium haemodialysis reduces interdialytic fluid consumption but paradoxically increases post-dialysis thirst. *Nephrology, Dialysis, Transplantation*. Vol.19, No.11, (November, 2004), pp. 2883-2885, ISSN 0931-0509

Petitclerc, T. (1999). Festschrift for Professor Claude Jacobs. Recent developments in conductivity monitoring of haemodialysis session. *Nephrology, Dialysis, Transplantation*. Vol.14, No.11, (November 1999), pp. 2607-2613, ISSN 0931-0509

Polaschegg, H. (1993). Automatic, noninvasive intradialytic clearance measurement. *The International Journal of Artificial Organs*. Vol.16, No.4, (April 1993), pp. 185-91, ISSN 0391-3988

Rockwell Medical. (September 2009). Hemodialysis Concentrates. April 17, 2011, Available from: <http://www.rockwellmed.com/dialysis-products-hemodialysis-concentrates.htm>

Sarkar, S., Kotanko, P. & Levin N. (2006). Interdialytic Weight Gain: Implications in Hemodialysis Patients. *Seminars in Dialysis*. Vol.19, No.5, (September 2006), pp. 429–433, ISSN 0894-0959

Sayarlioglu, H., Erkoc, R., Tuncer, M., Soyoral, Y., Esen, R., Gumrukcuoglu, H., Dogan, E. & Sayarlioglu, M. (2007). Effects of low sodium dialysate in chronic hemodialysis patients: an echocardiographic study. *Renal Failure*. Vol.29, No.2, (May 2007), pp. 143-6, ISSN 0886-022X

Schubert, M. (1964). Intercellular Macromolecules Containing Polysaccharides. *Biophysical Journal*. Vol.4, supplement (January 1964), pp. 119-38, ISSN 0006-3495

Selby, N., Taal, M. & McIntyre C. (2007). Comparison of progressive conductivity reduction with diacontrol and standard dialysis. *ASAIO Journal*. Vol.53, No.2, (March 2007), pp. 194-200, ISSN 1058-2916

Song, J., Lee, S., Suh, C. & Kim, M. (2002). Time-averaged concentration of dialysate sodium relates with sodium load and interdialytic weight gain during sodium-profiling hemodialysis. *American Journal of Kidney Diseases*. Vol.40, No.2, (August 2002), pp. 291–301, ISSN 1523-6838

Stewart, W., Fleming L. & Manuel, M. (1972) Muscle Cramps During Maintenance Haemodialysis. *Lancet*, Vol.1, No.7759, (May 1972), pp. 1049-51, ISSN 0140-6736

Thein, H., Haloob, I. & Marshall, M. (2007). Associations of a facility level decrease in dialysate sodium concentration with blood pressure and interdialytic weight gain. *Nephrology Dialysis Transplantation*. Vol.22, No.9, (September 2007), pp. 2630-2639, ISSN 0931-0509

Titze, J., Shakibaei, M., Schafflhuber, M., Schulze-Tanzil, G., Porst, M., Schwind, K., Dietsch, P. & Hilgers, K. (2004). Glycosaminoglycan polymerization may enable osmotically inactive Na+ storage in the skin. *American Journal of Physiology. Heart and Circulatory Physiology*. Vol.287, No.1, (July 2004) pp. H203–H208, ISSN 0363-6135

Titze, J. & Machnik, A. (2010) Sodium sensing in the interstitium and relationship to hypertension. *Current Opinion in Nephrology and Hypertension*. Vol.19, No.4, (July 2010), pp. 385-392, ISSN 1535-3842

Tobain, L., Janecek, J., Tomboulain, A. & Ferreira, D. (1961). Sodium and potassium in the walls of arterioles in experimental renal hypertension. *The Journal of Clinical Investigation*. Vol.40, (October, 1961), pp. 1922-1925, ISSN 0021-9738

Wilkinson, R., Barber, S. & Robson, V. (1977). Cramps, thirst and hypertension in hemodialysis patients -- the influence of dialysate sodium concentration. *Clinical Nephrology*. Vol.7, No.3, (March 1977), pp. 101-105, ISSN 0301-0430

Woodbury, D. (1956). Effect of acute hyponatremia on distribution of water and electrolytes in various tissues of the rat. *The American Journal of Physiology*. Vol.185, No.2, (May 1956), pp. 281-286, ISSN 0002-9513

4

Polyethersulfone Hollow Fiber Membranes for Hemodialysis

Baihai Su[1,2], Shudong Sun[2] and Changsheng Zhao[2]
[1]*Department of Nephrology, West China Hospital, Sichuan University,*
[2]*College of Polymer Science and Engineering, State Key Laboratory of Polymer Materials Engineering, Sichuan University,*
PR China

1. Introduction

Polyethersulfone (PES) is one of the most important polymeric materials and is widely used in separation fields. PES and PES-based membranes show outstanding oxidative, thermal and hydrolytic stability as well as good mechanical and film-forming properties. PES membranes could endure many kinds of sterilized methods, including epoxy ethane gas, steam, and γ-ray. Furthermore, PES-based membranes show high permeability for low molecular weight proteins when used as hemodialysis membranes. Thus, PES membranes are also widely employed in biomedical fields such as artificial organs and medical devices used for blood purification, e.g., hemodialysis, hemodiafiltration, hemofiltration, plasmapheresis and plasma collection (Zhao et al., 2001; Tullis, et al., 2002; Samtleben et al., 2003; Werner et al., 1995), especially in recent years.

However, when contacting with blood, proteins will be rapidly adsorbed onto the surface of PES membrane and the adsorbed protein layer may lead to further undesirable results, such as platelet adhesion, aggregation and coagulation. As a consequence, the blood compatibility of PES membrane is not adequate, and injections of anti-coagulants are needed during its clinical application (Liu et al., 2009).

The main disadvantage is related to the relatively hydrophobic character of PES membrane. And many studies have concluded that membrane fouling (as caused by protein adsorption) is directly related to hydrophobicity as reviewed by Van der Bruggen (Van der Bruggen, 2009) and Khulbe et al. (Khulbe et al., 2010), although the opposite has also been reported (Yu et al., 2008). Membrane fouling is mainly caused by adsorption of nonpolar solutes, hydrophobic particles or bacteria (Van der Bruggen, 2009; Koh et al., 2005). It is a serious problem in membrane filtration, resulting in a higher energy demand, shorter membrane lifetime, and unpredictable separation performance (Agenson & Urase, 2007). Thus, PES hollow fiber membranes used in hemodialysis are usually modified by hydrophilic polymers.

For the modification of PES membranes, there are three approaches: (1) bulk modification of PES material, and then to prepare modified membrane; (2) surface modification of prepared PES membrane; and (3) blending, which can also be regarded as a surface modification. The modification procedures allow finding a compromise between the hydrophobicity and hydrophilicity, and localize the hydrophilic material specifically in the membrane pores, where they have a positive effect on flux and fouling reduction, and on the membrane surface to improve blood compatibility. However, not all the methods are suitable for the modification of PES hemodialysis membranes.

For hemodialysis membranes, safety and efficiency should be evaluated firstly in vitro before clinical application, and simulation solutions are used. Through the experiments in vitro, many results, which are useful for clinical applications, could be obtained, including protein adsorption, platelet adhesion, ultrafiltration (UF) coefficient, and solute clearances (such as for urea, creatinine, and phosphate, and so on). For high-flux hemodialysis membranes, the clearance of β_2-microglobin should be investigated. When the membranes are applied for patients, the safety and efficiency are also very important.

In the present chapter, preparation and characterization of PES hemodialysis hollow fiber membranes are discussed firstly, and then the safety and efficiency in vitro and in vivo are discussed.

2. Preparation and modification of polyethersulfone hollow fiber membranes

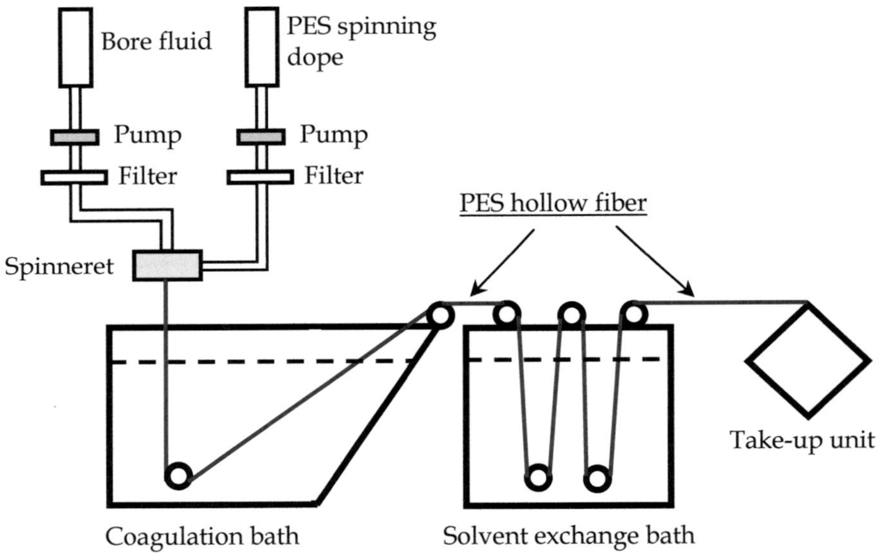

Fig. 1. PES hollow fiber spinning line

PES hollow fiber membranes for hemodialysis are usually spun by dry-wet spinning technique based on liquid-liquid phase separation method, see Figure 1. The cross-section view of the PES hollow fiber membrane is shown in Figure 2. After post-treatment, PES hollow fiber hemodialyzer is prepared by using polyurethane resin as the potting material. However, the blood compatibility of the PES membrane is not adequate, and injections of anticoagulants are needed during hemodialysis. Thus, all the PES membranes used for hemodialysis are not the pristine PES membranes. As a hydrophilic additive and a membrane forming agent, poly (vinyl pyrrolidone) (PVP) is most widely used for the modification of PES membranes by blending. Many other methods can also be used for modifying PES membranes. The aim of the modification is to improve the biocompatibility and protein antifouling property of the membranes, thus different sections are separated based on the methods and the modification objective.

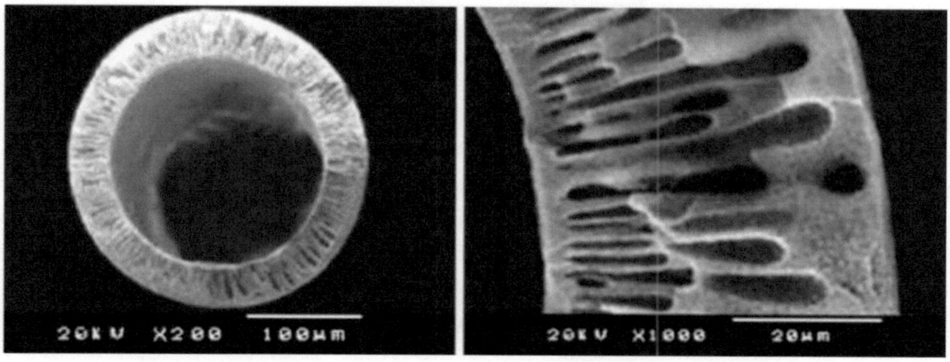

Fig. 2. SEM images of PES hollow fiber membrane (From reference, Su et al., 2008)

2.1 Blending

Blending is the simplest and most widely used method to modify PES membranes both for flat-sheet and hollow fiber membranes, though sometimes the results might be not very well. By directly blending with hydrophilic polymers, such as polyvinylpyrrolidone (PVP) (Barzin et al., 2004; Mosqueda-Jimenez et al., 2006; Su BH, et al., 2008; Wang et al., 2009) and polyethyleneglycol (PEG) (Wang et al., 2006), PES membranes are easy to be modified; here PVP and PEG also are also used as pore-forming agents. The hydrophilicity of the membranes increased, the antifouling property and blood compatibility are also increased (Su BH, et al., 2008; Wang et al., 2006). However, the elution of the blended hydrophilic polymer is unavoidable. Thus, amphiphilic copolymers are synthesized recently and used for blending with PES to prepare membranes (Zhu et al.; 2008a, 2008b; Zhao et al., 2008; Peng et al., 2009). For hemodialysis membranes, the objective of blending is to improve the membrane hydrophilicity, biocompatibility, and other properties, such as protein antifouling property.

2.1.1 Improve biocompatibility

In our recent study (Su BH, et al., 2008), larger molecular weight PVP was used to blend with PES to prepare hollow fiber hemodialysis membrane, and the performance was evaluated in vitro and in vivo. The biocompatibility profiles of the membranes showed slight neutropenia and platelet adhesion at the initial stage of the hemodialysis. The clearance and the reduction ratio after the hemodialysis of small molecules (urea, creatinine, phosphate) for the PES membrane were higher in vitro than that in vivo.

Barzin et al. (Barzin et al., 2004) prepared two kinds of PES hollow fiber membranes for hemodialysis by blending two ratios of PES to PVP (PES/PVP = 18/3 and 18/6 by weight). It was observed that the water flux of the hollow fiber increased significantly when heat-treated in water, while decreased when heat-treated in air. On the other hand, the molecular weight cutoff of the hollow fiber increased slightly when heat-treated in water, while decreased drastically when heat-treated in air. SEM images also showed that the surface morphology of the membranes was different before and after heat-treatment. The performance data of the hollow fiber heated in air at 150 °C was found to be the most appropriate for hemodialysis application. It was also found that the hollow fiber membrane prepared from the blend ratio of PES/PVP = 18/3 showed slightly higher flux than that prepared from a solution with PES/PVP ratio of 18/6. Of course, PVP could also be used to modify PES hollow fiber membranes for hemofiltration (Yang et al., 2009). Gholami et al. (Gholami et al.; 2003) found that the hollow fiber membranes shrank by heat treatment, as evidenced by a decrease in flux and an increase in solute separation, although there was no visible change in the hollow-fiber dimension. However, for flat-sheet PES membranes, the membrane surface altered, and surface parameters (such as surface roughness) have been changed after non-contact heating (microwave irradiation) (Mansourpanah et al., 2009).

Erlenkotter and coworkers (Erlenkotter et al, 2008) evaluated the dialysis membrane hemocompatibility. In order to compare different polymers used in the manufacturing of dialysis membranes, a set of the following hemocompatibility parameters was assessed and assembled to an overall score: generation of complement factor 5a, thrombin-antithrombin III-complex, release of platelet factor 4, generation and release of elastase from polymorphonuclear granulocytes, and platelet count. By blending polyarylate with PES, the membrane hemocompatibility improved. They also provided a score model to facilitate the selection of membrane polymers with an appropriate hemocompatibility pattern for dialysis therapy.

2.1.2 Improve antifouling property

Membrane fouling is still a crucial problem for hollow fiber membrane. When fouling takes place on membrane surfaces, it causes flux decline, leading to an increase in production cost due to increased energy demand. Qin et al. (Qin et al., 2004) selected solvent-resistant hollow-fiber UF membranes by measurement of fiber swelling and treatability studies on spent solvent cleaning rinse. The results indicated that the membranes made of both cellulose acetate (CA) and polyacrylonitrile (PAN) materials could tolerate the solvent present and were suitable or treating the spent solvent rinses, whereas PES and PSF membranes were not suitable. The CA membrane had the lowest fouling tendency when treating the spent solvent rinse. Nakatsuka et al. (Nakatsuka et al., 1996) also found that the permeate flux for the hydrophilic CA membranes was much higher than that of the hydrophobic PES membrane, a phenomenon which was explained by membrane fouling due to the adsorption of substances in raw water on and in the pores of the membranes. Xu et al. (Xu et al., 2009) observed that the fouling layer grew faster on the inside surface of the PES hollow fiber at a lower flow rate than that at a higher flow rate due to the lower shear stress. These results suggested that PES hollow fiber membrane should be modified to improve antifouling property by increasing hydrophilicity.

Arahman et al. (Arahman et al., 2009) modified PES hollow-fiber membrane by blending with hydrophilic surfactant Tetronic 1307. The fouling of the PES membrane with blending Tetronic 1307 was lower than that of the original PES membrane in the case of BSA filtration. A functional terpolymer of poly (methyl methacrylate–acrylic acid–vinyl pyrrolidone) (PMMA-AA-VP) was synthesized via free radical solution polymerization using DMAC as the solvent in our recent study (Zou et al., 2010). The terpolymer can be directly blended with PES using the solvent to prepare modified PES hollow fiber membrane. The hydrophilicity of the blended membranes increased, and the membranes showed good protein antifouling property. The antifouling property is always expressed as the time-dependent flux during the ultrafiltration process (PBS solution and BSA solution alternatively switched), as shown in Figure 3.

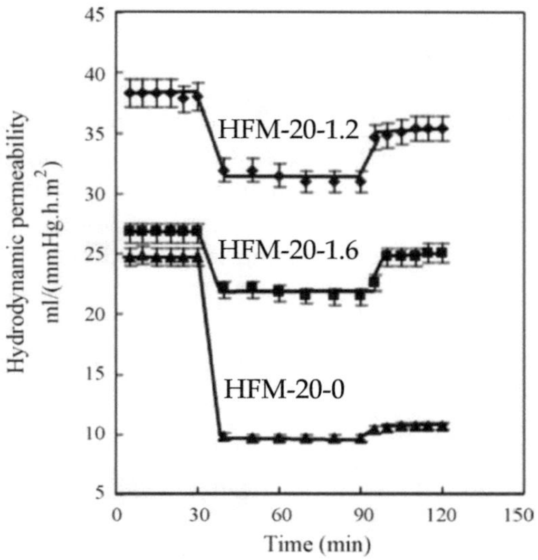

Fig. 3. Time-dependent flux of PMMA-AA-VP modified PES membranes during the ultrafiltration process.
For the membranes: HFM-20-1.2 (The amounts of PES and the terpolymer are 20 and 1.2 wt.%, respectively); HFM-20-1.6 (The amounts of PES and the terpolymer are 20 and 1.6 wt.%, respectively); HFM-20-0 (20wt.% PES).
PBS solution: 0–30 and 95–120 min; BSA solution: 40–90 min. n=3.
(From reference, Zou et al., 2010)

2.2 Other methods

Many other methods can also be used for the modification of PES hollow fiber, the following reviewed the methods. Though not all of them are discussed for hemodialysis membranes, some of the methods can be used for the modification of PES hemodialysis membranes.

2.2.1 Surface-coating

Torto and coworkers (Torto et al., 2004) provided a method for the in situ modification of hollow fiber membranes used as sampling units for microdialysis probes. The method consisted of adsorption-coating of high-molecular-weight PEI onto membranes, already fitted on microdialysis probes. Modification of membranes was designed to specifically explore the so-called Andrade effects and thus enhance the interaction of membranes with enzyme. Such a procedure can be modified and employed to either promote or reduce membrane-protein interaction for hollow fibers used as microdialysis sampling units or other similar membrane applications.

2.2.2 Photo-induced surface grafting

To modify PES membranes, photochemical surface technique is attractive, and has several advantages. Mild reaction conditions and low temperature may be applied; and high selectivity is possible by choosing the reactive groups or monomers and respective excitation wavelength; and it can be easily incorporated into the end stages of a manufacturing process (Zhao et al., 2003). However, the method is always applied to modify flat-sheet membrane; it is difficult to modify hollow fiber membranes, especially to modify the internal surface of hollow fiber membrane.

Few studies focused on the modification of PES hollow fiber membranes by photo-induced grafting method, since it is difficult to apply irradiation on internal surface of hollow fiber membrane. Bequet and coworkers (Bequet et al., 2002) developed a way to prepare nanofiltration hollow fiber from ultrafiltration membranes, consisting of in-line external modification of the skin of a polysulfone (PSF) ultrafiltration hollow fiber by grafting AA under UV irradiation. The continuous photo-grafting set-up is shown in Figure 4. As shown in the figure, the modification is applied on the outer surface of the hollow fiber membrane. As mentioned above, AA and MA could be grafted on the surfaces of PES membranes by the photochemical method. It should be noticed that due to the present of carboxyl groups, these modified membranes showed pH-sensitivity.

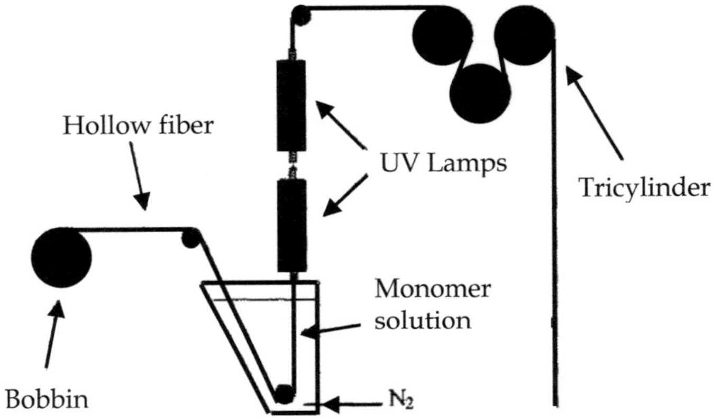

Fig. 4. Schema for the experimental continuous photo-grafting set-up.
(From reference, Bequet et al., 2002)

Shen et al. (Shen et al., 2005) modified the inner-surface of PSF hollow fiber UF membranes by using gas-initiation under UV and liquid-polymerization, which aimed to adjust the diameter of the pores in the membranes. Benzophenone (BP) was in a gaseous condition as photo-initiator, AM as graft monomer, the polyacrylamide (PAM) chain was grafted on the surface of the membranes. After the membrane surface being modified, the water flux and retention altered, and thus it could be seen that the diameter of the pores in the membrane was altered. Of course, the method could also be used to produce the PES hollow fiber membrane with small pore size.

Goma-Bilongo and co-workers (Goma-Bilongo et al., 2006) developed a numerical model to represent the process by which hollow-fiber membranes could undergo continuous surface modification by UV photo-grafting, which was the same as reported by Bequet (Bequet et al., 2002). The model took into account the coupled effects of radiation, mass transfer with polymerization reaction and heat transfer with evaporation. Then, they modified PSF hollow fiber membranes using sodium p-styrene sulfonate (NaSS) as a vinyl monomer, for treatment of anionic dye solutions (Akbari et al., 2007). However, till now, no report for the modification of PES hollow fiber membranes was found.

Hollow fiber scaffolds that compartmentalize axonal processes from their cell bodies can enable neuronal cultures with directed neurite outgrowth within a three-dimensional (3-D) space for controlling neuronal cell networking in vitro. Controllable 3-D neuronal networks in vitro could provide tools for studying neurobiological events. In order to create such a scaffold, PES micro-porous hollow fibers were ablated with a KrF excimer laser to generate specifically designed channels for directing neurite outgrowth into the luminal compartments of the fibers. These hollow fiber scaffolds can potentially be used in combination with perfusion and oxygenation hollow fiber membrane sets to construct a hollow fiber-based 3-D bioreactor for controlling and studying in vitro neuronal networking in three dimensions between compartmentalized cultures (Brayfield et al., 2008).

2.2.3 Plasma treatment and plasma-induced grafting polymerization

The same as other methods mentioned above, few study was reported on the modification of PES hollow fiber membranes by plasma treatment or plasma-induced grafting method. Only one study on the modification of PES hollow fibres by O2 plasma treatment (Batsch et al., 2005) was reported. After about one month of stable operation, the membrane samples were taken and also cleaned with chemical solutions, and the fouling could be prevented by the modification.

2.2.4 Thermal-induced grafting and immobilization

Thermal induced graft polymerization is a facile way to modify PES membranes. The method always uses chemical initiator or cleavage agent. Furthermore, many kinds of biomolecules, such as enzyme, protein and amino acid, could be covalently immobilized onto PES membranes by a simple chemical reaction.

Kroll et al. (Kroll et al., 2007) chemically modified commercially available PES and PSF hollow fiber membranes by reacting terminal hydroxyl groups with ethylene glycol diglycidyl ether (EGDGE) to produce terminal epoxy groups. For increasing loading capacity hydroxyethyl cellulose polymers were bound to the epoxy groups. Second epoxidation produced final polymers containing reactive epoxy groups on the hollow fiber surface. From this modified PES and PSF, respectively, a wide variety of N-containing reagents (e.g. iminodiacetic acid (IDA)) can be bound to the epoxy groups. The different reactions were proved by acid orange II assay and phenol sulfuric assay. The chelating IDA-membranes were complexed with different divalent metal ions (Cu^{2+}, Ni^{2+}, Co^{2+}, and Zn^{2+}). Immobilized metal ion affinity PES hollow fiber membranes were used for purification of a recombinant protein (GFP-His) from Escherichia coli, which carried a polyhistidine sequence.

3. Biocompatibility and separation performance of the membrane in vitro

The biocompatibility and separation performance of PES-based hemodialysis membranes in vitro are discussed. Protein adsorption on material surface is a common phenomenon during thrombogenic formation. Thus, the amount of protein adsorbed on the PES membrane is considered to be one of the important factors in evaluating the blood compatibility of the membrane. The adhesion of platelets to blood-contacting medical devices is a key event in thrombus formation on material surface. Thus, protein adsorption and platelet adhesion on PES membrane surface are studied. In addition, the clearance and the reduction ratio of small molecules (urea, creatinine, phosphate) during hemodialysis for the PES membrane in vitro are investigated.

3.1 Protein adsorption and platelet adhesion

3.1.1 Experimental

3.1.1.1 Protein adsorption

The protein adsorption experiments were made with BSA and FNG solutions. The concentrations of BSA and FNG were 4.0 g/dl and 0.3 g/dl in phosphate buffered saline (PBS, pH=7.4), respectively. The membrane with an area (for hollow fiber, it's the total surface areas of inside surface and outer surface) of 1 cm^2 was incubated in distilled water for 24 h, washed 3 times with PBS solution, and then immersed in the protein solution for 2 h. After protein adsorption, the membranes were carefully rinsed 3 times with PBS solution and then rinsed with distilled water. The adsorbed proteins were quantitatively eluted with 1.0 ml 2% SDS solution for 6 h. The amount of protein in the SDS solution was quantified by protein analysis (Micro BCA protein assay reagent kit).

3.1.1.2 Platelet adhesion

The platelet adhesion experiments were carried out using platelet-rich plasma (PRP). Healthy human fresh blood was collected using vacuum tubes (7 ml, Venoject II, Terumo, Co.), containing citrate/phosphate/dextrose/adenine-1 mixture solution (CPDA-1) as an anticoagulant (anticoagulant to blood ratio, 1:7). The blood was centrifuged at 1000 rpm for 10 min to obtain platelet-rich plasma (PRP) or at 2800 rpm for 15 min to obtain platelet-poor plasma (PPP). The fresh PRP sample was used for the platelet adsorption experiments.

The PES membranes (1×1 cm^2 each piece, always flat-sheet membranes) were immersed in PBS solution and equilibrated at 37 °C for 1 h. The PBS solution was removed and then 1ml of fresh PRP was introduced. The membranes were incubated with PRP at 37 °C for 2 h. PRP was decanted off and the membranes were rinsed 3 times with PBS solution. Finally, the membranes were treated with 2.5 wt% glutaraldehyde in saline for 2 days at 4 °C. The samples were washed with PBS solution, subjected to a drying process by passing them through a series of graded alcohol-saline solutions (0%, 25%, 50%, 75% and 100%) and then dried at room temperature. The dried membranes after gold coating were examined using a S-2500C scanning electron microscope (SEM, Hitachi, Japan). The number of adhering platelets on the membranes was calculated from four SEM pictures at a 500 magnification from different places on the same membranes. These procedures were performed on each membrane using four independent membranes (totally n=16), and the number was finally averaged to obtain reliable data.

3.1.2 Results and discussion

3.1.2.1 Protein adsorption

Non-specific protein adsorption is a dominant factor for membrane fouling. When membrane is used for blood purification, protein adsorption is the first stage of the interactions of membrane and blood, which may lead to further undesirable results. Protein adsorption has some relationship with the blood compatibility. There are many factors which affect the interaction between membrane surface and protein, such as surface charged character, surface free energy and topological structure, solution environment (e.g. pH, ionic strength), and protein characters (Leng et al., 2003; Okpalugo et al., 2004). The hydrophilic/hydrophobic character of membrane material plays a relatively important role in the interaction between protein and membrane. Since hydrophilic surface preferentially adsorbs water rather than solutes, many researchers have followed the idea of increasing the hydrophilicity of a membrane material with the goal of reducing protein fouling and/or protein adsorption (Mockel et al., 1999). Herein, the surfaces of the PES and some typical modified PES membranes (Copolymer of poly (acrylonitrile-co-acrylic acid), PAN-AA, modified PES membranes with the ratios of the copolymer to PES of 0/16, 0.4/16 and 0.6/16, respectively; and BSA grafted membranes following the copolymer/PES blended membranes) were studied in relation to the adsorption of BSA and FNG in vitro, data are shown in Fig. 5.

3.1.2.2 Platelet adhesion

The adhesion of platelets to blood-contacting medical devices is a key event in thrombus formation on material surface. After the platelet adhesion and activation, a series of actions could produce the thrombins which led further coagulant. Therefore, in vitro platelet adhesion assay could reflect the blood compatibility of material surface. To study the platelet adhesion, the morphology of the adhering platelet and the amounts of platelet adhesion on the membrane surfaces are always investigated through scanning electron microscopy (SEM).

Figure 6 shows the typical morphology of the platelets adhering to the PES and modified PES membranes. Herein, the membranes were modified by blending sulfonated PES and a terpolymer of poly (acrylonitrile-acrylic acid-N-vinyl pyrrolidinone) (P(AN-AA-VP)). To prepare the membranes, PES, SPES and P(AN-AA-VP) were dissolved in solvent NMP. The solution was vigorously stirred until clear homogeneous solution was obtained. The concentration of all the solute was 16 wt. %. In the experiment, different kinds of membranes were prepared by changing the ratios of PES, SPES and P(AN-AA-VP) in the casting solutions, and the ratios of PES, SPES and P(AN-AA-VP) were 16:0:0, 15:0:1, 14:0:2, 10:6:0,10:5:1, 10:4:2, respectively. After vacuum degassing, the casting solutions were prepared into membranes by spin-coating coupled with a liquid-liquid phase separation technique at room temperature. The obtained membranes were washed with distilled water thoroughly to remove the residual solvent, which were confirmed by UV scanning. All the prepared membranes were in a uniform thickness of about 60~70 μm, and the membranes were termed M-16-0-0, M-15-0-1, M-14-0-2, M-10-6-0, M-10-5-1, and M-10-4-2, respectively.

As shown in Figure 6, when compared the pictures in the same amplification multiple, it was observed that a large amount of platelets were adhered and aggregated on the PES membrane surface and the platelets formed circular or "pan-cake" shape, which suggested that the platelets were activated and already retracted the pseudopods. However, for the modified membranes, very sparse platelets were found; and the platelet expressed a rounded morphology with nearly no pseudopodium and deformation.

Figure 7 shows the amounts of the adhering platelets on the membranes from platelet-rich plasma. It could be observed that much lower number of the adhering platelets on the modified membranes compared with the PES membrane. Furthermore, the platelet

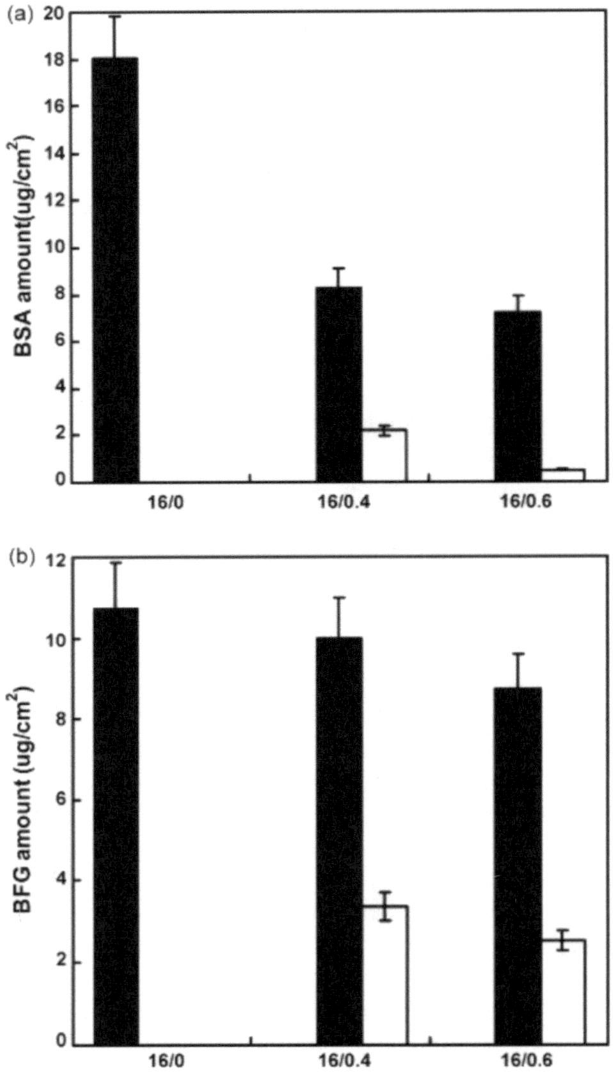

Fig. 5. (a). BSA adsorption on the membrane surfaces with the blending ratios of PES to PANAA as 16/0.2, 16/0.4, 16/0.6. (■) For the blended membranes; (□) for the BSA grafted membranes (each point represents the means±S.D. of three independent measurements.). (b) BFG adsorption on the membrane surfaces with the blending ratios of PES to PANAA as 16/0.2, 16/0.4, 16/0.6. (■) For the blended membranes; (□) for the BSA grafted membranes (each point represents the means±S.D. of three independent measurements.).
(From reference, Fang et al., 2009)

(a)

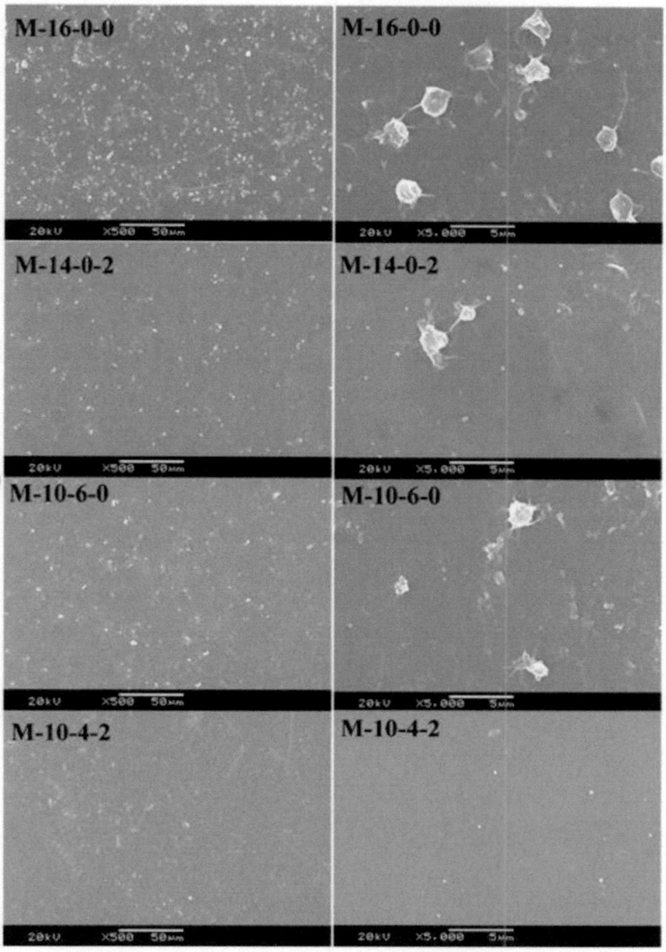

Fig. 6. Scanning electron micrographs of the platelets adhering to the membranes.

adhesion on the terpolymer modified membranes decreased with the increase of the content of the terpolymer P(AN-AA-VP). These results were consistent with those obtained from the protein adsorption, which demonstrated that the platelet adhesion had some relation with the carboxylic groups which were supplied by P(AN-AA-VP). It could also be observed that the platelet adhesion of the SPES modified membrane was significantly depressed, which was attributed to the sulfonic acid group provided by SPES.

Han et al. (Han et al., 1996) suggested that the sulfonic acid groups exhibited high adsorption of albumin and low adsorption of FBG, which might improve the blood compatibility. Thus, the platelet adhesion demonstrated the enhanced blood compatibility of SPES modified membrane. Furthermore, as the ratios of P(AN-AA-VP) to SPES changing, the different amounts of the platelet adhesion could be obtained, and no adhering platelet was found on the surface of the modified membrane M-10-4-2. The reduction of the platelet adhesion on the modified membranes was considered to be the introduction of the sulfonic acid and carboxylic groups which were supplied by SPES and P(AN-AA-VP), respectively.

The platelet adhesion results were consistent with FBG adsorption. It is well known that FBG adsorption from plasma onto a material surface might promote the adhesion of the platelets because it had the ability to bind specifically to the platelet membrane glycoprotein, GP IIb-IIIa (Phillips et al., 1988). Thus, the observed decreasing amounts of platelet adhesion might be attributed to the increased hydrophilicity, and decreased FBG adsorption. These results indicated that the surface heparin-like PES membranes modified by SPES and P(AN-AA-VP) had good blood compatibility for using as blood contacting devices.

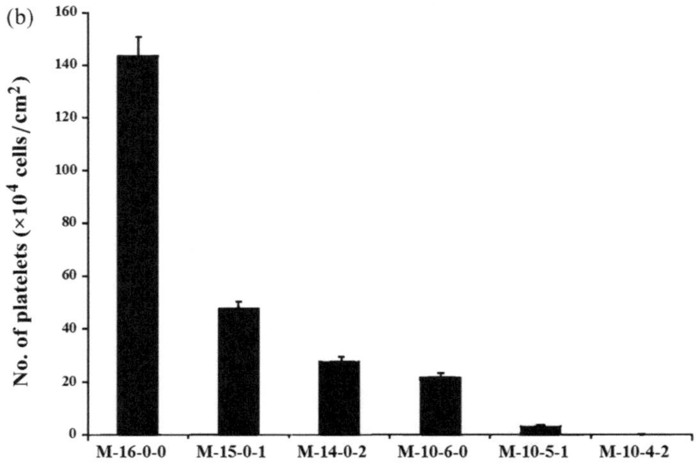

Fig. 7. The number of the adhering platelets on the membranes

3.2 Ultrafiltration and solute clearances

3.2.1 Experimental

3.2.1.1 Hemodialysis using a simulation solution

The test solutions were prepared according to the international standard ISO 8637. The molar concentrations of urea, creatinine and phosphate in the simulation solution were 15mmol/l, 500μmol/l and 1mmol/l, respectively. The test procedure was accordant to the procedure in ISO 8637. The ultrafiltration coefficient was calculated as the unit ml/mmHg.h. The clearance (K) of small molecules (urea, creatinine, phosphate) were established by sampling from the inlet and outlet segments of the extracorporeal circuit 1 h after the initiation of the treatment, and was calculated using the following formula.

$$K = \left(\frac{C_{BI} - C_{BO}}{C_{BI}}\right) Q_{BI} + \frac{C_{BO}}{C_{BI}} Q_F$$

where C_{BI} is the solute concentration in the blood (here is the simulation solution); I and O refer to the inlet and the outlet to the device, respectively; Q_{BI} is the blood flow rate at the dialyser inlet; Q_F is the filtration rate.

Urea was determined by a reagent Kit for Urea Determination (Diethyl-Monoxime, Beijing chemical regent factory, China); creatinine was quantified by the absorption at 235nm using an UV-VIS spectraphotometer U-200A (Hitachi Co., Ltd., Tokyo, Japan) through a standard curve. Phosphate was determined using the molybdate blue method: phosphate reacts with ammonium molybdate and is then reduced by stannous chloride to form a blue complex, and then measured at 670nm with the UV-VIS spectraphotometer U-200A.

3.2.1.2 Hemodialysis using swine blood in vitro

Fresh swine blood was collected using a glass tank, containing citrate/phosphate/dextrose/adenine-1 mixture solution (CPDA-1) as an anticoagulant (anticoagulant to blood ratio, 1:7). The dialysis procedure was the same as the section **3.2.1.1**, and the solute clearance was calculated using the same formula as described in the section 2.2. The concentrations of urea, creatinine and phosphate were determined using an Auto Biochemistry Analyzer 7170A (Hitachi Co., Ltd., Tokyo, Japan)

3.2.2 Results and discussion

Table 1 summarizes the clearance data and the reduction ratio after the dialysis for small molecules in vitro. It was clearly that the clearances and the reduction ratios for all the solutes were larger using the simulated solution than that for blood. The removal of small molecules during dialysis is governed by hydrodynamic conditions within the dialyser rather than membrane structure since the major resistance to transport from the blood into the dialysis fluid lies not in the membrane but boundary layers adjacent to the membrane. Thus, the data of clearance and the reduction ratio (Table 1) for the simulated solution were higher than that for the blood due to the proteins in the blood, which may induce concentration polarization.

Hemolysis ratio was determined for the swine blood in vitro and for the goat blood in vivo. Data showed that there was only a slightly hemodialysis phenomena (about 1.7%) in vitro.

	Clearance (ml/min)			Reduction ratio (%)	
	Urea	creatinine	phosphate	Urea	creatinine
Simulated solution	174.0±6.0	169.0±5.0	170.0±6.0	94.3±3.8	92.4±4.1
Blood in vitro	157.5±7.4	143.6±6.8	144.5±7.2	71.2±3.9	69.9±4.0
Blood in vivo	153.6±9.4	141.6±8.2	142.5±7.3	69.2±4.5	68.9±5.2

Data are expressed as the means±SD, n =3

Table 1. Small molecular clearance at a blood (or simulated solution) flow rate of 180 ml/min and dialysate flow rate of 500 ml/min

4. Performance evaluation in vivo

The biocompatibility and separation performance of PES-based hemodialysis membranes in vivo are also discussed. Animal experiments are carried out to evaluate the PES hollow fiber membranes firstly, and goat was selected as the experimental animal. Experiments were performed to evaluate the solute clearance and the blood compatibility. The blood compatibility and performance of the PES-based high-flux hemodialysis membrane in hemodialyzation were also clinically evaluated, and compared with those of two conventional high-flux membranes, polysulfone (PSF) and polyamide (PA) membranes. The PES and PSF membranes showed similar blood compatibility and solute clearance, and the blood compatibility for PES and PSF might be better than that of the PA membrane.

4.1 Evaluation by animal experiments

4.1.1 Experimental

4.1.1.1 Hemodialysis procedure

Adult hybrid goats (about 20 kg) were used in the experiment. All the animals underwent local anesthesia with 1.0% procaine hydrochloride by injection into the neck muscle. The hair on the neck was cleared away carefully. The animal was laid on its back and fixed on the experimental table.

Extracorporeal circuits were primed with 500ml normal saline solution to remove the bubbles in the circuits and in the dialyzer, then primed with 500ml saline solution containing 10000 IU heparin. 150mg urea and 50mg creatinine were injected to the animal blood before the treatment. At the initiation of the treatment goats received a loading dose (3000 IU) of heparin, and followed by continuous infusion (3000 IU/h). The infusion was terminated at 30 min prior to the end of the dialysis.

4.1.1.2 Solute transport

Extracorporeal circuits with left-right neck intravenous cannulation were created on the animal using B. Braun blood tubing lines for hemodialysis. The clearance (K) of small molecules (urea, creatinine, phosphate) were established by sampling from the inlet and outlet segments of the extracorporeal circuit 1 h after the initiation of the treatment, and was calculated using the formula described in section 3.2. The fluid removal ratio during these measurements was maintained at (3 ml/min).

Removal of β_2-microglobulin was established from the changes in plasma β_2-microglobulin levels during the treatment at different time intervals (30, 60, 120, 180 and 240mins). Plasma β_2-microglobulin levels were determined using a commercially produced ELISA assay (Cambridge Life Sciences, Cambridge, UK).

Electrolyte levels were determined before and after hemodialysis. K^+,Na^+ and Cl^- were determined using electrolyte analyzer (NOVA CRT-4, US), and Ca^{2+} was determined using an Auto Biochemistry Analyzer 7170A (Hitachi Co., Ltd., Tokyo, Japan).

4.1.1.3 Biocompatibility

The levels of urea, creatinine, phosphate, total proteins, albumin (ALB), alanine aminotransferase (ALT), aspartate aminotransferase (AST) and alkaline phosphatase (ALP) were determined using an Auto Biochemistry Analyzer 7170A (Hitachi Co., Ltd., Tokyo, Japan).

Blood cells including red blood cell (RBC) and white blood cell (WBC), and blood components including hemoglobin (HGB) and platelet were determined using a blood cell analyzer (BC-3000peus, Shenzhen Mairui Biomedical Device Co. Ltd., China). Blood gas was determined using a blood gas analyzer (CORNing 238, US).

For complement and WBC activation investigation, various membranes were used from different companies, Cuprophane (Nephross, Netherlands), Cellulose acetate (Nissho, Japan), Hemophane (Ningbo-Yatai, China), Polysulfone (PSF, Fresenius, Germany). Polycarbonate (PC) was obtained from BASF Co. Ltd., and the PC membrane was prepared in our Lab. Complement C_3 activation was determined in vitro by enzymelinked immunosorbent assays (ELISA) (Zwirner et al., 1995). For comparing the results, activation for Cuprophane membrane was used as control.

4.1.2 Results and discussion

4.1.2.1 Solute transport

Table 1 also summarizes the clearance data and the reduction ratio after the dialysis for small molecules in vivo. Changes in β_2-microglobulin during the dialysis for the goats are plotted in Figure 8. The reduction ratio was about 50% after the treatment for 4hrs.
The ultrafiltration coefficient was obtained by the hemodialysis process using the simulated solution with a value of 81ml/h.mmHg, from which we could conclude that the PES membrane was a high-flux hemodialysis membrane.
The PES membrane was able to reduce the plasma burden of β_2-microglobulin during the treatment, as shown in Figure 8. The data were analyzed by consideration of actual values and the percentage reductions achieved. The reduction ratio was about 50% after the treatment for 4 hrs; this value is comparable to that for PSF membrane and polyflux (Hoenich & Katopodis, 2002).
As shown in table 1, the reduction ratio for the β_2-microglobulin was smaller than that for the urea and creatinine due to the higher molecular weight ($p<0.05$). The alteration of β_2-microglobulin in plasma levels may not simply be a result of trans-membrane transport; the adsorption to the membrane may also play a role in the observed plasma changes (Hoenich & Katopodis, 2002). For the removal of β_2-microglobulin, cellulose derived membrane is impermeable to β_2- microglobulin due to its dense symmetrical structure which does not permit the easy diffusion or convection of proteins through the membrane, while polyacrylonitrile (PAN), polysulfone and polymethylmethacrylate (PMMA) membrane could be used (Moachona et al., 2002). The PMMA membrane could also adsorb β_2-microglobulin. To remove β_2-microglobulin more efficiently from plasma, hemodialysis membranes must therefore not simply be considered as filters of low-molecular-weight metabolites but should be equally assessed for their capacity to eliminate potentially deleterious low-molecular-weight plasma proteins. For the PES membrane, β_2-microglobulin adsorption is not an important mechanism of removal. The large solute removal by the membrane is mainly caused by the asymmetric structure and the higher ultra-filtration coefficient, which was presumably caused by the larger pore size and the hydrophilicity of the membrane.

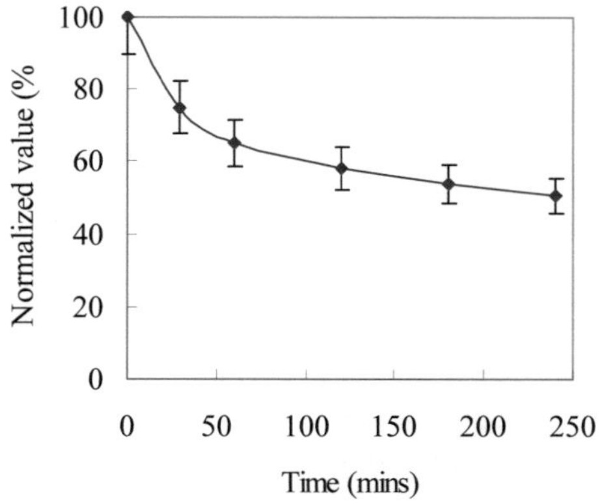

Fig. 8. Changes in β_2-microglobulin during the dialysis. Data are expressed as the means±SD, n =3 (From reference, Su et al., 2008)

Table 2 shows the electrolyte values in the goat blood before and after the dialysis process. Among the these ions, only the K^+ exhibited statistically significant decreases after the dialysis, whereas Na^+, Cl^- and Ca^{2+} did not change. As shown in the table, only the K^+ exhibited statistically significant decreases during the dialysis ($p<0.05$), whereas Na+, Cl- and Ca^{2+} did not change ($p>0.05$). The electrolyte balance could be adjusted by the dialysis fluid, and the accurate K^+ values are critically important for the management of patients with little or no residual kidney function (Barry 2003; Morgera et al., 2005).

	pre-dialysis	post-dialysis
K^+(mmol/L)	3.71±0.37	2.98±0.17
Na^+(mmol/L)	144.0±3.8	142.8±1.8
Cl^-(mmol/L)	105.1±4.1	101.0±1.2
Ca^{2+}(mmol/L)	2.12±0.16	2.02±0.11

* Data are expressed as the means±SD, n =3

Table 2. Electrolyte values pre- and post-dialysis

4.1.2.2 Biocompatibility

Figure 9 summarizes the changes in the goat blood observed during the dialysis in respect of white cells (WBC) and platelets. Both white blood cell and platelet counts have been normalized to pretreatment levels and expressed as a percentage of these values. A small decline in both was noted at the first 30 minutes, which returned to the initial levels after about 2 h. These phenomena have been reported frequently in hemodialysis, hemofiltration, and plasma separation.

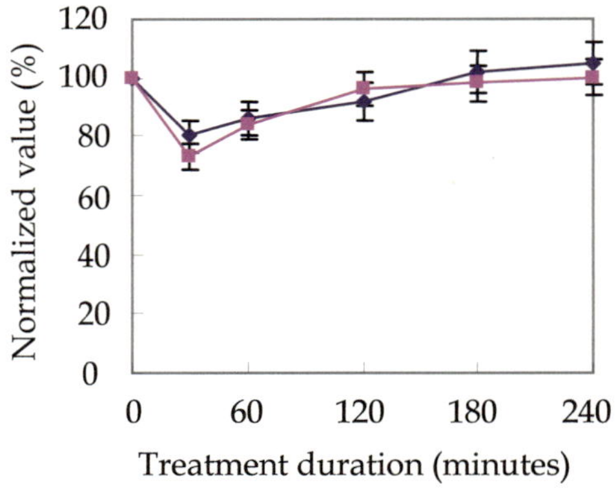

Fig. 9. Changes in WBC and platelet during the dialysis in vivo ♦ Platelet; ■ WBC; Data are expressed as the means±SD, n =3 (From reference, Su et al., 2008)

The complement and WBC activation for various membranes were investigated after contacting to blood for 1h. The data showed the correlation between the complement and WBC activation. We also found that the concentration of C3a increased rapidly at the beginning of the contact between the blood and the PES membrane and remained constant after 90 min, which was consistent with the decrease of white blood cells (Zhao et al., 2001). The decrease of WBC is caused by complement activation; the activation of complement system results in release of anaphylatoxins into the circulation which have potent physiological effects, thus complement activation has been the most widely used parameter to evaluate hemocompatibility.

Hemolysis ratio was determined for the swine blood in vitro and for the goat blood in vivo. Data showed that there was only a slightly hemolysis phenomena (about 1.7%) in vitro, while the hemolysis ratio was zero in vivo (The absorption value for (+) is 0.832, but for the sample is 0).

The red blood cell (RBC) and hemoglobin (RGB) levels were also determined during the dialysis. The RBC level was (2.04±0.12)×1012/L and (1.96±0.10)×1012/L respectively before and after the hemodialysis. And the HGB level was 115.0±8.0g/L and 110.5±8.0g/L before and after the hemodialysis, respectively.

Biochemistry for the blood was analyzed before and after the hemodialysis, and the data were summarized in Table 3. Only the alkaline phosphatase (ALP) level increased. And the others, including alanine aminotransferase (ALT), aspartate aminotransferase (AST), total protein (TP) and plasma albumin (ALB) were slightly decreased. The blood gas was also analyzed as shown in Table 4. The data showed no statistically change during the dialysis. The urine solution was also analyzed before and after the hemodialysis; the pH value, urine protein and urine glucose had no change before and after the hemodialysis. The concentrations of urobilinogen were 3.5mmol/L and 3.7mmol/L before and after the hemodialysis, respectively.

Red blood cells (RBC) and hemoglobins (HGB) levels decreased slightly after the treatment, and both of the reduction ratios were about 5%. Slightly decreases in alanine aminotransferase (ALT), aspartate aminotransferase (AST), total protein (TP) and plasma albumin (ALB) were also observed. The reduction ratios for all of them ranged 3-10%, which were presumably caused by the dilution of the blood by normal saline solution infused after the hemodialysis process. ALP is produced primarily in the liver and in bone, and the result for ALP indicts that the PES membrane has no effect on the liver.

	pre-dialysis	post-dialysis
ALT(IU/L)	29.0±3.0	26.5±1.5
AST(IU/L)	189.5±9.5	173.0±15.5
ALP(IU/L)	284.0±33.0	266.0±13.0
TP(g/L)	70.2±1.4	63.8±1.8
ALB(g/L)	29.2±0.4	27.6±0.4

* Data are expressed as the means±SD, n =3

Table 3. Data for biochemistry analysis pre- and post-dialysis

	pre-dialysis	post-dialysis
pH	7.43±0.0	7.47±0.02
PCO_2(Kpa)	4.5±0.7	4.3±0.1
PO_2 (Kpa)	9.7±0.4	9.2±0.3
HCO_3(mmol/L)	24.5±2.4	25.6±1.5

* Data are expressed as the means±SD, n =3

Table 4. Blood gas values pre- and post-dialysis

4.1.3 Summary

The PES hollow fiber hemodialysis membrane could effectively remove water and waste products, not only small molecular weight solute such as urea and creatinine, but also "middle" molecular solute as β_2-microglobulin. Slight neutropenia and platelet adhesion were observed at the initial stage of the hemodialysis and no significant differences were found in electrolyte, blood gas and blood biochemistry before and after the treatment. The results also suggested that the PES membrane hemodialyzer could be used for clinical application.

4.2 Clinical evaluation

4.2.1 Experimental

4.2.1.1 Hemodialysis procedure

Three groups of hemodialysis patients with mature functioning arteriovenous fistula participated in this study. Their mean age was 48 ± 12 yr, and they had been receiving dialysis treatments for 35 ± 14 months with an average frequency of 3 times per wk. For each patient, Hct was determined at the beginning of the hemodialysis session.

Standard midweek hemodialysis sessions were analyzed, and bicarbonate dialysate was used. The dialysate contained 140 mmol/L sodium, 2 mmol/L potassium, 108 mmol/L chloride, 1.50 mmol/L calcium, 0.5 mmol/L magnesium and 32 mmol/L bicarbonate. The blood flow was 200 ml/min and the dialysate flow was 500 ml/min. Three kinds of dialyzers (PES, polysulfone (PSF), and polyamide (PA)) were used for the three groups of patients, respectively.

4.2.1.2 Calculation of solute clearance

The levels of urea, creatinine, phosphate, total proteins, albumin (ALB), alanine aminotransferase (ALT), aspartate aminotransferase (AST) and alkaline phosphatase (ALP) were determined using an Auto Biochemistry Analyzer 7170A (Hitachi Co., Ltd., Tokyo, Japan).

The removal of β_2-microglobulin was established by the changes in plasma level during the treatment at different time intervals (30, 60, 120, 180 and 240mins). Plasma β_2-microglobulin levels were determined using a commercially produced ELISA assay (Cambridge Life Sciences, Cambridge, UK).

Electrolyte levels were determined before and after hemodialysis. The levels of K+, Na+ and Cl- were determined using electrolyte analyzer (NOVA CRT-4, US), and Ca2+ was determined using an Auto Biochemistry Analyzer 7170A (Hitachi Co., Ltd., Tokyo, Japan).

4.2.1.3 Evaluation of blood compatibility

In order to investigate the complement and immunoglobin activation, complement C3, C4 and immunoglobin G, A, M and E were determined by enzyme-linked immunosorbent assays (ELISA)

Blood cells including red blood cell (RBC) and white blood cell (WBC), and blood components including hemoglobin (HGB) and platelet were determined using a blood cell analyzer (BC-3000peus, Shenzhen Mairui Biomedical Device Co. Ltd., China). Blood gas was determined by a blood gas analyzer (CORNing 238, US).

4.2.1.4 Statistical analysis

The software of SPSS 13.0 was used for statistical analysis. The deviation between the three groups was calculated by analysis of one-factor variance (ANOVA), and the deviation between samples in one group was calculated by Student-Newman-Keuls (q-test). All the data are shown by mean values and standard deviations (m±s), $p<0.05$ is considered to have statistical difference.

4.2.2 Results and discussion

All the patients participated in the whole study period. The vital signs were stable with no adverse events during the dialysis, and there were no abnormal findings in laboratory security parameters. During the dialysis by PA membrane dialyzer, some clots were found after 175 minutes in the extracorporeal blood circuit of a male patient who was on a repeated bolus fraxiparine anticoagulation regimen (6000 IU in total), but the patient still finished the treatment. This was the only adverse event during the whole study. All of patients who were treated by PES, PA or PSF membrane dialyzers were performed without provoking any adverse symptoms, such as headache or hypotension.

4.2.2.1 Solute clearance

The clearance of small molecular and middle molecular toxins was expressed as the solute reduction ratio (RR) after 4 hours hemodialysis, and could be calculated by: RR (%) = (1-(post-solute concentration/pre-solute concentration))×100%. The blood flow was controlled at 200 ml/min and the dialysate flow was 500 ml/min. Figure 10 shows the RRs of urea, creatinine and β_2-microglobulin for the three kinds of hollow fiber dialyzers. As shown in the figure, large amount of the toxins were removed after the hemodialysis. The RRs of urea for PES, PA and PSF membranes were 61.2%, 63% and 62.3%, respectively. The RRs of creatinine were 51.3%, 54.5% and 54.7%, respectively. Meanwhile, the RRs of β_2-microglobulin were 60.8%, 51.3% and 57.7%, respectively. The RRs of urea and creatinine for the PES membrane were slightly smaller than that for the PA and PSF membranes, but no statistical difference. However, the RRs of β_2-microglobulin for the PES membrane were slightly larger than that for the PA and PSF membranes. It proved that the PES, PA and PSF hollow fiber hemodialysis membranes could effectively remove waste products including not only small molecular weight solutes such as urea and creatinine but also "middle" molecular solutes as β_2-microglobulin.

To increase the removal of large molecular solutes, the rates of diffusion and convection should be increased, and the membrane pore size and porosity should be increased. Pore size limitations arise from the concern over potential loss of blood proteins such as albumin. Given that dialysis patients are generally malnourished, and the relative risk of death of dialysis patients increases as the serum albumin concentration decreases, it is desirable to minimize the albumin loss to the dialysate. Furthermore, small albumin losses may be clinically insignificant to the patient, but may lead to practical problems in the dialysis clinic, such as the foam formation in the dialysate drains. An ideal dialysis membrane should have a uniform pore size large enough to allow the passage of β_2-microglobulin but small enough to retain albumin (66,000 daltons). Unfortunately, methods currently used to produce dialysis membranes resulted in a non-uniform pore size distribution. In the phase inversion membrane production process, polymer is dissolved in a solvent and then exposed to a non-solvent as it is extruded through an annular die. The breadth of the distribution produced by the phase inversion process resulted from the finite rate of molecular diffusion through the viscous polymer solution during the membrane coagulation phase (Qian et al., 2009). While previous membrane improvements have resulted from reducing the viscosity of the polymer solution, it is unlikely that the breadth of the pore size distribution can be significantly reduced by further modification of the phase inversion process. Given a fixed breadth of the pore size distribution, the requirement for albumin retention limited not only the maximum pore size but also the mean pore size. As a result, the sieving coefficient of β_2-microglobulin is generally 0.6 or less in order to maintain the albumin sieving coefficient at 0.01 or less. The PES membrane may be adequate to this requirement (Kim & Kim, 2005).

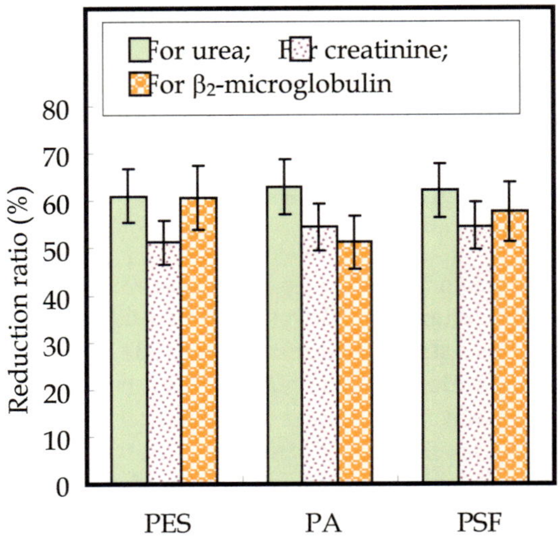

Fig. 10. Reduction ratios of small molecules urea and creatinine, as well as middle molecules β_2-microglobulin after four hours hemodialysis at a blood flow rate of 200 ml/min and dialysate flow rate of 500 ml/min. Data are expressed as the means±SD, n =3

4.2.2.2 Biocompatibility

Figure 11 shows the white cell (WBC) changes in the patient bloods during the dialysis for the three kinds of membranes. The blood cell counts have been normalized to pre-treatment levels and expressed as a percentage of these values. A small decline was noted at the first 30 minutes for all the membranes, and returned to the initial levels after about 1 h, and no significant difference was observed among the three membranes. The changes in platelet, complement factor C3, and complement C4 during the hemodialysis process for the three membranes were also investigated, and similar results were obtained as the change in WBC (Data not shown).

Retrospective analyses have shown that hemodialysis with synthetic dialysis membranes is associated with improved patient survival in ESRD (Kim & Kim, 2005). This observation was mainly attributed to membrane biocompatibility. Synthetic membranes are generally regarded as to be highly biocompatible, since they lead to low complement activation and leucopenia, which are the two classical parameters to characterizing biocompatibility in dialysis (Hakim et al., 1996). However, several other systems become altered during blood-membrane interaction. Among them are the coagulation system and imbalances of the oxidative and anti-oxidative system (Krieter et al., 2007; Klingel et al., 2004).

A slightly decrease in outlet leukocyte counts was observed for the three dialyzers, and significant difference was observed among them, as shown in Figure 11. The decrease of white blood cells was caused by complement activation, thus similar results were obtained in the changes of complement factor C3 and complement C4 during the hemodialysis process. When comparing PES, PA and PSF membranes, these change showed no significant difference, which indicated that the blood compatibility might be the same, though different membrane materials were used.

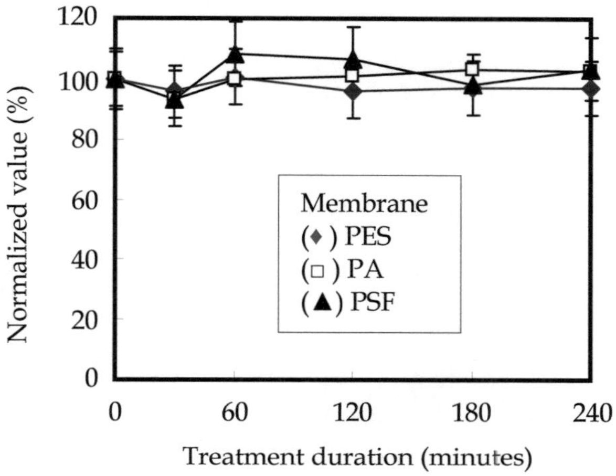

Fig. 11. Changes in WBC during the dialysis in vivo. Data are expressed as the means±SD, n =3

The concentration of albumin (ALB) and immunoglobin (GLB) slightly increased after 4 h hemodialysis, and no significant difference among the three membranes. Total protein adsorption of the membranes was also determined, and the amounts for PES, PA and PSF membranes were 12.2, 10.2, and 11.9 g/cm^2, respectively.

Total bilirubin (TBIL), direct bilirubin (DBIL), alanine aminotransferase (ALT), and aspartate aminotransferase (AST) levels were measured after 4 h hemodialysis, and compared with the initial levels for the three kinds of membranes, as shown in Figure 12. There are no significant differences in the changes of TBIL, DBIL, ALT, and AST for the PES and PSF membranes, and both the TBIL and DBIL levels increased compared to the initial levels. However, for the PA membrane, the TBIL, and AST levels decreased obviously.

In Figure 12, slightly changes in total bilirubin (TBIL), direct bilirubin (DBIL), alanine aminotransferase (ALT), and aspartate aminotransferase (AST) were also observed. The change ratios for all of them ranged 3-10%. There are no significant differences in the changes of TBIL, DBIL, ALT, and AST for the PES and PSF membranes, and both the TBIL and DBIL levels increased compared to the initial levels, which were presumably caused by the dilution of the blood by normal saline solution infused or pachemia after the hemodialysis process. However, for the PA membrane, the TBIL, and AST levels decreased obviously. TBIL, DBIL, ALT and AST are produced primarily in the liver; all of them are lipophilic and hydrophobic. The dialyzer permits diffusive clearance of non-protein-bound, water soluble uraemic solutes, such as urea and creatinine. The corollary is that the substances are tightly protein-bound and present in small quantities in the aqueous phase, or are lipophilic and removed by HD in negligible amounts, if at all. The results indicted that the PES and PSF membrane had no effect on the liver, and might have possibly higher hydrophilicity than PA membrane.

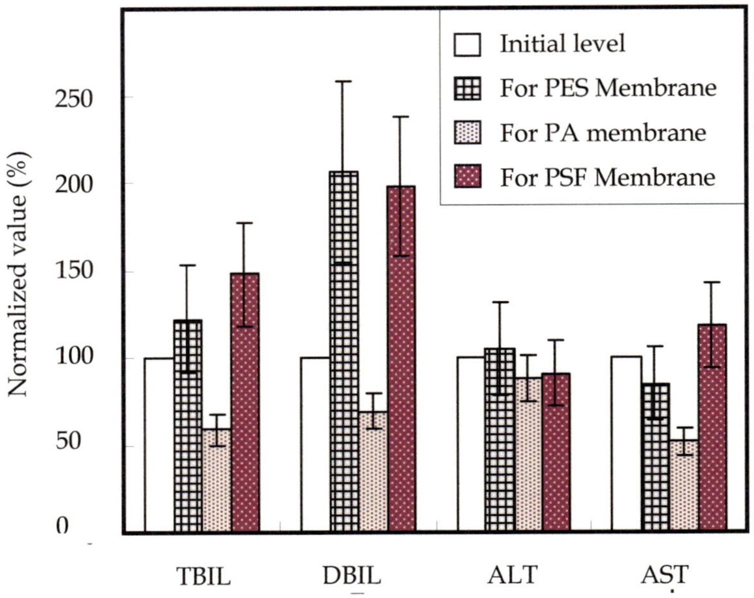

Fig. 12. *Total* bilirubin (TBIL), *direct* bilirubin (DBIL), alanine aminotransferase (ALT), and aspartate aminotransferase (AST) level changes after 4 h hemodialysis. Data are expressed as the means±SD, n =3

We speculated that the high-flux dialysis membrane might possibly let some biocompatibility markers enter dialysis solution so that the plasma levels of these markers could provide biased information. The plasma levels of biocompatibility markers may have also been influenced by adsorption to the membrane surface (Benz et al., 2007; Gotz et al., 2008). The adsorption to the membrane was not determined in our study. However, the protein adsorption capacity was investigated, and no difference was observed. On the basis of our results, we concluded that the designed modifications of the new high-flux PES dialyzer resultED in its higher middle molecule clearance efficacy, and had an effect on thrombogenicity as assessed by platelet behavior and fibrinolysis. Although coagulation system judged by one of the evaluated parameters was slightly higher compared with the other dialyzers, it was still within the biocompatible dialyzer range. In terms of complement activation and changes in leukocyte count, the new dialyzer is also comparable with the other biocompatible dialyzers. Besides the thrombogenicity, complement activation, and WBC count changes, other issues must be considered when evaluating bio(in)compatibility (Krieter et al., 2007; Klingel et al., 2004)

One further aspect merits consideration is that the PES membrane dialyzer series exhibits a higher permeability and thus, cytokine-inducing substances, possibly present in the dialysis fluid, might gain access to the blood stream through internal filtration (backfiltration). Therefore, investigations on the pyrogen permeability of PES membranes have been performed to the studies on the inflammatory response of the membrane. In the study, the dialysate compartment was deliberately contaminated with purified lipopolysaccharides (LPS) from Escherichia coli, as well as with LPS derived from Stenotrophomonas (Sten) maltophilia. No significant generation of interleukin 1 (IL-1), IL-6 or tumor necrosis factor (TNF) was found in the blood compartment for the PES dialyzer and Fresenius PSF series of dialyzers as compared with sterile controls. However, significant induction of IL-1, IL-6, and TNF was observed for the highly permeable polysulfone membrane DIAPES, suggesting that not all of the polysulfone membranes were alike with regard to their pyrogen permeability due to the different modification methods. The PES, PA, and PSF dialyzers offered important safety features with regard to a possible contamination of the dialysis fluid (Wang et al., 1996; Schiffl & Lang, 2010).

4.2.3 Summary

The PES hollow fiber membrane hemodialyzer was effective and safe in the therapy for uremic patients. The PES hollow fiber hemodialysis membrane could effectively remove water and waste products including not only small molecular weight solutes such as urea and creatinine but also "middle" molecular solute as β_2-microglobulin. Slight neutropenia and platelet adhesion were observed at the initial stage of the hemodialysis and no significant difference was found in electrolyte or blood biochemistry before or after the treatment. The data indicated that the performances of PES, PSF and PA hemodialyzers in the clinical setting were comparable and the PES hemodialyzer might be better than the others. The results indicated that PES hollow fiber membrane had a potentially wide application for hemodialysis.

5. Conclusions

Polyethersulfone (PES) is one of the most important polymeric materials and is widely used in separation fields. PES and PES-based membranes show outstanding oxidative, thermal and hydrolytic stability as well as good mechanical and film-forming properties. Furthermore, PES-based membranes show high permeability for low molecular weight proteins when used as hemodialysis membranes. However, the blood compatibility of the PES membrane is not adequate, and injections of anti-coagulants are needed during its clinical application.

Thus, all the PES membranes used for hemodialysis are not the pristine PES membranes, and most widely used modification method for hemodialysis PES membranes is blending. Poly (vinyl pyrrolidone) (PVP) is the most widely used for the modification of PES membranes by blending, and PVP also acts used as a hydrophilic additive and a membrane forming agent. Surface-coating and grafting methods can also be used for the modification of PES hollow fiber membranes. All the modifications are based on the premise that the materials used in the modification give inherently more hydrophilicity and adsorb less protein than the underlying substrate.

Protein adsorption on material surface is a common phenomenon during thrombogenic formation. Thus, the amount of protein adsorbed on the PES membrane is considered to be one of the important factors in evaluating the blood compatibility. The adhesion of platelets to blood-contacting medical devices is a key event in thrombus formation on material surface. The clearances and the reduction ratios of small molecules (urea, creatinine, phosphate) for the PES membrane after the hemodialysis in vitro were larger than those in vivo. Animal experiments and clinical experiments indicated that the PES-based high-flux hemodialysis membrane had good blood compatibility, and could effectively remove "middle" molecular solute as β_2-microglobulin.

The blood compatibility and performance in hemodialyzation were compared with two conventional high-flux membranes, polysulfone (PSF) and polyamide (PA) membranes. The PES and PSF membranes showed similar blood compatibility and solute clearance, and the blood compatibility for PES and PSF might be better than the PA membrane.

In conclusion, PES-based hollow fiber membranes have good blood compatibility and solute clearance, and the PES hollow fiber membrane hemodialyzer might be a good commercial product in the future.

6. Acknowledgment

These works were financially sponsored by the National Natural Science Foundation of China (No. 50973070, 51073105 and 30900691), and State Education Ministry of China (Doctoral Program for High Education, No. JS 20100181110031). We should also thank our laboratory members for their generous help, and gratefully acknowledge the help of Ms. H. Wang, of the Analytical and Testing Center at Sichuan University, for the SEM, and Ms Liang, of the Department of Nephrology at West China Hospital, for the human fresh blood collection.

7. References

Agenson KO & Urase T. (2007). Change in membrane performance due to organic fouling in nanofiltration (NF)/reverse osmosis (RO) applications. *Separation and Purification Technology*, Vol. 55, No. 2, (June 2007), pp. 147-156, ISSN 1383-5866

Akbari A, et al. (2007). Application of nanofiltration hollow fiber membranes, developed by photografting, to treatment of anionic dye solutions. *Journal of Membrane Science*, Vol. 297, No. 1-2 (July 2007), pp. 243-252, ISSN 0376-7388

Arahman N, et al. (2009). Fouling Reduction of a Poly(ether sulfone) Hollow-Fiber Membrane with a Hydrophilic Surfactant Prepared via Non-Solvent-Induced Phase Separation. *Journal of Applied Polymer Science*, Vol. 111, No. 3 (February 2009), pp. 1653-1658, ISSN 0021-8995

Barry K. (2003). The effect of hemodialysis on electrolytes and acid-base parameters. *Clinica Chimica Acta*, Vol. 336, No. 1-2 (October 2003), pp. 109-113, ISSN 0009-8981

Barzin J, et al. (2004). Characterization of polyethersulfone hemodialysis membrane by ultrafiltration and atomic force microscopy. *Journal of Membrane Science*, Vol. 237, No. 1-2, (July 2004), pp. 77-85, ISSN 0376-7388

Batsch A, et al. (2005). Foulant analysis of modified and unmodified membranes for water and wastewater treatment with LC-OCD. *Desalination*, Vol. 178, No. 1-3 (July 2005), pp. 63-72, ISSN 0011-9164

Benz K, et al. (2007). Hemofiltration of Recombinant Hirudin by Different Hemodialyzer Membranes: Implications for Clinical Use. *Clinical Journal of the American Society Of Nephrology*, Vol. 2, No. 3 (May 2007), pp. 470-476, ISSN 1555-905X

Bequet S, et al. (2002). From ultrafiltration to nanofiltration hollow fiber membranes: a continuous UV-photografting process. *Desalination*, Vol. 144, No. 1-3 (September 2002), pp. 9-14, ISSN 0011-9164

Brayfield CA, et al. (2008). Excimer laser channel creation in polyethersulfone hollow fibers for compartmentalized in vitro neuronal cell culture scaffolds. *Acta Biomaterialia*, Vol. 4, No. 2 (March 2008), pp. 244-255, ISSN 1742-7061

Erlenkotter A, et al. (2008). Score Model for the Evaluation of Dialysis Membrane Hemocompatibility. *Artificial Organs*, Vol. 32, No. 12 (December 2008), pp. 962-969, ISSN 0160-564X

Fang BH, et al. (2009). Modification of polyethersulfone membrane by grafting bovine serum albumin on the surface of polyethersulfone/poly(acrylonitrile-co-acrylic acid) blended membrane, *Journal of Membrane Science*, Vol. 329, No. 1-2 (March 2009), pp. 46-55, ISSN 0376-7388

Gholami M, et al. (2003). The effect of heat-treatment on the ultrafiltration performance of polyethersulfone (PES) hollow-fiber membranes. *Desalination*, Vol. 155, No. 3 (July 2003), pp. 293-301, ISSN 0011-9164

Goma-Bilongo T, et al. (2006). Numerical simulation of a UV photografting process for hollow-fiber membranes. *Journal of Membrane Science*, Vol. 278, No. 1-2 (July 2006), pp. 308-317, ISSN 0376-7388

Gotz AK, et al. (2008). Effect of membrane flux and dialyzer biocompatibility on survival in end-stage diabetic nephropathy. *Nephron Clinical Practice*, Vol. 109, No. 3 (March 2008), pp. 154-160, ISSN 1660-2110

Hakim RM, et al. (1996). Effect of the dialysis membrane on mortality of chronic hemodialysis patients. *Kidney International*, Vol. 50, No. 2 (August 1996), pp. 566–570, ISSN 0085-2538

Han DK, et al. (1996). Plasma protein adsorption to sulfonated poly(ethylene oxide)-grafted polyurethane surface. *Journal of Biomedical Materials Research*, Vol. 30, No. 1 (January 1996), pp. 23-30, ISSN 0021-9304

Hoenich NA & Katopodis KP. (2002). Clinical characterization of a new polymeric membrane for use in renal replacement therapy. *Biomaterials*, Vol. 23, No. 18 (September 2002), pp. 3853-3858, ISSN 0142-9612

Khulbe KC, Feng C & Matsuura T. (2010). The Art of Surface Modification of Synthetic Polymeric Membranes. *Journal of Applied Polymer Science*, Vol. 115, No. 2, (January 2010), pp. 855-895, ISSN 0021-8995

Kim JH & Kim CK. (2005). Ultrafiltration membranes prepared from blends of polyethersulfone and poly(1-vinylpyrrolidone-co-styrene) copolymers. *Journal of Membrane Science*, Vol. 262, No. 1-2 (October 2005), pp. 60-68, ISSN 0376-7388

Klingel R, et al. (2004). Comparative analysis of procoagulatory activity of haemodialysis, haemofiltration and haemodiafiltration with a polysulfone membrane (APS) and with different modes of enoxaparin anticoagulation. *Nephrology Dialysis Transplantation*,

Vol. 19, No. 1 (January 2004), pp. 164-170, ISSN 0931-0509

Koh M, Clark MM & Howe KJ. (2005). Filtration of lake natural organic matter: Adsorption capacity of a polypropylene microfilter. *Journal of Membrane Science*, Vol. 256, No. 1-2, (July 2005), pp. 169-175, ISSN 0376-7388

Krieter DH, et al. (2007). Effects of a polyelectrolyte additive on the selective dialysis membrane permeability for low-molecular-weight proteins, *Nephrology Dialysis Transplantation*, Vol. 22, No. 2 (February 2007), pp. 491-499, ISSN 0931-0509

Kroll S, et al. (2007). Heterogeneous surface modification of hollow fiber membranes for use in micro-reactor systems. *Journal of Membrane Science*, Vol. 299, No. 1-2 (August 2007), pp. 181-199, ISSN 0376-7388

Leng YX, et al. (2003). Mechanical properties and platelet adhesion behavior of diamond-like carbon films synthesized by pulsed vacuum arc plasma deposition. *Surface Science*, Vol. 531, No. 2 (May 2003), pp. 177-184, ISSN 0039-6028

Liu ZB, et al. (2009). BSA-Modified Polyethersulfone Membrane: Preparation, Characterization and Biocompatibility. *Journal of Biomaterials Science-Polymer Edition*, Vol. 20, No. 3, (March 2009), pp. 377-397, ISSN 0920-5063

Mansourpanah Y, et al. (2009). The effect of non-contact heating (microwave irradiation) and contact heating (annealing process) on properties and performance of polyethersulfone nanofiltration membranes. *Applied Surface Science* Vol. 255, No. 20 (July 2009), pp. 8395-8402, ISSN 0169-4332

Moachona N, et al. (2002). Influence of the charge of low molecular weight proteins on their efficacy of filtration and/or adsorption on dialysis membranes with different intrinsic properties. *Biomaterials*, Vol. 23, No. 3 (February 2002), pp. 651-658, ISSN 0142-9612

Mockel D, Staude E & Guiver MD. (1999). Static protein adsorption, ultrafiltration behavior and cleanability of hydrophilized polysulfone membranes. *Journal of Membrane Science*, Vol. 158, No. 1-2 (June 1999), pp. 63-75, ISSN 0376-7388

Morgera S, et al. (2005). Regional citrate anticoagulation in continuous hemodialysis–acid-base and electrolyte balance at an increased dose of dialysis. *Nephrol Clin Practice*, Vol. 101, No. 4 (September 2005), pp. 211-219, ISSN 1660-2110

Mosqueda-Jimenez DB, Narbaitz RM & Matsuura T. (2006). Effects of preparation conditions on the surface modification and performance of polyethersulfone ultrafiltration membranes. *Journal of Applied Polymer Science*, Vol. 99, No. 6, (March 2006), pp. 2978-2988, ISSN 0021-8995

Nakatsuka S, Nakate I & Miyano T. (1996). Drinking water treatment by using ultrafiltration hollow fiber membranes. *Desalination*, Vol. 106, No. 1-3 (August 1996), pp. 55-61, ISSN 0011-9164

Okpalugo TIT, et al. (2004). Platelet adhesion on silicon modified hydrogenated amorphous carbon films. *Biomaterials*, Vol. 25, No. 2 (January 2004), pp. 239-245, ISSN 0142-9612

Peng JM, et al. (2009). Separation of oil/water emulsion using Pluronic F127 modified polyethersulfone ultrafiltration membranes. *Separation and Purification Technology*, Vol. 66, No. 3 (May 2009), pp. 591-597, ISSN 1383-5866

Phillips DR, et al. (1988). The platelet membrane glycoprotein IIb-IIIa complex. *Blood*, Vol. 71, No. 4 (April 1988), pp. 831-843, ISSN 0006-4971

Qian BS, Fang BH & Zhao CS. (2009). Preparation and characterization of pH-sensitive polyethersulfone hollow fiber membrane for flux control. *Journal of Membrane Science*, Vol. 344, No. 1-2 (November 2009), pp. 297-303, ISSN 0376-7388

Qin JJ, et al. (2004). The use of ultrafiltration for treatment of spent solvent cleaning rinses from nickel-plating operations: membrane material selection study. *Desalination*, Vol. 170, No. 2 (October 2004), pp. 169-175, ISSN 0011-9164

Samtleben W, et al. (2003). Comparison of the new polyethersulfone high-flux membrane DIAPES® HF800 with conventional high-flux membranes during on-line haemodiafiltration. *Nephrology Dialysis Transplantation*, Vol. 18, No. 11, (November 2003), pp. 2382-2386, ISSN 0931-0509

Schiffl H & Lang SM. (2010). Effects of Dialysis Purity on Uremic Dyslipidemia. *Therapeutic Apheresis and Dialysis*, Vol. 14, No. 1 (February 2010), pp. 5-11, ISSN 1744-9979

Shen YJ, et al. (2005). Gas-initiation under UV and liquid-grafting polymerization on the surface of polysulfone hollow fiber ultrafiltration membrane by dynamic method. *Journal of Environmental Sciences-China*, Vol. 17, No.3 (March 2005), pp. 465-468, ISSN 1001-0742

Su BH, et al. (2008). Evaluation of polyethersulfone highflux hemodialysis membrane in vitro and in vivo. *Journal of Materials Science: Materials in Medicine*, Vol. 19, No. 2 (February 2008), pp. 745-751, ISSN 0957-4530

Torto N, et al. (2004). In situ poly(ethylene imine) coating of hollow fiber membranes used for microdialysis sampling. *Pure and Applied Chemistry*, Vol. 76, No. 4 (April 2004), pp. 879-888, ISSN 0033-4545

Tullis RH, et al. (2002). Affinity Hemodialysis for Antiviral Therapy. I. Removal of HIV-1 from cell culture supernatants, plasma, and blood. *Therapeutic Apheresis*, Vol. 6, No. 3, (June 2002), pp. 213-220, ISSN 1091-6660

Van der Bruggen B. (2009). Chemical Modification of Polyethersulfone Nanofiltration Membranes: A Review. *Journal of Applied Polymer Science*, Vol. 114, No. 1, (October 2009), pp. 630-642, ISSN 0021-8995

Wang DL, Li K & Teo WK. (1996). Polyethersulfone hollow fiber gas separation membranes prepared from NMP/alcohol solvent systems. *Journal of Membrane Science*, Vol. 115, No. 1 (June 1996), pp. 85-108, ISSN 0376-7388

Wang HT, et al. (2009). Improvement of hydrophilicity and blood compatibility on polyethersulfone membrane by adding polyvinylpyrrolidone. *Fibers and Polymers*, Vol. 10, No. 1 (February 2009), pp. 1-5, ISSN 1229-9197

Wang YQ, et al. (2006). Protein-adsorption-resistance and permeation property of polyethersulfone and soybean phosphatidylcholine blend ultrafiltration membranes. *Journal of Membrane Science*, Vol. 270, No. 1-2 (February 2006), pp. 108-114, ISSN 0376-7388

Werner C, Jacobasch HJ & Reichelt G. (1995). Surface characterization of hemodialysis membranes based on streaming potential measurements. *Journal of Biomaterials Science-Polymer Edition*, Vol. 7, No. 1, (January 1995), pp. 61-76, ISSN 0920-5063

Xu XC, et al. (2009). Non-invasive monitoring of fouling in hollow fiber membrane via UTDR. *Journal of Membrane Science*, Vol. 326, No. 1 (January 2009), pp. 103-110, ISSN 0376-7388

Yang Q, Chung TS & Weber M. (2009). Microscopic behavior of polyvinylpyrrolidone hydrophilizing agents on phase inversion polyethersulfone hollow fiber membranes for hemofiltration. *Journal of Membrane Science*, Vol. 326, No. 2 (January 2009), pp. 322-331, ISSN 0376-7388

Yu CH, et al. (2008). Hydrophobicity and molecular weight of humic substances on ultrafiltration fouling and resistance. *Separation and Purification Technology*, Vol. 64, No. 2, (December 2008), pp. 206-212, ISSN 1383-5866

Zhao CS, et al. (2001). An Evaluation of a Polyethersulfone Hollow Fiber Plasma Separator by Animal Experiment. *Artificial Organs*, Vol. 25, No. 1, (January 2001), pp. 60-63, ISSN 0160-564X

Zhao CS, et al. (2003). Surface characterization of polysulfone membranes modified by DNA immobilization. *Journal of Membrane Science*, Vol. 214, No. 2 (April 2003), pp. 179-189, ISSN 0376-7388

Zhao W, et al. (2008). Fabrication of antifouling polyethersulfone ultrafiltration membranes using Pluronic F127 as both surface modifier and pore-forming agent. *Journal of Membrane Science*, Vol. 318, No. 1-2 (June 2008), pp. 405-412, ISSN 0376-7388

Zhu LP, et al. (2008a). Molecular design and synthesis of amphiphilic copolymers, and the performances of their blend membranes. *Acta Polymerica Sinica*, Vol. 1, No. 4 (April 2008), pp. 309-317, ISSN 1000-3304

Zhu LP, et al. (2008b). Amphiphilic graft copolymers based on ultrahigh molecular weight poly(styrene-alt-maleic anhydride) with poly(ethylene glycol) side chains for surface modification of polyethersulfone membranes. *European Polymer Journal*, Vol. 44, No. 6 (June 2008), pp. 1907-1914, ISSN 0014-3057

Zou W, et al. (2010). Poly (methyl methacrylate-acrylic acid-vinypyrrolidone) terpolymer modified polyethersulfone hollow fiber membrane with pH-sensitivity and protein antifouling property. *Journal of Membrane Science*, Vol. 358, No. 1-2 (August 2010), pp. 76-84, ISSN 0376-7388

Zwirner J, Dobos G & Gotze O. (1995). A novel elisa for the assessment of classical pathway of complement activation in-vivo by measurement of c4-c3 complexes. *Journal of Immunological Methods*, Vol. 186, No. 1 (October 1995), pp. 55-63, ISSN 0022-1759

5

The Evolution of Biocompatibility: From Microinflammation to Microvesiscles

Ciro Tetta[1,2], Stefano Maffei[3], Barbara Cisterna[4], Valentina Fonsato[4], Giorgio Triolo[3], Giuseppe Paolo Segoloni[5], Giovanni Camussi[4,5], Maria Chiara Deregibus[4] and Emanuele Gatti[1,6*]

1. Introduction

Haemodialysis (HD) is a life-saving treatment for patients with chronic kidney disease (CKD) stage 5. CKD persists as a chronic worldwide epidemic and HD is the more frequently (70%) adopted treatment modality. Exponential growth trend continues on a global scale. The HD population becomes every year increasingly older (average age: 75 yrs) and sicker due to the associated co-morbidities such as cardiovascular disease (heart failure, coronary heart disease, and peripheral vascular disease), diabetes, hypertension, and peripheral vascular disease. Most of the complications associated with HD involve the cardiovascular system (Go et al., 2004; Culleton et al., 1999, Goodkin et al., 2003, Foley 2004; Barret, 2002). The evolution in the history of HD technology has greatly helped to make the HD procedure a safe and more biocompatible extracorporeal therapy. However, it must be admitted that despite significant improvements in HD technology and in the management of patients due to a better understanding of uremia toxicity, improvements in dialysis technology, better correction of anaemia and metabolic abnormalities, implementation of best practice guidelines, no significant improvement has been achieved in patient survival over the last decade (Rayner et al., 2004). The extracorporeal circuit offers a large surface of contact of the blood with foreign materials, namely the dialysis membrane, the tubings and the large volumes of the dialysate. The concept of biocompatibility has greatly evolved in the last two decades. Initially, numerous studies focused on the blood-dialyzer membrane interaction, leading to the activation of plasma systems (complement, coagulation, fibrinolysis). These studies helped in the understanding of some unknown effects occurring in the early stages of the HD session leading to pulmonary sequestration of leukocytes (mainly neutrophils) that explained the profound neutropenia associated with the cuproammonium membranes. The availability of reliable testing of complement-activated

*[1]*Biologics Research, Intl Research and Development, Fresenius Medical Care, Bad Homburg, Germany.*
[2]*Doctoral School of Biotechnology, University of Torino, Torino, Italy.*
[3]*Department of Medicine, Nephrology and Dialysis Unit, CTO Hospital, Torino, Italy.*
[4]*Department of Internal Medicine, Centre for Molecular Biotechnology and Centre for Research in Experimental Medicine (CeRMS), Torino, Italy.*
[5]*Chair of Nephrology and Department of Nephrology, Dialysis and Transplantation, University of Torino, Italy*
[6]*Danube University, Center for Biomedical Technology, Krems, Austria.*

products (C3a and C5a and their desarginated products) guided the development of less neutropenia-inducing membranes and ultimately to the final development of fully synthetic membranes which have very low if at all capacity to induce complement activation. At that time, coagulation was an important reason for frequent interruptions and delays in the HD sessions. Due to the complex interplay known to occur between the activation of the complement and coagulation systems, it became of great interest to try to reduce the propensity for intravascular coagulation. The development of high-flux membranes and growing awareness of the benefits of convective and convective/diffusive under several contexts (intradialytic cardiovascular stability, better control or the uremic status and fluid control) gave impetus to a large number of enlightening studies on another mechanism of HD bio**IN**compatibility. The contamination by bacterial products, particularly with the widespread use of bicarbonate-based dialysates opened a new era in the field of biocompatibility. The formulation of the "interleukin hypothesis" was *a posteriori* not only the basis for further studies on the monocyte stimulation during HD, but also provided a link between biocompatibility and chronic inflammation. Basically, the evolution of biocompatibility has led us to consider two sides of the same coin: on one side, the biological responses at the blood-membrane interface; on the other hand, the consequences derived from the contact on the membrane performances (e.g. hydraulic permeability and sieving coefficients).

In this review, we will summarize the most important steps in the evolution from the concept of the blood-dialyzer membrane interaction to that of the whole HD system compatibility. In face of very recent developments of cell-to-cell communication and signal transduction, we will also discuss the new hypothesis for a role of microvesicles (MVs) in cell activation, as well as in tissue and vascular repair. We will not deal with other important aspects of biocompatibility such as the oxidant stress, the relevant role of additives in dialyzer manufacturing, and of leachables and the effects of different sterilization modes.

2. Blood-membrane interaction: the role of complement, coagulation, kinin-kallikrein systems and soluble mediators

2.1 Activation of the complement alternative pathway

Early studies on biocompatibility focused on acute hypersensitivity-like reactions which in some cases were fatal. Various mechanisms were elucidated. Activation of complement was shown by Craddock *et al* in 1977 (Craddock et al, 1977). Hydroxyl radicals, present on the surface of cellulosic membranes, bind with the C3b in the blood and activate the alternative pathway leading to the release of potent anaphylatoxins, C3a and C5a. Both C3a and C5a and their relative desarginated products induce prompt activation and aggregation of polymorphonuclear neutrophils (PMNs) and leukopenia. This is a very rapid process reaching a nadir from 15 to 30 min after initiation of dialysis. Aggregates of PMNs are sequestered particularly in the lung capillaries. Although the extent of the anaphylatoxin generation and of the neutropenia is also patient-dependent, these studies failed to find a relationship with chronic clinical trade-offs despite the hypothesis that recurrent pulmonary sequestration could induce pulmonary fibrosis. Reduction of the hydroxyl groups on the membrane surface or new synthetic polymers reduced the activation of the alternative pathway of the complement cascade. Temperature could also reduce complement activation (*Maggiore Q, personal communication, 1988*). Testing complement activation (C3a or C5a plasma levels) by highly sensitive ELISA tests has become a standard requirement for the evaluation of biocompatibility ever since along with the precise characterization of the polymer structure (Krieter et al, 2008). It also became clear that synthetic polymers had a very low neutropenia-inducing effect. In some cases such as the polyacrylonitrile membrane, this was also due to the capacity of the membrane to adsorb C3b and the anaphylytoxins thus masking in fact complement activation (Pascual et al 1993) (**Figure 1**).

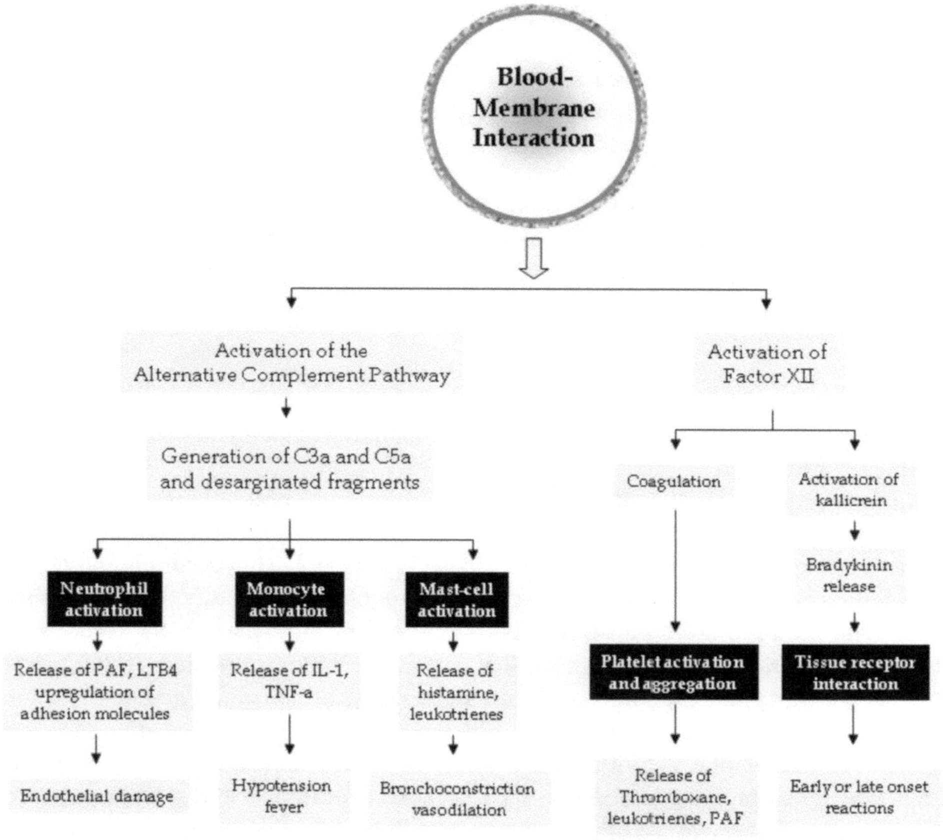

Fig. 1. Pathways involved in blood-membrane interactions. LTB4 denotes leukotriene B4, PAF, platelet-activating factor, IL-1, interleukin-1, TNF-α, tumor necrosis factor.

2.2 Activation of the coagulation system

Numerous acquired hemostatic abnormalities have been identified in chronic renal failure. HD adds to these disturbances as it repetitively implies turbulent blood flow, high shear stress, and contact of blood to artificial surfaces. Anticoagulation in HD is targeted to prevent activation of coagulation during the procedure. Most anticoagulant agents inhibit the plasmatic coagulation cascade. Still commonly used is unfractionated heparin, followed by low-molecular-weight heparin preparations with distinct advantages. Immune-mediated heparin-induced thrombocytopenia constitutes a potentially life-threatening complication of heparin therapy requiring immediate switch to nonheparin alternative anticoagulants. Danaparoid, lepirudin, and argatroban are currently being used for alternative anticoagulation, all of which possess both advantages and limitations. Recently citrate has been proposed as anticoagulant in maintenance HD (Wright et al, 2010). In the past, empirical strategies reducing or avoiding heparin were applied for patients at bleeding risk, whereas nowadays regional citrate anticoagulation is increasingly used to prevent bleeding by allowing procedures without any systemic anticoagulation. Avoidance of clotting within the whole hemodialyzer circuit is not granted. Specific knowledge of the mechanisms of coagulation, the targets of the anticoagulants in use, and their respective characteristics constitutes the basis for individualized anticoagulation aimed at achieving full patency of the circuit throughout the procedure. Patency of the circuit is an important prerequisite for optimal HD quality. Intrinsic coagulation Hageman factor XII as well as other coagulation factors are also activated (Fischer, 2007). However, the activation of the coagulation is a very complex phenomenon that may be enhanced by different independent factors other than the membrane surface *per se* such as: the dynamics at the dialyzer heads, defects in the hollow fibre cutting of the polyurethane, any condition that predisposes for blood to be stagnant. The activation of coagulation by a membrane in a dialyzer is difficult to assess given the above-mentioned factors and the host's response to the anticoagulation regime put in place (**Figure 1**).

2.3 Activation of the kinin-kallikrein system

Surface activation of Factor XII induces the kinin-kallikrein that ensues in the generation of bradykinin (**Figure 2**).

Bradykinin is physiologically under the tight control of very potent kinases that are able to promptly lyse the molecule and inactivate its potent vasodilator activity. In certain conditions, however, the lytic effect of this kinase is deficient. This occurs in patients under therapy with angiotensin converting enzyme enzyme (ACE) inhibitors. However, there are patients who experience hypersensitivity-like phenomena, that can be reconducted to bradykinin generation, even in the absence of concomitant therapy with ACE inhibitors. The explanation of this phenomenon came from pioneering studies on angio-edema, a rare but potentially fatal condition (Adam et al., 2002). These reactions are mainly associated to defects in the enzymatic activity of the aminopeptidase P (**Figure 2**). Bradykinin acts through two types of tissue receptors: R1 are mostly located in the skin and respiratory tissues (lungs and bronchi), while R2 are mostly found in the gastrointestinal tract. The overproduction of bradykinin may lead to two different clinical presentations: the first is mainly characterized by a rapid developing skin flushing, hypotension, and dyspnoea. These reactions may be mild but very severe, fatal episodes of shock have been described. In the second instance, these reactions, which were for some time unexplained, occur after 1 h-2 hr of HD treatment, may but may be not associated with the use of ACE inhibitors. The patient has severe diarrhoea which requires immediate interruption of the extracorporeal treatment. This manifestation may unpredictably recur and disappears upon disconnection. Bradykinin-induced reaction, may in principle occur following the contact with any foreign surface. Their potential, unpredictable severity should call for immediate action even in patients with mild forms. The commonest causes have been the use of strongly negative surfaces such as AN-69 membranes (Tielemans et al., 1990), or adsorbents used in LDL apheresis (Owen et al., 1994) or in Hemodiafiltration (HDF) with regeneration of the ultrafiltrate (Tetta C, Wratten ML, unpublished observation, 2001). The appearance of signs and symptoms of a hypersensitivity-related event can be dramatic in the practice of HD. The complexity of the causal factors and the underlying mechanisms are often difficult to unveil (Arenas et al., 2006). The majority of reported cases have been due to ethylene oxide (ETO) (Poothullil et al., 1975), triggered by both immunoglobulin E (IgE) and non-IgE factors (Johansson et al., 2001). However, a considerable number of publications have focused on other HD substances and materials such as heparins, different dialyser membranes, iron, erythropoietin, polyacrylonitrile AN69® high flux membranes, latex, antiseptic or formaldehyde (Ebo et al, 2006). Many different underlying mechanisms have been postulated. Hypersensitivity reactions have been estimated to occur in ~4/100000 dialysis treatments. A postal survey of all HD centres in the UK suggested that 1/20 to 1/50 patients may be susceptible to anaphylactoid reaction to a new hemodialyser at some time in between, while the risk of reaction occurring with any single HD session is~1/1000 to 1/5000. Although it is likely that many reactions are unrecognized or unreported, the scale of the problem is larger than many nephrologists have suspected (Nicholls et al., 1987).

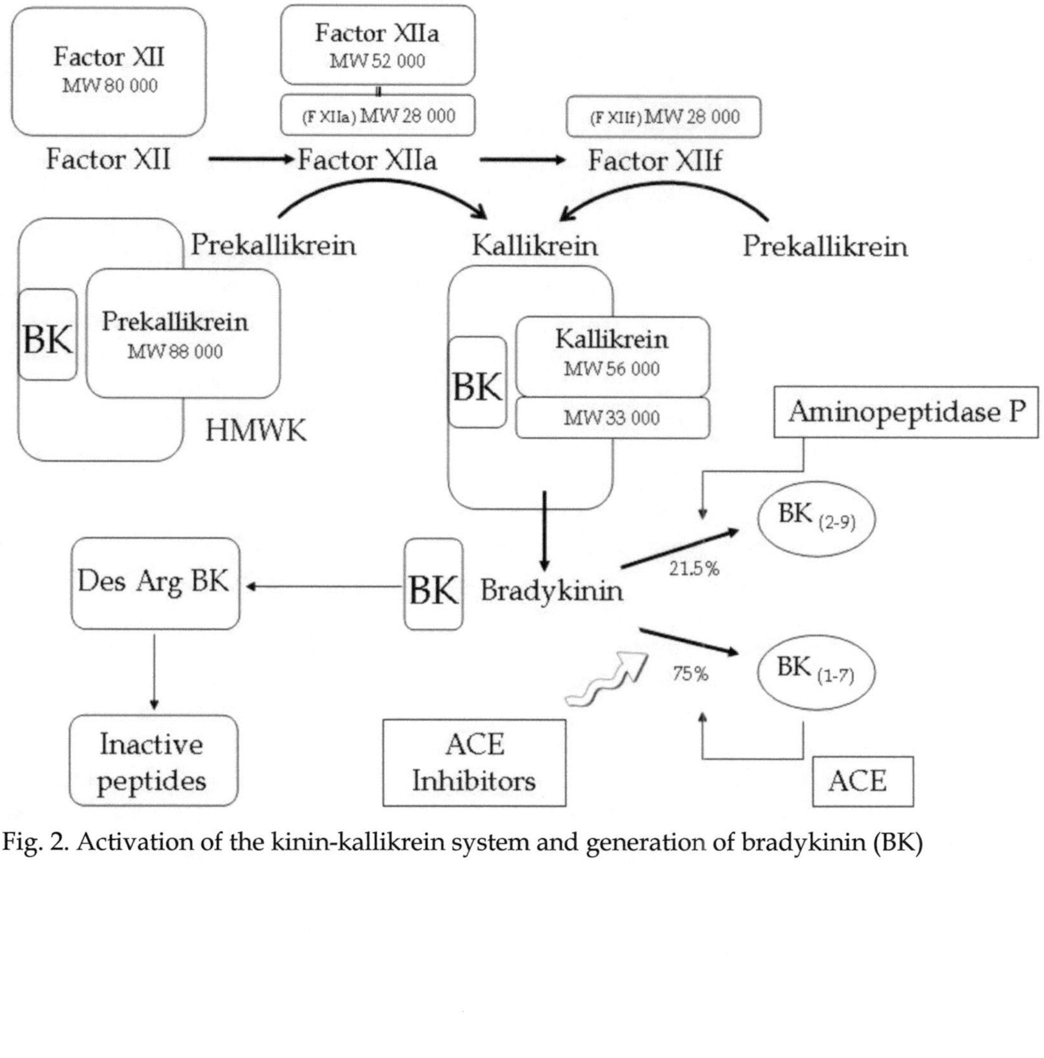

Fig. 2. Activation of the kinin-kallikrein system and generation of bradykinin (BK)

2.3.1 Soluble mediators

Many soluble mediators are produced and released following the blood-membrane interaction. Products of the phospholipase A2 such as platelet-activating factor (PAF) and leukotrienes are released by the direct interaction of PMNs and platelets with complement-activating membranes. Although in the presence of blood, the mechanisms of production of PAF and leukotrienes can not be readily differentiated from the activation, as they follow the same kinetics, we could show that for PAF for example, its production and release could be observed in complement-independent conditions such as in the absence of plasma by purified cells incubated with flat HD membranes (Tetta et al., 1996). A large number of studies have also suggested the occurrence in the plasma of lytic enzymes normally present in the vacuoles of inflammatory cells such as elastases, and metalloenzymes. The release of these lytic enzymes is caused by a phenomenon named by cell physiologists as "frustrated phagocytosis".

3. The effect of blood on dialyzer performances

When blood enters the HD system *via* the arterial line, a complex interplay of factors alters membrane performances *e.g.* clearances, ultrafiltration rates and sieving coefficients. These factors are patient- and system- dependent.

3.1 Patient-dependent factors

3.1.1 Albumin: Relevant amount of albumin fragments are detectable in the serum of patients undergoing HD. Uremia appears to facilitate the fragmentation of albumin and/or the retention of albumin fragments in blood (Donadio et al., 2009). Depending on their molecular weight, albumin fragments may be either lost in the dialysate or remain trapped in the wall of the hollow fibre. More in general, plasma proteins may cause a phenomenon names as "protein fouling".

3.1.2 Plasma viscosity which is related (but not exclusively) to albumin, fibrinogen and lipids.

3.1.3 Free hemoglobin: *In vitro* data have shown that blood circulation produces an increase of up to 280% in free hemoglobin levels and an increase of 320% in electronegative LDL (LDL(-) subfraction, a highly atherogenic form of oxidized LDL. The significant correlation between LDL(-) and free hemoglobin levels shows the oxidative activity of free hemoglobin (Ziouzenkova et al., 1999) (**Figure 3**).

3.1.4 System-dependent factors

3.1.4.1 Several factors are here involved such as the **vascular access flow rate**, and **the pump rate** and the response of the dialyzer depending on the membrane resistance and geometry. As seen from a kinetic perspective, the blood flow, and pressures are on-off events which are reflected in a "push-pull" effect on the dialyzer hollow fibre. Although these effects are still not completely known, they seem to be relevant on the shear rates, the erythrocyte orientation, leading in the worst conditions to predispose to their agglutination and clogging of the hollow fibre. Calculating clearances, ultrafiltration rates and sieving coefficient using aqueous solution can lead to an overestimate of 30%and is therefore hardly informative of the dialyzer behaviour in vivo. Finally, it was shown that sieving coefficients may change over the time of treatment rendering the calculation of clearances on the basis of the quantization of urea on the ultrafiltrate may also lead to an overestimation of the dialyzer performances (Claure-Del Granado et al., 2010).

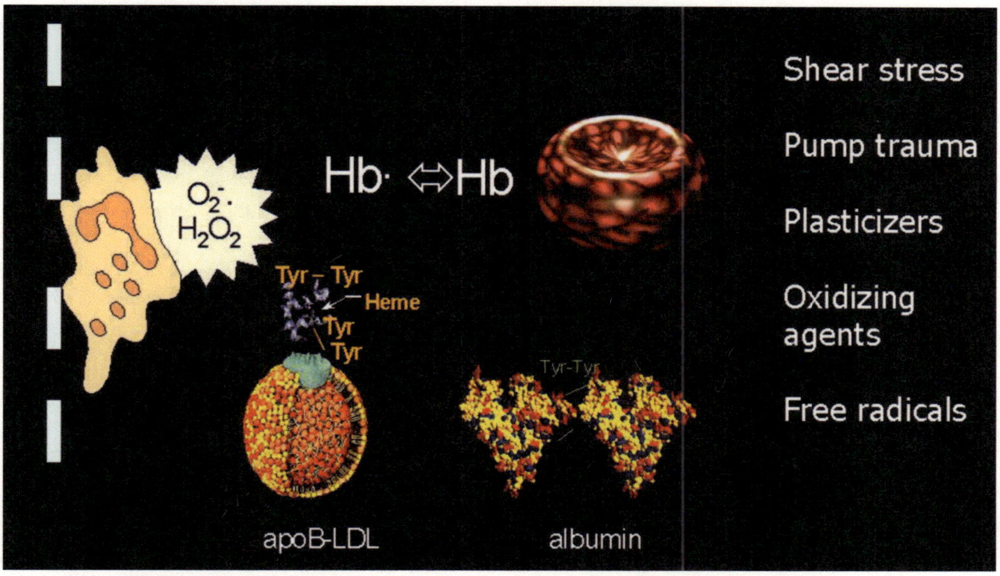

Fig. 3. Microhemolysis is the release of small quantities of hemoglobin (micro- or nanomolar) from erythrocytes. The tyrosine of a hemoglobin molecule can undergo a transition to a reactive free radical. This can react with other protein tyrosine residues to form a dityrosine molecule. Microhemolysis occurs during the HD procedure in which the erythrocytes are slightly damaged and tend to „leak" very small quantities of hemoglobin. This is a very common phenomena in HD and should not be confused with gross hemolysis.

4. The evolution of treatment biocompatibility

4.1 From system biocompatibility to systemic chronic inflammation

The concept that inflammation underlines many diseases once considered to be linked to degenerative processes has revolutionized the approach to the research into the pathogenesis and new therapeutics alike. In the field of cardiovascular disease, the process of endothelial dysfunction, vascular damage and atherosclerosis is now seen as a continuum (Libby et al., 2002). Cardiovascular disease is among the leading cause of morbidity and mortality in CKD patients on maintenance HD (US Renal Data System, 1997; Parfey & Foley, 1999). Even before reaching the state of chronic kidney disease Stage 5, patients with chronic renal failure present signs of chronic inflammation. Once patients are on HD, the risk of cardiovascular death is approximately 30 times higher than in the general population, and still remains 10 to 20 times higher after stratification for age, gender, and presence of diabetes. Traditional risk factors seem inadequate to explain the remarkable prevalence of cardiovascular disease observed in the uremic population (Foley et al 1998).

4.1.1.1 Systemic Chronic Inflammation

Inflammatory mechanisms play a relevant role in the development and progression of atherosclerosis (Ross, 1999) and heart failure (Vasan et al., 2003). Epidemiological studies in the general population have shown that even minor elevations of C-reactive protein (CRP), an acute phase reactant that markedly increases during an inflammatory response (Ridker PM, et al., 1997) predict the development of coronary heart disease and cardiac failure

(Liuzzo et al 1994, Lagrand et al., 1999, Badht et al, 2002). C-reactive protein may directly promote the development of atherosclerosis, through complement activation, tissue damage and activation of endothelial cells. Recent studies performed in CKD patients have shown that CRP is a strong predictor of cardiovascular death (Stenvinkel, 2001, Kaysen, 2005). The link between CRP and cardiovascular risk was initially thought to be indirect, reflecting circulating CRP only to the extent of the acute phase reaction in response to nonspecific stimuli such as confounding risk factors, atherosclerosis, vascular injury, ischemia and necrosis. **(Figure 4).**

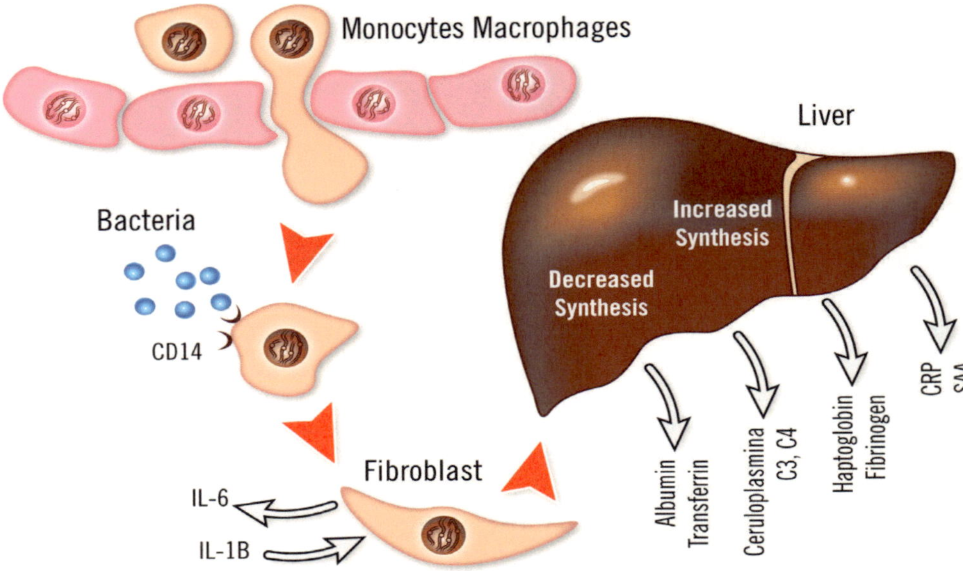

Fig. 4. Acute phase response is a defence response which occurs as a consequence of an inflammatory stimulus occurring in the blood or at tissue level. The enhanced production of interleukin-6 (IL-6), the most potent inducer of this reaction at the level of the liver, triggers the synthesis of newly synthesized proteins, e.g., C-reactive protein (which plasma levels may increase up to 50-to 100-fold the normal levels) as well as to the shut-down of the translation of genes coding for proteins, e.g., albumin.

Stenvinkel et al (1999) first convincingly showed that the malnutrition-inflammation complex syndrome described as MIA syndrome is associated with the highest mortality rates in ESRD. Their results were confirmed and extended (Panichi et al. 2008). As reviewed by Stenvinkel & Barany (2002), there is consensus on a link between CKD and inflammation. A number of studies have highlighted the association between increased inflammatory indexes and a reduced response to Erythropoietin-stimulating agents (ESAs), in particular, high CRP levels were found in HD patients requiring higher ESAs doses (Singh et al., 2007; Bradbury et al. 2009). However, the association between ESAs resistance and increased CRP levels (Barany et al. 1997; Gunnell et al. 1999) is unclear. Plasma IL-6 rather than CRP seem to better predict outcomes in CKD patients (Panichi et al., 2004). Various possible explanations may underline the advantage of IL-6 over CRP as a predictor of ESAs resistance. One possibility is that IL-6, being located upstream in the cascade of events which lead to the synthesis of many acute-phase reactants, is a better marker for the inflammatory burden affecting the development of CVD (Panichi et al., 2011). A frequently asked question is what is the contribution of HD bioincompatibility to the chronic inflammatory state. In this context, the evolution of HD technology has moved the focus from membrane bioincompatibility only to a more complex and integrated view of the HD system. The possibility that HD may be shift to a "cardioprotective" therapy is inherent to new technologies in machines, water treatment, dialysis fluids and blood tubings.

4.1.1.2 The Interleukin Hypothesis

Originally introduced as an elegant concept in 1986 (Bingel et al., 1986), the "interleukin hypothesis" was first coined to indicate the production of interleukin-1, the endogenous pyrogen as produced by the result of complement-activated mononuclear cells. Indeed, the interleukin hypothesis explained much more than was initially predictable. Several studies have ever since reported an increased cytokine production secondary to blood interaction with contaminated dialysate. Interleukin-1 (IL-1), tumor necrosis factor-a (TNF-a) and mainly IL-6 are the 3 proinflammatory cytokines that are involved in the pathogenetic aspects of HD-related disease (as reviewed by Lonnemann, 2004, Panichi et al., 2000 (**Figure 5**).

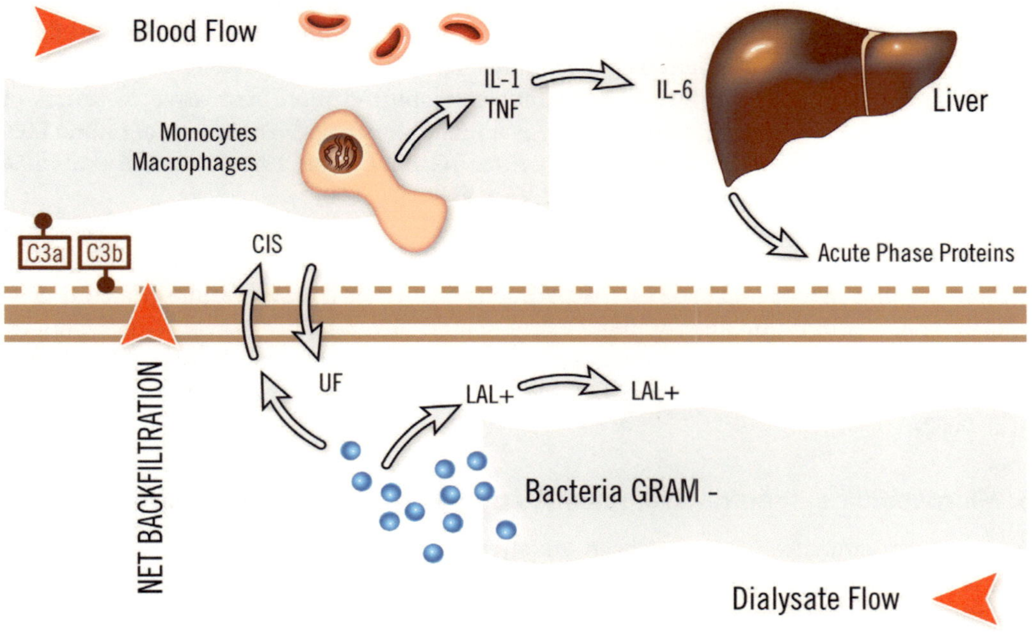

Fig. 5. Here are schematically depicted the mechanisms related to the backdiffusion/backfiltration of bacteria-derived contaminants from the dialysate into the blood. Their interaction with circulating monocytes/macrophages leads to the activation of innate immunity and to the attendant triggering of proinflammatory cytokines (interleukin-1 (IL-1), tumor necrosis factor-α. Abbreviations: CIS, cytokine-inducing substances; LAL, *Limulus amoebocyte* lysate, UF, ultrafiltrate.

The proposed mechanisms include blood interaction with endotoxins from the contaminated dialysate through HD membranes. A large number of studies have greatly contributed to increasing our knowledge in the mechanisms of endotoxin transfer across the membrane In fact, when using high permeability membranes, backfiltration and backdiffusion occur and have ebeen extensively described (Fiore & Ronco, 2007, Ronco, 2007). Thus, the transmembrane passage of endotoxins or other cytokine stimulating substances (CIS) occurs during HD (Schindler et al., 2004, Tetta et al., 2006). The reduction of backfiltration of standard dialysate may reduce the plasma concentration of IL-1ra, a sensitive indicator of inflammation in HD patients (*Dinarello personal communication, 2004*), and IL-1 (Panichi et al., 1998). Studies on large groups of patients have shown that high-volume exchange HDF, a treatment in which dialysate backfiltration is minimal, if any, is associated with significantly lower CRP plasma values (Panichi et. 1998). Comparing in a double cross-over study patients treated with high-flux and on line HDF using ultrapure dialysate and infusate, it was shown that a significant reduction of pro-inflammatory CD14+/CD16+ mononuclear subset (Carracedo et al., 2006) occurs in on line HDF. These studies emphasize that the convective component has an additional anti-inflammatory effects (Ramirez et al., 2007).

The new technology of pyrogen-adsorbing, non-complement activating, high-permeability synthetic membrane and dedicated machines (Tetta et al., 2011), as well as the awareness of the deleterious effects derived from contamination of dialysis fluids has reduced the clinical impact to a periodic microinflammatory stimulus. Undoubtedly, the availability of monitors for on-line HDF and its increased popularity have spurred more restrictive measures on safety issues and monitoring. Water quality is a mandatory issue. The safety of online HDF has been shown repeatedly in several monocenter (Canaud et al., 1998, Pizzarelli et al., 1998 and multicenter studies (Canaud et al., 2001,Vaslaki et al., 2000).

Nowadays, the philosophy of "ultrapure dialysate"is in common practice (Kessler et al., 2002). The clinical, consolidated experience on line HDF warrants well-defined procedures and leaves no space for "experiments" in what is now routine (Canaud et al, 2011). The "hemocompatibility network" should eventually prevent the periodic microinflammation induction through the implementation of rigid protocols of disinfection and maintenance of water-treatment systems and HD monitors (Cappelli et al., 2006; Kessler et al. 2002).

5. Microvesicles: their nature, release and pathophysiological relevance

A chronic inflammatory state has been widely documented since the early stages of CKD and becomes more pronounced in those with CKD stage V undergoing HD. Oxidant stress (Wratten et al., 2000, Morena et al. 2011), endothelial dysfunction (Recio-Mayoral et al., 2011), high circulating cytokine-producing monocyte subpopulation (Ramirez et al., 2006), reduced number and/or impaired function of endothelial progenitor cells (Krenning et al., 2009), are today considered as hallmarks of vascular damage and defective repair. Uremia also causes telomere shortening and premature cellular senescence of immunocompetent cells (Jimenez et al, 2005). In recent years, increasing attention has been drawn by the awareness of the pathophysiologic role of small, circular membrane fragments named as Microvesiscles (MVs) (Ratajczak et al., 2006) (**Figure 6**).

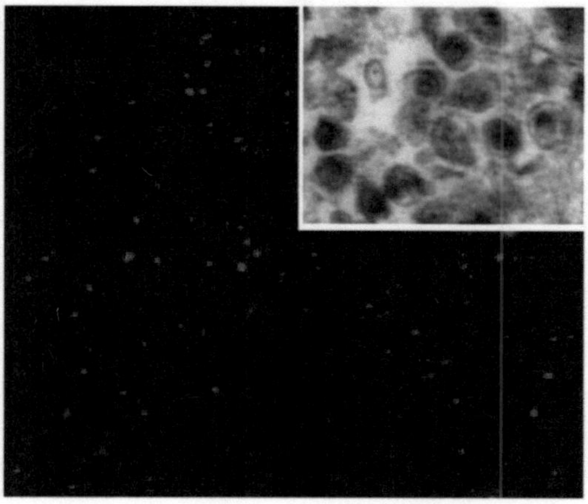

Representative micrograph showing purified MV labelled with the fluorescent dye PKH26 observed by confocal microscope (original magnification X630). The inset shows the transmission electronmicroscope appearence of purified MV (original magnification X25,000).

Fig. 6.

For long time MVs were considered to be inert cellular debris. The frequently observed vesicles by electron microscopy in the interstitial space of tissues or in blood were considered as the consequence of cell damage or the result of dynamic plasma membrane turnover (Siekevitz et al., 1972). As the vesicle population detectable both *in vitro* and *in vivo* is a mixed population of exosomes and shedding vesicles, we will refer to them collectively as MVs. Released MVs may remain in the extracellular space in proximity of the place of origin or may enter into the biological fluids reaching distant sites. This may explain the presence of MVs in plasma, urine, milk and cerebrospinal fluid. The bulk of MVs present in the circulation is derived from platelets (George, 1982), and in less extent from other blood cells and endothelial cells (Martinez et al., 2005). The MVs derived from platelets are also designed as microparticles while those derived from polymorphonuclear leukocytes are also named ectosomes (Hess et al., 1999). Finally, MVs released during morphogenesis of multicellular organisms are indicated as argosomes (Greco et al., 2001). Besides normal cells, also tumor cells may release MVs and in patients suffering for neoplastic diseases tumor-derived MVs may be detected within the biological fluids (Kim et al, 2003, Iero et al., 2008). Therefore, MVs are an assorted population, differing in cellular origin, number, size and antigenic composition (Diamant et al., 2004) shed by various cell types in physiological and pathological conditions. The release of MVs may be constitutive or consequent to cell activation by soluble agonists, by physical or chemical stress such as the oxidative stress and hypoxia, and by shear stress (Ratajczak et al., 2006). Exosomes have an endosome origin and are a rather homogenous population with a size ranging from 30 to 120nm (7). They are stored as intraluminal vesicles within multivesicular bodies of the late-endosome and are released when these multivesicular bodies fuse with the cell membrane. Our knowledge on the mechanism of assembly and sorting of the exosomes is only partial, due to the fact that a common sorting signal for all cell types has not so far been identified (Johnstone et al., 2006). Shedding vesicles are usually larger than exosomes with size ranging from 100nm to 1μm. Formation of shedding vesicles takes place from the budding of small cytoplasmic protrusions followed by their detachment from the cell surface. This process is dependent on calcium influx, calpain and cytoskeleton reorganization.

5.1 MV biological activities

It is now recognized that MVs are an integral part of the intercellular microenvironment and may act as regulators of cell-to-cell communication. This concept is based on the observation that MVs released from a given cell type may interact through specific receptor-ligands with other cells leading to target cell stimulation directly or by transferring surface receptors (Janowska-Wieczorek et al., 2001, Morel et al., 2004). This interaction may either be limited to a receptor-mediated binding to the surface of target cells forming a platform for assembly of multimolecular complexes or leading to cell signaling, either be followed by internalization as result of direct fusion or endocytic uptake by target cells (Cocucci et al., 2008). Once internalized, MVs can fuse their membranes with those of endosomes, thus leading to a horizontal transfer of their content in the cytosol of target cells. Alternatively, they may remain segregated within endosomes and be transferred to lysosomes or dismissed by the cells following the fusion with the plasmamembrane, thus leading to a process of transcytosis. It was proposed that MV-mediated cell-to-cell communication emerged very early during evolution as a template for the development of further more refined mechanisms of cell communication (Ratajczak et al., 2006). MVs may influence the behavior of target cells in multiple ways.

5.1.1 MVs may act as signaling complexes by direct stimulation of target cells (Ratajczak et al., 2006, Cocucci et al., 2008). MVs derived from platelets, for instance, play an important role in coagulation as their phosphatidylserine-enriched membranes provide a surface for assembly of clotting factors (Zwaal et al., 2004). After activation, platelets shed MVs coated with tissue factor which may interact with macrophages, neutrophils and other platelets by ligation with molecules expressed on the surface of these cells such as P-selectin (Polgar et al., 2005). On the other hand, MVs released from neutrophils express activated Mac-1 able to induce platelet activation (Andrews & Berndt, 2004). Moreover, platelet-derived MVs, besides coagulation, trigger various cell responses as they activate endothelial cells (Barry et al., 1997), polymorphonuclear neutrophils (Miyhamoto et al., 1988) and monocytes (Barry et al., 1999). .

5.1.2 MVs may act by transferring receptors between cells. The transferring of receptors between cells is supported by the observation that bystander B cells rapidly acquire antigen receptors from activated B cells by a membrane transfer (Quah et al., 2008).

5.1.3 MVs may deliver proteins within the target cells. An example of this mechanism is the recently reported MV-mediated transfer of a cell death message via encapsulated caspase-1 (Sarkar et al., 2009). It has been found that endotoxin stimulated monocytes induce the cell death of vascular smooth muscle cells by releasing MVs containing caspase-1. This trans-cellular apoptosis induction pathway depends on the function of the delivered caspase-1 within the target cells. It has been also suggested that MVs may contribute to dissemination of certain infective agents, such as HIV or prions (Facler & Peterlin, 2000, Fevrier et al., 2004).

5.1.4 MVs may mediate a horizontal transfer of genetic information. The occurrence of epigenetic changes has been frequently reported in co-culture conditions. An explanation of this phenomenon is the transfer of genetic information between cells. We demonstrated that MVs derived from human endothelial progenitors (EPC) can also act as a vehicle for mRNA transport among cells (Deregibus et al., 2007). MVs generated from EPC were incorporated in normal endothelial cells by interaction with α4- and β1-integrins expressed on their surface and activated an angiogenic program. Besides mRNA, MVs may transfer microRNAs (miRNA) to target cells (Yuan et al., 2009). Since miRNAs are naturally occurring regulators of protein translation, this observation opens the possibility that stem cells can alter the expression of genes in neighbouring cells by transferring microRNAs contained in MVs. We recently characterized miRNA shuttled by MVs released by human adult mesenchymal stem cells (MSCs) (Collino et al., 2010). Hierarchical clustering and similarity analysis of microRNAs showed that microRNA compartmentalization and secretion by MVs are both highly regulated processes.

5.2 Microvesicles in CKD

The biologic role of MVs and their implication in pathophysiology depends on the several factors namely the cell of origin, their phenotype, the genetic material (mRNA and microRNA) and the target cells. In CKD, several studies have accrued evidence that MVs or MPs could participate to the vascular damage and the evolution of the atherosclerotic lesion.

5.2.1 Circulating platelet-derived microparticles (PMPs) with procoagulant activity are considered a potential cause of thrombosis in uremic patients undergoing HD (Ando et al., 2002). Elevated counts of circulating PMPs have been reported in association with thrombotic disorders, such as cerebrovascular accidents (Katopodis et al., 1997), unstable angina (Katopodis et al., 1997), and acute myocardial infarction (Gawaz et al., 1996). In addition, PMPs that adhered to vascular endothelium and leukocytes activate such cells and transport their chemical mediators to those cells, potentially leading to the development of thrombosis and atherosclerosis (Mallat et al., 1999, Barry et al., 1997).

5.2.2 Endothelial MVs (EMVs) - Treatment modalities that reduce the inflammatory potential of the cells originating MVs have interestingly been correlated with a decreased number of endothelial microparticles (Carracedo et al., 2005, Ramirez et al., 2005). Circulating EMPs have recently been reported to correlate with impaired vascular function in HD patients (Faure et al., 2006). A recent study showed an increase in the percentage of CD14+CD16+ monocytes in CKD-NonD and HD patients. In PD patients, regardless of RRF, the percentage of CD14+CD16+ was similar to controls (Merino et al., 2010). It is interesting to note that HD patients displayed significantly higher apoptotic EMPs and VEGF levels than the two PD and CKD-non dialyszed groups. In contrast, there were no differences between CKD-NonD and PD groups. In CKD-non dialyszed and HD patients, the percentage of CD14+CD16+ was correlated with endothelial damage. It appears that PD, compared with HD, reduces but does not fully prevent the endothelial damage induced by uremia, in spite of presenting a microinflammatory status similar to that of the controls. The role of EMVs is still to be elucidated in the complex unbalance observed in CKD patients between circulating endothelial cells and endothelial progenitor cells.

5.2.3 MVs in treatment modalities

Preliminary studies in our laboratory have shown an interesting trend in the reduction of total MVs in a cross-over clinical study when patients shifted from high-flux HD to on-line HDF (**Figure 7**).

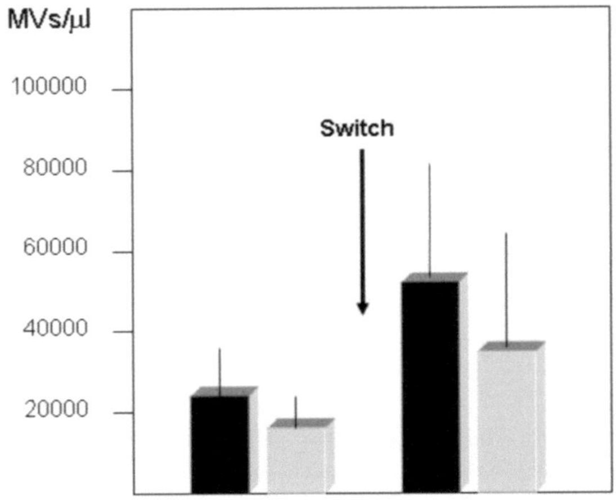

Fig. 7. Total MVs count in patients on maintenance HD. In a cross-over design, 8 patients were started on bicarbonate HD (black columns) and 8 patients on on-line HDF (grey columns). MVs were counted by cytofluorimetry. MVs were also characterized (data not shown) by the following specific markers: CD62P, CD41, CD42, CD31, for platelets; CD45, for leukocytes; CD31, CD146, CD144 for the endothelium: CD235 and CD242 (ICAM 4), for erythrocytes.

More studies are needed to better assess the relevance of these observations and to better characterize the type and biological effects of the MVs. It is still to be fully elucidated whether MVs are a consequence or a cause of disease. Increasing evidence for their pathophysiologic role in other human diseases such as sepsis and tumors (Camussi et al., 2011) is rapidly accruing. Many points require further investigation. i. The stimuli and the molecular pathways that regulate the assembly within MVs of the biological active molecules that they shuttle. ii. The stimuli that trigger their release. iii. The surface receptors that may confer selective specificity. iv. The full diagnostic potential of MVs in different pathological conditions. v. The strategy to inhibit formation or to remove from circulation potentially harmful MVs. The recognition of MVs has opened a new era and new perspectives of investigation also in biocompatibility of extracorporeal treatments.

6. Conclusions

The outlook of more biocompatible and physiological dialysis is today confronted with a older and sicker population in need of maintenance HD. The knowledge of biological mechanisms operating at the system level will be approached with the help of improved technologies hopefully able to reduce the deleterious effect of the repetitive contact with a foreign surface and to insure optimal performances for the elimination of small and middle molecule solutes. Advances in dialyzer membranes and geometries, as well as blood tubings together with new concepts in machine technology have already shown their great potential to improve survival and cardiovascular stability.

7. Conflict of interest

Ciro Tetta and Emanuele Gatti are full-time employees of Fresenius Medical Care.

8. Acknowledgement

The authors thank Dr Sudhir Bowry for critically reviewing the manuscript.

9. References

Adam A, Cugno M, Molinaro G, Perez M, Lepage Y, & Agostoni A. (2002). Aminopeptidase P in individuals with a history of angio-oedema on ACE inhibitors. *Lancet.* 359(9323):2088-9.

Ando M, Iwata A, Ozeki Y, Tsuchiya K, Akiba T, & Nihei H (2002). Circulating platelet-derived microparticles with procoagulant activity may be a potential cause of thrombosis in uremic patients *Kidney Int*, 62:1757–1763

Arenas MD, Niveiro E, Moledous A, Gil MT, Albiach B, & Carretón MA (2006) .Fatal acute systemic hypersensitivity reaction during haemodialysis. *Nephrol Dial Transplant.* 21(10):2966-70

Barret BJ. (2002). Reducing the burden of cardiovascular disease in patients on dialysis. *Dial Transplant* 31: 155–163

Barry OP, Pratico D, Lawson JA, & FitzGerald GA (1997). Transcellular activation of platelets and endothelial cells by bioactive lipids in platelet microparticles. *J Clin Invest* 99: 2118-2127.

Barry OP, Kazanietz MG, Praticò D, & Fitzgerald GA(1999). Arachidonic acid in platelet microparticles up-regulates cyclooxygenase-2-dependent prostaglandin formation via a protein kinase C/mitogen-activated protein kinase-dependent pathway. *J Biol Chem* 274: 7545-7556.

Bhatt DL, & Topol EJ. (2002). Need to test the arterial Inflammation hypothesis. *Circulation* 106:136–140.

Bingel M, Lonnemann G, Shaldon S, Koch KM, & Dinarello CA. (1986). Human interleukin-1 production during hemodialysis. *Nephron.* 1986;43(3):161-3

Bradbury BD, Critchlow CV, Weir MR Stewart R, Krishnan M, & Hakim RH (2009). Impact of elevated C-reactive protein levels on Erythropoiesis-stimulating agent (ESA) dose and responsiveness in naemodialysis patients. *Nephrol Dial Transplant* 24: 919-925.

Camussi G, Deregibus MC, Bruno S, Grange C, Fonsato V, & Tetta C (2011). Exosome / microvesicle - mediated epigenetic reprogramming of cells *Am J Cancer Res* 1(1):98-110

Canaud B, Bosc JY, Leray H, Stec F, Argiles A, Leblanc M, & Mion C.(1998). On line hemodiafiltration: State of the art. *Nephrol Dial Transplant.* 5:3–11

Canaud B, Wizemann V, Pizzarelli F, Greenwood R, Schultze G, Weber C, & Falkenhagen D (2001). Cellular interleukin- 1 receptor antagonist production in patients receiving on-line haemodiafiltration therapy. *Nephrol Dial Transplant.* 16:2181–2187.

Canaud B, Chenine L, Renaud S, & Leray H. (2011). Optimal therapeutic conditions for online hemodiafiltration. *Contrib Nephrol.* 168:28-38.

Cappelli G, Riccardi M, Perrone S, Bondi M, Ligabue G, & Albertazzi A (2006). Water treatment and monitor disinfection. *Hemodialysis Int.* 10, Suppl 1: S13–S18.

Cocucci E, Racchetti G, & Meldolesi J (2008). Shedding microvesicles: artefacts no more. *Trends Cell Biol* 19: 43-51.

Carracedo J, Ramirez R, Soriano S, Alvarez de Lara MA, Rodriguez M, Martin-Malo A, & Aljama P. (2005). Monocytes from dialysis patients exhibit characteristics of senescent cells: does it really mean inflammation? *Contrib Nephrol.* 149:208-18.

Carracedo J, Merino A, Nogueras S, Carretero D, Berdud I, Ramírez R, Tetta C, Rodríguez M, Martín-Malo A, & Aljama P (2006). On-line hemodiafiltration reduces the proinflammatory CD14+CD16+ monocyte-derived dendritic cells: A prospective, crossover study. *J Am Soc Nephrol.* 17(8):2315-21.

Claure-Del Granado R, Macedo E, Chertow GM, Soroko S, Himmelfarb J, Ikizler TA, Paganini EP, & Metha RL (2010).. Effulent volume in continuous renal replacement therapy overestimates the delived dose of dialysis. *Clin J Am Soc Nephrol* epub november 29,

Collino F, Deregibus MC, Bruno S, Sterpone L, Aghemo G, Viltono L, Tetta C, & Camussi G (2010): Microvesicles derived from adult human bone marrow and tissue specific mesenchymal stem cells shuttle selected pattern of miRNAs. *PLoS One* 5: e11803.

Craddock PR, Fehr J, Dalmasso AP, Brighan KL, & Jacob HS. (1977) Hemodialysis leukopenia. Pulmonary vascular leukostasis resulting from complement activation by dialyzer cellophane membranes. *J Clin Invest.* 59(5):879-88.

Culleton BF, Larson MG, Wilson PW, Evans JC, Parfrey PS, & Levy D. (1999). Cardiovascular disease and mortality in a community- based cohort with mild renal insufficiency. *Kidney Int* 56: 2214–2219

Deregibus MC, Cantaluppi V, Calogero R, Lo Iacono M, Tetta C, Biancone L, & Bruno S (2007). Endothelial progenitor cell derived microvesicles activate an angiogenic program in endothelial cells by a horizontal transfer of mRNA. *Blood.* 110: 2440-2448.

Diamant M,, Tushuizen ME, Sturk A, & Nieuwland R (2004). Cellular microparticles: new players in the field of vascular disease? *Eur. J. Clin. Invest.* 34: 392-401.

Donadio E, Piccolomini F, Dimuccio V, Felicioli A, Balestreri E, Cianti R, Armini A, Bini L, Felicioli R, & Donadio C (2009). Serum albumin fragmentation in end-stage renal disease patients: a pilot study. *Clin Chem Lab Med.* 47(11):1373-9.

Kaysen GA (2002). Role of inflammation and its treatment in ESRD patients. *Blood Purif.* 20:70–80

Ebo DG, Bosmans JL, Counttenye MM, & Stevens WJ. (2006) Haemodialysis–associated anaphylactic and anaphylactoid reactions. *Allergy* 61:211–220.

Facler OT, & Peterlin BM. Endocytic entry of HIV-1 (2000). *Curr Biol* 10: 1005-1008.

Faure V, Dou L, Sabatier F, Cerini C, Sampol J, Berland Y, Brunet P, & Dignat-George F (2006). Elevation of circulating endothelial microparticles in patients with chronic renal failure. *J Thromb Haemost.* 4(3):566-73. Epub 2005 Dec 23.

Fevrier B, Vilette D, Archer F, Loew D, Faigle W, Vidal M, Laude H, & Raposo G. (2004). Cells release prions in association with exosomes. *Proc. Natl Acad Sci USA* 101: 9683-9688.

Fiore GB, & Ronco C. (2007) Principles and practice of internal hemodiafiltration. *Contrib Nephrol.* 158:177-84.

Fischer KG. (2007). Essentials of anticoagulation in hemodialysis. *Hemodial Int.* 11(2):178-89.

Foley RN, Parfrey PS, & Sarnak MJ (1998). Clinical epidemiology of cardiovascular disease in chronic renal failure. *Am J Kidney Dis.* 32(Suppl 5):S112–S119.

Foley RN (2004). Cardiac disease in chronic uremia: can it explain the reverse epidemiology of hypertension and survival in dialysis patients? *Semin Dial* 17: 275–278

Hess C, Sadallah S, Hefti A, Landmann R, & Schifferli JA (1999). Ectosomes released by human neutrophils are specialized functional units. *J Immunol* 163: 4564-4573.

Gawaz M, Neumann JF, Ott I, Schliessler A, & Schoemig A (1996). Platelet function in acute myocardial infarction treated with direct angioplasty. *Circulation*.3493:229–237.

George JN, Thoi LL, McManus LM, & Reinmann TA (1982). Isolation of human platelet membrane microparticles from plasma and serum. *Blood* 60:834-840.

Go AS, Chertow GM, Fan D, McCulloch CE, & Hsu CY (2004). Chronic kidney disease and the risks of death, cardiovascular events, and hospitalization. *N Engl J Med* 351: 1296–1305

Greco V, Hannus M, & Eaton S (2001). Argosomes: a potential vehicle for the spread of morphogens through epithelia. Cell 106: 633-645.

Katopodis JN, Kolodny L, Jy W, Horstman LL, Dearchena EJ, Tao JG, Haynes DH, & Ahn Ys (1997): Platelet microparticles and calcium hemostasis in acute coronary ischemias. *Am J Hematol* 33;54:95–101,

Kessler M on behalf of the EBPG Working Group (2002). Section IV. Dialysis fluid purity. European Best Practice Guidelines for Haemodialysis (Part 1). European Dialysis and Transplant Association. *Nephrol Dial Transplant* 17 Suppl 7:45.-54

Kim HK, Song KS, Park YS, Kang YH, Lee YJ, Lee KR, Kim HK, Ryu KW, Bae JM, & Kim S. (2003). Elevated levels of circulating platelet microparticles, VEGF, IL-6 and RANTES in patients with gastric cancer: possible role of a metastasis predictor. *Eur J Cancer* 39: 184-91.

Krenning G, Dankers PY, Drouven JW, Waanders F, Franssen CF, van Luyn MJ, Harmsen MC, & Popa ER. (2009). Endothelial progenitor cell dysfunction in patients with progressive chronic kidney disease. *Am J Physiol Renal Physiol*. 296(6):F1314-22.

Krieter DH, Lemke HD, & Wanner C (2008). A new synthetic dialyzer with advanced permselectivity for enhanced low-molecular weight protein removal. *Artif Organs*. 32(7):547-54.

Iero M, Valenti R, Huber V, Filipazi P, Parmiani G, Fais S, & Rivoltini L. (2008). Tumour-released exosomes and their implications in cancer immunity. *Cell Death Differ* 15: 80-88.

Goodkin DA, Bragg-Gresham JL, Koenig KG, Woolfe RA, Akiba T, Andreucci VE, Saito A, Rayner HC, Kurokawa K, Port FK, Held PJ, & Young EW. (2003). Association of comorbid conditions and mortality in hemodialysis patients in Europe, Japan, and the United States; the Dialysis Outcomes and Practice Patterns Study (DOPPS). *J Am Soc Nephrol* 14:3270–3277

Janowska-Wieczorek A, Majka M, Kijowski J, Baj-Krzyworzeka M, Reca R, Turner AR, Ratajczak J, Emerson SG, Kowalska MA, & Ratajczak MZ. (2001) Platelet-derived microparticles bind to hematopoietic progenitor cells and enhance their engraftment. *Blood* 98: 3143-3149

Jimenez R, Carracedo J, Santamaría R, Soriano S, Madueño JA, Ramírez R, Rodríguez M, Martín-Malo A, & Aljama P. (2005). Replicative senescence in patients with chronic kidney failure. *Kidney Int* .Suppl. 99:S11-5.

Johansson SG, Hourihane JO, Bousquet J, Bruijnzeel-Koomen C, Dreborg S, Haahtela T, Kowalski ML, Mygind N, Ring J, van Cauwenberge P, van Hage-Hamsten M, & Wüthrich B. (2001) EAACI (the European Academy of Allergology and Cinical Immunology) nomenclature task force. A revised nomenclature for allergy. An EAACI position statement from the EAACI nomenclature task force. Allergy 56:813–824.

Johnstone RM. (2006). Exosomes biological significance: A concise review. *Blood Cells Mol Dis*. 36: 315-321.

Lagrand WK, Visser CA, Hermens WT, Niesssen HW, Verheught FW, Wolbink GJ, & Hack CE. (1999). C-reactive protein as a cardiovascular risk: More than an epiphenomenon? *Circulation* 100:96–102.

Libby P, Ridker PM, & Maseri A. (2002). Inflammation and atherosclerosis. *Circulation*. 3:187–197.

Liuzzo G, Biasucci LM, Gallimore JR, Grillo RL, Rebuzzi AG, Pepys MB, & Maseri A. (1994) . The prognostic value of C-reactive protein and serum amyloid a protein in severe unstable angina. *New Engl J Med*. 331:417–424.

Lonnemann G. (2004) When good water goes bad: How it happens, clinical consequences and possibile solutions. *Blood Purif.* 22:124–129.

Morel O, Toti F, Hugel B, & Freyssinet JM (2004) Cellular microparticles: a disseminated storage pool of bioactive vascular effectors. *Curr Opin Hematol*. 11: 156-164.

Mallat Z, Hugel B, Ohan J, Leseche G, Freyssinet JM, & Tedqui A. (1999) Shed membrane microparticles with procoagulant potential in human atherosclerotic plaques. A role for apoptosis in plaque thrombogenicity. *Circulation* 99:348–353.

Martinez MC, Tesse A, Zobairi F, & Andriantsihohaina R. (2005). Shed membrane microparticles from circulating and vascular cells in regulating vascular function. *Am J Physiol Hearth Circ Physiol* 288: H1004-H1009.

Merino A, Portolés J, Selgas R, Ojeda R, Buendia P, Ocaña J, Bajo MA, del Peso G, Carracedo J, Ramírez R, Martín-Malo A, & Aljama P. (2010) Effect of different dialysis modalities on microinflammatory status and endothelial damage. *Clin J Am Soc Nephrol*. 5(2):227-34.

Meziani F, Delabranche X, Asfar P, & Toti F. (2010). Bench-to-bedside review: Circulating microparticles - a new player in sepsis? *Critical Care* 14:236-244.

Miyamoto S, Kowalska MA, Marcinkiewicz C, Marcinkiewicz MM, Mosser D, Edmunds LH, & Niewiaroswski S. (1998) Interaction of leukocytes with platelet microparticles derived from outdated platelet concentrates. *Thromb Haemost* 80: 982-988.

Morena M, Patrier L, Jaussent I, Bargnoux AS, Dupuy AM, Badiou S, Leray-Moragues H, Klouche K, Canaud B, & Cristol JP (2011). Reduced glomerular filtration rate, inflammation and HDL cholesterol as main determinants of superoxide production in non-dialysis chronic kidney disease patients. *Free Radic Res. 45*(6):735-45.

Nicholls AJ. (1987) Hypersensitivity to haemodialysis: the United Kingdom experience. *Artif Organs* 11:87–89.

Owen HG, Brecher ME (1994). Atypical reactions associated with use of angiotensin-converting enzyme inhibitors and apheresis. *Transfusion* 94; 891–894,

Panichi V, De Pietro S, Andreini B, Migliori M, Tessore V, Taccola D, Rindi P, Palla R, & Tetta C. (1998). Cytokine production in hemodiafiltration: A multicentre study. *Nephrol Dial Transplant*. 13:1452–1459.

Panichi V, Migliori M, De Pietro S, Taccola D, Andreini B, Metelli MR, Giovannini L, & Palla R. (2000). The link of biocompatibility to cytokine production. Kidney Int. 59, Suppl 76: 96–103.

Panichi V, Tetta C, Rindi P, Palla R, & Lonnemann G. Plasma C-reactive protein is linked to ackfiltration associated interleukin 6 production. ASAIO J. 1998; 744: M415–M417.

Panichi V, Maggiore U, Taccola D, Migliori M, Rizza GM, Consani C, Bertini A, Sposini-Garcia R, Rindi P, Palla R, & Tetta C. (2004). Interleukin-6 is a stronger predictor of total and cardiovascular mortality than C-reactive protein in hemodialysis patients. *Nephrol Dial Transplant* 19:1154-60.

Panichi V, Rizza GM, Paoletti S, Bigazzi R, Aloisi M, Barsotti G, Rindi P, Donati G, Antonelli A, Panicucci E, Tripepi G, Tetta C, & Palla R; RISCAVID Study Group (2008) Chronic inflammation and mortality in haemodialysis: effect of different renal replacement therapies. Results from the RISCAVID study. *Nephrol Dial Transplant.* 23(7):2337-43.

Panichi V, Rosati A, Bigazzi R, Paoletti S, Mantuano E, Beati S, Marchetti V, Bernabini G, Grazi G, Rizza GM, Migliori M, Giusti R, Lippi A, Casani A, Barsotti G, & Tetta C; on behalf of the RISCAVID Study. (2011). Group.Anaemia and resistance to erythropoiesis-stimulating agents as prognostic factors in haemodialysis patients: results from the RISCAVID study. *Nephrol Dial Transplant. Feb 16. [Epub ahead of print]*

Pascual M, Schifferli JA. (1993). Adsorption of complement factor D by polyacrylonitrile dialysis membranes. *Kidney Int.* 43(4):903-11.

* Parfey PS, & Foley RN. (1999) The clinical epidemiology of cardiac disease in chronic renal failure. *J Am Soc Nephrol.* 10:1606–1615.

Pizzarelli F, Cerrai T, Dattolo P, Tetta C, & Maggiore Q. (1998) Convective treatments with on line production of replacement fluid: A clinical experience lasting 6 years. *Nephrol Dial Transplant.* 13:363–369.

Polgar J, Matuskova J, & Wagner DD. (2005) The P-selectin, tissue factor, coagulation triad. J *Thromb Haemost;* 3: 1590-1596.

* Poothullil J, Shimizu A, Day RP, & Dolovich J. (1975) Anaphylaxis from the product(s) of ethylene oxide gas. *Ann Intern Med* 82:58–60.

Quah BJ, Barlow VP, McPhun V, Matthaei KI, Hulett MD, & Parish CR. (2008). Bystander B cells rapidly acquire antigen receptors from activated B cells by membrane transfer. *Proc Natl Acad Sci USA* 105: 4259-4264.

Ramirez R, Carracedo J, Berdud I, Carretero D, Merino A, Rodríguez M, Tetta C, Martín-Malo A, & Aljama P. (2006). Microinflammation in hemodialysis is related to a preactivated subset of monocytes. *Hemodial Int.,* Suppl 1:S24-7.

Ramirez R, Carracedo J, Merino A, Nogueras S, Alvarez-Lara MA, Rodríguez M, Martin-Malo A, Tetta C, & Aljama P. (2007) Microinflammation induces endothelial damage in hemodialysis patients: the role of convective transport. *Kidney Int.* 72(1):108-13.

Ratajczak J, Wysoczynski M, Hayek F, Janowska-Wieczorek A, & Ratajczak MZ. (2006) Membrane-derived microvesicles: important and underappreciated mediators of cell-to-cell communication. *Leukemia;* 20: 1487-1495.

* Rayner HC, Pisoni RL, Bommer J, Canaud B, Hecking E, Locatelli F, Piera L, Bragg-Gresham JL, Feldman HI, Goodkin DA, Gillespie B, Wolfe RA, Held PJ, & Port FK. (2004). Mortality and hospitalization in haemodialysis patients in five European countries: results from the Dialysis Outcomes and Practice Patterns Study (DOPPS). *Nephrol Dial Transplant.* 19(1):108-20.

Ramírez R, Carracedo J, Soriano S, Jiménez R, Martín-Malo A, Rodríguez M, Blasco M, & Aljama P. (2005). Stress-induced premature senescence in mononuclear cells from patients on long-term hemodialysis. *Am J Kidney Dis.* 45(2):353-9.

Recio-Mayoral A, Beneriee D, Streather C, & Kaski JC. (2011). Endothelial dysfunction, inflammation and atherosclerosis in chronic kidney disease - a cross-sectional study of predialysis, dialysis and kidney-transplantation patients. *Atherosclerosis.* Feb. 18 [Epub ahead of print].

Ridker PM, Cushman M, Stampfer MJ, Tracy RP, & Hennekens CH.(1997). Inflammation, aspirin and the risk of cardiovascular disease in apparently healthy men. *N Engl J Med.* 336: 973–979.

Ronco C. (2007) Fluid mechanics and crossfiltration in hollow-fiber hemodialyzers. *Contrib Nephrol.* 158:34-49.

Ross R. (1999) Atherosclerosis: An inflammatory disease. *N Engl J Med.* 340:115–126.

Sarkar A, Mitra S, Mehta S, Raices R, & Wewers MD. (2009). Monocyte derived microvesicles deliver a cell death message via encapsulated caspase-1. *PLoS One* 4: e7140.

Schindler R, Beck W, Deppisch R, Aussieker M, Wilde A, Goehl H, & Frei U. (2004). Short bacterial DNA fragments: Detection in dialysate and induction of cytokines. *J Am Soc Nephrol.* 15:3207–3214.

Siekevitz P. (1972) Biological membranes: the dynamics of their organization. *Annu Rev Physiol* 34: 117-140.

Singh AK, Coyne DW, Shapiro W, Rizkala AR. (2007). Predictors of the response to treatment in anemic haemodialysis patients with high serum ferritin and low transferring saturation. *Kidney Int* 71: 1163-1171.

Stenvinkel P, Heinburger O, Paultre F, Diczfalusy U, Wang T, Berglund L, & Jogestrand T.. (1999). Strong associations between malnutrition, inflammation and atherosclerosis in chronic renal failure. *Kidney Int* 55: 1899-1911,

Stenvinkel P. (2001). Malnutrition and chronic inflammation as risk factors for cardiovascular disease in chronic renal failure. *Blood Purif.* 19:143–151.

Tetta C, Haeffner-Cavaillon N, Navino C, David S, Franceschi C, Mariano F, & Camussi G (1996). The role of platelet-activating actor in the biocompatibility of hemodialysis membranes. *Adv Exp Med Biol.* 416:243-8.

* Tetta C, David S, Marcelli D, Cogliati P, Formica M, Inguaggiato P, & Panichi V. (2006). Clinical effects of online dialysate and infusion fluids. *Hemodial Int* 10: S60–S66

Tetta C, Roy T, Gatti E, & Cerutti S. (2011). The rise of hemodialysis machines: new technologies in minimizing cardiovascular complications. Expert Rev. Cardiovasc. Ther. 9(2), 155–164.

Tielemans C, Madhoun P, Lenaers M, Schandene L, Goldman M, Vanherweghem JL. (1990). Anaphylactoid reactions during hemodialysis on AN69 membranes in patients receiving ACE inhibitors. *Kidney Int.* 38(5):982-4.

US Renal Data System. Excerpts from the USRDS 1997 annual data report. (1997) *Am J Kidney Dis.* 30:S1–S195.

Vasan RS, Sullivan LM, Roubenoff R, Dinarello CA, Harris T, Benjamin EJ, Sawyer DB, Wilson PW, D'Agostino RB: Framingham Heart Study (2003). Inflammatory markers and risk of heart failure in erderly subjects without prior myocardial infarction: The Framingham Heart Study. *Circulation* 107:1486–1491.

Vaslaki L, Karatzon A, Voros P, Maior L, Pethoe F, Ladanyi E, Weber C, Mitteregger R, & Falkengagen D. (2000). Can sterile and pyrogen-free on-line substitution fluid be rotuineley delivered? A multicentre study on the microbiological safety of on-line hemodiafiltration. *Nephrol Dial Transplant.* 15, Suppl 1: 74–78.

Wratten ML, Tetta C, Ursini F, & Sevanian A. (2000). Oxidant stress in hemodialysis: prevention and treatment strategies. Kidney Int. Suppl. 2000, 76: S126-32.

Wright S, Steinwandel U, & Ferrari P. (2010) Citrate anticoagulation during long-term haemodialysis. Nephrology (Carlton). Nov 3. [Epub ahead of print]

Yuan A, Farber EL, Rapoport AL, Tejada D, Deniskin R, Akhmedov NB, & Farber DB. (2009). Transfer of microRNAs by embryonic stem cell microvesicles. *PLoS One* 4: e4722

Ziouzenkova O, Asatryan L, Akmal M, Tetta C, Wratten ML, Loseto-Wich G, Jürgens G, Heinecke J, & Sevanian A. (1999). Oxidative cross-linking of ApoB100 and hemoglobin results in low density lipoprotein modification in blood. Relevance to atherogenesis caused by hemodialysis. *J Biol Chem.* 274(27):18916-24.

Zwaal RF, Comfurius P, & Bevers EM, Scott syndrome, a bleeding disorder caused by defective scrambling of membrane phospholipids. *Biochim Biophys Act* 1636: 119-128.

6

Pulse Push/Pull Hemodialysis: Convective Renal Replacement Therapy

Lee, Kyungsoo
University of Michigan, Ann Arbor, and AnC Bio Inc.
USA

1. Introduction

The incidence of kidney disease is rapidly increasing worldwide, fueled by the increasing incidences of diabetes and obesity (Centers for Disease Control and Prevention, 2010), and thus, more patients with hypertension and diabetes develop end-stage renal disease (ESRD). Maintenance hemodialysis has become an established protocol for treating ESRD patients. This process is facilitated by two physical phenomena that facilitate mass transfer in purifying blood during maintenance hemodialysis. Diffusion caused by a concentration gradient between blood and dialysate contributes to the removal of uremic solutes, particularly small-size molecules. The removal of excess body water and mid-size molecules depends primarily on convective mass transfer, which results from hydraulic and osmotic pressure gradients (Daugirdas & Van Stone, 2000).

Remarkable improvements have been made in the technologies used for renal supportive dialysis treatment in ESRD patients. Polymeric membranes better prevent the transfer of pyrogenic substances into the blood stream and membrane biocompatibilities are much improved (Weber et al., 2004). The sharp molecular cut-offs of these membranes also prevent further loss of albumin during high-dose convective treatment (Ahrenholz et al., 2004). Narrow pore size distributions and improved hydraulic properties in the membrane field are matched by the evolution of various modalities for renal supportive treatment. Furthermore, better outcomes achieved by convective treatment have encouraged the use of synthetic membranes with high water permeability and sieving characteristics in clinical setups (Woods & Nandakumar, 2000), to the extent that hemodiafiltration (HDF) and volume-controlled high-flux hemodialysis (HD) are now regarded as preferred forms of convective therapy, because the retention of middle to large-sized molecules by chronic renal failure patients is closely related to renal-failure associated mortality (Leypoldt et al., 1999).

Volume-controlled high-flux HD adequately clears mid-size solutes without sterile fluid infusion. Forward filtration exceeding desired volume removal is compensated for by backfiltration (Ofsthun & Leypoldt, 1995), and thus, this modality can provide a simpler form of dialysis treatment than other treatment methods. The convective dose delivered during high-flux HD has been shown to reduce mortality in patients at risk, as defined by a serum albumin level of <4 g/dl (Locatelli et al., 2009). However, overall patient survival remains comparable to that of low-flux HD (Eknoyan et al., 2002), which presumably is caused by the limited amount of internal filtration involved due to limitations imposed by fluid dynamics and the geometric nature of the hemodialyzer.

Therefore, HDF is considered the gold standard for high-dose convective therapy, and has even been reported to reduce mortality risk as compared with high-flux HD (Canaud et al., 2006). HDF, which describes an intermittent renal supportive therapy of combined simultaneous diffusive and convective solute transport, is characterized by a large filtration volume that far exceeds the desired volume removal, and hence, external substitution is essential. In early HDF trials, a large number of sterile bags were used to supply substitution fluid, which was costly and complicated (Ledebo, 2007). However, technical advances made in the production of pyrogen-free ultrapure water allow sterile dialysate to be readily produced, which enables on-line based HDF to be used on a clinical basis. Several types of on-line HDF are clinically available that differ in terms of the ways in which external replacement fluid is administered, such as, by pre- or post-dilution. Due to their unique benefits, mixed forms of pre- and post-infusion have also been devised, such as, mixed-dilution or mid-dilution HDF (Krieter & Canaud, 2008, Pedrini & De Cristofaro, 2003). However, the inevitable complexities associated with HDF machines and patient monitoring, and the requirement for the exogenous infusion of replacement fluid is still problematic. Therefore, various modifications of HDF strategies have been proposed to integrate HDF and HD modes, that is, to increase convective dose without the requirement for external infusion. These modifications can be classified into three developmental categories; (1) to increase the internal filtration rate by increasing pressure gradients along the hemodialyzer, (2) to use independent domains for forward filtration and backfiltration, or ultrafiltration and diffusion, and (3) to alternate forward and backward filtration procedures.

In this chapter, the trials on HDF strategies undertaken without exogenous substitution infusion will be discussed in terms of their technical aspects, *in vivo* and *in vitro* efficacies and applicabilities for clinical use. This is followed by an in-depth review on pulse push/pull hemodialysis (PPPHD), a recently introduced pulsatile technique that provides infusion-free HDF.

2. HDF strategies that do not require exogenous substitution infusion

Hemodiafiltration is an intermittent renal supportive therapy that involves the process of convection and diffusion. Total filtration volumes invariably exceed desired amounts and this dehydration must be corrected in real time. Despite various modifications of the HDF techniques based on infusion modes, the need for external replacement fluid infusion has not been eliminated. Accordingly, efforts continue to be made to eliminate exogenous sterile fluid infusion during HDF sessions. This is achieved by spontaneous fluid reinfusion at a rate that matches convection. Backfiltration and regenerated ultrafiltrate can be the methods of spontaneous fluid restoration.

2.1 Internal Filtration Enhanced HDF (internal HDF or iHDF)

Internal filtration (IF) is defined as the total water flux across membranes within the closed blood and dialysate compartments of a dialyzer (Dellanna et al., 1996). Volume controlled high-flux HD is a representative modality to use the internal filtration phenomenon, and provides a straightforward means of achieving enhanced convection by augmenting internal filtration rates. The amount of internal filtration is directly regulated by pressure gradients through the hemodialyzer. A pressure drop is inevitable, as fluid flows through a cylindrical tube, and it is expressed by Poiseuille's equation:

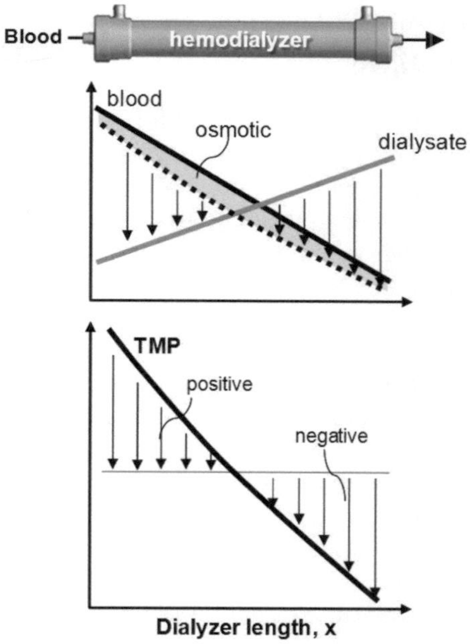

Fig. 1. Blood and Dialysate Pressure Gradient along Dialyzer Length. The sum of hydraulic and osmotic pressures is termed TMP, as TMP = ΔPb- ΔPd-Δπ. Here, ΔPb represents the average value of arterial and venous blood pressure, ΔPd for average hydraulic dialysate pressures, and Δπ is oncotic pressures.

$$\Delta P \propto \frac{\mu L}{d^4} Q \tag{1}$$

Where, ΔP is the pressure drop, μ is the fluid viscosity, L and d are the length and diameter of the flow path, and Q the flow rates. Thus, blood and dialysate pressures drop along the dialyzers. However, because blood and dialysate flow in opposite directions, these pressure drops occur with opposing gradients, and in some region, hydraulic blood and dialysate pressures overlap (Fig. 1). In a normal countercurrent dialysis setup, the sum of hydraulic and osmotic pressures, termed transmembrane pressure (TMP), is positive in the proximal region of a hollow fiber dialyzer, and plasma moves to the dialysate compartment across the membranes (forward filtration). However, fluid movement occurs in the opposite direction in the distal region, because hydraulic blood pressures are below the sum of dialysate compartment pressure and osmotic pressure, and thus, backward filtration occurs and compensates for fluid loss in the proximal region.

2.1.1 Factors influencing internal HDF

Even though forward and backward filtration rates are highly dependent on membrane permeabilities and the degree of membrane fouling, they remain directly proportional to the positive and negative TMPs, respectively. As shown in Fig. 1, resulting TMP gradients can be readily increased by increasing blood and/or dialysate pressure drops (Fiore & Ronco, 2004, 2007). For blood, the pressure drop is proportional to blood viscosity and tube length in accord with Poiseuille's equation (Eq. 1), which shows that tube length increases pressure differential. Likewise, blood hematocrit and total protein levels also affect the pressure drop through viscosity.

The diameter of the flow path is another important factor. Poiseuille's equation shows that the pressure drop is inversely proportional to the 4th power of tube diameter, which means that membrane (a bundle of hollow fibers) lumen diameter is the predominant factor for governing blood pressure drops, and therefore, many investigations of internal HDF have focused on dialytic efficiencies using hemodialyzers with smaller membrane diameters. In early clinical studies, beta-2 microglobulin (β2M) removal was found to be significantly increased when membrane diameter was reduced. A 175 μm diameter dialyzer was found to enhance β2M clearances by factors of two and four, respectively, over 200 and 250 μm diameter hemodialyzers (Dellanna et al., 1996). Clearances of inulin and vitamin b12 were also significantly greater with 175 μm dialyzer than a 200 μm dialyzer, without changing the clearances of low molecular weight solutes (Ronco et al., 2000). In addition, a mathematical model showed that internal filtration rates increase rapidly with membrane diameter, and this theoretical result was also confirmed experimentally (Mineshima, 2004, Mineshima et al., 2000). Myoglobin clearance was increased by 34% when a membrane of diameter 150 μm, rather than 200 μm, with the same surface area was used at the same blood flow rates. These benefits in dialytic efficiency afforded by reducing membrane lumen diameter allow internal filtration enhanced hemodialyzers to be used clinically (Lucchi et al., 2004, Righetti et al., 2010).

However, the underlying risk of hemoconcentration due to high levels of forward filtration may not be negligible. Pressure-driven filtration causes large volume losses from blood and promptly increases blood viscosity, which deteriorates membrane sieving and hydraulic capabilities. Membrane-binding by blood components is a major cause of permeability reductions, and inevitably diminish membranes efficiencies, particularly in the forward filtration region. Nevertheless, membrane fouling, which tends to be more of an issue during the early stage of iHDF treatment, tends to have little effect on overall membrane transfer capacity during iHDF (Yamamoto et al., 2005).

Dialysate pressure is also regulated by increasing the flow resistance on the dialysate stream. Several techniques can be used to increase dialysate flow resistances, such as increasing membrane packing density, lengthening the hemodialyzer, or placing obstacles in the dialysate flow path. Obviously, dialyzer length effectively regulates dialysate pressure drops. In one study conducted to clarify the effect of dialyzer length on solute clearance, middle-to-large uremic molecules, such as β2M and alpha-1 microglobulin (α1M), were shown to be better cleared by a 250 mm dialyzer than a 195 mm dialyzer (Sato et al., 2003). Dialysate pressure drop can also be manipulated by modulating membrane packing density. The higher the packing density of membrane fibers, the greater the resistance to dialysate flow, because the effective cross-sectional area available for dialysate flow decreases. Analytical and experimental studies revealed myoglobin clearances using a hemodialyzer with 71.3% packing density were slightly higher than hemodialyzers with packing densities of 52% or 60.1% (Mineshima, 2004). However, high hemodialyzer packing densities cause substantial degrees of dialysate channeling and flow mismatch between blood and dialysate. This unmatched flow distribution leads to a loss of effective surface area and impairs the diffusion process (Gastaldon et al., 2003). Flow visualization studies in a dialyzer with a high packing density (75%) reconfirmed this disproportionate flow pattern of dialysate, as compared with standard packing density dialyzers (68%), and consequent reductions in urea clearance (Fujimura et al., 2004, Yamamoto et al., 2005). Nevertheless, a unique design of housing wall, involving addition of a short taper to the inner housing surface effectively prevented the dialysate from being channeled (Fujimura et al., 2004).

2.1.2 Internal filtration quantification

The beneficial effects of internal HDF, such as increased middle-size solute clearances, may be quantified by evaluating internal filtration rates, because the internal filtration level is directly related to delivered convective dose. The flux across a membrane (Q) at a local region of the hemodialyzer (x) can be expressed by membrane hydraulic permeability (Kuf measured in ml/h/mmHg) and TMP (mmHg), as follows:

$$Q(x) = Kuf(x) * TMP(x) = Kuf(x) * (\Delta Pb - \Delta Pd - \Delta\pi) \tag{2}$$

Where, Pb, Pd and π represent the blood, dialysate and osmotic pressures. However, the flow dynamics inside the hemodialyzer are so complex that precise determinations of internal filtration rates are not available clinically. This is principally because Kuf across membranes is neither linearly related to the pressure gradient, nor constant at any position in the hemodialyzer (Ficheux et al., 2010). Kuf values are also substantially lowered by membrane fouling, which is remarkably affected by blood viscosity, coagulation, the abilities of membrane materials to bind plasma proteins, and treatment modalities. Hence, fluxes and permeabilities across membranes become parameters beyond the operator's control. Alternatively, a semi-empirical model based on clinical data has been developed to determine internal filtration rates. Using this model, internal filtration volumes and reinfusion rates were determined during internal HDF and post-dilution HDF modes, and revealed that differences between total convections (4.1 and 5.4 L/h for iHDF and HDF) well reflected differences between β2M clearance rates (123±11 and 149±26 ml/min for iHDF and HDF, respectively) (Lucchi et al., 2004). In a study conducted using *in vitro* scintigraphy method to verify this semi-empirical model, the model was found to show excellent accuracies of around 97% and a prediction error of only 3% (Fiore et al., 2006).
In addition to the mathematical model, methods for performing indirect measurements of the internal filtration have also been proposed. Changes in non-permeable molecular concentrations occur in response to the water content of blood, and thus, the kinetics of water transport across membrane can be evaluated by measuring the cumulative concentration changes of non-permeable molecules (Ronco et al., 1992). Radiolabeled albumin (a non-permeable molecule) has been employed to determine the amounts of convection for hemodialyzers with reduced fiber diameters or an obstacle in dialysate stream (Ronco et al., 2000, 1998). A series of *in vitro* experiments proved that this scintigraphic method was accurate for measuring internal filtration rates, but despite its precision, its clinical application is not plausible due to the safety issue raised by the use of radio-labeled molecules and the complexities of the procedures and equipment.
Another approach to determine internal filtration is offered by Doppler ultrasonography, which measures changes in blood velocity within dialyzers. In the absence of net-filtration, blood volume depletion in the proximal portion of a hemodialyzer leads to a reduction in blood flow velocity, and after the lowest point has been reached, the blood velocity gradually increases due to backfiltration. Thus, changes in blood velocity along a dialyzer provide information on blood volume changes and on amounts of forward and backward filtration. In one study, the internal filtration rate of a 250 mm dialyzer was found to be 37.7

ml/min by Doppler ultrasonography, but only 11.1 ml/min for a standard 195 mm dialyzer (Sato et al., 2003). Doppler ultrasonography is straightforward, non-invasive, and easily used at bedside (Mineshima, 2011). However, the method is still incapable of measuring blood flow velocity precisely, particularly blood velocity deep within the membrane fiber bundle. In other words, this method is based on velocities measured in peripheral membranes, which are quite different from velocities within centrally located fibers, and as a result, deviations from true values are unavoidable.

Other techniques have also been explored in an effort to quantify the filtration phenomena, or to visualize flow distributions inside hemodialyzers, these techniques include magnetic resonance imaging (Hardy et al., 2002), computed tomography (Frank et al., 2000, J. C. Kim et al., 2008) and a computerized scanning technique (Ronco et al., 2000, 2002). However, the quantification of internal filtration using these techniques is not available clinically, due to concerns of patient safety and technical requirements.

Summarizing, internal HDF can provide a means of convective treatment by increasing internal filtration rates using specifically designed hemodialyzers, and at the same time spontaneous backfiltration compensates for fluid loss, and hence, this technique is simpler than other modalities. The hemodialyzer design for internal HDF must be optimized based on specified structural factors and on the filtration characteristics of membrane fibers. The literature suggests superior dialysis outcomes for iHDF, but the precise quantification of internal filtration remains to be determined.

2.2 Double high-flux HDF

Solute removal during extracorporeal hemodialysis, particularly for low-flux HD, is mainly facilitated by diffusion which is driven by the concentration gradient across membrane. Thus, solute clearances are highly dependent on their molecular weights. On the other hand, hemofiltration (HF) is purely convective. Thus, it could be speculated that HF delivers higher middle- to large-size solutes clearances than HD, but poorer small-size mass transfer. The additional advantages of this convective treatment include better maintenance of cardiovascular instability in ESRD patients or in ICUs. These benefits of hemofiltration encouraged investigations aimed at compensating for the inferior diffusive clearances of HF, and a hybrid configuration based on multiple membranes was introduced (Cheung et al., 1982).

Double high-flux HDF was first introduced in the early 1980's as a means of combining HD and HF. This technique was particularly aimed at significantly increasing small (diffusion) and middle-size molecular removal (convection) in order to shorten overall treatment time, and therefore, much larger surface areas were used by arranging two high-flux hemodialyzers in series, in conjunction with a extremely high blood (400-500 ml/min) and dialysate flow rate (800-1000 ml/min) and a bicarbonate dialysate (Miller et al., 1984, von Albertini et al., 1984).

This arrangement of two hemodialyzers enabled flow resistances through the two hemodialyzers to be manipulated, which permitted TMP gradients (both positive and negative) to be adjusted. A flow restrictor, placed on the intermediate blood line of two hemodialyzers, serves as a means of increasing blood pressures in the arterial-side hemodialyzer, which cause positive TMPs through this dialyzer and ultrafiltration (Fig. 2). On the other hand, blood pressure drops below dialysate pressures at the venous-side dialyzer and TMPs become negative, which leads to backfiltration (Shinzato et al., 1982).

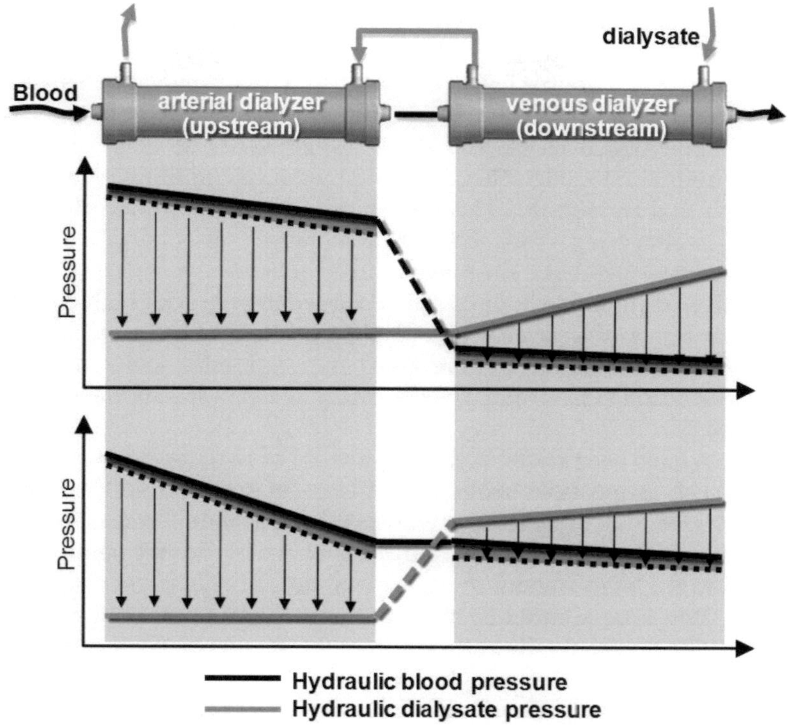

Fig. 2. Schematic Pressure Profiles during Double HDF, when a flow restrictor is placed on blood tube (upper) and on dialysate tube (below) of the two hemodialyzers.

TMP regulation is also achieved by regulating dialysate pressure. Flow resistance applied to the dialysate tubing between the two dialyzers promptly increases dialysate pressures at the venous dialyzer because blood and dialysate flow in opposing directions. Hydraulic dialysate pressures exceed blood pressures, which leads to backfiltration in the venous dialyzer. However, dialysate pressures rapidly fall in the arterial dialyzer due to flow restriction, which causes ultrafiltration in the arterial dialyzer. In addition, the high blood and dialysate flow rates used are also associated with larger pressure gradients. Hence, ultrafiltration at the arterial dialyzer at levels of exceeding those required can be promptly compensated for by backfiltration at the venous dialyzer, and thus, exogenous replacement infusion is not required for this method.

The flow resistance placed on the dialysate stream was originally made from a gauge needle assembled with a bypass line in parallel. A clamp on the bypass line forced the dialysate into the gauge needle, and created flow resistance in dialysate stream. The flow resistance in this configuration is fixed, and the amounts of ultrafiltration and backfiltration cannot be adjustable externally. Hence, the means of creating resistance to dialysate flow was improved in the advanced version, termed convection-controlled double high-flux HDF, in which variable and controllable flow resistances were integrated (Pisitkun et al., 2004).

Therefore, together with these features, this modality achieved unmatched depurative outcomes, as demonstrated by far higher uremic molecular clearances regardless of molecular size (Cheung et al., 1982, Shinzato et al., 1982, von Albertini et al., 1985). Furthermore, increased clearances allowed treatment times to be shortened (Miller et al.,

1984, von Albertini et al., 1984). Solute removal in a relatively short time (e.g., 2 hours) may cause greater rebound of uremic solute levels after post-dialysis equilibrium, thus solute removal rates in trials of double HDF far surpassed the removal rates desired during hemodialysis, achieving two and half times higher clearances over 2 hours as was achieved over 4 hours in conventional HD mode. These results were also confirmed by comparing treatment modalities. Double high-flux HDF attained significantly greater β2M reduction and Kt/V_{UREA} values than high-flux HD, and showed comparable β2M clearance to that of on-line HDF (Susantitaphong et al., 2010, Tiranathanagul et al., 2007). Furthermore, the beneficial effect of this technique on patient survival was also suggested in a long-term assessment. In this study, double high-flux HDF was compared with high-efficiency or high-flux HD modes in terms of treatment time, Kt/V and standardized mortality ratio over 6 years. Kaplan-Meier Survival analysis revealed a significantly lower mortality ratio for double HDF versus USRDS (0.41 and 1, respectively) despite the shortened treatment time (Bosch et al., 2006).

However, concerns have been raised regarding the use of two hemodialyzers in this double HDF technique, such as, possible increases in treatment cost and system complexity. One possible way of overcoming these issues involves the reuse of dialyzers, although regulatory guidelines on renal replacement practices in some countries do not permit reuse. Another concern arises from the large amount of cross-membrane flux. In particular, a large quantity of backfiltration should be assured by the strict and regular verification of water quality (Bosch & Mishkin, 1998. One positive aspect is that the venous dialyzer acts as a final barrier to pyrogen transfer.

Double high-flux HDF emerged as a result of an effort to increase treatment efficiencies and shorten treatment times by maximizing both diffusive and convective mass transfer. Many observations have confirmed the high solutes clearances across a wide spectrum of molecular weights, which are the results of the unique features of this method. In particular, the unique control of hydraulic pressures possibly gives this unit the ability to regulate convective dose. However, the widespread implementation of this technique may require the identification of patients capable of tolerating treatment and the overcoming of the above-mentioned underlying concerns.

2.3 Paired filtration dialysis with endogenous reinfusion (HFR)

Another two-chamber technique for obtaining short and efficient HDF treatment is the so-called paired filtration dialysis (PFD). Like double HDF, PFD is also a strategy of simultaneous HD and HF treatment aimed at increasing both diffusive and convective clearances, but its design principles separate convection from diffusion (Ghezzi et al., 1989, 1987, Ronco et al., 1990). A hemofilter with a relatively small surface area is combined with a hemodialyzer in this sequence (Fig. 3). Ultrafiltration purely occurs at the hemofilter and then blood is dialyzed continually through the hemodialyzer.

The convection, which is not connected with diffusion, can minimize interactions between diffusion and convection (Ghezzi et al., 1987). Total resulting clearances during HDF are always lower than the sum of convective and diffusive clearances, which is attributed to the reciprocal interactions of these two processes (Gupta & Jaffrin, 1984, Sprenger et al., 1985). As diffusion and convection occur within the same membranes, the contribution made by convection to total clearances is diminished by the presence of diffusion, particularly for highly diffusive molecules. This is because the concentrations of these molecules

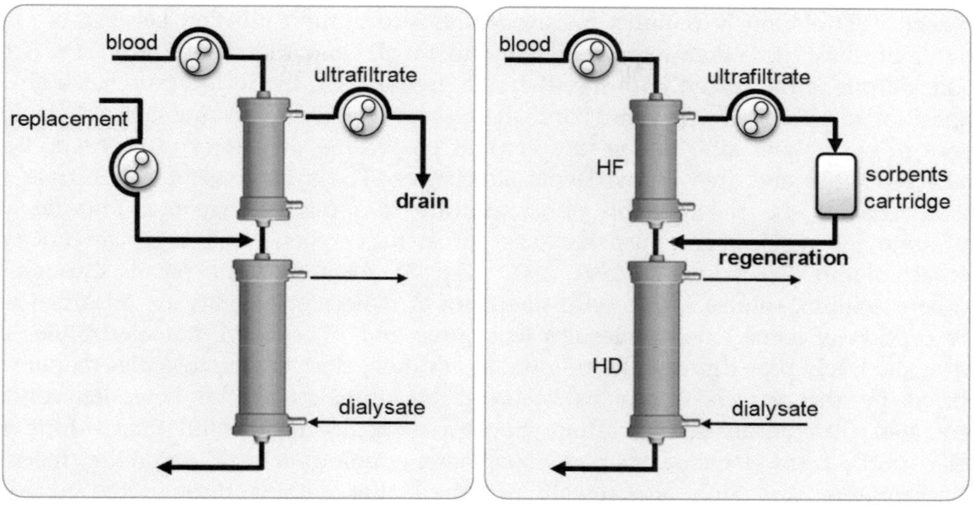

Fig. 3. PFD (left) and HFR (right)

promptly decreases along the dialyzer length due to diffusion, and in this situation, solute concentrations in ultrafiltrate are reduced. Likewise, diffusive mass transfer is also disrupted by the presence of convection. High filtration rates throughout the entire membrane causes the formation of protein gel layer, which acts as secondary resistance; that is, the membrane fouling decreases membrane permeability and filtration rates, and consequently, convective clearances are substantially diminished. Furthermore, molecular sieving coefficients are also reduced because of protein binding, which eventually reduces membrane diffusivity (Morti & Zydney, 1998). In the PFD technique, however, convection occurs in a separate region from diffusion and theoretically, no interference between diffusion and convection occurs.

In addition, independent convection allows ultrafiltrate volume to be regulated. The total amount of ultrafiltration surpasses desired volume removal, and sterile replacement fluid is administered at the mid-point between the hemofilter and hemodialyzer shown in the Fig. 3. In addition, desired net-volume removal by PFD can be achieved either by balancing ultrafiltration and reinfusion through the hemofilter, or by balancing internal filtration in the hemodialyzer.

Likewise, as for other convective treatments, simultaneous but separate convection of PFD permitted higher depurative outcomes than standard HD mode, and even allowed treatment times to be reduced (Vanholder et al., 1991). Dialysis times could be reduced to as little as 150 minutes per session in patients with a body weight of < 61 kg without compromising dialytic tolerance and efficiency (Botella et al., 1991). PFD also achieves dialytic efficiencies comparable with HDF despite significantly lower filtration rates (40 versus 75 ml/min, respectively) (Bufano et al., 1991), which is primarily due to minimal interference between diffusion and convection. However, β2M removal is smaller than in HF mode (Marangoni et al., 1992). Other benefits of PFD may include the minimal use of backfiltration in the hemodialyzer and superior biocompatibility (Panichi et al., 1998). Since convection is achieved at the hemofilter, dialysis can be accomplished with minimal internal filtration and pressure gradients.

However, PFD obviously requires the exogenous substitution infusion because of larger amounts of ultrafiltrate than required volume removal. One unique feature of PDF is that the ultrafiltrate is not mixed with the dialysate. In addition, the ultrafiltrate has a similar composition of plasma. On the other hand, the replacement fluid must possess a physiologic balance of electrolytes after taking into account preexisting deficits or excesses, and also should be sterile and free of pyrogenic substances. These features of ultrafiltrate and infusate enables the regeneration of ultrafiltrate to replace exogenous infusate, and ultrafiltrate for replacement purposes was successfully regenerated using an uncoated charcoal column (Ghezzi et al., 1991, 1992) (Fig. 3). As ultrafiltrate passes through the adsorbent column, solutes with a wide spectrum of molecular weights are adsorbed with the exception of some small molecules (e.g., urea and phosphate), but electrolytes and bicarbonate freely pass through the column. In addition, since small molecules that are not captured by the adsorbent can be removed by diffusion at the hemodialyzer, the regenerated ultrafiltrate is successfully applied as replacement fluid (Sanz-Moreno & Botella, 1995). Trace elements, such as manganese, selenium, arsenic, cadmium, mercury, lead, chromium, and zinc, also remain unaltered after passing through the adsorbent column, whereas copper is completely retained by the charcoal (de Francisco et al., 1997). Adsorption capacities were further increased by combining hydrophobic styrenic resin along with uncoated charcoal, because the resin has a high binding affinity for several mid molecular weight species, such as, β2M (Marinez de Francisco et al., 2000) and homocysteine (Splendiani et al., 2004), or free immunoglobulin light chains (Testa et al., 2010).

The other benefits of this regenerated ultrafiltrate include a better acid-base balance due to the reinfusion of endogenous bicarbonate (de Francisco et al., 1997), and also the not inconsiderable advantage of combining high convection without compromising physiologic molecule loss. Ultrafiltrate has a composition similar to that of plasma and contains huge numbers of polypeptides and other beneficial substances, such as, hormones, amino acids, and vitamins (Weissinger et al., 2004), and ultrafiltrate regeneration allows these beneficial nutrients to be reinfused (La Greca et al., 1998). In terms of plasma amino acid levels, no significant changes in their intradialytic levels occur during HFR, whereas a ~25% reduction occur during acetate-free biofiltration (Borrelli et al., 2010).

A number of clinical studies on ESRD patients have revealed that HFR remarkably improve dialytic efficiencies and solute removal over a wide molecular weight ranges, such as, the removal of uremic marker molecules (β2M, leptin and free immunoglobulin light chains) (Bolasco et al., 2006, S. Kim et al., 2009, Testa et al., 2006), cardiovascular risk factors (homocysteine) (Splendiani et al., 2004), inflammatory cytokines (CRP, IL-1, IL-6), and biomarkers of oxidative stress (ox-LDL, IL-1β) (Calo et al., 2011, Testa et al., 2006). In a comparison between HFR and on-line HDF, both were found to be highly biocompatible and to considerably reduce inflammatory markers, such as, CRP and IL-6 (Panichi et al., 2006). One technical variance of HFR is the repositioning of convection and diffusion. The change of sequence during HFR significantly enhanced reductions in urea and β2M, possibly due to the less saturated use of adsorbents, and also reduced cytokine levels, e.g., IL6 and TNFα, more than conventional HFR (Meloni et al., 2004, 2005).

In addition, HFR appears to be more beneficial at reducing oxidative stress and the risk of atherosclerotic cardiovascular disease than standard HD mode. A comparative study of HFR and low-flux bicarbonate HD revealed that HFR reduced not only the plasma level of oxidized low-density lipoprotein (LDL), but also the mRNA production of p22phox and PAI-1 (palsminogen activator inhibitor 1), whose protein expressions are known to be closely related to inflammation and oxidative stress (Calo et al., 2007). Furthermore, plasma total antioxidant capacity (TAC) and antioxidant enzymes activities were found to be lower for HFR than high-flux HD (Gonzalez-Diez et al., 2008).

However, contrary results have also been presented. For ESRD patients who undertook bicarbonate HD and then were switched to HFR, nutritional and inflammatory parameters remained unchanged over a year. Neither serum β2M nor PTH levels varied over the course of time, which led to the conclusion that although the change to HFR from bicarbonate HD is safe and tolerated, it is not associated with an improvement in nutritional or inflammatory parameters, or a reduction in β2M levels (Bossola et al., 2005). Prolonged, larger-scale clinical studies for HFR are warranted.

More recently, a significant decrease was observed in cardiac troponin (cTnT) levels, a marker of myocardial damage and cardiac hypertrophy, throughout HFR sessions when using acetate-free dialysate, but cTnT increased after HFR using dialysate containing acetate. These results show that further explanation is required for the correlation between cTnT and acetate (Bolasco et al., 2011). However, both hemoglobin (Hb) levels and erythropoietic-stimulating agent (ESA) doses were not related to the presence of acetate. Hb levels increased, but ESA requirements tended to reduce continually during the 9-month study period (Bolasco et al., 2011).

In summary, PFD is a HDF technique whereby ultrafiltrate is isolated from dialysate. Renal replacement therapies, facilitated by convection and diffusion, are still unsatisfactory for removing uremic toxins, and thus, adsorption as a third mechanism has been employed in HFR units. Adsorption during HFR allows convective treatments to be performed by the endogenous reinfusion of ultrafiltrate. Even if the loss of beneficial substances during HDF is inevitable, ultrafiltrate reinfusion reduces these losses to a minimum, like low-flux HD. Another feature of ultrafiltrate regeneration is the guaranteed purity of substitution fluid. Substitution is continuously obtained from ultrafiltrate, but the ultrafiltration, adsorption, and reinfusion system is totally closed during HFR, and therefore, excludes any possibility of contamination and ensures superior biocompatibility. However, despite these outstanding features, this unit has complications and associated costs. Furthermore, technical improvements in the preparation of ultrapure dialysate are expected to further cut the cost of preparing sterile, ultrapure replacement fluid, and this could increase the cost gap between HFR and on-line HDF.

2.4 Push/Pull Hemodiafiltration

A similar but simpler HDF strategy has been also introduced. This system relies on alternate repetitions of forward and backward filtration during dialysis treatment, and thus, it was named push/pull HDF. When the infusion-free HDF technique using a serial arrangement of two hemodiafilters was described in the early 1980's, the push/pull concept was devised to eliminate the need for two hemodiafilters. It is obvious that repetitive ultrafiltration can increase total filtration volume, but such a system also requires a means of repeating backfiltration (Usuda et al., 1982). Thus, a redundant dialysate bag is integrated downstream of the hemodialyzer, which is connected to the dialysate stream by a bidirectional peristaltic pump. The push/pull action that is accomplished by this bi-direction pump is responsible for alternating the evacuation and replenishment of the bag. During normal operation, inlet and outlet dialysate flow rates are equally maintained and the desired volume removal is achieved by a separate ultrafiltration pump. In this situation, when the bidirectional pump pulls a portion of dialysate into the bag (70 ml/min for 3 minutes), hydrostatic pressures through the dialysate compartment decrease, because the dialysate compartment is closed and has a fixed volume, and water flux occurs from blood to the dialysate compartment (ultrafiltration) at the same level as dialysate removal from the dialysate compartment. Soon after the ultrafiltration completes, the pump operates in reverse and pushes the dialysate in the bag into the dialysate stream, which causes a volume overload in the dialysate compartment. The surplus dialysate in the closed dialysate compartment is then moved to the blood compartment (backfiltration). In the same manner, another bag and an additional bidirectional peristaltic pump is also integrated into the venous chamber, and conducts the pulling and pushing of blood, although in this case, the actions of the blood-side pump are 180° out of phase with those of the dialysate side pump to keep blood flow returning to the patient constant.

When pure dialysate is pushed into the blood stream, solute concentrations in blood are immediately equilibrated and decreased by dilution. Soon after, the blood-to-dialysate pressure gradient reverses from negative to positive, and plasma fluid in blood is forced to move into the dialysate compartment, which removes various molecules from plasma. This repetitive ultrafiltration obviously contributes to convective mass transfer and increases the reductions of small-sized (urea) or mid-sized (β2M) molecules as compared with HF or HD, respectively (Shinzato et al., 1989). On the other hand, repetitive backfiltration during push/pull HDF prevents volume depletion. In addition, the repetitive backflushing of dialysate also helps prevent membrane binding (Usuda et al., 1982).

However, disposable bags and separate bidirectional peristaltic pumps make this unit complicated and increase treatment costs. Instead, a double-chamber cylinder pump was devised with two independent chambers and a reciprocal piston; that is, each chamber is connected to either dialysate or the blood stream (Tsuruta et al., 1994), as seen in Fig. 4.

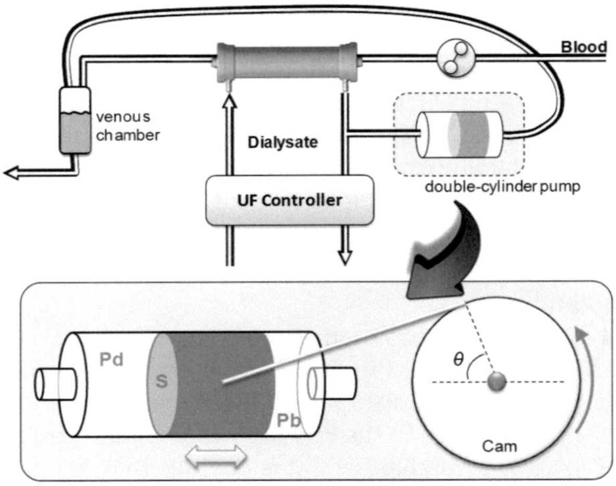

Fig. 4. Push/Pull HDF and Double-Chamber Cylinder Pump

When the piston squeezes the chamber on the dialysate side, the dialysate compartment, which has a fixed volume, is pressurized and backfiltration begins. At this time, the chamber on the blood side expands and blood in the venous chamber starts flowing in the direction of the double-chambered pump. Since the blood volume that returns to the blood-side chamber of the pump is equal to the backfiltration volume, blood flow returning to patients remains constant. The piston then moves in the opposite direction and squeezes the blood-side chamber, the dialysate compartment begins to expand, and the dialysate compartment becomes depressurized, which leads ultrafiltration. However, despite the large amount of ultrafiltration, blood flow in the venous line is maintained, because the ultrafiltrate removed in the hemodialyzer is replenished in the venous chamber.

Furthermore, the reciprocating movement of the piston is regulated by pressure differences between the two chambers of the cylinder pump (i.e., Pb-Pd). The rotation torque of the driving motor attached to the piston can be expressed in accord with TMP (i.e., torque = TMPxSxLxsinθ). Voltage applied to the motor is adjusted so that the TMP is set at 400 mmHg during forward filtration, but at -400 mmHg during the backward filtration phase, that is, pressure-controlled push/pull HDF can maintain transmembrane pressures at the maximum permissible level throughout treatment (Shinzato et al., 1994). In addition, contrary to the original push/pull HDF, in which one cycle of filtration and backfiltration takes approximate 4~5 minutes, the pressure controlled push/pull HDF unit can repeat one cycle in 1.5~1.7 seconds.

This optimized use of transmembrane pressure and more frequent alternations of forward and backward filtration in the revised push/pull HDF unit are obviously accompanied with a markedly larger total filtration volumes and higher solutes clearances (Shinzato et al., 1994). Push/pull HDF tends to relieve symptoms like arthralgia (joint pain), irritability, pruritus, and insomnia more rapidly than conventional HD (Maeda et al., 1990, Maeda & Shinzato, 1995, Shinzato et al., 1995). Furthermore, the optimal maintenance of membrane permeabilities by prompt backfiltration has the added benefit of considerably inhibiting albumin loss in addition to increasing convection and diffusion (Shinzato et al., 1996). Albumin loss is inevitable when using membranes with high water permeabilities and sieving characteristics (Combarnous et al., 2002). Since convective therapy is based on larger amounts of fluid exchange and solvent drag during fluid exchange occurs randomly, albumin permeation becomes more worrisome during convective treatments (Ahrenholz et al., 2004). In addition, filtration-induced elevated albumin concentration at the inner membrane wall also aggravates the albumin loss (Miwa & Shinzato, 1999). Protein concentration polarization develops quickly after sudden TMP development and the hydraulic permeabilities of the membrane decrease rapidly in about 2 seconds. However, during push/pull HDF, backward flushing of dialysate takes place within the time frame required for the protein layer to fully develop (i.e., 1.5~1.7 seconds), and thus, it can effectively wash out the inner lumen and inhibit excessive albumin leakage (Shinzato et al., 1996).

However, this modality still requires the use of a separate device so that dialysate pressures are regulated instantaneously. In addition, no clinical observation has been conducted to examine the long-term clinical effect of pressure-controlled push/pull HDF versus on-line HDF. Push/pull HDF is based on repetitive dilution at a rate of approximate 15 ml per 1.7s cycle, which exceeds blood flow rates (3.3~5 ml/s). Hence, push/pull HDF is assumed to be close to pre-dilution mode HDF (Shinzato & Maeda, 2007). Even though post-dilution HDF is more efficient in terms of solute removal, the substantial amount of total filtration and the optimal use of membrane offered by the push/pull HDF technique probably translate to outstanding hemodialytic outcomes.

Push/pull HDF was developed in an effort to perform infusion-free, simultaneous HD and HF by using a single hemodialyzer. Thus, it alternates between forward filtration and backfiltration instead of dividing ultrafiltration and backfiltration regions. Pressure-controlled push/pull HDF using a double-chambered cylinder pump can maintain TMPs at maximal levels and the total filtration volumes achieved are far greater than that of any other treatment modality. In addition to the filtration quantity, repetitive cycles in a shorter time than the time required for a protein layer to be established ensure superior membrane use throughout treatment, which further inhibits albumin loss. However, given the advances represented by membranes with high β2M sieving coefficients (>0.8), but very small albumin sieving coefficients (<0.01) (Ronco et al., 2002), the differences between push/pull HDF and high-flux HD with respect to β2M removal may be reduced, and albumin leakage less problematic. To an extent in modern dialysis practice, albumin permeable membranes are even considered to remove non-soluble and/or much larger molecules (De Smet et al., 2007, Samtleben et al., 2003). Therefore, a prolonged prospective study on push/pull HDF may be worthwhile to determine the benefits of this modality versus other forms of convective renal replacement.

3. Pulse Push/Pull Hemodialysis (PPPHD)

Flow patterns, that is, pulsatile versus non-pulsatile, remain topics of research for treatments requiring extracorporeal blood circulation. Despite controversy, blood pulsation has been accepted to have a benefit during cardiopulmonary bypass, because it achieves greater perfusion to peripheral vessels and end-organs (Dapper et al., 1992, Orime et al., 1999). Furthermore, blood pulsation in a pediatric CRRT[1] animal model was found to deliver adequate performance over a 2-hour period in terms of ultrafiltration rates and cross-filter blood pressure drops (Lopez-Herce et al., 2006, Ruperez et al., 2003). In addition, it was also found that the pulsatile flow tends to enhance ultrafiltration rates versus non-pulsatile flow (Lim et al., 2009, Runge et al., 1993), which attributed to an increased rheological power of pulsatile flow. However, little clinical or experimental evidence is available that explains the efficacy of pulsatile flow during dialysis. Pulse push/pull HD is a convection enhanced dialysis treatment, based on the use of pulsatile flows to achieve a cyclic repetition of forward and backward filtration. As explained in the previous section, the repetitive manner of ultrafiltration and backfiltration contributes substantially to total volume exchange and convective mass transfer.

3.1 Pulse push/pull HD

Repetitive procedures of ultrafiltration and backfiltration during PPPHD are achieved by replacing conventional roller pumps with pulsatile pumps for both blood and dialysate. During an early trial, a T-PLS pump (Twin Pulse Life Supporter, AnC Bio Inc., Seoul, Korea) was used as pulsatile pumps for blood and dialysate (K. Lee et al., 2008). The T-PLS consists of blood and dialysate sacs, a reciprocating actuator, and a motor-cam assembly (J. J. Lee et al., 2005). The actuator is located between blood and dialysate sacs (Fig. 5). When the actuator squeezes the blood sac, blood in the sac can move only in the forward direction due to the presence of one-way check valves. At the same time, the dialysate sac expands and is filled with fresh dialysate. In the same manner, dialysate also moves forward when the sac is squeezed, and these reciprocating movements create pulsatile flow. By setting their phase difference at 180° degrees, the respective pushing phases of blood and dialysate pumps alternate, and TMPs cycle between positive and negative, which drive consecutive periods of ultrafiltration and backfiltration.

[1] Continuous Renal Replacement Therapy

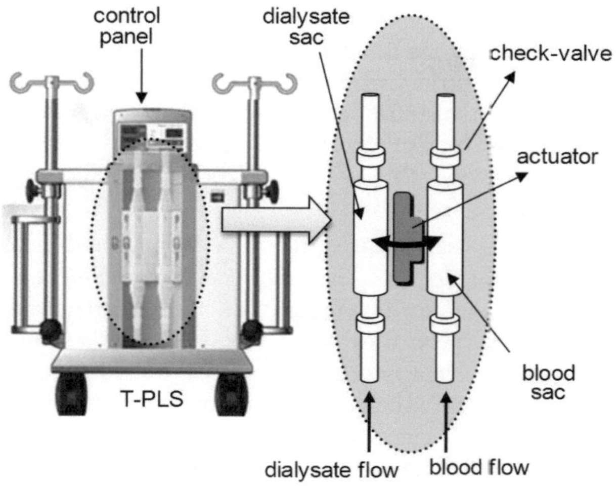

Fig. 5. T-PLS pump for the original PPPHD

The hemodialytic efficiencies of PPPHD have been demonstrated *in vitro* and also *in vivo*, and these studies have shown that PPPHD substantially improves the clearances of uremic marker molecules, particularly for mid-sized molecules (Table 1) (K. Lee et al., 2008), which is believed to be due to a higher level of total filtration. Pressure profiles also showed obvious oscillations of TMPs throughout treatment, and their magnitudes were significantly larger than those observed in conventional hemodialysis (CHD) mode.

Group	BPM	QB	QD	Clearance (ml/min)			
				BUN	Creatinine	Vitamin b12	Inulin
CHD	-	236±3.6	420±3	161.1±4.3	127.2±3.9	37.5±6.3	25.3±5.1
PPPHD	40	234±3.1	419±3	166.2±3.8	136.9±4.2	55.7±5.0	37.8±3.9
% Increase		-	-	3.2	7.6	48	49
P-value		NS	NS	0.053	<0.05	<0.001	<0.001

Table 1. Solutes Clearances. (CHD, conventional high-flux HD; PPPHD, pulse push/pull HD; BPM, beats per minute; QB, blood flowrate; QD, dialysate flowrate; BUN, blood urea nitrogen; NS, not significant)

Increased filtration volumes in the PPPHD unit may also be due to reduced membrane fouling. In an *in vivo* setup on PPPHD, one cycle of ultrafiltration and backfiltration took 3 seconds at a pulse frequency of 20 bpm (K. Lee et al., 2008). When ultrafiltration and backfiltration times were defined as the durations of positive and negative TMPs, respectively, ultrafiltration and backfiltration times for the PPPHD unit were 1.68±0.02 and 1.31±0.03 seconds, respectively. Since protein concentration polarization on the blood-side membrane develops during the forward filtration phase and it is reduced by backfiltration, membrane convective capacity might be better maintained during PPPHD than during CHD, showing smaller reductions in post-dialysis hydraulic permeabilities (K. Lee et al., 2008). Furthermore, PPPHD-treated animals were tolerably sustained and their physiologic parameters were stable.

Pulse push/pull HD is conceptually similar to push/pull HDF. Both modalities were devised to increase total filtration level by alternating forward and backward filtration. However, the underlying design of PPPHD differs from push/pull HDF, and thus, the supplementary component required to switch from ultrafiltration to backfiltration phases or vice versa used in push/pull HDF was eliminated for PPPHD and the entire system was remarkably simplified.

3.2 Modification of PPPHD

Repetitive ultrafiltration and backfiltration offers a simple and efficient HDF strategy. However, the pulsatile circulation of blood during extracorporeal renal replacement treatment appears to be potentially problematic. In particular, instant suction generated by a pulse pump through a narrow needle or catheter may cause blood damage, vessel narrowing, or vessel collapse. In addition, instantaneous negative pressures generated upstream of a pulsatile blood pump not only introduce the risk of circuit aeration, but also lead to a failure to maintain predetermined blood flow rates (Depner et al., 1990, Teruel et al., 2000).

Hence, we revised PPPHD and many aspects of the original PPPHD were retained in the revised version, including an alternating water flux across the membrane, but blood pulsation was excluded. This was achieved by employing dual pulsation in the dialysate stream, that is, pulsatile devices in the dialysate stream both upstream (a dialysate pump) and downstream (an effluent pump) of the dialyzer. Backfiltration occurs when the sum of the cross-membrane pressures is negative, but ultrafiltration when the sum is positive. The hydraulic pressures of blood and dialysate were both manipulated in the original PPPHD, but since blood pulsation was eliminated, the dialysate pressure is the only variable that regulates TMP in the revised unit. Therefore, an assumption was made; (1) dialysate compartment pressures must be far higher than blood-side pressures when pure dialysate is forced into the dialyzer (that is, when the dialysate sac is squeezed), but (2) dialysate pressures drop to lower than blood pressures during effluent pump expansion. For this purpose, the dialysate and effluent pumps are replaced with a dual pulse pump (K. Lee et al., 2008).

The dual pulse pump (DPP) is a pulsatile device that was developed to eliminate the one-way valves that are generally required for pulsatile devices to prevent retrograde flow; instead, time-delayed tube openings and closings constitutes a cycle of pulse generation (Fig. 6). In other words, two separate silicone tubes in the DPP are periodically opened or closed. Pulse generation with DPP can be described in terms of four phases as determined by cam rotation, which translates motor rotation to actuator linear displacement. As the cam rotates, the four actuators periodically push on the tubing segments at the positions shown in the Fig. 6. Actuator 1 pushes on the tubing segments at positions 1 and 6 (p1 and p6) simultaneously, and actuator 3 squeezes the tubing segments at positions 3 and 4. Actuators 2 and 4 squeeze tubing segments at p 2 and p5, respectively, and caused the dialysate in the tube to move in the required direction. The first phase was defined as a cam rotation angle (θ) between 0 and 90°. Likewise, the 2nd and 3rd phases were defined as cam rotation angles between 90°~180° and 180°~270°, respectively. For pulse generation by the dialysate pump, as the cam rotates from θ=0° to 90°, the p2 tubing segment opens and p1 closes, and these processes overlap such that pure dialysate fills p2 tubing. While p2 expands, p3 remains closed, acting as an upstream valve to prevent retrograde dialysate. These tube openings and closings are also depicted in the tube openness diagram in Fig. 7. Tube openness is defined as the ratio of compressed tube diameter to the original internal diameter, as described elsewhere (K. Lee et al., 2008). During the first phase, with p3 closed, p2 tube

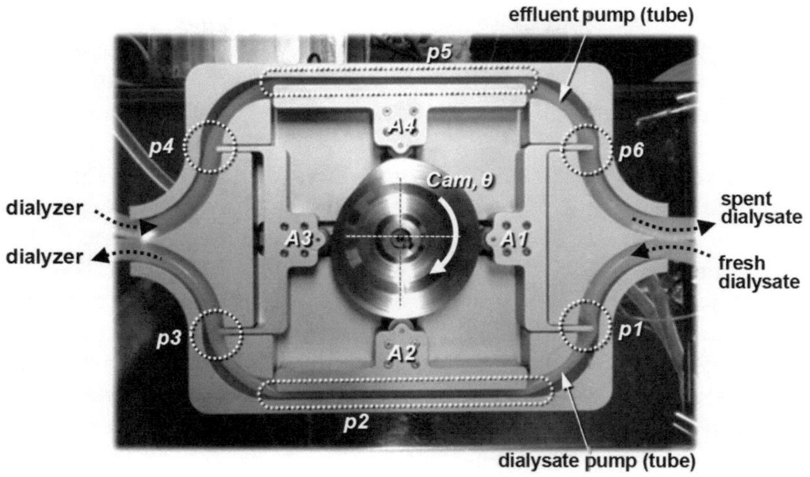

Fig. 6. Dual Pulse Pump (DPP). Its body is made of an aluminum alloy, and comprises a base plate, a unidirectional electric motor (not seen), a cam, and four actuators. It can also contain two separate silicone tubes. Pulsatile flow is generated by squeezing each dialysate and effluent tubing segments. (A1~A4, actuators 1 to 4; p1~p6, silicone tubing segments at positions 1 to 6, respectively)

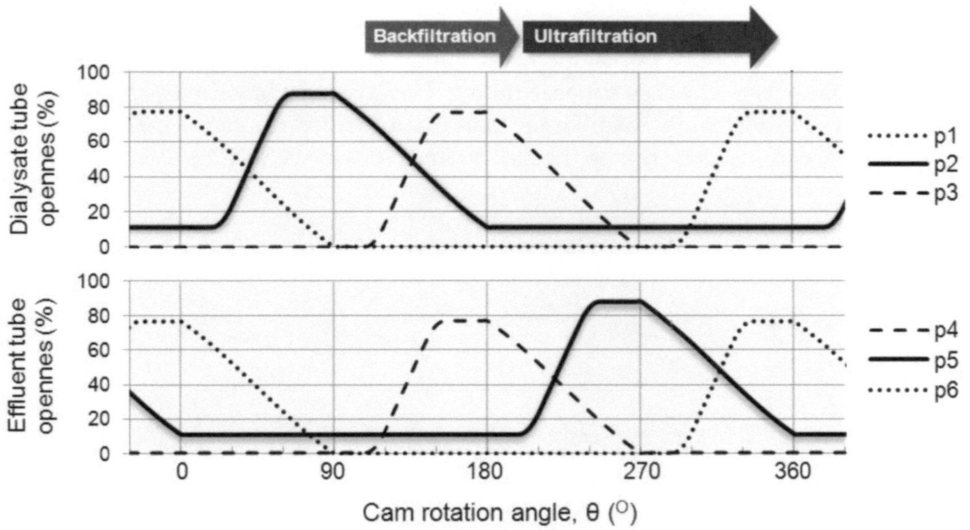

Fig. 7. Tube Openness Diagram for Dialysate (upper) and Effluent Pump (below) of DPP.

openness increases whereas p1 tube openness decreases. During the 2nd phase (θ=90°~180°), with p1 closed, p2 begins to be squeezed and simultaneously p3 begins to open, and pure dialysate is driven into the hemodialyzer. Closure of p1 fulfills the same function as atrioventricular valve closure during left ventricular systole, which prevents retrograde flow. During the 3rd phase (θ=180°~270°), p3 is closed, while p1 and p2 remain closed and in the final phase (θ=270°~360°), p1 is open, and p2 and p3 remain closed in preparedness for the next filling phase. These time-delayed tube openings and closures constitute one cycle of pulse generation. In the same manner, effluent pulsations were also generated through the effluent tube, although in this case, the actions of actuators 1 and 3 were reversed, and the pulsatile flow pattern was 180° out of phase with that in the dialysate tube.

Theoretically, forward and backward filtration rates during one cycle of PPPHD are identical to effluent and dialysate flow rates, respectively. The moment when pure dialysate is driven to the dialyzer (i.e., during p2 squeezing), the effluent dialysate path is closed at p6. At the same time, p1 is also closed, and thus, the pure dialysate pushed into dialyzer should move into the blood stream (backfiltration), because the whole dialysate compartment is fixed and closed. Immediately after the backfiltration is completed, the effluent tubing (p5) begins to expand (i.e., p5 expansion), and since the dialysate and effluent pathways are still closed at p1 and p6, respectively, dialysate pressures in the hemodialyzer drop steeply and ultrafiltration takes place at a rate determined by effluent stroke volume.

During animal experiments using the PPPHD, in which we used an acute canine renal failure model (achieved by ligating renal arteries and veins), the animals remained stable without any procedurally related complications. Molecular removals were satisfactory, and total protein levels, albumin concentrations, and glucose levels were preserved uniformly throughout PPPHD sessions (Table 2). Furthermore, TMPs clearly cycled positive and negative due to huge fluctuations in hydraulic dialysate pressures (Fig. 8). In addition, despite the use of a peristaltic roller pump for blood, the blood pressures acquired during PPPHD showed an obvious fluctuation which was perfectly synchronized with dialysate pressure pulsation. Generally, peristaltic roller pumps create small fluctuations in flow and pressure, because of the way they squeeze tubing. However, the blood pressure fluctuations acquired during PPPHD were much larger than that observed for conventional HD, which provides evidence of dialysate flux to the blood stream or vice versa (Fig. 8).

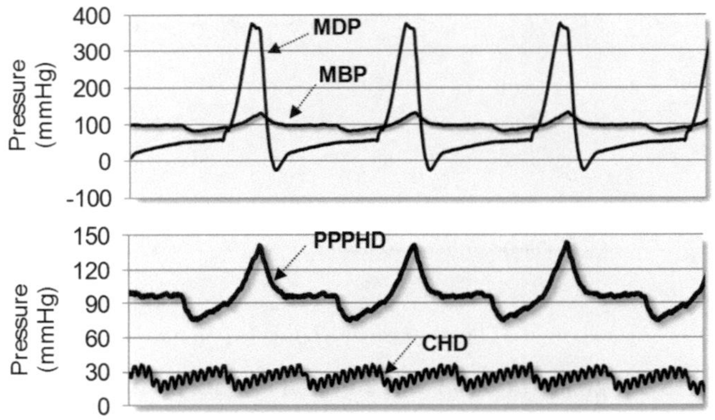

Fig. 8. Pressure Profiles during PPPHD treatment (upper), and Changes in Blood Pressures for PPPHD and CHD (below). (MDP, mean dialysate pressure; MBP, mean blood pressure; CHD, conventional HD)

In addition, as stated before, the DPP is characterized by a lack of valves, which makes the pulsatile device simple and inexpensive, and thus, any medical-grade silicone tubes can be used as dialysate and effluent sacs. Furthermore, with the exception of small tubing sections at p1, p3, p4, and p5, most of the tubing is operated non-occlusively, which reduces the probabilities of tubing rupture and spallation (W. G. Kim & Yoon, 1998, Leong et al., 1982).

PPPHD

(h)	PCV	TP	ALB	Glu	Ca2+	Na+	K+	BUN	Crea
0	28.5±4.6	5.3±0.4	3.1±0.1	119±7	12.4±0.8	136±5.7	5.7±0.6	90.3±12.7	6.5±0.9
2	28.0±3.6	5.6±0.7	3.1±0.2	111±4	11.5±0.8	134±4.2	5.1±0.6	63.7±5.7	4.6±0.7
4	27.3±3.5	5.3±0.4	3.1±0.2	126±44	10.8±0.5	132±3.1	4.3±0.5	47±7.2	3.8±0.4

Table 2. Animal Experiment Results. PCV, packed cell volume (%); TP, total protein (g/dl); ALB, albumin (g/dl) ; Glu, glucose (mg/dl); BUN, blood urea nitrogen (mg/dl); Crea, creatinine (mg/dl)

3.3 Fluid management in PPPHD

Recently, the dual pulsatile pump integrated into the dialysate stream has been remarkably ameliorated to achieve a substantial increase in the accuracy of volume control. Maintaining pre-determined flow rates and precise volume control are pre-requisites of extracorporeal renal replacement treatments for ESRD patients, particularly when using membranes with high-water permeability. Therefore, the dual pulsation system acting on the PPPHD dialysate compartment was replaced with a dual piston pump, as shown in Fig. 9. This modification allows pulse generation and push/pull to be achieved, not only by the novel design of the piston pump, but also by the unique control of piston movements offered (Fig. 10). As the dialysate piston compresses the cylinder, pure dialysate is forced into the dialyzer, but at this time, the effluent stream is functionally closed at the effluent piston pump, and thus, dialysate compartment pressures increase rapidly and backfiltration occurs (Phase 1).The effluent piston then begins to expand and dialysate moves into the effluent cylinder, while the dialysate supply line is still closed at the dialysate pump. Because of effluent suction, dialysate compartment pressures fall sharply and water flux from blood lumen to dialysate occurs (Phase 2). During the final step, pure dialysate fills the dialysate cylinder, and simultaneously used dialysate is drained (Phase 3).

In an *in vitro* test of PPPHD with the dual piston pump, in which bovine blood was circulated through the blood lumen of the hemodialyzer at 200 ml/min and isotonic saline solution was used as dialysate at the rate of 400 ml/min, the phenomena of push (backfiltration) and pull (ultrafiltration) were well sustained throughout sessions, and their levels perfectly matched those of stroke volumes of the dialysate and effluent pumps, respectively. In addition, as was expected, dialysate and effluent piston pumps served as a flow equalizer, and controlled isovolumetic dialysate flow rates upstream and downstream of the dialyzer. Hydrostatic dialysate pressures were maintained at 520~700 mmHg during the backfiltration phase (Phase 1) and at -400~-540 mmHg during the ultrafiltration phase (Phase 2).

In addition, PPPHD is also versatile and can be easily converted to conventional high-flux HD. Time-controlled piston operations perform the push and pull operations, but when the two piston movements are synchronized alternately (that is, dialysate piston compression and effluent piston expansion or dialysate piston expansion and effluent piston compression

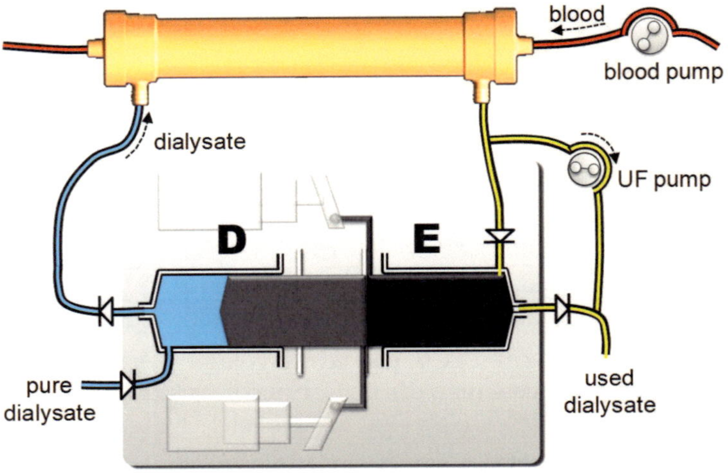

Fig. 9. Schematic Diagram of PPPHD with Dual Piston Pump. (D, dialysate pump; E, effluent pump)

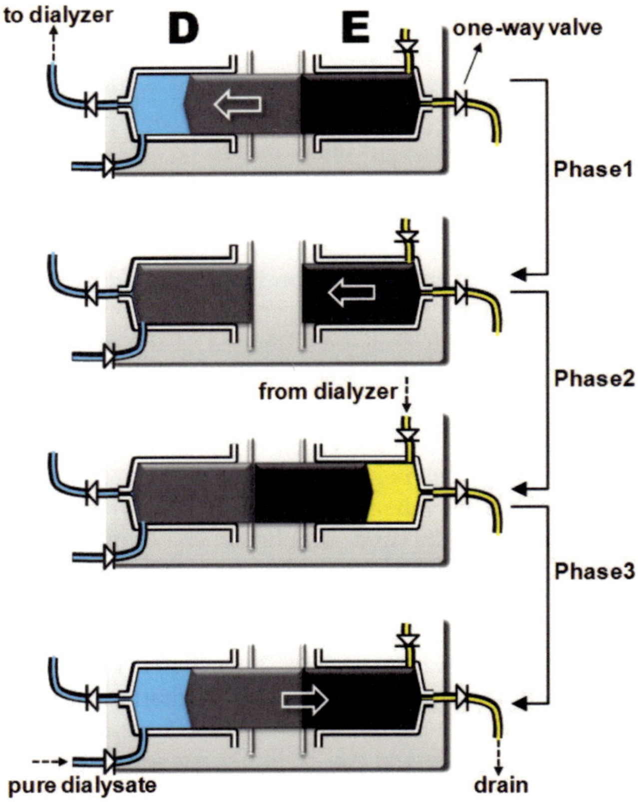

Fig. 10. Pulse Generation and Push/Pull during PPPHD with Dual Piston Pump. (D, dialysate pump; E, effluent pump)

occur simultaneously), dialysate passes through the hemodialyzer without significant flow into blood lumen. In this situation, the two piston pumps serve as a flow equalizer and dialysis is largely achieved by diffusive mass transfer.

The PPPHD unit presented was developed recently, and thus, it requires further investigation. Convective volume attained during PPPHD was equal to the accumulated total dialysate volume, and consequently, this unit delivered the maximally permissible level of total volume exchange. This encourages us to speculate on the capability of this unit in terms of removing mid-sized uremic toxins. Another issue regarding the enormous fluid exchange is the quantification of the contribution made by convection to dialytic efficiency. Backfiltration and ultrafiltration repeat in a relatively short time, and despite a large amount of filtration, the probability that some ultrafiltrate comes directly from dialysate backfiltered during a previous phase cannot be excluded, because that portion of ultrafiltrate does not contribute to depurative efficiency. In addition, forward filtration and backfiltration rates exceed the blood flow rate, which implies a reduction in solute concentrations due to dilution. As is the case for pre-dilution HDF, this repeated dilution may be expressed by an efficiency drop. Finally, although convection commonly inhibits diffusion during HDF, this inhibition is expected to be small for PPPHD due to repetitive backfiltration. Although an *in vitro* or *in vivo* setup revealed that alternate backfiltration has a positive influence on inhibiting concentration polarization and permeability reduction, it is believed that optimizations, in terms of pulse frequencies and stroke volumes, will further benefit the optimal use of membrane convective capacities throughout PPPHD treatments.

4. Conclusion

Much evidence shows that HDF delivers better dialysis outcomes than high-flux HD; for example, HDF has been shown to improve middle-to-large size molecular removal, allow better EPO control, reduce oxidative stress and inflammation (Lornoy et al., 2000, Vaslaki et al., 2006, Ward et al., 2000), and even to positively influence patient mortality (Canaud et al., 2006, Jirka et al., 2006). These benefits have been attributed to the higher convective doses permitted during HDF. Furthermore, ultrapure dialysate, required due to the large amount of substitution infusion, further inhibits the inflammation risk (Lonnemann, 2000).

In this chapter, we review HDF techniques that do not require exogenous substitution infusion. These techniques must be accompanied by spontaneous fluid restoration, such as, backfiltration or ultrafiltrate regeneration (Table 3). A simpler way might be to increase forward and backward filtration rates during HD sessions, although this can only be done to a limited extent. Much higher efficiencies can be achieved by the two-chamber techniques, that is, double high-flux HDF and HFR, which were developed in an effort to increase solute removal and shorten treatment times, by separating ultrafiltration and backfiltration, or convection and diffusion domains. However, these modalities appear to unavoidably increase overall system complexity. Push/pull HDF, which uses a single hemodialyzer, was derived by considering phases, rather than physical regions, for forward and backward filtration. The pulse push/pull HD described here is also based on the phase-separated use of forward filtration and backfiltration using a single high-flux dialyzer. This strategy was devised as a result of efforts to modulate flow patterns for extracorporeal dialysis treatment, and thus, a unique design for managing dual pulsation through the dialysate compartment allows the whole unit to be as simple as the conventional HD unit.

As these novel HDF strategies evolved, remarkable improvements have been achieved in dialysis technologies. Modern dialysis machines offer HDF and HD as default therapies, and are also equipped with outstanding monitoring facilities not only for patients (BTM, BVM, OCM[2]), but also for treatments (fail-safe design and high-precision balancing) (Polaschegg, 2010). In particular, advances in water treatment allow ultrapure replacement fluid to be prepared in real time. These technical advancements are certainly lowering the barriers to higher convective HDF therapies.

Modality	Filter(s)	Additional components	TFV §	Filtration	Reinfusion
Internal HDF	1	-	+	proximal part of dialyzer	BF
Double HDF	2	flow restrictor	++	hemodialyzer (upstream)	BF
HFR	2	adsorbent column, filtrate pump	+	hemofilter (upstream)	FR
PP HDF	1	double-chamber pump	+++	whole membrane	BF
Pulse PP HD	1	-	+++	whole membrane	BF

§ Total filtration volume per session (4 hours, L); +, low (<20L); ++, moderate (20-40L); +++ high (>60L)

Table 3. Infusion-free HDF modalities. (HFR, hemofiltrate reinfusion; TFV, total filtration volume; PP, push/pull; FR, filtrate regeneration; BF, backfiltration)

Therefore, in addition to convective clearances, we believe the PPPHD system should be equipped by features that simplify overall treatment and enable dialysis to be performed in outside clinics, because this unit allows simple and efficient operation. Future development targets designed to accomplish these features include; greater user friendliness (that is, intuitive control and operation, fail-safe operations and treatment automation), readily available sterile dialysate, accessible maintenance, and a miniaturized unit that is both light and portable (without compromising depurative efficiency). A dialysis unit equipped with these features may also provide treatment alternatives beyond the current thrice weekly 4-h practice, and perhaps allow even daily dialysis for ESRD patients.

5. References

Ahrenholz, P. G., Winkler, R. E., & Michelsen, A. (2004). Dialysis membrane-dependent removal of middle molecules during hemodiafiltration: the beta2-microglobulin/albumin relationship. *Clin Nephrol,* Vol.62, No.1, (Jul), pp.(21-28), 0301-0430

Bolasco, P. G., Ghezzi, P. M., & Ferrara, R. (2006). Effect of on-line hemodiafiltration with endogenous reinfusion (HFR) on the calcium-phosphorus metabolism: medium-term effects. *Int J Artif Organs,* Vol.29, No.11, (Nov), pp.(1042-1052), 0391-3988,1724-6040(e)

[2] Body Temperature Monitor, Body Volume Monitor, and Online Clearance Monitor

Bolasco, P. G., Ghezzi, P. M., & Serra, A. (2011). Effects of acetate-free haemodiafiltration (HDF) with endogenous reinfusion (HFR) on cardiac troponin levels. *Nephrol Dial Transplant,* Vol.26, No.1, (Jan), pp.(258-263), 0931-0509,1460-2385(e)

Bolasco, P. G., Ghezzi, P. M., & Serra, A. (2011). Hemodiafiltration with Endogenous Reinfusion with and without Acetate-Free Dialysis Solutions: Effect on ESA Requirement. *Blood Purif,* Vol.31, No.4, (Jan 14), pp.(235-242), 0253-5068,1421-9735(e)

Borrelli, S., Minutolo, R., & De Nicola, L. (2010). Intradialytic changes of plasma amino acid levels: effect of hemodiafiltration with endogenous reinfusion versus acetate-free biofiltration. *Blood Purif,* Vol.30, No.3, pp.(166-171), 0253-5068,1421-9735(e)

Bosch, J. P., Lew, S. Q., & Barlee, V. (2006). Clinical use of high-efficiency hemodialysis treatments: long-term assessment. *Hemodial Int,* Vol.10, No.1, (Jan), pp.(73-81), 1492-7535

Bosch, J. P. & Mishkin, G. J. (1998). Hemofiltration and double high flux dialysis: risks and benefits. *Curr Opin Nephrol Hypertens,* Vol.7, No.6, (Nov), pp.(643-647), 1062-4821

Bossola, M., Muscaritoli, M., & Tazza, L. (2005). Switch from bicarbonate hemodialysis to hemodiafiltration with online regeneration of the ultrafiltrate (HFR): effects on nutritional status, microinflammation, and beta-microglobulin. *Artif Organs,* Vol.29, No.3, (Mar), pp.(259-263), 0160-564X,1525-1594(e)

Botella, J., Ghezzi, P., & Sanz-Moreno, C. (1991). Multicentric study on paired filtration dialysis as a short, highly efficient dialysis technique. *Nephrol Dial Transplant,* Vol.6, No.10, pp.(715-721), 0931-0509,1460-2385(e)

Bufano, G., Ariano, R., & Pecchini, P. (1991). Haemodiafiltration versus paired filtration dialysis: evaluation of in vivo solute removal. *Nephrol Dial Transplant,* Vol.6 Suppl 2, pp.(82-83), 0931-0509,1460-2385(e)

Calo, L. A., Naso, A., & Carraro, G. (2007). Effect of haemodiafiltration with online regeneration of ultrafiltrate on oxidative stress in dialysis patients. *Nephrol Dial Transplant,* Vol.22, No.5, (May), pp.(1413-1419), 0931-0509,1460-2385(e)

Calo, L. A., Naso, A., & Davis, P. A. (2011). Hemodiafiltration with online regeneration of ultrafiltrate: effect on heme-oxygenase-1 and inducible subunit of nitric oxide synthase and implication for oxidative stress and inflammation. *Artif Organs,* Vol.35, No.2, (Feb), pp.(183-187), 0160-564X,1525-1594(e)

Canaud, B., Bragg-Gresham, J. L., & Marshall, M. R. (2006). Mortality risk for patients receiving hemodiafiltration versus hemodialysis: European results from the DOPPS. *Kidney Int,* Vol.69, No.11, (Jun), pp.(2087-2093), 0085-2538,1523-1755(e)

Centers for Disease Control and Prevention. (2010). Incidence of end-stage renal disease attributed to diabetes among persons with diagnosed diabetes --- United States and Puerto Rico, 1996-2007. *MMWR Morb Mortal Wkly Rep,* Vol.59, No.42, (Oct 29), pp.(1361-1366), 0149-2195 ,1545-861X(e)

Cheung, A. C., Kato, Y., & Leypoldt, J. K. (1982). Hemodiafiltration using a hybrid membrane system for self-generation of diluting fluid. *Trans Am Soc Artif Intern Organs,* Vol.28, pp.(61-65), 0066-0078

Combarnous, F., Tetta, C., & Cellier, C. C. (2002). Albumin loss in on-line hemodiafiltration. *Int J Artif Organs,* Vol.25, No.3, (Mar), pp.(203-209), 0391-3988,1724-6040(e)

Dapper, F., Neppl, H., & Wozniak, G. (1992). Effects of pulsatile and nonpulsatile perfusion mode during extracorporeal circulation--a comparative clinical study. *Thorac Cardiovasc Surg,* Vol.40, No.6, (Dec), pp.(345-351), 0022-5223

Daugirdas, J. T. & Van Stone, J. C. (2000). In: *Handbook of Dialysis,* Daugirdas, J. T., Blake, P. G. & Ing, T. S., pp. (15-45), Lippincott Williams & Wilkins, 9780781752534

de Francisco, A. L., Botella, J., & Escallada, R. (1997). Haemodiafiltration with sorbent-regenerated ultrafiltrate as replacement fluid: a multicenter study. *Nephrol Dial Transplant,* Vol.12, No.3, (Mar), pp.(528-534), 0931-0509,1460-2385(e)

De Smet, R., Dhondt, A., & Eloot, S. (2007). Effect of the super-flux cellulose triacetate dialyser membrane on the removal of non-protein-bound and protein-bound uraemic solutes. *Nephrol Dial Transplant,* Vol.22, No.7, (Jul), pp.(2006-2012), 0931-0509,1460-2385(e)

Dellanna, F., Wuepper, A. & Baldamus, C. A. (1996). Internal filtration--advantage in haemodialysis? *Nephrol Dial Transplant,* Vol.11 Suppl 2, pp.(83-86), 0931-0509,1460-2385(e)

Depner, T. A., Rizwan, S. & Stasi, T. A. (1990). Pressure effects on roller pump blood flow during hemodialysis. *ASAIO Trans,* Vol.36, No.3, (Jul-Sep), pp.(M456-459), 0889-7190

Eknoyan, G., Beck, G. J., & Cheung, A. K. (2002). Effect of dialysis dose and membrane flux in maintenance hemodialysis. *N Engl J Med,* Vol.347, No.25, (Dec 19), pp.(2010-2019), 0028-4793,1533-4406(e)

Ficheux, A., Kerr, P. G., & Brunet, P. (2010). The ultrafiltration coefficient of a dialyser (KUF) is not a fixed value, and it follows a parabolic function: the new concept of KUF max. *Nephrol Dial Transplant,* (Sep 8), 0931-0509,1460-2385(e)

Fiore, G. B., Guadagni, G., & Lupi, A. (2006). A new semiempirical mathematical model for prediction of internal filtration in hollow fiber hemodialyzers. *Blood Purif,* Vol.24, No.5-6, pp.(555-568), 0253-5068,1421-9735(e)

Fiore, G. B. & Ronco, C. (2004). Internal hemodiafiltration (iHDF): a possible option to expand hemodiafiltration therapy. *Int J Artif Organs,* Vol.27, No.5, (May), pp.(420-423), 0391-3988,1724-6040(e)

Fiore, G. B. & Ronco, C. (2007). Principles and practice of internal hemodiafiltration. *Contrib Nephrol,* Vol.158, pp.(177-184), 0302-5144,1662-2782(e)

Frank, A., Lipscomb, G. G. & Dennis, M. (2000). Visualization of concentration fields in hemodialyzers by computed tomography. *J Memb Sci,* Vol.175, pp.(239-251), 0376-7388

Fujimura, T., Uchi, Y., & Fukuda, M. (2004). Development of a dialyzer with enhanced internal filtration to increase the clearance of low molecular weight proteins. *J Artif Organs,* Vol.7, No.3, pp.(149-154), 1434-7229

Gastaldon, F., Brendolan, A., & Crepaldi, C. (2003). Effects of novel manufacturing technology on blood and dialysate flow distribution in a new low flux "alpha Polysulfone" hemodialyzer. *Int J Artif Organs,* Vol.26, No.2, (Feb), pp.(105-112), 0391-3988,1724-6040(e)

Ghezzi, P. M., Botella, J., & Sartoris, A. M. (1991). Use of the ultrafiltrate obtained in two-chamber (PFD) hemodiafiltration as replacement fluid. Experimental ex vivo and in vitro study. *Int J Artif Organs,* Vol.14, No.6, (Jun), pp.(327-334), 0391-3988,1724-6040(e)

Ghezzi, P. M., Dutto, A., & Gervasio, R. (1989). Hemodiafiltration with separate convection and diffusion: paired filtration dialysis. *Contrib Nephrol,* Vol.69, pp.(141-161; discussion 162-147), 0302-5144,1662-2782(e)

Ghezzi, P. M., Gervasio, R., & Tessore, V. (1992). Hemodiafiltration without replacement fluid. An experimental study. *Asaio J,* Vol.38, No.1, (Jan-Mar), pp.(61-65), 1058-2916,1538-943X(e)

Ghezzi, P. M., Sanz-Moreno, C., & Gervasio, R. (1987). Technical requirements for rapid high-efficiency therapy in uremic patients. Paired filtration-dialysis (PFD) with a two-chamber technique. *ASAIO Trans,* Vol.33, No.3, (Jul), pp.(546-550), 0889-7190

Ghezzi, P. M., Zucchelli, P., & Ringoir, S. (1987). Paired filtration-dialysis (PFD): a separate convective-diffusive system for extracorporeal blood purification in uraemic patients. *Adv Exp Med Biol,* Vol.223, pp.(267-275), 0065-2598

Gonzalez-Diez, B., Cavia, M., & Torres, G. (2008). Effect of a hemodiafiltration session with on-line regeneration of the ultrafiltrate on oxidative stress. Comparative study with conventional hemodialysis with polysulfone. *Blood Purif,* Vol.26, No.6, pp.(505-510), 0253-5068,1421-9735(e)

Gupta, B. B. & Jaffrin, M. Y. (1984). In vitro study of combined convection- diffusion mass transfer in hemodialysers. *Int J Artif Organs,* Vol.7, No.5, (Sep), pp.(263-268), 0391-3988,1724-6040(e)

Hardy, P. A., Poh, C. K., & Liao, Z. (2002). The use of magnetic resonance imaging to measure the local ultrafiltration rate in hemodialyzers. *J Memb Sci,* Vol.204, pp.(195-205), 0376-7388

Jirka, T., Cesare, S., & Di Benedetto, A. (2006). Mortality risk for patients receiving hemodiafiltration versus hemodialysis. *Kidney Int,* Vol.70, No.8, (Oct), pp.(1524; author reply 1524-1525), 0085-2538,1523-1755(e)

Kim, J. C., Kim, J. H., & Kim, H. C. (2008). Effect of fiber structure on dialysate flow profile and hollow-fiber hemodialyzer reliability: CT perfusion study. *Int J Artif Organs,* Vol.31, No.11, (Nov), pp.(944-950), 0391-3988,1724-6040(e)

Kim, S., Oh, K. H., & Chin, H. J. (2009). Effective removal of leptin via hemodiafiltration with on-line endogenous reinfusion therapy. *Clin Nephrol,* Vol.72, No.6, (Dec), pp.(442-448), 0301-0430

Kim, W. G. & Yoon, C. J. (1998). Roller pump induced tubing wear of polyvinylchloride and silicone rubber tubing: phase contrast and scanning electron microscopic studies. *Artif Organs,* Vol.22, No.10, (Oct), pp.(892-897), 0160-564X,1525-1594(e)

Krieter, D. H. & Canaud, B. (2008). New strategies in haemodialfiltration (HDF)--prospective comparative analysis between online mixed HDF and mid-dilution HDF. *Nephrol Dial Transplant,* Vol.23, No.4, (Apr), pp.(1465-1466; author reply 1466), 0931-0509,1460-2385(e)

La Greca, G., Brendolan, A., & Ghezzi, P. M. (1998). The concept of sorbent in hemodialysis. *Int J Artif Organs,* Vol.21, No.6, (Jun), pp.(303-308), 0391-3988,1724-6040(e)

Ledebo, I. (2007). Fluids in bags for hemodiafiltration. *Contrib Nephrol,* Vol.158, pp.(87-93), 0302-5144,1662-2782(e)

Lee, J. J., Lim, C. H., & Son, H. S. (2005). In vitro evaluation of the performance of Korean pulsatile ECLS (T-PLS) using precise quantification of pressure-flow waveforms. *Asaio J,* Vol.51, No.5, (Sep-Oct), pp.(604-608), 1058-2916,1538-943X(e)

Lee, K., Lee, S. R. & Min, B. G. (2008). Pulse push/pull hemodialysis: in vitro study on new dialysis modality with higher convective efficiency. *Artif Organs,* Vol.32, No.5, (May), pp.(406-411), 0160-564X,1525-1594(e)

Lee, K., Min, B. G., & Mun, C. H. (2008). Pulse push/pull hemodialysis in a canine renal failure model. *Blood Purif,* Vol.26, No.6, pp.(491-497), 0253-5068,1421-9735(e)

Lee, K., Mun, C. H., & Lee, S. R. (2008). Hemodialysis using a valveless pulsatile blood pump. *Asaio J,* Vol.54, No.2, (Mar-Apr), pp.(191-196), 1058-2916,1538-943X(e)

Leong, A. S., Disney, A. P. & Gove, D. W. (1982). Spallation and migration of silicone from blood-pump tubing in patients on hemodialysis. *N Engl J Med,* Vol.306, No.3, (Jan 21), pp.(135-140), 0028-4793,1533-4406(e)

Leypoldt, J. K., Cheung, A. K., & Carroll, C. E. (1999). Effect of dialysis membranes and middle molecule removal on chronic hemodialysis patient survival. *Am J Kidney Dis,* Vol.33, No.2, (Feb), pp.(349-355), 0272-6386,1523-6838(e)

Lim, K. M., Park, J. Y., & Lee, J. C. (2009). Quantitative analysis of pulsatile flow contribution to ultrafiltration. *Artif Organs,* Vol.33, No.1, (Jan), pp.(69-73), 0160-564X,1525-1594(e)

Locatelli, F., Martin-Malo, A., & Hannedouche, T. (2009). Effect of membrane permeability on survival of hemodialysis patients. *J Am Soc Nephrol,* Vol.20, No.3, (Mar), pp.(645-654), 1046-6673,1533-3450(e)

Lonnemann, G. (2000). Chronic inflammation in hemodialysis: the role of contaminated dialysate. *Blood Purif,* Vol.18, No.3, pp.(214-223), 0253-5068,1421-9735(e)

Lopez-Herce, J., Ruperez, M., & Sanchez, C. (2006). Continuous venovenous renal replacement therapy with a pulsatile tubular blood pump: analysis of efficacy parameters. *Artif Organs,* Vol.30, No.1, (Jan), pp.(64-69), 0160-564X,1525-1594(e)

Lornoy, W., Becaus, I., & Billiouw, J. M. (2000). On-line haemodiafiltration. Remarkable removal of beta2-microglobulin. Long-term clinical observations. *Nephrol Dial Transplant,* Vol.15 Suppl 1, pp.(49-54), 0931-0509,1460-2385(e)

Lucchi, L., Fiore, G. B., & Guadagni, G. (2004). Clinical evaluation of internal hemodiafiltration (iHDF): a diffusive-convective technique performed with internal filtration enhanced high-flux dialyzers. *Int J Artif Organs,* Vol.27, No.5, (May), pp.(414-419), 0391-3988,1724-6040(e)

Maeda, K., Kobayakawa, H., & Fujita, Y. (1990). Effectiveness of push/pull hemodiafiltration using large-pore membrane for shoulder joint pain in long-term dialysis patients. *Artif Organs,* Vol.14, No.5, (Oct), pp.(321-327), 0160-564X

Maeda, K. & Shinzato, T. (1995). Push/pull hemodiafiltration: technical aspects and clinical effectiveness. *Nephron,* Vol.71, No.1, pp.(1-9), 0028-2766

Marangoni, R., Savino, R., & Colombo, R. (1992). Short time treatment with high-efficiency paired filtration dialysis for chronic renal failure. *Artif Organs,* Vol.16, No.6, (Dec), pp.(547-552), 0160-564X,1525-1594(e)

Marinez de Francisco, A. L., & Ghezzi, P. M., Brendolan, A. (2000). Hemodiafiltration with online regeneration of the ultrafiltrate. *Kidney Int Suppl,* Vol.76, (Aug), pp.(S66-71), 0098-6577

Meloni, C., Ghezzi, P. M., & Cipriani, S. (2004). One year of clinical experience in postdilution hemofiltration with online reinfusion of regenerated ultrafiltrate. *Blood Purif,* Vol.22, No.6, pp.(505-509), 0253-5068,1421-9735(e)

Meloni, C., Ghezzi, P. M., & Cipriani, S. (2005). Hemodiafiltration with post-dilution reinfusion of the regenerated ultrafiltrate: a new on-line technique. *Clin Nephrol,* Vol.63, No.2, (Feb), pp.(106-112), 0301-0430

Miller, J. H., von Albertini, B., & Gardner, P. W. (1984). Technical aspects of high-flux hemodiafiltration for adequate short (under 2 hours) treatment. *Trans Am Soc Artif Intern Organs,* Vol.30, pp.(377-381), 0066-0078

Mineshima, M. (2011). Estimation of internal filtration flow rate in high-flux dialyzers by Doppler ultrasonography. *Contrib Nephrol,* Vol.168, pp.(153-161), 0302-5144,1662-2782(e)

Mineshima, M. (2004). New trends in HDF therapies: validity of internal filtration-enhanced hemodialysis. *Blood Purif,* Vol.22 Suppl 2, pp.(60-66), 0253-5068,1421-9735(e)

Mineshima, M., Ishimori, I., & Ishida, K. (2000). Effects of internal filtration on the solute removal efficiency of a dialyzer. *ASAIO J,* Vol.46, No.4, (Jul-Aug), pp.(456-460), 1058-2916,1538-943X(e)

Miwa, M. & Shinzato, T. (1999). Push/pull hemodiafiltration: technical aspects and clinical effectiveness. *Artif Organs,* Vol.23, No.12, (Dec), pp.(1123-1126), 0160-564X,1525-1594(e)

Morti, S. M. & Zydney, A. L. (1998). Protein-membrane interactions during hemodialysis: effects on solute transport. *Asaio J,* Vol.44, No.4, (Jul-Aug), pp.(319-326), 1058-2916,1538-943X(e)

Ofsthun, N. J. & Leypoldt, J. K. (1995). Ultrafiltration and backfiltration during hemodialysis. *Artif Organs,* Vol.19, No.11, (Nov), pp.(1143-1161), 0160-564X,1525-1594(e)

Orime, Y., Shiono, M., & Hata, H. (1999). Cytokine and endothelial damage in pulsatile and nonpulsatile cardiopulmonary bypass. *Artif Organs,* Vol.23, (Jun), pp.(508-512), 0160-564X,1525-1594(e)

Panichi, V., De Pietro, S., & Andreini, B. (1998). Cytokine production in haemodiafiltration: a multicentre study. *Nephrol Dial Transplant,* Vol.13, No.7, (Jul), pp.(1737-1744), 0931-0509,1460-2385(e)

Panichi, V., Manca-Rizza, G., & Paoletti, S. (2006). Effects on inflammatory and nutritional markers of haemodiafiltration with online regeneration of ultrafiltrate (HFR) vs online haemodiafiltration: a cross-over randomized multicentre trial. *Nephrol Dial Transplant,* Vol.21, No.3, (Mar), pp.(756-762), 0931-0509,1460-2385(e)

Pedrini, L. A. & De Cristofaro, V. (2003). On-line mixed hemodiafiltration with a feedback for ultrafiltration control: effect on middle-molecule removal. *Kidney Int,* Vol.64, No.4, (Oct), pp.(1505-1513), 0085-2538,1523-1755(e)

Pisitkun, T., Eiam-Ong, S., & Tiranathanagul, K. (2004). Convective-controlled double high flux hemodiafiltration: a novel blood purification modality. *Int J Artif Organs,* Vol.27, No.3, (Mar), pp.(195-204), 0391-3988,1724-6040(e)

Polaschegg, H. D. (2010). Hemodialysis machine technology: a global overview. *Expert Rev Med Devices,* Vol.7, No.6, (Nov), pp.(793-810), 1743-4440,1745-2422(e)

Righetti, M., Filiberti, O., & Ranghino, A. (2010). Internal hemodiafiltration versus low-flux bicarbonate dialysis: Results from a long-term prospective study. *Int J Artif Organs,* Vol.33, No.11, (Dec 1), pp.(796-802), 0391-3988,1724-6040(e)

Ronco, C., Bowry, S. K., & Brendolan, A. (2002). Hemodialyzer: from macro-design to membrane nanostructure; the case of the FX-class of hemodialyzers. *Kidney Int Suppl,* No.80, (May), pp.(126-142), 0098-6577

Ronco, C., Brendolan, A., & Crepaldi, C. (2000). Dialysate flow distribution in hollow fiber hemodialyzers with different dialysate pathway configurations. *Int J Artif Organs,* Vol.23, No.9, (Sep), pp.(601-609), 0391-3988,1724-6040(e)

Ronco, C., Brendolan, A., & Crepaldi, C. (2002). Blood and dialysate flow distributions in hollow-fiber hemodialyzers analyzed by computerized helical scanning technique. *J Am Soc Nephrol,* Vol.13 Suppl 1, (Jan), pp.(S53-61), 1046-6673,1533-3450(e)

Ronco, C., Brendolan, A., & Feriani, M. (1992). A new scintigraphic method to characterize ultrafiltration in hollow fiber dialyzers. *Kidney Int,* Vol.41, No.5, (May), pp.(1383-1393), 0085-2538,1523-1755(e)

Ronco, C., Brendolan, A., & Lupi, A. (2000). Effects of a reduced inner diameter of hollow fibers in hemodialyzers. *Kidney Int,* Vol.58, No.2, (Aug), pp.(809-817), 0085-2538,1523-1755(e)

Ronco, C., Feriani, M., & Brendolan, A. (1990). Paired filtration dialysis: studies on efficiency, flow dynamics and hydraulic properties of the system. *Blood Purif,* Vol.8, No.3, pp.(126-140), 0253-5068,1421-9735(e)

Ronco, C., Orlandini, G., & Brendolan, A. (1998). Enhancement of convective transport by internal filtration in a modified experimental hemodialyzer: technical note. *Kidney Int,* Vol.54, No.3, (Sep), pp.(979-985), 0085-2538,1523-1755(e)

Runge, T. M., Briceno, J. C., & Sheller, M. E. (1993). Hemodialysis: evidence of enhanced molecular clearance and ultrafiltration volume by using pulsatile flow. *Int J Artif Organs,* Vol.16, No.9, (Sep), pp.(645-652), 0391-3988,1724-6040(e)

Ruperez, M., Sanchez, C., & Garcia, C. (2003). Continuous venovenous renal replacement therapy using a pulsatile blood pump. *Pediatr Nephrol,* Vol.18, No.1, (Jan), pp.(29-32), 0931-041X

Samtleben, W., Dengler, C., & Reinhardt, B. (2003). Comparison of the new polyethersulfone high-flux membrane DIAPES HF800 with conventional high-flux membranes during on-line haemodiafiltration. *Nephrol Dial Transplant,* Vol.18, No.11, (Nov), pp.(2382-2386), 0931-0509,1460-2385(e)

Sanz-Moreno, C. & Botella, J. (1995). Hemodiafiltration in two chambers without replacement fluid: a clinical study. *Artif Organs,* Vol.19, No.5, (May), pp.(407-410), 0160-564X,1525-1594(e)

Sato, Y., Mineshima, M., & Ishimori, I. (2003). Effect of hollow fiber length on solute removal and quantification of internal filtration rate by Doppler ultrasound. *Int J Artif Organs,* Vol.26, No.2, (Feb), pp.(129-134), 0391-3988,1724-6040(e)

Shinzato, T., Fujisawa, K., & Nakai, S. (1994). Newly developed economical and efficient push/pull hemodiafiltration. *Contrib Nephrol,* Vol.108, pp.(79-86), 0302-5144,1662-2782(e)

Shinzato, T., Kobayakawa, H. & Maeda, K. (1989). Comparison of various treatment modes in terms of beta 2-microglobulin removal: hemodialysis, hemofiltration, and push/pull HDF. *Artif Organs,* Vol.13, No.1, (Feb), pp.(66-70), 0160-564X,1525-1594(e)

Shinzato, T. & Maeda, K. (2007). Push/pull hemodiafiltration. *Contrib Nephrol,* Vol.158, pp.(169-176), 0302-5144,1662-2782(e)

Shinzato, T., Miwa, M., & Kobayakawa, H. (1995). Effectiveness of new push/pull hemodiafiltration for arthralgia in long-term hemodialysis patients. *Contrib Nephrol,* Vol.112, pp.(111-118), 0302-5144,1662-2782(e)

Shinzato, T., Miwa, M., & Nakai, S. (1996). Alternate repetition of short fore- and backfiltrations reduces convective albumin loss. *Kidney Int,* Vol.50, No.2, (Aug), pp.(432-435), 0085-2538,1523-1755(e)

Shinzato, T., Sezaki, R., & Usuda, M. (1982). Infusion-free hemodiafiltration: simultaneous hemofiltration and dialysis with no need for infusion fluid. *Artif Organs,* Vol.6, No.4, (Nov), pp.(453-456), 0160-564X,1525-1594(e)

Splendiani, G., De Angelis, S., & Tullio, T. (2004). Selective adsorption of homocysteine using an HFR-ON LINE technique. *Artif Organs,* Vol.28, No.6, (Jun), pp.(592-595), 0160-564X,1525-1594(e)

Sprenger, K. G., Stephan, H., & Kratz, W. (1985). Optimising of hemodiafiltration with modern membranes? *Contrib Nephrol,* Vol.46, pp.(43-60), 0302-5144,1662-2782(e)

Susantitaphong, P., Tiranathanagul, K., & Katavetin, P. (2010). Efficacy of convective-controlled double high-flux hemodiafiltration versus on-line hemodiafiltration: 1-year prospective study. *Blood Purif,* Vol.29, No.1, pp.(35-43), 0253-5068,1421-9735(e)

Teruel, J. L., Fernandez Lucas, M., & Marcen, R. (2000). Differences between blood flow as indicated by the hemodialysis blood roller pump and blood flow measured by an ultrasonic sensor. *Nephron,* Vol.85, No.2, (Jun), pp.(142-147), 0028-2766

Testa, A., Dejoie, T., & Lecarrer, D. (2010). Reduction of free immunoglobulin light chains using adsorption properties of hemodiafiltration with endogenous reinfusion. *Blood Purif,* Vol.30, No.1, pp.(34-36), 0253-5068,1421-9735(e)

Testa, A., Gentilhomme, H., & Le Carrer, D. (2006). In vivo removal of high- and low-molecular-weight compounds in hemodiafiltration with on-line regeneration of ultrafiltrate. *Nephron Clin Pract,* Vol.104, No.1, pp.(c55-60), 1660-2110,1660-2110(e)

Tiranathanagul, K., Yossundharakul, C., & Techawathanawanna, N. (2007). Comparison of middle-molecule clearance between convective control double high-flux hemodiafiltration and on-line hemodiafiltration. *Int J Artif Organs,* Vol.30, No.12, (Dec), pp.(1090-1097), 0391-3988,1724-6040(e)

Tsuruta, K., Andoh, F., & Kurahara, I. (1994). A simple method for clinical application of push/pull hemodiafiltration. *Contrib Nephrol,* Vol.108, pp.(71-78), 0302-5144,1662-2782(e)

Usuda, M., Shinzato, T., & Sezaki, R. (1982). New simultaneous HF and HD with no infusion fluid. *Trans Am Soc Artif Intern Organs,* Vol.28, pp.(24-27), 0066-0078

Vanholder, R., De Smet, R., & Gervasio, R. (1991). In vivo solute elimination of paired filtration dialysis. *Int J Artif Organs,* Vol.14, No.1, (Jan), pp.(23-27), 0391-3988

Vaslaki, L., Major, L., & Berta, K. (2006). On-line haemodiafiltration versus haemodialysis: stable haematocrit with less erythropoietin and improvement of other relevant blood parameters. *Blood Purif,* Vol.24, No.2, pp.(163-173), 0253-5068,1421-9735(e)

von Albertini, B., Miller, J. H., & Gardner, P. W. (1984). High-flux hemodiafiltration: under six hours/week treatment. *Trans Am Soc Artif Intern Organs,* Vol.30, pp.(227-231), 0066-0078

von Albertini, B., Miller, J. H., & Gardner, P. W. (1985). Performance characteristics of the hemoflow F 60 in high-flux hemodiafiltration. *Contrib Nephrol,* Vol.46, pp.(169-173), 0302-5144,1662-2782(e)

Ward, R. A., Schmidt, B., & Hullin, J. (2000). A comparison of on-line hemodiafiltration and high-flux hemodialysis: a prospective clinical study. *J Am Soc Nephrol,* Vol.11, No.12, (Dec), pp.(2344-2350), 1046-6673,1533-3450(e)

Weber, V., Linsberger, I., & Rossmanith, E. (2004). Pyrogen transfer across high- and low-flux hemodialysis membranes. *Artif Organs,* Vol.28, No.2, (Feb), pp.(210-217), 0160-564X,1525-1594(e)

Weissinger, E. M., Kaiser, T., & Meert, N. (2004). Proteomics: a novel tool to unravel the patho-physiology of uraemia. *Nephrol Dial Transplant,* Vol.19, No.12, (Dec), pp.(3068-3077), 0931-0509,1460-2385(e)

Woods, H. F. & Nandakumar, M. (2000). Improved outcome for haemodialysis patients treated with high-flux membranes. *Nephrol Dial Transplant,* Vol.15 Suppl 1, pp.(36-42), 0931-0509,1460-2385(e)

Yamamoto, K., Hiwatari, M., & Kohori, F. (2005). Membrane fouling and dialysate flow pattern in an internal filtration-enhancing dialyzer. *J Artif Organs,* Vol.8, No.3, pp.(198-205), 1434-7229

7

Optical Dialysis Adequacy Monitoring: Small Uremic Toxins and Contribution to UV-Absorbance Studied by HPLC

Kai Lauri[1], Jürgen Arund[1], Jana Holmar[1], Risto Tanner[1,2], Merike Luman[3] and Ivo Fridolin[1]

[1]Department of Biomedical Engineering, Technomedicum, Tallinn University of Technology,
[2]Laboratory of Chemical Physics, National Institute of Chemical Physics and Biophysics,
[3]Department of Dialysis and Nephrology, North Estonia Medical Centre,
Estonia

1. Introduction

Uremic toxicity is described as a clinical picture resulting from impaired renal elimination and accumulation of uremic toxins in the body. Uremic toxins can be classified as small water-soluble compounds, middle molecules and protein-bound compounds. A long list of possible uremic toxins has been identified in recent decades. Under normal conditions these compounds are excreted by healthy kidneys. If kidney function fails, waste products accumulate in the blood and in the body. Dialysis treatment replaces some kidney functions through diffusion (waste removal) and ultrafiltration of fluid across a semi-permeable membrane, which is a thin layer of material with holes or pores of various sizes. A deeper understanding about the accumulation and removal mechanisms of the retained solutes during care of renal insufficiency is needed (Eloot, 2008; Eloot, 2007). This understanding would be especially informative with respect to predicting the mode of action of uremic toxins and their specific role in complications associated with dialysis or ureamia, but also with cardiovascular disease and inflammation (Vanholder, et al., 2008; Vanholder, 2003). The methods contributing to the identification, characterisation and evaluation of uremic retention solutes could be assessed in order to ensure dialysis adequacy and quality (Vanholder, 2005). The choice of the correct concentration of potential uremic toxins is still an unresolved issue (Vanholder, 2003). In everyday clinical practice, uremic components are not examined due to the measurement of most uremic components using the available laboratory methods being difficult and complex. A number of standard biochemical techniques are used in clinical laboratories, but there is no universal methodology. In addition, some chromatographic methods have been developed which explore uremic retention solutes.

Dialysis efficiency and quality has been an important issue accompanied by optimisation and the best outcome of the treatment of chronic end stage renal disease for many years. In connection to this, online monitoring of the dialysis dose has been suggested as an effective way of improving treatment quality. The concept of online monitoring is based on the real-time measurement of chemical signals coming from the patient. This enables the early recognition of signs of intolerance and allows for early intervention. Despite the first online monitors of dialysis doses being available today, it is essential to monitor the patient's condition during the dialysis session and, if necessary, change some conditions of dialysis treatment (e.g. time) more specifically considering uremic toxins with various characteristics and elimination profiles.

The aim of this chapter is to describe and assess performance of optical dialysis adequacy monitoring technique related to the removal of uremic retention solutes during dialysis. The assessment is based on the high performance liquid chromatography (HPLC) profiles of the serum and the spent dialysate connected to the origin of the cumulative and integrated UV absorbance arising from the contribution of uremic retention solutes - chromophores, among them probably several uremic toxins.

2. Dialysis adequacy and online monitoring

Dialysis adequacy means providing a sufficient amount of dialysis treatment to maintain a uremic patient in the best condition. The goal of qualitatively treated dialysis is to prevent complications due to uremic toxicity.

Some recent studies are reviewed suggesting that uremic toxins are involved in the progression of renal failure and are at least partially removed by hemodialysis (Lesaffer, 2000; Eloot, 2008; Vanholder, 2003). The efficiency of a dialysis session has been estimated through concentration of uremic toxins measured before and after the dialysis session. A classic marker of the dialysis dose and adequacy is a small molecule urea.

Two methods are generally used to assess dialysis adequacy: URR and Kt/V. The urea reduction ratio (URR) is based on tests of blood urea, by measuring the levels before and after treatment to show how much has been removed. The Kt/V is mathematically related to the URR and can be derived from it (NKF-DOQI, 2006). In a simplified model of urea removal from a fixed volume with no urea generation, Kt/V is related to URR as follows:

$$Kt/V = -\ln (1 - URR) \tag{1}$$

In general, this method of dialysis adequacy is based on pre- and post-dialysis measurements of urea concentration. Online methods are considered to be more accurate than methods based on pre- and post-dialysis urea concentrations and have been found to be better suited to clinical routines. Online monitoring of the dialysis dose has been suggested as a valuable tool in ensuring adequate dialysis prescription (Locatelli, 2005).

3. Optical dialysis online monitoring

Two optical techniques have made progress toward clinical use over the past ten years – namely the ultraviolet (UV) absorbance and near infrared (NIR) techniques. The experimental results indicate very good correlation between UV absorbance and several small solutes such as urea, creatinine and uric acid in the spent dialysate and in the blood for every individual treatment at a fixed wavelength of 285 nm (Fridolin, 2002). Good correlation between UV absorbance and a small removed waste solute such as urea enables the determination of Kt/V for urea (Fridolin, 2003). The NIR method can measure urea directly using signal processing of the raw NIR spectra (Cho, 2008; Eddy, 2001; Eddy, 2003).

To implement NIR technology as a simple and robust sensor based on Fourier transform near-infrared (FT-NIR) spectrometer or acousto optical tunable filter (AOFT) based spectrometer is far more complicated because of the underlying optical principle, in which interference or diffraction is utilised (Jensen, 2002; Cho, 2008). The UV method is more straightforward and is not as demanding considering the source and detector characteristics and other technological modules. The UV method has recently been commercialised as a monitoring tool for dialysis dose in terms of the urea-based parameters, Kt/V and URR. Validation studies of the system have shown that the results with UV technology are indistinguishable from blood based Kt/V (Castellarnau, 2010).

An optical dialysis online monitoring system utilising UV absorbance has been developed for the continuous monitoring of the toxins eliminated by the spent dialysate. This system represents a spectrophotometer connected to the fluid outlet of the dialysis machine. All spent dialysate passes through a specially designed optical cuvette. The transmitted light intensity of the spent dialysate is measured. All substances - chromophores - absorbing the UV-radiation at a particular wavelength, give the total online UV absorbance curve. The schematic clinical set-up of online monitoring experiments is shown in Figure 1.

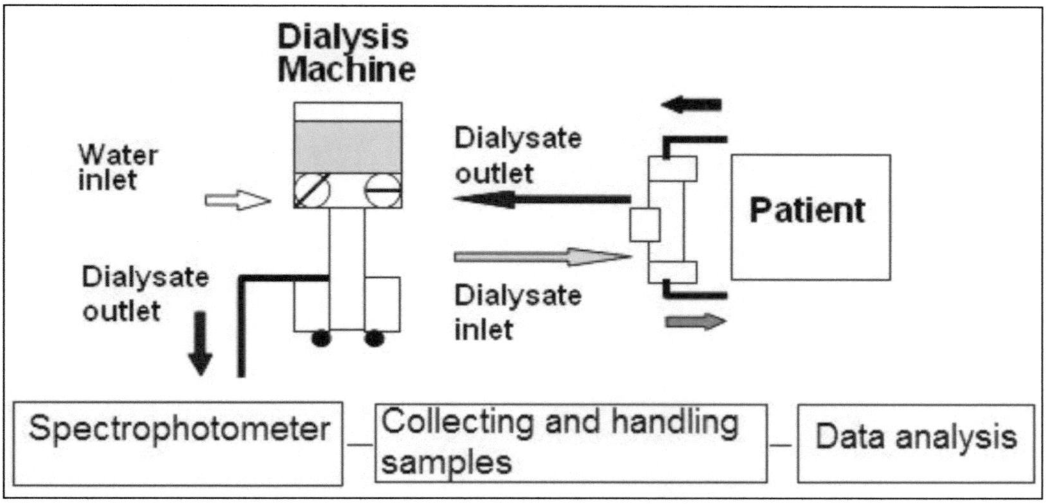

Fig. 1. Clinical experimental set-up and sample analysis

The obtained UV absorbance values are processed and presented on the computer screen by a PC incorporated in the spectrophotometer using special software. The absorbance A of a solution, obtained by the spectrophotometer using the pure dialysate as the reference solution, is determined as:

$$A = \log \frac{I_r}{I_{r+s}} \tag{2}$$

where I_r is the intensity of transmitted light through the reference solution (pure dialysate) and I_{r+s} is the summated intensity of transmitted light through the reference solution containing the solutions under study (pure dialysate + waste products from the blood). The absorbance is measured in arbitrary units (a.u.). A sampling frequency at two samples per minute is usually sufficient, but can be much higher (e.g. if a more detailed curve is desired or noise reduction is necessary).

The examples of two online signals measured at 280 nm from two different dialysis treatments are shown in Figure 2. The UV absorbance is higher at the beginning of treatment because of the high concentration of metabolic waste products in the body fluids. When the waste products are removed from the blood the UV absorbance decreases during the dialysis session. The times at which the blood and dialysate samples were collected are also shown in this figure. Blood samples were drawn before the start of dialysis treatment (B_{start}) and immediately after the treatment (B_{end}). Dialysate samples were taken 10 minutes after the start of the dialysis session (D_{start}) and at the end of the treatment (D_{end}) (210 or 240 minutes).

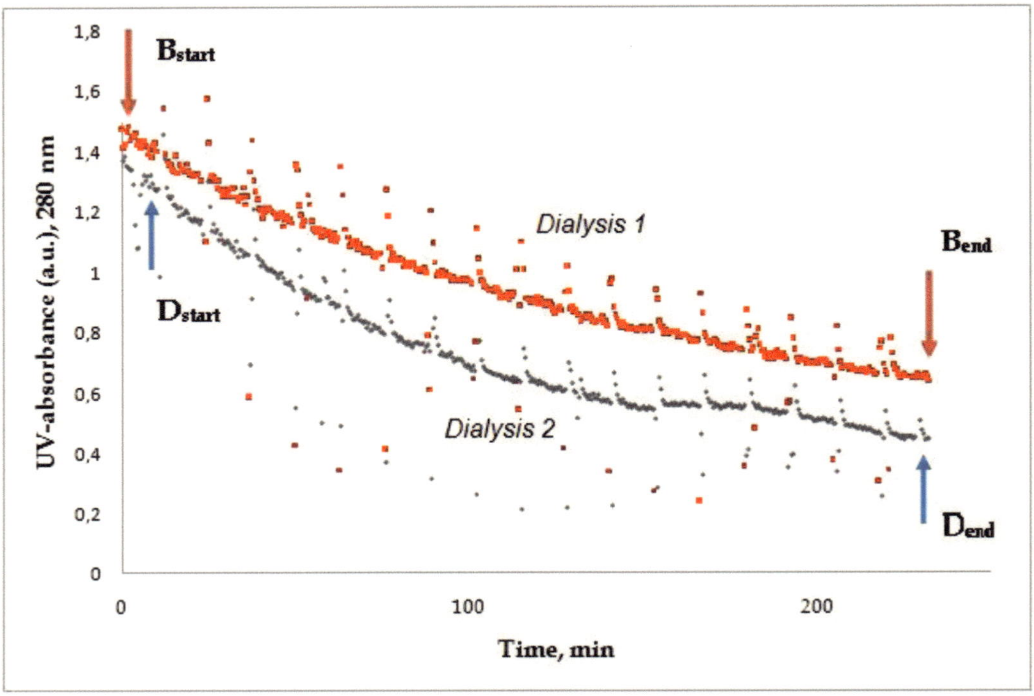

Fig. 2. Example of two different online UV absorbance measurements (at 280 nm). Time points when the samples were taken for later analysis are as follows: D_{start} - dialysate sample collected 10 minutes after start of hemodialysis, D_{end}- dialysate sample collected at the end of hemodialysis, B_{start} – blood sample collected before dialysis session, B_{end} – blood sample collected at the end of hemodialysis

This figure presents a classic picture of UV absorbance signals obtained by the optical online dialysis dose monitor, which can be used for estimation of uremic solutes removal.

As seen from Figure 2, the UV absorbance curves are somewhat different. The exponential decrease of the UV absorbance curve represents the elimination rate of the all UV-absorbing compounds - chromophores - which varies from patient to patient and from treatment to treatment. Good correlation between the UV absorbance measured in the spent dialysate and the concentration of several uremic retention solutes, both in the spent dialysate and in the blood of the dialysis patients, has been previously shown (Fridolin, 2002). For these reasons the origin of the cumulative and integrated UV absorbance arising from the contribution of uremic retention solutes, among them probably several uremic toxins, should be investigated.

4. HPLC as an analysis tool for biological samples

High performance liquid chromatography (HPLC) is a technique of analytical chemistry which can separate and identify the components of a mixture of different chemical compounds in liquid solution. The reversed-phase HPLC technique is the most commonly used form of HPLC. This method is recommended as a sensitive, accurate and reproducible tool for qualitative and quantitative analysis of aqueous samples (Vanholder, 2001). Furthermore, the use of ambient temperature in reversed-phase columns makes it possible to investigate the many non-volatile or thermally unstable compounds commonly found in biological samples. The principle involved in HPLC testing enables the separation of compounds in a mixture more efficiently and faster than that of traditional column chromatography.

In general, the HPLC system consists of two essential components - a stationary phase and a mobile phase. The stationary phase is a column packed with small solid sorbent particles and where the separation of different compounds takes place. The mobile phase is a flowing liquid (solvent) that transports the compounds from the sample through the stationary phase. Thus, the compounds of the mixture travel at different rates due to their relative affinities with the solvent and stationary phase. Separation of compounds in the stationary phase occurs with slight differences in chemical properties, such as chemical polarity and size of non-polar groups.

Figure 3 is a simple block diagram illustrating the main components of a modern HPLC. A system consists of several units: pumping, sample-injection, separation (column), detection and data-processing.

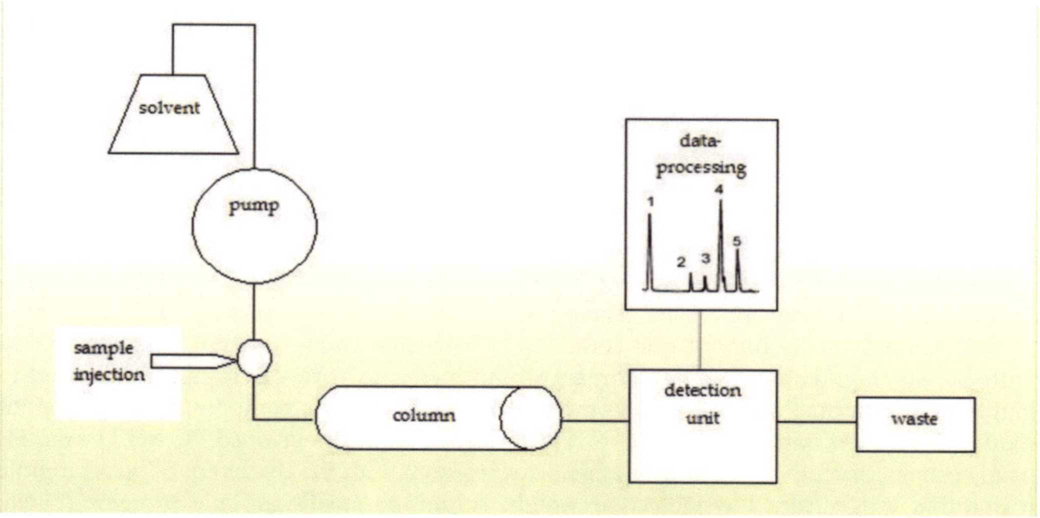

Fig. 3. Schematic reversed-phase HPLC method principle

The results of chromatographic analysis are known as chromatograms, where the signal intensity from the detector is recorded on the time axis. For HPLC there are several different detection methods; the most popular are optical. An ultraviolet-visual light (UV-VIS) absorption detector is the main optical detection method. This detector is effective in the detection of components with an absorption wavelength of 400 nm or less in the ultraviolet region. There are three types of UV-VIS detectors: a fixed wavelength detector; a variable wavelength detector; and a diode array detector (DAD). However, in modern HPLC systems DAD is commonly used, which in addition to the UV-VIS signal offers the ability to produce an absorption spectrum for every time slice during the chromatogram. A DAD detects the absorption in the UV to VIS region. Using the DAD, absorption on a large number of wavelengths can be measured simultaneously. This enables us to select the best wavelengths for actual analysis. Additionally, one of the advantages of DAD is that it allows us to detect sufficiently pure peaks. Often the peak shape itself does not reveal that it actually corresponds to two or even more components. In such a case, absorbance rationing on several wavelengths is particularly helpful in deciding whether the peak represents a single compound or a composite peak. However, compared with a UV-VIS detector, the DAD is susceptible to changes, such as lamp fluctuations, and noise is large because the amount of light is small.

For those compounds which fluoresce or which exhibit an appropriate fluorescence due to derivatisation, a fluorescence detector is the most sensitive of the existing modern HPLC detectors. Its sensitivity is 10-1000 times higher than that of the UV detector for strong UV-absorbing materials. Fluorescence detectors are very specific and selective compared to other optical detectors. A universal detector, but the least sensitive for non-ionic compound monitoring, is the refractive index detector. To estimate oxidisable and reducible compounds, the most suitable is the electrochemical detector.

Reversed-phase HPLC has been found to be useful in the analysis of uremic biofluids. A number of authors have reported the application of the HPLC method in the analysis of dialysate and serum samples already in several decades ago (Schoots, 1989; Schoots, 1982). Different detectors have been used. Some naturally fluorescent compounds have been separated and identified with a fluorescence detector, in both serum and haemodialysate (Niwa, 1993; Barnett, 1985; Swan, 1983). A liquid chromatographic method including a UV detector for detection of UV-absorbing solutes in uremic serum has been developed (Schoots, 1985; Senftleber, 1976; Knudson 1978). A fixed wavelength at 254 nm was mainly used in these studies. Additionally, several types of chromatographic methods, such as gas chromatography mass spectrometry (GC-MS), for the detection of uremic toxins has also been developed (Niwa, 1997; Niwa, 2009). Mass spectrometry (MS) has been applied to the identification and quantification of uremic toxins and uremia-associated modified proteins (Niwa, 2009). However, GC-MS cannot analyse highly polar, thermally labile and high-molecular weight compounds and usually requires sample preparation, such as extraction or derivation to make non-volatile compounds thermally stable and volatile. Compared with GC-MS, liquid chromatography mass spectrometry (LC-MS) can separate and identify highly polar, thermally labile or high-molecular weight mixture compounds and does not require derivation; sample preparation is also simple. Newly developed LC-MS techniques have been successfully applied to uremic toxin research with the discovery of novel uremic toxins that range from low-molecular weight solutes to small-molecule proteins (Niwa, 2011). This new analytical method is available today, opening up new horizons for uremic toxin identification detected earlier as unidentified HPLC peaks.

5. HPLC study of UV absorbance profiles

In order to explain the origin and potential of the online UV absorbance dialysis dose monitoring method, the HPLC method of analysing UV absorbance profiles was developed.

Ten uremic patients - three females and seven males (mean age 62.6 ± 18.6 years) - participated in the study. All of the patients were investigated over a course of 30 hemodialysis treatments. Three different polysulphone dialysers were used (Fresenius Medical Care, Germany): a low flux membrane dialyser F8 HPS (N=14), a low flux membrane dialyser F10 HPS (N=3) and a high flux membrane dialyser FX 80 (N=11). The elimination of toxins by the different types of semi-permeable membranes was also estimated.

Blood samples were drawn before the start of dialysis treatment (B_{start}) and immediately after the treatment (B_{end}) (Figure 2) using the slow flow/stop pump sampling technique. Blood was sampled into BD Vacutainer® Glass Serum Tube (red cup, Beckton Dickinson) and was allowed to clot. After centrifugation at 3000 r.p.m. the serum was ready for clinical chemistry analysis. Small molecules - creatinine (MW=113.12 Da), uric acid (MW=168.11 Da) and urea (MW=60.06 Da) - were measured at the Clinical Chemistry Laboratory of the North Estonia Medical Centre using standardised methods (Hitachi 912 autoanalyser, Roche, Switzerland). The accuracy for creatinine was 5%, for uric acid 2% and for urea 4%.

For HPLC analysis the additional pre-treatment of the centrifugated serum was necessary to release the blood proteins. The serum samples were purified from proteins by centrifuging with two different Microcon centrifugal filters (Millipore, USA): a YM-3 with cut-off 3 kDa and a YM-100 with cut-off 70 kDa. The aim of using different filters was to estimate the presence of different-sized molecules in the serum.

Dialysate samples were taken 10 minutes after the start of the dialysis session (D_{start}) and immediately after the treatment (D_{end}) (210 or 240 minutes) (Figure 2). Also, pure dialysate, used as the reference solution, was collected before each dialysis session, when the dialysis machine was being prepared and the conductivity was stable. For HPLC analysis, the dialysate samples were acidified with formic acid to pH 4.0. Sample sizes of 50 μL or 100 μL were used for chromatographic separation. Figure 4 presents a block diagram illustrating the collection and handling of blood and dialysate samples.

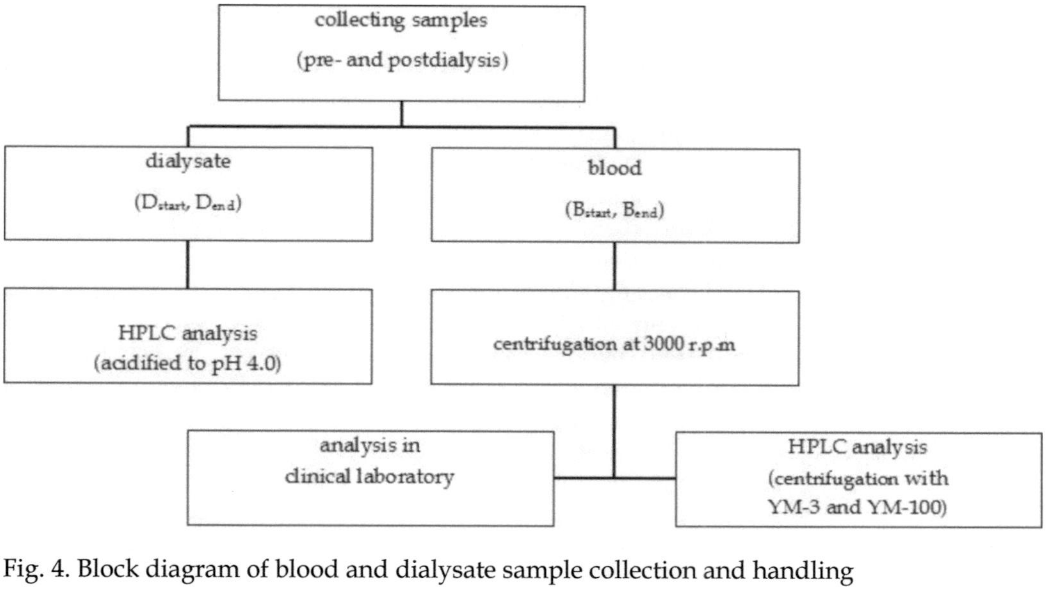

Fig. 4. Block diagram of blood and dialysate sample collection and handling

The HPLC instrumentation and tools were as follows: a diode array spectrophotometric detector (DAD, Perkin Elmer, USA); a manual injector (Rheodyne, USA); and a Zorbax C8 4.6 x 250 mm column (Du Pont Instruments, USA) with security guard KJO-4282 (Phenomenex, USA). The eluent was mixed with 0.05 M formic acid (pH 4.0), HPLC grade methanol and HPLC-S grade acetonitrile (Rathburn, Scotland), with a six-step gradient programme. The total flow rate of 1 mL/min was used continuously and the column temperature was adjusted to 30°C. The method followed has been described previously (Lauri, 2010). The chromatographic peaks were detected by the UV detector at wavelengths of 254 and 280 nm. The data was processed by means of Turbochrom WS and Turboscan 200 software from Perkin Elmer.

The decrease of the uremic retention solutes was estimated as the reduction ratio (RR) and assessed as a percentage (%). Thus, the RR of compounds was defined as a function of pre-dialysis concentration (C_{pre}) and concentration at the end of hemodialysis (C_{post}) and calculated as:

$$RR = \frac{C_{pre} - C_{post}}{C_{pre}} 100\% \tag{3}$$

5.1 Results

The results from the studies obtained by the HPLC method in order to analyse the UV absorbance profiles of the serum and dialysate samples are presented below. The results are presented as mean ± standard deviation (SD). A student's t-test was used to compare groups of values wherein $p < 0.05$ was considered significant. Pearson's correlation coefficient (r) between the UV absorbance from HPLC and online monitoring versus concentration of the substances in the blood was investigated. Samples taken at times coinciding with the self-tests or alarms of the dialysis machine were excluded (3 of 60 dialysate samples). Some sessions were excluded due to the technical failure of the spectrophotometer (3 of 30 sessions) and due to laboratory errors (3 of 30 sessions). The data analyses were performed in Microsoft Excel 2003 (for Windows).

The characteristic HPLC profiles of the spent dialysate at the start of the dialysis session (D_{start}) and at the end (D_{end}) are presented in Figure 5. When comparing the start and end values, the decrease in the height of the peaks (due to solute removal from the blood and into dialysate during dialysis) can be clearly seen.

As can be seen from this figure, a number of higher prevalent peaks can be observed from the HPLC profiles indicating the presence of chromophores, which are the main cause of cumulative and integrated UV absorbance. The highest peak on the HPLC profile is detected as uric acid causing a substantial amount of UV absorbance.

Figure 6 shows the HPLC chromatograms of the serum (filter YM-3 with cut-off 3 kDa) measured on wavelengths of 254 nm and 280 nm. Identified HPLC peaks, such as creatinine, uric acid (the highest contribution), hypoxanthine, indoxyl sulphate and hippuric acid, are shown. Absorbing spectra of two unknown persistent peaks (P1 and P2) were identified at retention times (RT) of 15.46 and 15.82 min.

Some chromophores, such as P2, creatinine, hypoxanthine and hippuric acid, give higher peaks on a wavelength of 254 nm, while P1 and indoxyl sulphate are better identified on a wavelength of 280 nm. This is due to the absorbing spectrum characteristics of the UV chromophores. This confirms the results obtained by the spectrophotometric analysis in this UV region.

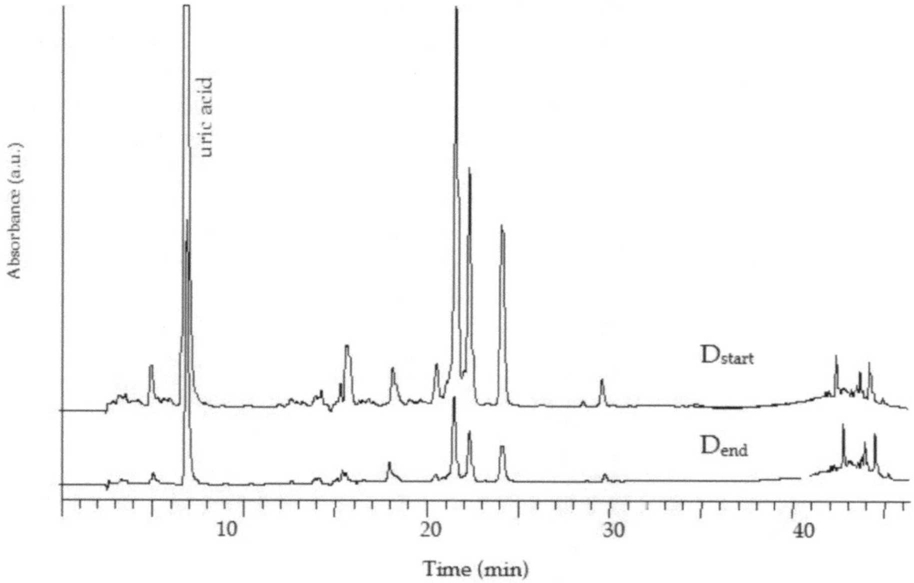

Fig. 5. Characteristic HPLC profiles of spent dialysate monitored on a wavelength of 280 nm; D_{start} - dialysate sample collected 10 minutes after start of hemodialysis, D_{end} - dialysate sample collected at the end of hemodialysis

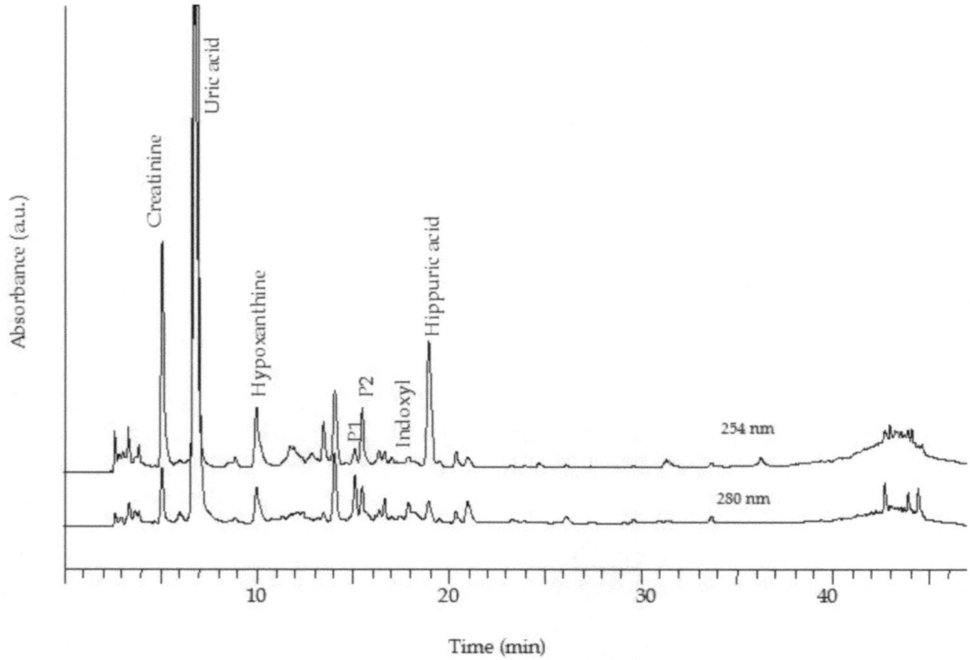

Fig. 6. Characteristic HPLC profiles of serum monitored on different wavelengths. Blood samples were collected before the dialysis session (B_{start}) and monitored on wavelengths of 254 nm and 280 nm. Detected HPLC peaks - uremic toxins - are presented.

As seen from Figure 6, around ten peaks on the HPLC profiles can be selected forming the major part of the total HPLC signal. As a result of this, the total area of the ten main peaks (Top 10 area %) was estimated. The comparison for Top 10 area % in the serum and dialysate is presented in Figure 7. The contribution of ten main peaks forms approximately 80-90% of all HPLC peaks in both spent dialysate and serum. However, there is a difference in the number of peaks on different wavelengths. In comparison with the 254 nm wavelength, the Top 10 area % on the 280 nm wavelength is higher. According to the HPLC profiles obtained (Figure 5 and 6), the largest contribution to Top 10 area % on the 280 nm wavelength originates from the small water-soluble non-protein-bound uremic toxin uric acid. Additionally, there was no significant difference between the serum results filtered with different type of filter cut-off (3 kDa and 70 kDa) ($p < 0.05$).

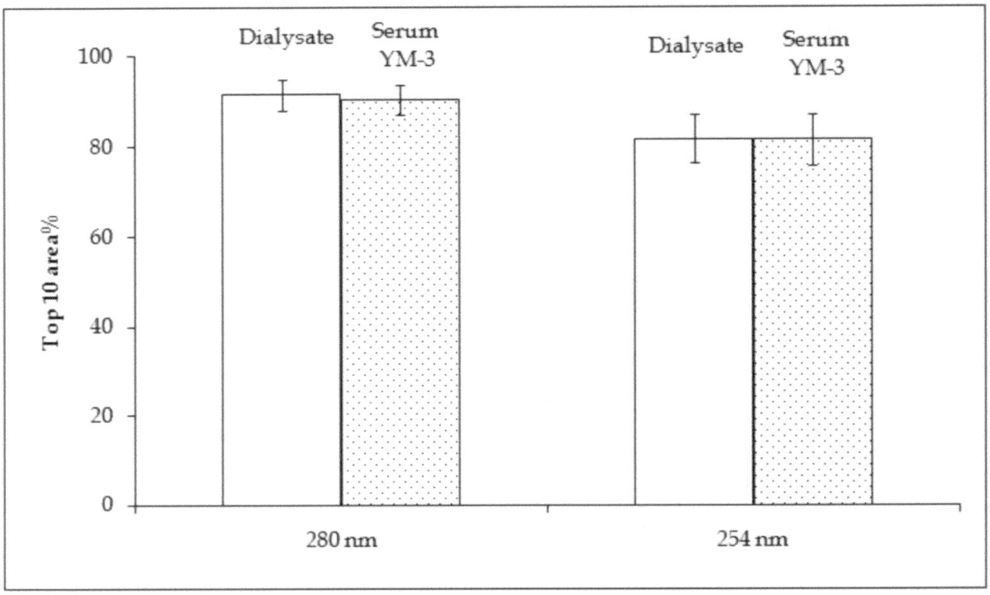

Fig. 7. Comparison of Top 10 area % on wavelengths of 254 nm and 280 nm in serum (filter YM-3 with cut-off 3 kDa) and spent dialysate

The RR of the detected chromatographic solutes was estimated. Table 1 presents the comparison of the RR (%) of solutes and all HPLC UV absorbance peaks on wavelengths of 254 nm and 280 nm in serum and for the online UV absorbance at 280 nm in the spent dialysate for different types of membranes: low flux (F8 HPS, F10 HPS) and high flux (FX80). There was no significant difference between the results for RR of low flux and high flux membranes ($p < 0.05$).

Hippuric acid had the highest RR, while the small water-soluble compound hypoxanthine and protein-bound solute indoxyl sulphate had the lowest RR. The RR of all HPLC Ppeaks at 280 nm was similar to uric acid and urea and higher than the RR of online UV absorbance at 280 nm and creatinine. At the same time, the RR of all HPLC peaks at 254 nm and P2 were lower than uric acid and urea. Online UV absorbance at 280 nm, creatinine and P2 were all removed in a statistically similar way ($p < 0.05$) and had lower RR than uric acid, urea and all HPLC peaks at 280 nm.

	RR (%)	
	Low flux	High flux
Hippuric acid	75.1 ± 11.5 (N=15)	68.1 ± 9.4 (N=10)
Uric acid	67.7 ± 8.5 (N=15)	65.6 ± 6.7 (N=15)
Urea	67.0 ± 8.7 (N=15)	63.2 ± 5.07 (N=15)
All HPLC peaks, 280 nm	65.2 ± 9.6 (N=15)	60.6 ± 7.9 (N=14)
P1	62.1 ± 13.0 (N=12)	61.0 ± 5.3 (N=7)
All HPLC peaks, 254 nm	60.2 ± 12.5 (N=14)	57.2 ± 7.7 (N=13)
P2	59.2 ± 17.5 (N=13)	51.6 ± 5.9 (N=12)
Online UV absorbance, 280 nm	58.1 ± 8.3 (N=15)	57.0 ± 10.4 (N=13)
Creatinine	58.2 ± 7.7 (N=15)	56.6 ± 5.4 (N=15)
Hypoxanthine	42.6 ± 16.0 (N=10)	46.1 ± 18.5 (N=8)
Indoxyl sulphate	42.1 ± 18.0 (N=13)	47.8 ± 14.0 (N=12)

Table 1. RR (%) of solutes and total area of all HPLC UV absorbance peaks on wavelengths of 254 nm and 280 nm in serum and RR of online UV absorbance at 280 nm in spent dialysate for different types of membranes

As the low flux and high flux membranes showed similar RR for every uremic solute, the results can be combined. Figure 8 present an illustrative comparison between the RR of serum uric acid, urea and creatinine measured in the clinical laboratory using standardised methods, all HPLC peaks measured on two different wavelengths (254 and 280 nm) and dialysate online UV absorbance measurement (280 nm).

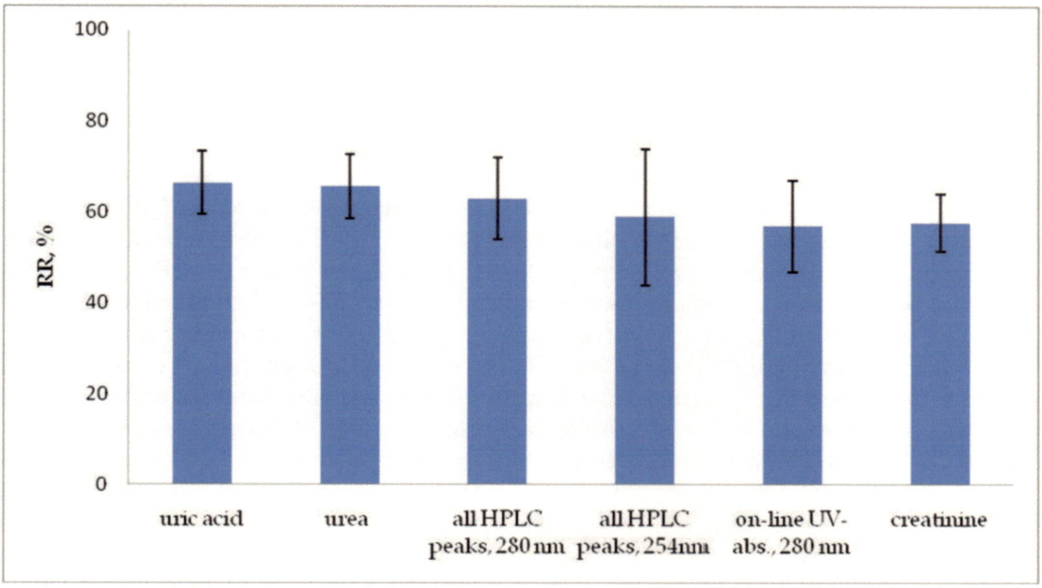

Fig. 8. Comparison of RR of small molecular uremic retention solutes (uric acid, urea and creatinine) in serum, RR of all HPLC serum peaks on two different wavelengths (254 and 280 nm) and spent dialysate online UV absorbance (280 nm)

The RR of urea and uric acid and the RR of all HPLC peaks at 280 nm are > 60%, while the RR of all HPLC peaks at 254 nm, of online UV absorbance measurement and creatinine are < 60%. Interestingly, the removal of urea and uric acid was statistically undifferentiated ($p > 0.05$). Figure 8 shows that the RR of serum creatinine is statistically different ($p < 0.05$) from the RR of serum urea and uric acid concentrations and from the RR of all HPLC peaks in the serum (at 280 nm), but not different from that of 254 nm. The RR of online measurement is comparable with the RR of creatinine and of all HPLC peaks at 254 nm and lower than the RR of urea, uric acid and all HPLC peaks at 280 nm ($p < 0.05$). At the same time, the RR of serum urea and uric acid are not statistically different; neither are they different from the RR of all HPLC peaks at 254 nm and 280 nm ($p < 0.05$).
The correlation coefficients between RR UV absorbance at 254 nm and at 280 nm from the total area of the HPLC peaks, from online monitoring at 280 nm and RR for certain substances with different molecular weights in spent dialysate and serum are shown in Table 2.

	Uric acid	Urea	Creatinine
RR of all HPLC peaks, 254 nm	0.755	0.811	0.812
RR of all HPLC peaks, 280 nm	0.933	0.881	0.926
Online UV absorbance, 280 nm	0.890	0.873	0.888

Table 2. Pearson correlation coefficients between RR of all HPLC peaks (254 nm and 280 nm), online absorbance at 280 nm and RR of uric acid, urea and creatinine in serum. The significance level of the results is $P<0.01$.

A high correlation for uric acid, urea and creatinine was obtained in both spent dialysate and serum. Some differences regarding 254 nm and 280 nm can be observed. However, urea does not represent as good a correlation as uric acid.

6. Discussion

From the investigations presented in this chapter we can conclude the following: (i) UV absorbance decreases during the dialysis session as the waste products are removed; (ii) a number of higher prevalent peaks can be detected in the HPLC profiles; (iii) some low-molecular-weight uremic solutes were identified from the HPLC profiles contributing to UV absorbance, and the main solute responsible for the UV absorbance is uric acid; (iv) a difference between HPLC profiles on wavelengths of 254 and 280 nm was found; (v) a higher number of detected HPLC peaks in the serum comparing to spent dialysate has been detected; (vi) the low flux and high flux membranes showed similar RR for all studied uremic solutes; and (vii) the classic dialysis adequacy marker urea and the uremic solute uric acid have good correlation with uremic retention solute elimination forming the UV absorbance curve.
Figures 2 and 5 show how the concentration of the uremic retention solutes - chromophores - decreases during a dialysis session in spent dialysate. UV absorbance as well as the height of the HPLC peaks are higher at the beginning of the treatment because of the high concentration of metabolic waste products in the body fluids and UV absorbance is lower at the end of the dialysis session. This demonstrates the possibility of following a single dialysis session continuously and to monitor deviations during treatment using a UV absorbance online monitor. This enables us to estimate the dialysis efficiency and adjust the treatment settings if needed.

A number of higher prevalent HPLC peaks representing chromophores can be observed (Figure 5 and 6). This indicates that there is a group of compounds, among them several uremic toxins, which are the main cause of cumulative and integrated UV absorbance. The 10 main peaks formed app. 80-90% of the total area of all HPLC peaks; some of these are small molecular weight uremic toxins such as uric acid, creatinine, hippuric acid and indoxyl sulphate. The variations in the number of HPLC peaks depending on hemodialysis treatments and patients have been demonstrated in earlier studies (Schoots, 1982; Vanholder, 1992). The difference between two dialysis sessions may arise as shown in Figure 2, because of the different composition and removal of the uremic retention solutes contained in spent dialysate. When comparing the HPLC profiles of the spent dialysate in Figure 5 and those of the serum in Figure 6, more peaks are detected in the serum. Thus, not all solutes in serum are transported to dialysate and removed through the semi-permeable membrane.

The number of detected HPLC peaks at 254 nm and 280 nm is also demonstrated in Figure 6 and 7. The difference in the number of detected HPLC peaks on the wavelengths of 254 nm and 280 nm arises due to the characteristic absorbing spectra of the UV chromophores. The absorption of many components is higher on the wavelength of 254 nm than 280 nm. This confirms the results obtained via the spectrophotometric analysis in this UV region (Fridolin, 2003). However, the studies of relations between UV and small water soluble molecules such as urea and uric acid indicated that the wavelength of 280 nm may be preferred for online measurements when small water soluble molecules should be estimated. On this wavelength a relatively strong linear relationship exists between UV absorbance and concentrations of urea, creatinine and uric acid (Fridolin, 2002; Uhlin, 2003). While the contribution of uric acid forms a considerable part of the total area of HPLC peaks, uric acid plays an important role in online UV absorbance dialysis dose monitoring. Interestingly, the removal of urea and uric acid was statistically undifferentiated ($p > 0.05$). This information gives us alternative possibilities to use other components and methods to monitor urea reduction (URR) in a single hemodialysis session.

Additionally, the low flux and high flux membranes showed no different removal of the studied small molecule uremic toxins as presented in earlier studies (Lesaffer, 2000). In this study it was found that the cellulose triacetate and polysulphone HF membranes removed similarly classical markers and protein-bound liphophilic solutes as an LF polysulphone membrane. Parallel results were obtained even with the concentrations corrected using a correction factor based on the total protein concentration at the start and at the end of dialysis as used by Lesaffer et al. (Lesaffer, 2000). Furthermore, there was no statistical difference between intradialytic start-end values, and removal efficiency for the LF and HF membranes estimated by the total area of HPLC peaks at 254 nm and 280 nm in the serum and online UV absorbance at 280 nm in the spent dialysate. This indicates that UV absorbance follows the behaviour of UV-absorbing compounds - uremic toxins - which are the origin of total UV absorbance in serum and spent dialysate.

The RR values of different identified compounds, the total area of all HPLC UV absorbance peaks on the wavelengths of 254 nm and 280 nm in the serum and the RR of online UV absorbance at 280 nm in spent dialysate are presented in Table 1 and Figure 8. Taking into account the removal efficiency, a difference can be observed in the relation of UV absorbance to small water-soluble non-protein-bound solutes and to small protein-bound solutes such as indoxyl sulphate. The small non-protein-bound solutes uric acid and urea showed a far more substantial decrease of concentration than creatinine being statistically different ($p < 0.05$) from the RR of serum uric acid and urea. The similar removal of urea and uric acid makes it possible to use other components and methods to monitor urea reduction during a single hemodialysis session. At the same time, the RR of creatinine is statistically different ($p < 0.05$) from the RR of all HPLC peaks in the serum at 280 nm, but not different from that of 254 nm. The RR for online UV absorbance is lower compared to urea. Considering that RR (URR) is correlated to Kt/V (NKF-DOQI, 2006), this tendency is reported earlier, as the dialysis dose estimated by online UV absorbance was lower than Kt/V urea (Uhlin, 2003). The difference between the RR of all HPLC peaks in serum and online UV absorbance measurement (at 280 nm) in spent dialysate could be due to different chromophores in the serum and spent dialysate and because the serum was collected before and the dialysate sample 10 minutes after the start of dialysis. Moreover, the different binding of individual uremic retention solutes to serum proteins may modify percentage concentration changes of individual solutes in the course of haemodialytic treatment (Vanholder, 1992), supported by observations of decreased drug/protein interactions in uremic serum (De Smet, 1999).

The correlation analysis also provides additional insights into the removal characteristics of solutes and UV absorbance monitoring (Table 2). The RR of uric acid has the highest correlation for RR at 280 nm in both serum and spent dialysate, but not at 254 nm in serum. The explanation is the highest contribution of uric acid to UV absorbance compared to other chromophores at 280 nm (Figures 5 and 6). However, there are several other strong contributions from other compounds beside uric acid at 254 nm, and therefore the correlation is lower. The outcome in Table 2 is confirmed by comparing the millimolar extinction coefficients versus wavelengths for uric acid (Vasilevsky, 2005). A higher value of the extinction coefficient corresponds to the higher correlation for RR of uric acid at 280 nm.

The RR of urea is more related to RR at 280 nm both in serum and spent dialysate, but less so at 254 nm in serum (Fridolin, 2003). This means that relatively good correlation between the RR of UV absorbance and a particular solute may be achieved when the removal rate of a non-absorbing solute (e.g. urea) is similar to that of UV-absorbing substances during haemodialysis. This is also confirmed by very good correlation between several small molecular weight waste products and UV absorbance (Fridolin, 2002) and similar concentration changes during dialysis for several azotemic markers (e.g. urea, creatinine and uric acid) (Vanholder, 1992). The dominance of small molecular weight waste products among chromophores in serum and spent dialysate can be concluded because the number of detected HPLC peaks is not significantly different for serum filtered with a filter in cut-off 3 kDa and 70 kDa. Furthermore, it seems that the UV-absorbing solutes can be subject to similar corrections regarding distribution volume and intercompartmental equilibration rates, similar to urea, although not with exactly the same distribution and equilibration intercompartmental rates in the body as urea. This makes it possible to estimate the delivered dialysis dose in terms of Kt/V by monitoring UV absorbance in spent dialysate online (Uhlin, 2003).

The RR of creatinine demonstrates a high correlation for RR at 280 nm in both serum and spent dialysate. The reason could be similar removal of creatinine and other chromophores at 280 nm, where creatinine does not contribute significantly to UV absorbance (Figure 5).

As previous studies have shown, and as is confirmed by this work, the HPLC is a method which has its own place for the detection of uremic solutes in biological solutes. This is an effective method of studying accumulated metabolites in patients' blood and removed in dialysis. Identification of these metabolites gives us the opportunity to understand the cumulative and integrated UV absorbance curve utilised during optical dialysis dose online monitoring. The online methods are felt to be more accurate than methods based on pre- and post-dialysis urea concentrations, and to be better suited to clinical routine. Continuous monitoring of uremic retention solute concentrations during a dialysis session could be beneficial for the prevention of intradialytic morbidity and for the confirmation of dialysis adequacy.

7. Conclusions

This chapter contributes new information about the removal of uremic retention solutes during hemodialysis and the origin of the optical dialysis adequacy monitoring signal. The relationship between characteristics of the online UV absorbance curve measured during dialysis and the identified HPLC peaks in spent dialysate was investigated. It was demonstrated that the absorbance signal reflects the contribution of several UV-absorbing compounds in spent dialysate, with the strongest influence coming from the low-molecular-weight water-soluble non-protein bound compounds. Moreover, UV absorbance behaves more like small water-soluble non-protein-bound solutes than small protein-bound solutes. Monitoring the removal of compounds with different properties and elimination characteristics during various dialysis strategies adds knowledge of dialysis treatment and would be useful for future research in order to decrease complications related to dialysis quality and cardiovascular risk factors. Hopefully the online methods will add a new technique and methodology to the wide discussion about the quality and adequacy of dialysis, uremic toxicity and kidney functionality.

8. Acknowledgements

The authors wish to thank the nurses and technical staff who assisted us during our clinical experiments as well as the dialysis patients who kindly participated in the experiments. This study was supported by the Estonian Science Foundation (grant no. 8621), the Estonian targeted financing project SF0140027s07 and the European Union through the European Regional Development Fund.

9. References

Barnett, A.L. & Veening, H. (1985) Liquid-chromatographic study of fluorescent compounds in haemodialysate solutions, *Clinical Chemistry*, Jan.31(1), pp. 127-130

Castellarnau, A., Werner, M., Günthner, R. & Jakob, M. (2010). Real-time Kt/V determination by ultraviolet absorbance in spent dialysate: technique validation, *Kidney International*, 78, November (1), pp. 920-925

Cho, D. S., Olesberg, J.T., Flanigan, M.J. & Arnold, M. (2008). Online Near-Infrared Spectrometer to Monitor Urea Removal in Real Time During Hemodialysis, *Applied Spectroscopy*, Vol. 62, Issue 8, pp. 866-872

De Smet, R., Vogeleere, P. et al. (1999). Study by means of high-performance liquid chromatography of solutes that decrease theophylline protein binding in the serum of uremic patients, *Journal of Chromatography A.*, 847(1-2), pp. 141-153

De Smet, R., Dhondt, A., Galli, F., Waterloos, M.A. & Vanholder, R. (2007). Effect of the super-flux cellulose triacetate dialyser membrane on the removal of non-protein-bound and protein-bound uraemic solutes, *Nephrol Dial Transplant*, 22, pp. 2006-2012

Eddy, C.M. & Arnold, M.A. (2001). Near-infrared spectroscopy for measuring urea in hemodialysis fluids, *Clin Chem.*, 47 (7), pp. 1279-1286

Eddy, C. V., Flanigan, M. et al. (2003). Near-Infrared Spectroscopic Measurement of Urea in Dialysate Samples Collected During Hemodialysis Treatments, *Applied Spectroscopy*, 57(10), pp. 1230-6

Eloot, S., Torremans, A., De Smet, R., Marescau, B., De Deyn, PP., Verdonck, P. & Vanholder, R. (2007). Complex compartmental behavior of small water-soluble uremic retention solutes: evaluation by direct measurements in plasma and erythrocytes, *Am J Kidney Dis.*, 50, pp. 279-288

Eloot, S., Van Biesen, W., Dhondt, A., Van de Wynkele, H., Glorieux, G., Verdonck, P. & Vanholder, R. (2008). Impact of hemodialysis duration on the removal of uremic retention solutes, *Kidney International*, 73, pp. 765–770

Eknoyan, G., Beck, G.J., Cheung, A.K., et al. (2002). Effect of dialysis dose and membrane flux in maintenance hemodialysis, *N Engl J Med*, 347, pp. 2010–2019

Ficheux, A., Gayrard, N., et al. (2010). The use of SDS-PAGE scanning of spent dialysate to assess uraemic toxin removal by dialysis, *Nephrol Dial Transplan,* Dec 10

Fridolin, I., Magnusson, M. & Lindberg, L.-G. (2002). Online monitoring of solutes in dialysate using absorption of ultraviolet radiation: technique description, *Int J Artif Organs*, 25, pp. 748-761

Fridolin, I. & Lindberg, L.G. (2003). Online monitoring of solutes in dialysate using absorption of ultraviolet radiation - wavelength dependence, *Medical & Biological Engineering & Computing,* 41, pp. 263-270

Jensen, P. S. & Bak, J. (2002). Measurements of urea and glucose in aqueous solutions with dual-beam near-infrared Fourier transform spectroscopy, *Applied Spectroscopy*, 56(12), pp. 1593-1599

Kaplan, B., Cojocaru, M., Unsworth, E., Knecht, A. & Martin, B.M. (2003). Search for peptidic "middle molecules" in uremic sera: Isolation and chemical identification of fibrinogen fragments, *J Chromatogr B.*, 796, pp. 141–153

Knudson, E.J., Lau, Y.C., Veening, H. & Dayton, D.A. (1978). Time-concentration studies by high-performance liquid chromatography of metabolites removed during hemodialysis, *Clinical Chemistry,* Apr. 24(4), pp.686-91

Lauri, K., Tanner, R., Jerotskaja, J., Luman, M. & Fridolin, I. (2010). HPLC study of uremic fluids related to optical dialysis adequacy monitoring, *Int J Artif Organs,* 33 (2), pp. 96-104

Lesaffer, G., De Smet, R., Lameire, N., Dhondt, A., Duym, P. & Vanholder, R. (2000). Intradialytic removal of protein-bound uraemic toxins: role of solute characteristics and of dialyser membrane, *Nephrol Dial Transplant,* 15, pp. 50-57

Locatelli, F., Buoneristiani, U., Canaud, B., Khler, H., Petitclerc, T. & Zucchelli, P. (2005). Hemodialysis with online monitoring equipment: tools or toys?, *Nephrol Dial Transplant*, 20, pp. 22-33

Niwa, T. (1993). Phenol and p-cresol accumulated in uremic serum measured by HPLC with fluorescence detection, *Clinical Chemistry*, Vol 39, pp. 108-111

Niwa, T. (1997). Mass spectrometry in the search for uremic toxins. *Mass Spectrom Rev,*. Nov-Dec,16(6), pp. 307-32

Niwa, T. (2009). Recent progress in the analysis of uremic toxins by mass spectrometry, *J Chromatogr B Analyt Technol Biomed Life Sci.*, Sep 1, 877(25), pp. 2600-2606

Niwa, T. (2011). Update of uremic toxin research by mass spectrometry, *Mass Spectrometry Reviews*, 30 (3), pp. 510–521

NKF-DOQI (2006). Clinical practice guidelines for hemodialysis adequacy, *Am J Kidney Dis.*, 48, pp. 13-97

Olesberg, J.T., Arnold, M.A., et al. (2004). Online Measurement of Urea Concentration in Spent Dialysate during Haemodialysis,. *Clin Chem.*, 50(1), pp. 175-81

Schoots, A.C., Mikkers, F.E.P., et al. (1982). Characterization of Uremic "Middle Molecular" Fractions by Gas Chromatography, Mass Spectrometry, Isotachophoresis, and Liquid Chromatography, *Clin Chem.*, 28/1, pp. 45-49

Schoots, Ad.C., Homan, H.R., Gladdines, M.M, Cramers, C.A.M.G, De Smet, R. & Ringoir Severin, M. G. (1985). Screening of UV-absorbing solutes in uremic serum by reversed phase HPLC – Change of blood levels in different therapies, *Clinica Chimica Acta*, Volume 146, Issue 1, 28 February, pp. 37-51

Schoots, A.C, Peeters, J.A. & Gerlag, P.G. (1989). Effect of hemodialysis on serum concentrations of HPLC-analyzed accumulating solutes in uremia, *Nephron*, 53(3), pp. 208-217

Senftleber, F., Halline, A.G., Veenlng, H. & Dayton, D.A. (1976). Reversed-Phase Liquid-Chromatographic Analysis of Haemodialysate from Uremic Patients, *Clinical Chemistry*, 22 (9), pp. 1522-1527

Stiller, S., Al-Bashir A. & Mann H. (2001). Online Urea Monitoring during Hemodialysis: A Review, *Saudi Journal of Kidney Diseases and Transplantation*, 12 (3), pp- 364-374

Swan, J.S., Kragten, E.Y. & Veening, H. (1983). Liquid-chromatographic study of fluorescent materials in uremic fluids, *Clinical Chemistry*, Jul, 29(6), pp. 1082-1084

Uhlin, F., Fridolin, I., Lindberg, L.-G. & Magnusson, M. (2003). Estimation of delivered dialysis dose by online monitoring of the UV absorbance in the spent dialysate, *Am J Kidney Dis*, 41, pp. 1026-1036

Vanholder, R., De Smet, R.V. & Ringoir, S.M. (1992). Assessment of urea and other uremic markers for quantification of dialysis efficacy, *Clin Chem*, vol. 38, pp. 1429-1436

Vasilevsky, A.M. & Konoplyov, G.A.. (2005). Peculiar character of dialysate ultraviolet extinction spectra as an indicator of nucleic acid metabolism in humans, *Journal of Biomedical Optics*, 10(4), pp. 044026/1-7

Vanholder, R., De Smet, R. & Lameire, N.H. (2001). Redesigning the map of uremic toxins, *Contr. Nephrol.*, 133, pp. 42-70

Vanholder R., De Smet R., et al. (2003). Survival of Hemodialysis Patients and Uremic Toxin Removal, *Artificial Organs*, 27(3), pp. 218-223

Vanholder, R. et al. (2008). A Bench to Bedside View of Uremic Toxins, *J Am Soc Nephrol*, 19, pp. 863-870

Vanholder, R., Laecke, S. V., Verbeke, F., Glorieux, G. & Biesen, W.V. (2008). Uraemic toxins and cardiovascular disease: in vitro research versus clinical outcome studies, *NDT Plus*, 1, pp. 2-10

Vanholder, R. (2009). Effect of membrane permeability on survival of hemodialysis patients, *J Am Soc Nephrol*, 20, pp. 645–654

8

Influence of Online Hemodiafiltration on Hemoglobin Level, ESA-Dosage and Serum Albumin – A Retrospective, Multicenter Analysis

Roland E. Winkler, Peter Ahrenholz and Klaus Freivogel
Praxisverbund für Dialyse und Apherese, Rostock,
BioArtProducts GmbH, Rostock,
Analytica International GmbH, Lörrach,
Germany

1. Introduction

In renal replacement therapy (RRT) a wide range of uremic toxins have to be removed (Vanholder et al., 2003; Vanholder et al., 2008). It is well known that the combination of diffusive and convective dialysis strategies (online hemodiafiltration, olHDF) improves the removal of uremic toxins, i.e. middle molecules, hydrophobic substances and protein (albumin) bound materials (Krieter et al., 2005; Ahrenholz et al., 2004; Ronco et al., 1999; Kim, 1994; Testa et al., 2006; Meyer et al., 2005; Mandolfo et al., 2006; Kanter et al., 2008). In the presence of ultrapure dialysis fluid which is ultrafiltrated by endotoxin restraint systems (Weber et al., 2000; Canaud et al., 2001; Minetti et al., 1985; Hakim et al., 1984) and biocompatible high flux dialysis membranes the convective diffusive treatment significantly prevents the complement activation (Braun et al., 1995; Savica et al., 2006; Jorres et al, 1999; Hörl et al., 1986) in the first minutes of olHDF session and removes proinflammatory substances (cytokines) too (Bellomo et al., 1991; Filiopoulos et al., 2008; Haas et al., 2007; Libetta et al., 2007; Mariano et al., 2005). The intra and interdialytic inflammations are reduced (Ramirez et al., 2007; Ramirez et al., 2007; Carracedo et al., 2006). The suppressed inflammatory process during olHDF leads to an increasing serum albumin concentration via an increased synthesis rate. In spite of a varying albumin removal caused by different dialysis membranes with/without adsorptive character and pore size (Pichaiwong et al., 2006; Yamashita, 2007; Tomo et al., 2008; Winchester et al.,2003; Winchester et al., 2004) the albumin synthesis rate increases by absent inflammation (Giordano et al., 2001). It is shown that in olHDF the ESA dosage needed to reach the hemoglobin goal is reduced (Vaslaki et al., 2006; Bonforte et al., 2002; Eiselt et al., 2000). The efficacy of dialysis measured by single pool Kt/V could be improved (Ahrenholz et al., 1997; Ding et al., 2002). There is evidence of longer survival of patients treated by olHDF versus hemodialysis (HD) independently of dialysis dosage (Canaud et al., 2008; Panicchi et al., 2008). The cycling of hemoglobin levels depends on inflammatory episodes and malnutrition (Del et al., 2005; Brimble et al., 2005). This retrospective, non randomized, multicentre, descriptive clinical evaluation examined the influence of olHDF on hemoglobin concentration (Hb), ESA dosage (ESA), Hb variability (Hbvar), albumin and CRP.

2. Materials and methods

233 chronic hemodialysis patients were included in this clinical evaluation (dialysis center 1 (D1) n= 94, D2 n= 35, D3 n= 104 patients). 54.9% were male; the mean age was 63.8 years (range 22 - 89). The patients in all three centers were comparable with regard to gender distribution, mean age, mean time on dialysis, and distribution of underlying kidney disease. The clinical evaluation was carried out for 12 months retrospectively. Laborchemical parameters were estimated for hemoglobin (Hb) every 2 weeks (labanalyzer), CRP (turbidometry), albumin (alb; nephelometry) and ferritin (chemiluminescence technique) every three months. Serum iron (photometry) and transferrin (turbidometry) were necessary to calculate the transferrin saturation (every 4 weeks). Single pool kt/V was evaluated every 3 months with the Daugirdas technique (Daugirdas, 1993). Intraindividual variability of hemoglobin (Hbvar) was defined as the difference between minimal and maximal concentration (range) and by time to reach the target between Hb 6.8 mmol/l and 8.0 mmol/l within 9 months. Relevant changes in ESA dosages were defined as an elevation greater than two fold and lowering of a half of the ESA dosage, the end of ESA application or the start with more than 4200 U/week.
Hemodialysis (HD) was performed by MTS 5008 (Fresenius Medical Care), low flux dialyser FX8, FX10 (helixone, Fresenius Medical Care), Q_B 300 ml/min, Q_D 500 ml/min, ultrapure dialysis fluid, online hemodiafiltration (olHDF) by MTS 5008 (Fresenius Medical Care; automatic procedure with factor 1.2), high flux dialyser FX 60, FX80 (helixone, Fresenius Medical Care), Q_B 300 ml/min, Q_D 350.....360 ml/min, Q_S 51....60 ml/min, ultrapure dialysis fluid and Nikkiso DBB 05 (Nikkiso Medical Ltd.), high flux dialyser FDY 15 G (PEPA, Nikkiso Medical Ltd.), Q_B 300 ml/min, Q_D 700 ml/min, Q_S 60 ml/min, ultrapure dialysis fluid (Q_B... blood flow; Q_D...dialysate flow; Q_s...substitution flow). The group "mixed" contained patients started with HD and switched to olHDF (at least 6 months olHDF). We compared the mean values of collected serum parameters three times a month. Descriptive statistical evaluation was calculated by mean, standard deviation and significance by Wilcoxon test, correlation by Spearman rang correlation. The level of significance was defined as $p < 0.05$.

3. Results

The distribution of ESA applications in the three observed dialysis centers can be seen in table 1. Totally 185 of 233 patients received at least one ESA dosage. The mean value of ferritin was 538 mg/L. The transferrin saturation (TSAT) did not differ significantly in the observed dialysis units.

	Dialysis unit						Total	
	1		2		3			
	N	%	N	%	N	%	N	%
Application of ESA without ESA	37	39.4	4	11.4	7	6.7	48	**20.6**
At least 1 ESA dosage	57	60.6	31	88.6	97	93.3	185	**79.4**

Table 1. Application of ESA per dialysis unit and overall.

The mean weekly ESA dosage can be seen in table 2:

		Dialysis unit 1	2	3	Total
All patients	N	94	35	104	233
	Mean	3550	5934	9177	6420
	SD	4443	5316	8487	7129
	Min	0	0	0	0
	Median	1577	5077	6500	4692
	Max	18667	26769	46538	46538
Patients with at least one ESA dosage	N	57	31	97	185
	Mean	5855	6700	9840	8086
	SD	4365	5170	8409	7109
	Min	231	167	308	167
	Median	4714	5538	6769	6231
	Max	18667	26769	46538	46538

Table 2. Mean weekly ESA dosage

In nearly all patients (98.9%) an adjustment of ESA dosage was essential. Relevant changes in ESA dosages were defined as an elevation greater than two fold and lowering of a half of the ESA dosage, the end of ESA application or the start with more than 4200 U/week.
The mean value of Hb (measured per patient over the whole study time) was 7.35 mmol/l (Table 3). In patients without ESA application during the 12 months study the mean value of Hb was larger (7.66 mmol/l) in comparison to patients with ESA dosage (7.27 mmol/l).

			Dialysis unit 1	2	3	Total
Patients without ESA	Mean Hb	N	37	4	7	48
		Mean	7.63	7.76	7.74	**7.66**
		SD	0.46	0.61	0.63	0.49
		Min	6.7	6.9	7.2	6.7
		Median	7.5	8.0	7.5	7.5
		Max	8.8	8.3	8.8	8.8
At least one ESA dosage	Mean Hb	N	57	31	97	185
		Mean	7.38	7.09	7.25	**7.27**
		SD	0.41	0.52	0.53	0.50
		Min	6.2	6.0	5.1	5.1
		Median	7.5	7.2	7.4	7.4
		Max	8.6	8.4	8.3	8.6
Total	Mean Hb	N	94	35	104	233
		Mean	7.48	7.17	7.29	**7.35**
		SD	0.44	0.57	0.55	0.52
		Min	6.2	6.0	5.1	5.1
		Median	7.5	7.2	7.4	7.4
mmol/l		Max	8.8	8.4	8.8	8.8

Table 3. Mean Hb concentrations

Table 4 shows the intra-individual variability of hemoglobin (Hbvar):

			Dialysis unit			
			1	2	3	Total
ESA without ESA	Hb range (min-max)	N	37	4	7	48
		Mean	1.98	1.35	1.93	**1.92**
		SD	0.92	0.68	1.11	0.93
at least one ESA dosage	Hb range (min-max)	N	57	31	97	185
		Mean	2.20	1.74	2.41	**2.23**
		SD	0.73	0.85	0.88	0.86
Total	Hb range (min-max)	N	94	35	104	233
		Mean	2.11	1.70	2.37	**2.17**
		SD	0.81	0.83	0.90	0.88

Table 4. Means of haemoglobin variability

The relation between the treatment mode (HD, olHDF) and ESA dosage as well as Hb is shown in the tables 5 and 6:

			Dialysis unit			
			1	2	3	Total
HD	All patients	N	40	32	74	146
		Mean	3608	6132	8833	**6809**
		SD	5058	5511	8313	7293
	Patients with at least one ESA dosage	N	22	28	69	119
		Mean	6560	7009	9473	**8354**
		SD	5217	5339	8248	7234
HDF	All patients	N	15	.	4	19
		Mean	3515	.	7750	**4407**
		SD	4160	.	5535	4660
	Patients with at least one ESA dosage	N	9	.	4	13
		Mean	5859	.	7750	**6441**
		SD	3853	.	5535	4287
Mixed	All patients	N	39	3	26	68
		Mean	3505	3821	10378	**6147**
		SD	3960	1500	9441	7313
	Patients with at least one ESA dosage	N	26	3	24	53
		Mean	5257	3821	11243	**7887**
		SD	3775	1500	9314	7410

Table 5. Relationship between treatment mode and required weekly ESA dosage

Hb was larger in the olHDF group and the required ESA dosage to reach the Hb concentration lower (Hb olHDF 7.56± 0.35 mmol/l, HD 7.25± 0.52 mmol/l, p= 0.01; ESA/week olHDF 4407± 4660 U/l, HD 6809±7293 U/l, p= 0.1): Table 6.

			Dialysis unit			
			1	2	3	Total
Treatment mode						
HD	**Mean Hb [mmol/L]**	**N**	40	32	74	146
		Mean	7.37	7.16	7.23	**7.25**
		SD	0.43	0.59	0.53	0.52
HDF	**Mean Hb [mmol/L]**	**N**	15	.	4	19
		Mean	7.58	.	7.50	**7.56**
		SD	0.38	.	0.25	0.35
Mixed	**Mean Hb [mmol/L]**	**N**	39	3	26	68
		Mean	7.56	7.22	7.41	**7.49**
		SD	0.46	0.11	0.61	0.52
Total	**Mean Hb [mmol/L]**	**N**	94	35	104	233
		Mean	7.48	7.17	7.29	**7.35**
		SD	0.44	0.57	0.55	0.52

Table 6. Relationship between treatment mode and Hb value

In the olHDF group the intraindividual Hbvar was significantly lower than in HD (HD 0.66±0.28 mmol/l vs olHDF 0.53±0.16 mmol/l, p<= 0.05): Table 7.

				Dialysis unit			
				1	2	3	Total
HD	**All patients**	**Intra-individual standard deviation of the Hb-value**	**N**	40	32	74	146
			Mean	0.69	0.51	0.71	**0.66**
			SD	0.29	0.24	0.26	0.28
HDF	**All patients**	**Intra-individual standard deviation of the Hb-value**	**N**	15	.	4	19
			Mean	0.52	.	0.57	**0.53**
			SD	0.11	.	0.30	0.16

Table 7. Intra-individual standard deviation of the Hb-values as a function of the treatment mode

In the subanalysis the single pool Kt/V (spkt/V) was >1.2 on average in all centers. But there is a significant improvement of spKt/V for olHDF compared to HD (p = 0.04): Table 8:

			Dialysis unit			
			1	2	3	
HD	**Mean treatment efficacy (spkt/V)**	**N**				**Total**
		Mean	1.46	1.32	1.55	**1.48**
		SD	0.60	0.29	0.38	0.44
HDF	**Mean treatment efficacy (spkt/V)**	**N**	15	.	4	19
		Mean	1.57	.	1.82	**1.62**
		SD	0.17	.	0.52	0.28
Mixed	**Mean treatment efficacy (spkt/V)**	**N**	38	3	26	67
		Mean	1.48	1.16	1.45	**1.45**
		SD	0.24	0.04	0.31	0.27

Table 8. Single Pool Kt/V as a function of the treatment mode

Further analyses regarded the relationship between CRP and albumin. The tables 9 and 10 show the mean levels of CRP and albumin:

		Dialysis units			
		1	2	3	Total
Mean CRP [mg/l]	**N**	87	33	98	218
	Mean	15.82	14.77	13.58	**14.65**
	SD	19.48	8.75	9.67	14.30
	Min	3.6	4.5	3.1	3.1
	Median	10.2	13.1	10.4	10.6
	Max	160	47.6	40.5	160

Table 9. Mean CRP level per dialysis unit and overall

		Dialysis unit			
		1	2	3	Total
Mean albumin [g/l]	**N**	93	35	104	232
	Mean	40.28	39.44	38.81	**39.49**
	SD	3.10	2.17	2.84	2.93
	Min	30.4	35.8	31.0	30.4
	Median	40.5	39.6	39.0	39.6
	Max	47.1	43.7	45.9	47.1

Table 10. Mean albumin level per dialysis unit and overall

For all patients the Hb level was negatively correlated to CRP (r= - 0.24, p< 0.0005) and positively to Albumin (r= 0.30, p< 0.0001) and TSAT (r= 0.20, p< 0.005): see table 11:

Spearman Correlation Coefficients Prob > |r| under H0: Rho=0 Number of Observations		
	esamean	**hbmean**
crpmean CRP	0.08497 0.2115 218	-0.23764 0.0004 218
albmean Albumin	-0.23495 0.0003 232	0.30050 <.0001 232
tsatmean TSAT	-0.12875 0.0497 233	0.19808 0.0024 233

Table 11. Correlation of the total values for CRP, Albumin and TSAT with Hemoglobin

In a subanalysis we found significantly larger albumin levels and lower CRP concentrations in olHDF vs HD (albumin olHDF 40.63+/-2.23 g/l, HD 39.11± 2.76 g/l, p< 0.05; CRP olHDF 9.96± 8.28 mg/l, HD 16.07 ± 16.26 mg/l, p< 0.05): Tables 12 and 13:

			Dialysis unit			
			1	2	3	Total
Mode						
HD	albumin [g/l]	N	40	32	74	146
		Mean	39.89	39.35	38.58	**39.11**
		SD	3.10	2.11	2.72	2.76
HDF	albumin [g/l]	N	14	.	4	18
		Mean	40.74	.	40.24	**40.63**
		SD	2.32	.	2.17	2.23
Mixed	albumin [g/l]	N	39	3	26	68
		Mean	40.51	40.35	39.24	**40.02**
		SD	3.35	3.06	3.21	3.30

Table 12. Relationship between albumin levels and treatment mode

			Dialysis unit			
			1	2	3	Total
Mode						
HD	CRP [mg/l]	N	39	30	71	140
		Mean	18.56	15.52	14.94	**16.07**
		SD	26.70	8.82	10.05	16.26
HDF	CRP [mg/l]	N	12	.	2	14
		Mean	10.81	.	4.81	**9.96**
		SD	8.68	.	0.22	8.28
Mixed	CRP [mg/l]	N	36	3	25	64
		Mean	14.52	7.36	10.43	**12.59**
		SD	10.79	2.55	7.81	9.66

Table 13. Relationship between CRP levels and treatment mode

4. Discussion

Our retrospective analysis was performed in three different dialysis centers for 12 months. The D1 center had the largest percentage of patients treated with olHDF (olHDF+"mixed") (57 % in D1 vs. 9 % in D2, 29 % in D3). In D1 the lowest dosage of ESA to reach the Hb target was used (Table 2; D1 vs D2 $p= 0.003$; D1 vs D3 $p< 0.0001$), the smallest number of D1 patients were treated with ESA and the time in target was longer than in D2 and D3. In addition, it could be demonstrated that in D1 patients the frequency of adaptation of ESA dosage and Hbvar were reduced in comparison to the other centers.

Concerning the ferritin values and the transferrrin saturation (TSAT) there were no noticeable differences between the observed centers. But the subanalysis shows a positive correlation of the overall TSAT values with the Hb values ($p = 0.002$, see Table 11) and a negative one with the mean ESA consumption ($p = 0.05$). These results comply with the expectation because an improved Hb value is connected with a larger TSAT level and reduced ESA needs.

The treatment efficacy (single pool and equilibrated Kt/V; spKt/V, eKt/V), which was measured periodically in the 3 dialysis units, did not show any significant influence on ESA

dosage and Hb levels. But the subanalysis calculating the impact of the different treatment modes on Kt/V resulted in a significant increased spKt/V for olHDF treatments compared with HD (1.62±0.28 for olHDF versus 1.48±0.44 for HD; Table 8).
Interestingly the correlation analysis also shows a highly significant positive correlation of the mean albumin level with the mean Hb values ($p < 0.001$, Table 11) and a negative one with the mean ESA dosage ($p = 0.0003$). Simultaneously CRP is negatively correlated with Hb ($p = 0.0004$, Table 11).
The significant difference in albumin concentration most likely played the decisive role for ESA dosage and Hb level (Ward, 2005). It is known that in patients who underwent convective-diffusive treatment the ESA dosage could be reduced (Vaslaki et al., 2006; Bonforte et al., 2002; Eiselt et al., 2000). That observation was confirmed by our results, reaching an economically interesting level of savings in ESA costs: Fig. 1.

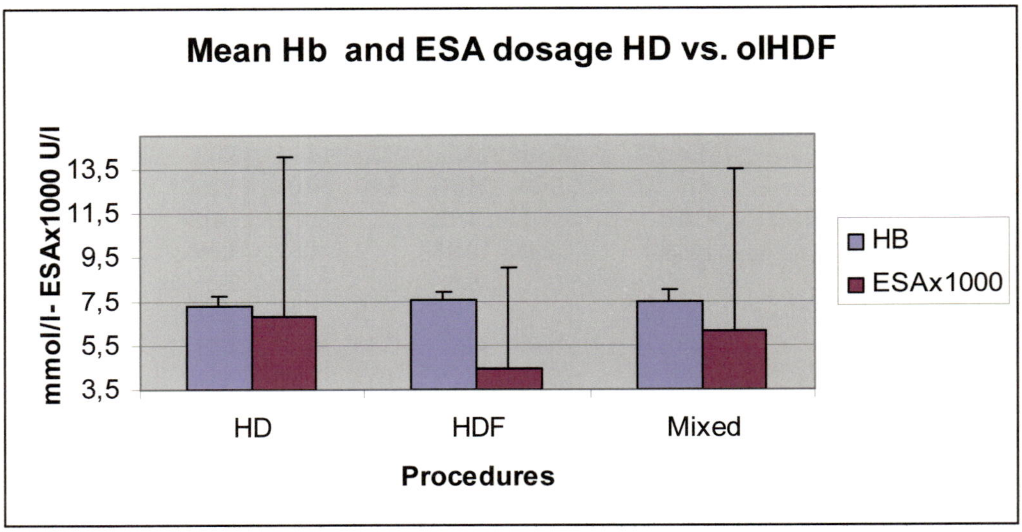

Fig. 1. Mean Hb level and ESA dosage HD vs. HDF (ESA: p=0.1, ns., Hb: p=0.01)

Typically, convective diffusive procedures are characterized by an additional removal of hydrophobic middle molecules and protein (albumin) bound uremic toxins depending on the membrane characteristics (hydrophobic areas, pore size, adsorptive properties, biocompatibility) (Ahrenholz et al., 2004; Panicchi et al., 2008). The loss of protein bound substances leads to a membrane determined loss of albumin during olHDF sessions (Ahrenholz et al., 2004; Samtleben et al., 2003; Combarnous et al., 2002). In low flux dialysis protein removal only occurs with adsorptive membranes (PMMA, polyacrilonitrile) with decreasing dialysis efficacy for water soluble toxins (Parzer et al., 1993). This removal of albumin can be compensated after a time of about 12 weeks in the absence of relevant inflammation (Ding et al., 2002; Kaysen et al., 1997). In chronic ambulant peritoneal dialysis protein losses are in-between 6 to 10 g/d and albumin losses up to 5 g/d over the peritoneal membrane (Kaysen et al., 1984).

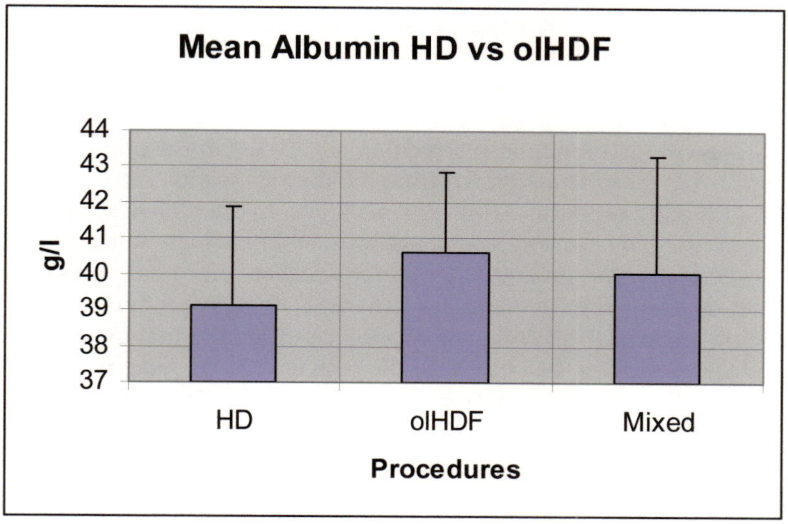

Fig. 2. Mean serum albumin concentration HD vs. olHDF (p=0.01)

Albumin losses during renal replacement procedures are generally thought of being unwanted, as low serum albumin correlates with poor outcome in dialysis patients. Therefore, olHDF, that technically spoken is an albumin-loosing therapy, might carry the danger of exposing the treated patients to threads associated with low albumin levels.

It is striking that in our analysis the olHDF group had the largest serum albumin concentration (Fig. 2, Table 12). All patients of the "mixed" group (containing patients that had switched from HD to olHDF) showed an increase in albumin level rather than a decrease.

Moreover, olHDF can remove proinflammatory substances such as cytokines (Bellomo et al., 1991; Lee et al., 2004). Again, we could confirm this phenomenon with lower CRP levels in the olHDF group vs. HD group (9.96+/- 8.28 mgl/l vs. HD 16.07+/- 16.26 mg/l, p=0.02), see Fig. 3, and Table 13:

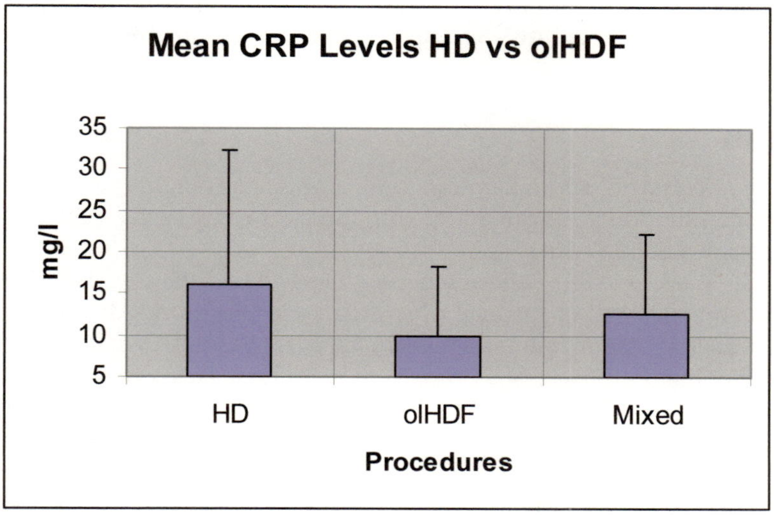

Fig. 3. Mean CRP concentration HD vs. olHDF (p=0.02)

Because albumin is a negative acute phase protein we can, in general, expect higher concentrations at lower inflammation (Panicchi et al., 2006; Kaysen et al., 1997). However, none-biocompatible membranes and partly low flux hemodialysis increases proinflammatory cytokines such as TNF-alpha. Ultrapure dialysis fluid is of relevant importance to prevent inflammation (Panicchi et al., 2008). On the other hand complement activation plays a role for inflammation during the dialysis sessions therefore biocompatible membranes are urgently necessary (Hakim et al., 1984). In the olHDF method as use in this study, both ultrapure dialysate and biocompatible membrane materials were used, enabling clear attenuation of procedure-associated inflammatory processes. This attenuation of inflammation to us seems the key factor for increased albumin production that even makes up for procedure-associated albumin losses. The nutritional situation (nPCR) has only a secondary influence (Savica et al., 2006; Stenvinkel, 2005). Hbvar also depends on inflammation and albumin concentration (Brimble et al., 2007). Hbvar in olHDF is lower than in HD because of less inflammation and higher concentration of albumin.

5. Conclusions

In a retrospective, descriptive, multicentre study the influence of olHDF on Hb Level, ESA dosage and Hbvar was evaluated. 233 patients were included in the clinical analysis in three dialysis departments (D1 n=94; D2 n= 35, D3 n= 104). Mean dialysis efficacy expressed as spkt/V by Daugirdas was comparable in all dialysis units. We found differences in the frequency of olHDF in the dialysis departments followed by varying parameters of inflammation (CRP) and nutrition (albumin). It can be demonstrated that patients who underwent olHDF showed the highest serum albumin levels and the lowest signs of inflammation (CRP). This combination leads to significantly higher Hb concentrations and surprisingly lower ESA dosages to reach the target Hb in ol HDF vs HD. Due to the reduced inflammation Hbvar was improved in olHDF vs HD. There is a correlation between serum albumin concentration, Hb level and ESA dosage. OlHDF could be the gold standard for prevention of inflammation because of removal of proinflammatory substances and hydrophobic and protein bound uremic toxins. OlHDF influences positively inflammation, nutrition, Hb level, Hb variability and required ESA dosage in chronic renal replacement therapy.

6. References

Ahrenholz, P., Winkler, R.E., Ramlow, W., Ties,s M., Müller, W. (1997). On-line hemodiafiltration with pre and post dilution: a comparison of efficacy, *Int J Artif Organs*. Vol.20(2):81-90

Ahrenholz, P., Winkler, R.E., Michelsen, A., Lang, D.A., Bowry, S.K.(2004). Dialysis membrane-dependent removal of middle molecules during hemodiafiltration: the beta2-microglobul.in/albumin relationship. *Clin Nephrol.* Vol.62(1):21-8

Bellomo, R., Tipping, P., Boyce, N. (1991). Tumor necrosis factor clearances during veno-venous hemodiafiltration in the critically ill. ASAIO Trans. Vol.37(3): M322- M323

Bonforte, G., Grillo, P., Zerb,i S., Surian, M. (2002). Improvement of anemia in hemodialysis patients treated by hemodiafiltration with high-volume on-line-prepared substitution fluid., *Blood Purif.* Vol. 20(4): 357- 363

Braun, N., Rosenfeld, S., Giolai, M., Banzhaf, W., Fretschner, R., Warth, H. et al. (1995). Effect of continuous hemodiafiltration on IL-6, TNF-alpha, C3a, and TCC in patients with SIRS septic shock using two different membranes, *Contrib. Nephrol.* Vol.116:89- 98

Brimble, K.S., Clase, C.M. (2007). Hemoglobin Variability in Dialysis Patients. *J Am Soc Nephrol*. Vol 18: 2219- 2220

Canaud, B., Wizemann, V., Pizzarelli, F., Greenwood, R., Schultze, G., Weber, C. et al. (2001). Cellular interleukin-1 receptor antagonist production in patients receiving on-line hemodiafiltration therapy. *Nephrol Dial Transplant* Vol.16(11): 2181- 2187

Canaud, B., Chenine, L., Henriet, D., Leray, H. (2008). Online Hemodiafiltration: A multipurpose therapy for improving quality of renal replacement therapy, *in*: Ronco C, Cruz DN. (eds) *Hemodialysis From Basic Research to Clinical Trials.* Contrib Nephrol. Basel, Karger, Vol. 161: 191- 198

Carracedo, J., Merino, A., Nogueras, S., Carretero, D., Berdud, I., Ramirez, R. et al. (2006). On-line hemodiafiltration reduces the proinflammatory CD14+CD16+ monocyte-derived dendritic cells: A prospective cross over study. *J Am Soc Nephrol.* Vol.17(8): 2315- 2321

Combarnous, F., Tetta, C., Cellier, C.C., Wratten, M.L., Custaud, De C.T. et al. (2002). Albumin loss in on-line hemodiafiltration. *Int J Artif Organs*. Vol.25(3): 203- 209

Daugirdas, J. (1993). Second generation logarithmic estimates of single-pool variable volume Kt/V: an analysis of error. *J Am Soc Nephrol*. Vol. 4: 1205-1213

Del, V.L., Pozzoni, P., Andrulli, S., Locatelli, F. (2005). Inflammation and resistance to treatment with recombinant human erythropoietin. *J Ren Nutr*. Vol.15-1: 137- 141

Ding, F., Ahrenholz, P., Winkler, R.E., Ramlow, W., Tiess, M., Michelsen, A., Pätow, W. (2002). Online hemodiafiltration versus acetate-free biofiltration: a prospective crossover study. *Artif Organs.* Vol.26(2):169-80

Eiselt, J., Racek, J., Opatrny, K., jr. (2000). The effect of hemodialysis and acetate-free biofiltration on anemia. *Int J Artif Organs.* Vol.23(3): 173- 180

Filiopoulos, V., Hadjiyannakos, D., Metaxaki, P., Sideris, V., Takouli, L., Anogiati, A. et al. (2008). Inflammation and oxidative stress in patients on hemodiafiltration. *Am J Nephrol.* Vol.28(6): 949- 957

Giordano, M., DeFeo, P., Lucidi, P., dePascale, E., Giordano, G., Infantone, L., Zoccolo, A.M,, Castellino, P. (2001). Increased Albumin and Fibrinogen Synthesis in hemodialysis patients with normal nutritional status. *J Am Soc Nephrol.* Vol.12: 349- 354

Haas, M., Bellomo, R., Morgera, S., Baldwin, I., Boyce, N. (2007). High cut-off-point membranes in septic acute renal failure: a systematic review. *Int J Artif Organs.* Vol. 30(12): 1031- 1041

Hakim, R.M., Fearon, D.T., Lazarus, J.M. (1984). Biocompatibility of dialysis membranes: effects of chronic complement activation. *Kidney Int.* Vol.26(2): 194- 200

Hörl, W.H., Riegel, W., Schollmeyer, P., Rautenberg, W., Neumann, S. (1986). Different complement and granulocyte activation in patients dialyzed with PMMA dialyzers. *Clin Nephrol*. Vol.25(6): 304- 307

Jorres, A., Gahl, G.M., Dobis, C., Polenakovic, M.H., Cakalaroski, K., Rutkowski, B. et al. (1999). Hemodialysis membrane biocompatibility and mortality of patients with dialysis dependent acute renal failure: a prospective randomised multicentre trial. International Multicentre Study Group. *Lancet.* Vol.354(9187):1337- 1341

Kanter, J., Puerta, M., Perez, G.R., Lopez, Gomez, J.M., Jofre, R., Rodriguez, P. (2008). On-line sequential hemodiafiltration (HDF-OL-S): a new therapeutic option. *Nefrologia.* Vol.28(4): 433- 438

Kaysen, G.A., Schoenfeld, P.Y. (1984). Albumin homeostasis in patients undergoing continuous ambulatory peritoneal dialysis. *Kidney Int.* Vol.25: 107- 114

Kaysen, G.A., Yeun, J., Depner, T. (1997). Albumin synthesis, catabolism and distribution in dialysis patients. Miner Electrolyte Metab. Vol.23(3-6): 218- 224

Kim, S.T. (1994). Characteristics of protein removal in hemodiafiltration. *Contrib Nephrol.* Vol.108: 23- 37

Krieter, D.H., Lemke, H.D., Canaud, B., Wanner, C. (2005). Beta(2)-microglobulin removal by extracorporeal renal replacement therapies. *Biochim Biophys Acta.* Vol.10 (1753(1)): 146-153

Lee, W.C., Uchino, S., Fealy, N., Baldwin, I., Panagiotopoulos, ., Goehl, H. et al. (2004). Super high flux hemodialysis at high dialysate flows: an ex vivo assessment. *Int J Artif Organs.* Vol 27(1): 24- 28

Libetta, C., Sepe, V., Zucchi, M., Pisacco, P., Cosmai, L., Melonie, F. et al. (2007). Intermittent hemodiafiltration in refractory congestive heart failure: BNP and balance of inflammatory cytokine. *Nephrol Dial Transplant.* Vol.22(7): 2013- 2019

Mandolfo, S., Borandelli, S., Imbasciati, E. (2006). Leptin and beta2-microglobulin kinetics with three different dialysis modalities. *Int J Artif Organs.* Vol.29(10): 949- 955

Mariano, F., Fonsato, V., Lanfranco, G., Pohlmeier, R., Ronco, C., Triolo, G. et al. (2005). Tailoring high-cut-off membranes and feasible application in sepsis-associated acute renal failure: in vitro studies. *Nephro Dial Transplant.* Vol.20(6): 1116- 1126

Meyer, T.W., Walthe,r J.L., Pagtalunan, M.E., Martinez, A.W., Torkamani, A., Fong, P.D. et al.(2005). The clearance of protein-bound solutes by hemofiltration and hemodiafiltration. *Kidney Int.* Vol.68(2): 867- 877

Minetti, L., Broggi, M.L., Civati, G., Guastoni, C., Teatini, U. (1985). Is the dialysate fluid source of complement activating factors? *Trans Am Soc Intern Organs.* Vol. 31: 673-677

Panicchi, V., Manza-Rizza, G., Paoletti, S., Taccola, D., Consani, C., Filippi, C. et al. (2006). Effects on inflammatory and nutritional markers of haemodiafiltration with online re generation of ultra filtrate (HFR) versus online haemodiafiltration: a cross-over randomized multicentre trial. *Nephrol Dial Transplant.* Vol.21(3): 756- 762

Panicchi, V., Rizz, G.M., Paoletti, S., Bigazzi, R., Aloisi, M., Barsotti, G. et al. (2008). Chronic inflammation and mortality in haemodialysis: effect of different replacement therapies. Results from the RISCAVID study. *Nephrol Dial Transplant.* Vol.23(7): 2337- 2343

Parzer, S., Balcke, P., Mannhalter, C. (1993). Plasma protein adsorption to hemodialysis membranes: studies in an in vitro model. *J Biomed Mater Res.* Vol.27(4): 455- 463

Pichaiwong, W., Leelahavanichkul, A., Eiam-ong, S. (2006). Efficacy of cellulose triacetate dialyzer and polysulfone synthetic hemofilter for continuous venovenous hemofiltration in acute renal failure. *J Med Assoc Thai.* Vol.89 (Suppl 2): S65- S72

Ramirez, R., Martin-Malo, A., Aljama, P. (1999). Inflammation and hemodiafiltration. *Contrib Nephrol.* Vol.158: 210- 215

Ramirez, R., Caracedo, J., Merino, A., Nogueras, S., Varez-Lara, M.A., Rodriguez, M. et al. (2007). Microinflammation induces endothelial damage in hemodialysis patients: the role of convective transport. *Kidney Int.* Vol.72(1): 108- 113

Ronco, C., Ghezzi, P., Bellomo, R., Brendolan, A. (1999). New perspectives in the treatment of acute renal failure. *Blood Purif.* Vol.17(2-3): 166- 172

Samtleben, W., Dengler, C., Reinhardt, B., Nothdurft, A., Lemke, H.D. (2003). Comparison of the new polyethersulfone high-flux membrane DIAPES HF800 with conventional high-flux membranes during on-line hemodiafiltration. *Nephrol Dial Transplant.* Vol.18(11): 2382- 2386

Savica, V., Ciolino, F., Monardo, P., Mallamace, A., Savica, R., Santoro, D. et al. (2006). Nutritional status in hemodialysis patients: options for on-line convective treatment. *J Ren Nutr.* Vol.6(3): 237- 240

Stenvinkel, P. (2005). Inflammation in end-stage renal disease a fire that burns within. Contrib Nephrol. Vol.149: 185- 199

Testa, A., Gentilhomme, H., Le, C.D., Orsonneau, J.L. (2006). In vitro removal of high and low molecular weight compounds in hemodiafiltration with on-line- regeneration of ultrafiltrate. *Nephron Clin Pract.* Vol.104(1): c55- c60

Tomo, T., Matsuyama, M., Nakata, T., Kadota, J., Toma, S., Koga, N. et al. (2008). Effect of high fiber densitiy ratio polysulphone dialyzer on protein removal. *Blood Purif.* Vol.26(4): 347- 353

Vanholder, R., deSmet, R., Glorieux, G,, Argiles, A., Bauermeister, U., Brunet, P., Clark, W., Cohen, G., deDeyn, P.P.,

Deppisch, R., Descam-Latscha, B., Henle, T., Jörres, A., Lemke, H.D,, Massy, Z.A., Passlick-Deetjen, J., Rodriguez, M., Stegmayr, B., Stenvinkel, P., Tetta, C., Wanner, C., Zidek, W. (2003). Review on uremic toxins: classification, concentration, and interindividual variability. *Kidney Int.* Vol.63:1934- 1943

Vanholder, R., Meert, N., Schepers, E., Glorieux, G. (2008). From Uremic Toxin Retention to Removal by Convection: Do We Know Enough?. In: Ronco C, Cruz DN. (eds) *Hemodialysis From Basic Research to Clinical Trials.* Contrib Nephrol. Basel, Karger, Vol.161: 125- 131

Vaslaki, L., Major, L., Berta, K., Karatson, A., Misz, M., Pethoe, F.,, Ladanyi, E., Fodor, B., Stein, G., Pischetsrieder, M., Zima, T., Wojke, R., Gauly, A., Passlick-Deetjen, J. (2006). On-line haemodiafiltration versus haemodialysis: stable haematocrit with less erythropoietin and improvement of other relevant blood parameters. *Blood Purif.* Vol.24(2):163-73

Ward, R.A. (2005). Protein leaking membranes for hemodialysis: a new class of membranes in search of an application? *J Am Soc Nephrol* . Vol.16(8): 2421- 2430

Weber, C., Groetsch, W., Schlotter, S., Mitteregger, R., Falkenhagen, D. (2000). Novel online infusate-assisted dialysis system performs microbiologically safely. *Artif Organs.* Vol.24(5): 323- 328

Winchester, J.F., Salsberg, J.A., Levin, N.W. (2003). Beta-2 microglobulin in ESRD: an in-depth review. *Adv ren Replace Ther.* Vol.10(4): 279- 309

Winchester, J..F., Silberzweig, J., Ronco, C., Kuntsevich, V., Levine, D., Parker, T. et al. (2004). Sorbents in acute renal failure and end-stage renal disease: middle molecule and cytokine removal. *Blood Purif.* Vol.22(1): 73- 77

Yamashita, A.C. (2007). Mechanisms of solute and fluid removal in hemodiafiltration. *Contrib Nephrol*. Vol.158: 50- 56

9

Leukocyte Function in High-Flux Hemodialysis

Jenny Olsson
Department of Nephrology and Transplantation
Skåne University Hospital, Malmö,
Sweden

1. Introduction

Patients with chronic kidney disease and patients on renal replacement therapy, such as hemodialysis and peritoneal dialysis, have an increased susceptibility to infectious diseases compared with healthy subjects (Sarnak & Jaber 2000; Allon et al. 2003). Infection is also the second most common cause of morbidity and mortality in patients with end-stage renal disease (Bloembergen & Port 1996; Powe et al. 1999; Graff et al. 2002).
One contributing factor could be the chronic inflammatory activation seen in patients with chronic kidney disease and patients on dialysis, which causes a refractoriness of leukocytes when confronted with invading microorganisms.

1.1 The innate and adaptive immune responses

The immune system is designed to defend us from invading microorganisms, such as viruses and bacteria. The first response is called the innate immune response, mostly dependent on recruitment and activation of neutrophils (Parkin & Cohen 2001). Complement activation occurs on the bacterial cell surface, triggering a cascade of proteolytic reactions that are specific in so far as they act on microbial surfaces but not on host cells. Neutrophils have receptors both for common bacterial constituents and for complement. Neutrophils become activated through complement (C3b and C5a) but can also get activated directly by bacterial peptides, such as lipopolysaccharide, lipotechoic acid, mannans and fMLP (N-formylmethionyl leucyl phenylalanine) (Parkin & Cohen 2001).
Activation of neutrophils occurs in several steps, comprising both priming and further activation, and is necessary for neutrophils to perform their specific actions at the inflammatory sites: phagocytosis and release of inflammatory mediators (Swain et al. 2002). Neutrophils are effector cells of great importance in the innate immune system. An impaired neutrophil function leads to several dysfunctions in the defense against invading microorganisms. Neutrophils have previously been regarded as wholly differentiated and static cells whose function is based on preformed receptors and soluble factors, and solely part of the innate immune system. This idea has been challenged by publications that show a high gene transcriptional activity following both activation and extravasation (Theilgaard-Monch et al. 2006). The transcriptional activation occurs at the inflammatory site and engages genes involved in multiple neutrophil functions, such as production of reactive oxygen species, hydrogen peroxide, cytokines and chemokines (Theilgaard-Monch et al. 2004; Coldren et al. 2006). Neutrophils direct both innate and adaptive immune responses,

by interacting with immune modulating cells (Cohen et al. 2001; Yamashiro et al. 2001; Cohen et al. 2003; Theilgaard-Monch et al. 2004). Neutrophil cytokine and chemokine production can be an important link between the innate and the adaptive immune responses. Cytokine-activated neutrophils produce and release multiple proinflammatory cytokines and chemokines, including IL-1, IL-8, monocyte chemotactic protein-1 (MCP-1/CCL2) and macrophage inflammatory protein-1α and 1β (MIP-1α/MIP-1β). MCP-1 and MIP-1α act as chemotactic and activating signals for mononuclear cells, especially monocytes, and for mobilization of other cell surface molecules involved in the adaptive immune response (Yamashiro et al. 2001; Kobayashi 2008).
Chemokines attract neutrophils and monocytes from the circulation to the inflammatory/infectious site by first making the endothelium more adhesive to the circulating cells and then through a chemokine gradient through the tissue leading the way to the site of inflammation (Janeway & Travers 2005). Circulating monocytes that extravasate and get activated rapidly develop into mature macrophages with the principal function of phagocyting microorganisms (Janeway & Travers 2005).

1.2 Adhesion molecules

The recruitment and accumulation of monocytes and neutrophils at inflammatory sites is an essential step in the defense against invading microorganisms. The process of extravasation, when leukocytes slip through the endothelial cells and basement membrane into the underlying interstitium and further to the inflammatory site requires the expression of adhesion molecules on the endothelium. This serves to initiate leukocyte adherence by interaction between adhesion molecules on leukocytes and vascular endothelial cells (Johnson-Leger et al. 2000; van Buul & Hordijk 2004). The main families of adhesion molecules are the intercellular adhesion molecules (ICAMs); integrins, selectins and cadherins (calcium-dependent adherins) (Parkin & Cohen 2001).
The selectins, P-selectin (PADGEM, CD62P) and E-selectin (ELAM-1, CD62E), are membrane glycoproteins with a lectin-like domain that binds transiently to oligosaccharide molecules on passing leukocytes after cytokine-mediated activation of the endothelial cells. CD62L is present on circulating leukocytes (Janeway & Travers 2005). Selectin binding leads to tethering, which allows leukocytes to search the endothelium for the presence of activating factors. In a second step, leukocytes bind firmly to the endothelium, followed by the process of diapedesis (Albelda et al. 1994). The tighter adhesion is mediated by β_2-integrins CD11a/CD18 (LFA-1) and CD11b (Mac-1 or CR3) expressed on leukocytes after a chemokine-mediated conformational change in the integrins. β_2-integrins bind to intercellular adhesion molecules (ICAM-2 on resting endothelium and ICAM-1 on activated endothelium) (Adams & Shaw 1994; Gonzalez-Amaro & Sanchez-Madrid 1999; Janeway & Travers 2005). The β_1- integrin very late antigen-4 (VLA-4) is present principally on mononuclear cells, mediating monocyte transmigration by binding to vascular adhesion molecules (VCAM-1) on activated endothelial cells (Chuluyan & Issekutz 1993).

1.3 Leukocyte adhesion and extravasation

Leukocyte adhesion is made possible by the action of chemokines: small, structurally related molecules that interact with G-protein-coupled receptors. They perform activation of integrins in order to confer tight adhesion between leukocytes and endothelial cells, and promote the migration of adherent leukocytes across the endothelium and through the extracellular matrix (Adams & Shaw 1994). Chemokines are small molecules, divided into

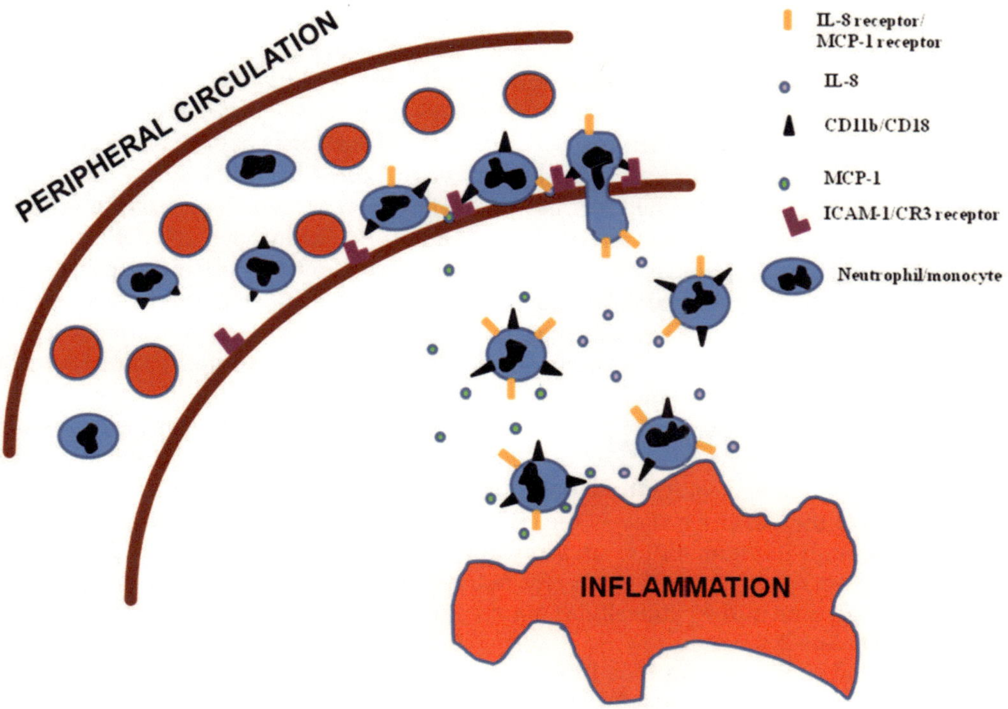

Fig. 1. Leukocyte adhesion to the endothelium, subsequent extravasation and transmigration through a chemotactic gradient in the interstitium towards a site of inflammation.

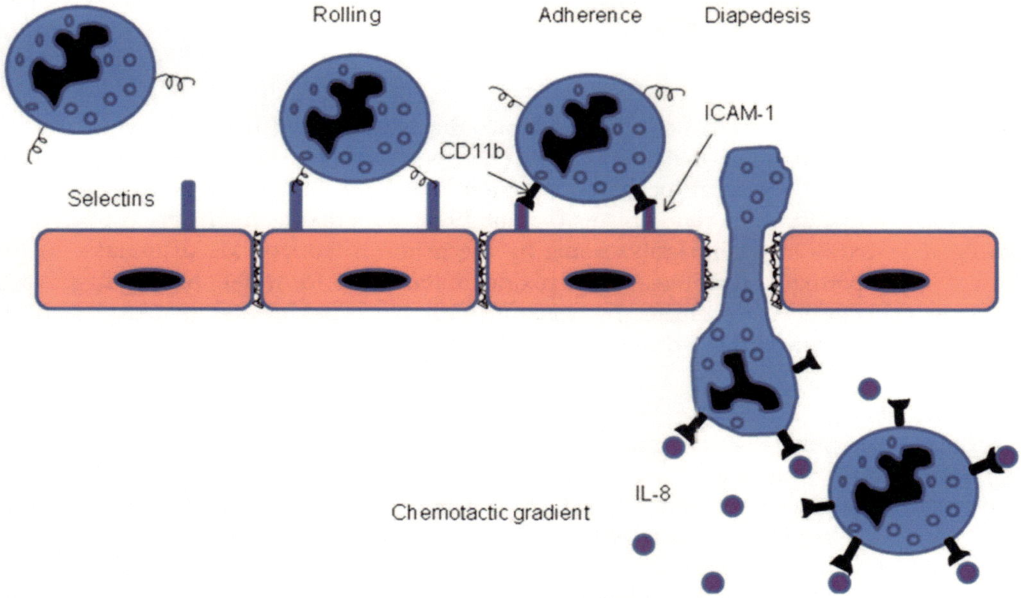

Fig. 2. Neutrophil adhesion, extravasation and transmigration.

CXC (α-chemokines) and CC (β-chemokines) depending on the positions of two cysteine residues (C) relative to other amino acids (X) (Charo & Ransohoff 2006). Chemokines are produced by inflammatory cells after stimulation with proinflammatory cytokines or bacterial products, and there are both soluble and membrane-bound chemokines, with various functions (Parkin & Cohen 2001). Some of the chemokines and cytokines analyzed in our study, and their respective functions, are listed in Table 1 and Table 2.

Leukocyte binding to endothelial cells induces production of signaling molecules in the endothelial cells and activation of NADPH oxidase in leukocytes. NADPH oxidase promotes production of reactive oxygen species that break down the barrier to leukocyte passage between the endothelial cells and through the basement membrane (van Buul & Hordijk 2004). PECAM-1 plays an important role in transendothelial migration of leukocytes, by inducing phosphorylation of tyrosine in junctional proteins which leads to loss of cell-cell adhesion (van Buul & Hordijk 2004).

When neutrophils extravasate, they produce enzymes (i.e. elastase and other proteases such as matrix metalloproteinase-9, MMP-9) that break down extracellular matrix proteins and in this way promote leukocyte migration through the interstitium (Hermant et al. 2003).

The final step of the transmigration is the chemokine concentration gradient, which guides leukocytes through the interstitium and towards the inflammatory site. CXCL8 (IL-8) and CCL2 (MCP-1) act as chemotactic factors for neutrophils and monocytes, respectively. They bind to proteoglycans in the extracellular matrix and to similar molecules on the leukocytes (Janeway & Travers 2005).

Neutrophils and monocytes in blood normally express a low amount of CD11b on their surface. Following chemokine-mediated activation of the cells, CD11b is mobilized on the cell surface and the molecules are activated in order to display their functions (Adams & Shaw 1994; Albelda et al. 1994; Adams & Lloyd 1997; Gonzalez-Amaro & Sanchez-Madrid 1999). Mobilization of CD11b is important in the process of leukocyte transmigration, phagocytosis and complement activation as a response to inflammation/infection (Bainton et al. 1987; Borregaard et al. 1987; Miller et al. 1987).

1.4 Respiratory burst

The enzyme complex NADPH oxidase promotes the generation of reactive oxygen species (e.g. superoxide anions) in leukocytes, in a process referred to as the respiratory burst. Respiratory burst is a central mechanism for the leukocyte function of phagocytosis and elimination of invading microorganisms (Babior 1999). Superoxide anions are converted to hydrogen peroxide in the phagolysosome by the action of superoxide dismutase. In the absence of superoxide dismutase, superoxide anions can form the highly aggressive oxidative substance peroxynitrite (by reacting with nitric oxide) and hydroxyl radicals (Dahlgren & Karlsson 1999; Johnson & Giulivi 2005).

1.5 Apoptosis

In early apoptosis, there is a reconformation of the cell membrane, with phosphatidyl serine (PS) translocated from the inner surface to the outer leaflet of the cell membrane. Fluorescein-conjugated Annexin V binds to PS with high affinity and identifies early apoptotic cells. Propidium iodide enters through damaged cell membranes after loss of membrane integrity and stains DNA, identifying late stages of apoptosis and secondary necrotic cells. PS is identified by phagocytes in the extracellular milieu in order to remove the dying cells by phagocytosis.

Chemokines		Receptor	Functions	References
IL-8 (interleukin-8)	**CXCL8**	IL-8 receptor α and β	Induces neutrophil CD11b/CD18 up-regulation, transmigration and activation. Stimulates the release of MMP-9/NGAL. Binding to the receptor causes a reconformation of integrins, which allows neutrophils to bind to the endothelial cells.	(Zeilhofer & Schorr 2000; Drost & MacNee 2002; Adams & Lloyd 1997)
MCP-1 (monocyte chemotactic protein-1)	**CCL2**	CCR2	Chemotactic factor and activator of monocytes and macrophages. Produced by many different inflammatory cells. Induces up-regulation of CD11b/CD18 and facilitates monocyte adhesion to endothelial cells. Associated with chronic and acute inflammation, as well as with the acute coronary syndrome.	(Adams & Lloyd 1997; Jiang et al. 1992; Jiang et al. 1994; Ikeda et al. 2002; de Lemos et al. 2003; Pawlak et al. 2004)
MIP-1α (macrophage inflammatory protein-1α)	**CCL3**	CCR1 and CCR5	Released from monocytes after trigging of CD11b/CD18. Promotes the recruitment of inflammatory cells. Chemotactic factor for both monocytes and neutrophils. Activates macrophages by up-regulation of CD11b/CD18.	(Rezzonico et al. 2001; Adams & Lloyd 1997; Ramos et al. 2005; Weber et al. 2000)
MMP-9/NGAL (matrix metalloproteinase-9 in complex with neutrophil gelatinase-associated lipocalin)			MMP-9 and proteolytic enzymes degrade the extracellular matrix and promote leukocyte transmigration. Marker of neutrophil activation and release of reactive oxygen species. Regulates chemokine activity by cleaving of chemokines and cytokines.	(Yan et al. 2001; Alberts et al. 2002; Brogden & Guthmiller 2002; Van Den Steen et al. 2003)

Table 1. Chemokines analyzed in our study and their respective functions.

Cytokines	Functions	References
TNF-α (tumor necrosis factor-α)	Produced by macrophages and monocytes in acute and chronic inflammation. Pro-apoptotic. Up-regulates adhesion molecules on endothelial cells. Chemotactic factor for monocytes and primes cells for phagocytosis. Increases vascular permeability and vasodilatation, promotes intravascular coagulation, and causes the septic syndrome and failure of vital organs.	(Idriss & Naismith 2000; Janeway & Travers 2005)
IL-6	Inflammatory marker, important role in acute inflammation and production of acute phase proteins from the liver.	(Adams & Lloyd 1997; Pupim et al. 2004; Pecoits-Filho et al. 2002; Panichi et al. 2004)

Table 2. Cytokines analyzed in our study and their respective functions.

1.6 Leukocyte dysfunction in chronic kidney disease

There is a complex state of leukocyte dysfunction in chronic kidney disease patients. The most important contributing factors are metabolic and functional abnormalities of leukocytes caused by the accumulation of uremic toxins that inhibit leukocyte function. In patients on dialysis, another factor influencing leukocyte function is bioincompatibility of the dialysis procedure resulting in a dysfunctional inflammatory activation (Lundberg et al. 1994; Vanholder et al. 1996; Cohen et al. 2001; Horl 2001; Cohen et al. 2003; Cheung et al. 2008).

In chronic kidney disease, there is an altered leukocyte adherence to endothelial cells, decreased activation of inflammatory cells, impaired phagocytosis and chemotaxis and an altered generation of reactive oxygen species and hydrogen peroxide (Gibbons et al. 1990; Haag-Weber & Horl 1996b; Horl 2001). Chemokine and cytokine dysregulation in chronic kidney disease gives rise to a dysfunctional activation of the immune system (Descamps-Latscha 1993; Malaponte et al. 2007; Carrero et al. 2008).

The comorbidity of the patient, such as a state of malnutrition and other chronic diseases, also plays an important role in this non-physiological inflammatory activity (Cohen et al. 1997; Stenvinkel et al. 2000; Pecoits-Filho et al. 2002). A study from our group has demonstrated that neutrophils and monocytes from patients with advanced chronic kidney disease have an impaired expression of CD11b in the interstitium compared with the corresponding cells from healthy subjects (Dadfar et al. 2004b, 2004a). The same result has been demonstrated for patients on peritoneal dialysis (Dadfar et al. 2004c).

1.6.1 Uremic toxins with effects on leukocytes

There are several uremic toxins that inhibit neutrophil functions, e.g. guanidino compounds, granulocyte inhibitory protein I and II, degranulation inhibitory protein I and II (identified as angiogenin and complement factor D), κ- and λ-light chains and chemotaxis inhibitory protein (Vanholder et al. 1994b; Haag-Weber & Horl 1996a; Kaysen 2001; Horl 2002; Kaysen & Kumar 2003; Cohen & Horl 2009b, 2009a).

1.6.2 Patients on hemodialysis

Historically, dialysis has contributed to saving many lives over the years. Without dialysis, a uremic patient unavoidably goes towards death. However, the life quality of patients on dialysis still has to be improved to develop an optimal treatment. In spite of the process in the last years to strive towards more biocompatible materials and methods, including high-flux dialysis treatment, patients on hemodialysis still display a high morbidity and mortality in infections (Bloembergen & Port 1996; Powe et al. 1999; Graff et al. 2002). Neutrophil dysfunction in dialysis patients is manifested by reduced chemotaxis, adherence, respiratory burst and glucose consumption in response to an inflammatory stimulus (Vanholder et al. 1993b; Vanholder et al. 1993a).

The dysfunctional state of inflammatory activation seen in dialysis patients could be caused by several different factors (Cheung et al. 1989; Haag-Weber et al. 1991; Descamps-Latscha 1993; Schindler et al. 2001; Carracedo et al. 2002; Horl 2002; Raj et al. 2002; Kosch et al. 2003; Koller et al. 2004). Fragments of bacterial products can be present in small amounts in the dialysate and enter the circulation by diffusion through the dialysis membrane (Horl 2002). These bacterial fragments activate proinflammatory cytokines such as IL-6, TNF-α and IL-1. There is also direct activation of complement factors and of leukocytes by contact with the dialysis membrane. Another aspect is the removal of cytokines and other inflammatory markers (lipopolysaccharide fragments, granulocyte inhibitory proteins 1 and 2, IL-1, TNF-α) and complement factors (C3a, C5a) by the hemodialysis procedure as well as the adsorption of substances to the hydrophobic high-flux membrane (e.g. factor D) (Clark et al. 1999; Schindler et al. 2006). Dialysis can reduce leukocyte-endothelial interactions and impair transmigration (Thylen et al. 1997). In patients on hemodialysis with cuprophane or polysulfone membranes, a significantly higher serum level of MCP-1 is seen compared with healthy subjects both before and after the hemodialysis session, independent of the membrane used (Jacobson et al. 2000; Thylen et al. 2000).

Biocompatibility of dialysis membranes probably plays an important role in determining leukocyte function in patients on hemodialysis (Himmelfarb et al. 1991; Himmelfarb et al. 1993; Hernandez et al. 2004; Schindler et al. 2006). High serum levels of cytokines and chemokines have been observed in patients on hemodialysis with modified cellulose membranes (Descamps-Latscha 1993; Pawlak et al. 2004; Muniz-Junqueira et al. 2005). High-flux hemodialysis causes lower levels of IL-6 and IL-1β than low-flux hemodialysis or dialysis with cuprophane membranes (Schindler et al. 2006). Our group has previously demonstrated that neutrophils and monocytes recruited to an induced interstitial inflammatory site in patients treated with low-flux bioincompatible hemodialysis have an impaired capacity of mobilizing CD11b in response to the induced inflammation, compared with the corresponding cells from healthy subjects (Thylen et al. 2000; Jacobson et al. 2002).

Chronic kidney disease is a state that induces apoptosis, but this is normalized with continuous and high-flux hemodialysis modalities (D'Intini et al. 2004; Bordoni et al. 2006). This is in accordance with studies showing that dialysis membrane characteristics affect leukocyte cell apoptosis (Martin-Malo et al. 2000; Sela et al. 2005; Sardenberg et al. 2006). The degree of spontaneous apoptosis of leukocytes is higher when bioincompatible membranes are used for hemodialysis, than when biocompatible membranes are used (Martin-Malo et al. 2000). This higher apoptotic activity in leukocytes is probably due to an antibody-dependent activation of the complement system caused by the material or structure of the dialysis filters. It has been shown that heat-inactivation of complement components results in significantly lower apoptosis rates and that bioincompatible membranes cause a higher degree of apoptosis than biocompatible membranes (Koller et al. 2004).

The dialysis membrane permeability and flux are also of importance in determining the acute and chronic effects of hemodialysis on the inflammatory system. High-flux polysulfone dialysis, as opposed to low-flux polysulfone and cuprophane treatment, has been shown to improve the transmigration of circulating neutrophils (Moshfegh et al. 2002). High-flux dialysis membranes decrease the levels of the two degranulation inhibitory proteins (angiogenin and complement factor D), which could contribute to the maintained respiratory burst and phagocytic capacity seen in patients on high-flux hemodialysis (Horl 2002). There are several molecules, mainly middle-sized molecules, that are cleared to a greater extent by convective therapies, such as hemofiltration or hemodiafiltration (Clark et al. 1999). Postdilution hemofiltration was the first convective therapy used, and this method provides a high clearance of middle- and large-sized molecules but a lower clearance of small molecules. Through predilution hemofiltration, with on-line ultrafiltration, the clearance of small molecules increased substantially. In hemodiafiltration, convection is combined with diffusion, and with this mechanism the clearance of small-, middle- and large-sized molecules can be achieved to more or less the same extent (Ledebo 1998).

A number of previous studies have suggested that the type of dialysis membrane (low-flux or high-flux) is associated with differences in long-term outcome of patients undergoing hemodialysis, both in terms of morbidity and mortality (Hornberger et al. 1992; Woods & Nandakumar 2000; Cheung et al. 2003; Locatelli 2003; Chauveau et al. 2005; Canaud et al. 2006). However, the results have been conflictive regarding different outcomes.

The HEMO study, which was the first large randomized clinical trial on patient outcome depending on membrane permeability, failed to show any difference in all-cause mortality between high-flux and low-flux hemodialysis, except in some subgroups of patients (Eknoyan et al. 2002; Cheung et al. 2003; Rocco et al. 2005). Some criticism regarding the generalizability of the results from the HEMO study has been raised (Locatelli 2003). Important results from the HEMO study indicate that middle-sized molecules, e.g. parathyreoid hormone, β_2-microglobulin, advanced glycosylation end products, granulocyte inhibitory proteins, advanced lipoxidation end products, advanced oxidation protein products and leptin (Horl 2002) are associated with systemic toxicity and that their accumulation predisposes dialysis patients to severe infections. An increased clearance of these molecules, e.g. β_2-microglobulin, by high-flux hemodialysis is associated with a lower mortality by infectious disease (Cheung et al. 2008). An increased removal of middle-sized molecules could also have positive effects of the cardiovascular system (Vanholder et al. 2001; Vanholder et al. 2008).

In a Cochrane database review by Rabindranath et al. in 2006, the authors were unable to demonstrate a significant advantage with convective therapies over low-flux hemodialysis with regard to clinical outcomes such as mortality, dialysis-related hypotension and hospitalization (Rabindranath et al. 2006).

The DOPPS study (Dialysis Outcomes and Practice Patterns Study) revealed that patients on high-flux hemodiafiltration had a 35 % lower mortality rate than patients on low-flux hemodialysis (Canaud et al. 2006; Canaud et al. 2008).

The MPO-study (Membrane Permeability Outcome) was a European randomized clinical trial on the effect of high-flux treatment in a large hemodialysis population. It was a prospective study which analyzed the long-term effects of membrane permeability on clinical outcomes such as mortality, morbidity, vascular access survival and nutritional status. The authors of the MPO-study did not find any significant survival benefit overall by high-flux hemodialysis versus low-flux hemodialysis. However, for some dialysis populations with low serum albumin and for patients with diabetes mellitus, a significantly lower mortality rate was observed using high-flux hemodialysis as compared with low-flux hemodialysis (Locatelli et al. 2009).

2. Leukocyte functional studies in patients on high-flux biocompatible hemodialysis

Our research group has described functions of *in vivo* extravasated monocytes and neutrophils from patients on high-flux hemodialysis/hemodiafiltration and healthy subjects (Olsson et al. 2007). The objective was to study leukocyte function and specifically, to study the up-regulation of CD11b, production of hydrogen peroxide and apoptosis of *in vivo* extravasated monocytes and neutrophils at the site of an induced interstitial inflammation in patients on high-flux hemodialysis/hemodiafiltration, compared with healthy subjects. Our group has also described the concentrations of important inflammatory mediators for neutrophils (IL-8 and MMP-9/NGAL) and monocytes (MCP-1 and MIP-1α) in the peripheral circulation and at sites of interstitial inflammation in patients on high-flux hemodialysis/hemodiafiltration, compared with healthy subjects (Olsson et al. 2009).

2.1 Methods for leukocyte functional studies

The method used was the skin chamber technique, which is well documented and has been used by a number of investigators to study transmigration and recruitment of leukocytes at the inflammatory site (Scheja & Forsgren 1985; Follin 1999; Thylen et al. 2000; Jacobson et al. 2002; Theilgaard-Monch et al. 2004; Dadfar et al. 2007; Paulsson et al. 2007). With the skin chamber technique, we measured leukocyte functions at time 0 (before the high-flux hemodialysis/hemodiafiltration session) and after 10 hours (within which time the high-flux hemodialysis/hemodiafiltration treatment was performed). The terms intermediate and intense inflammation were used to designate the blister stimulated with buffer and with autologous serum, respectively.

Leukocytes were measured with flow cytometry or FACS (fluorescence-activated cell sorting) a method in which cells are scanned by a laser and recognized as different cell populations through their light-scattering properties. Different leukocyte populations (lymphocytes, monocytes and neutrophils) can thus be counted and expressed as a percentage of the total leukocyte population. Mean fluorescence intensity (MFI) values for the different analyses of cell functions (CD11b expression, hydrogen peroxide formation and apoptosis) can also be measured and quantified.

The CD11b expression on leukocytes, both unstimulated and after stimulation with fMLP, was studied through immunostaining. Analysis of leukocyte hydrogen peroxide formation, after stimulation with fMLP or PMA, was performed using the 2′, 7′-dichlorofluorescein diacetate (DCFH-DA) method. We also stained leukocytes with Annexin V and propidium iodide (PI) to identify cells that were in an early or late apoptotic state.

Chemokines in skin blister fluids and serum from the peripheral circulation were analyzed with commercially available immunoassays (Quantikine®, R&D Systems Inc. Minneapolis, MN, USA). All immunoassays were used in accordance with the manufacturer's instructions. For further details, please review publications (Olsson et al. 2007 & Olsson et al. 2009).

2.2 Results

2.2.1 CD11b

There was a similar expression of CD11b on monocytes and neutrophils in patients on high-flux hemodialysis/hemodiafiltration and healthy subjects, both in the peripheral circulation and at the three sites of interstitial inflammation. *In vitro* activation with fMLP induced a significant increase in the expression of CD11b on monocytes and neutrophils in the peripheral circulation and at the sites of interstitial inflammation, both in patients on high-flux hemodialysis/hemodiafiltration and healthy subjects.

The preserved capacity of both monocytes and neutrophils to express CD11b at the sites of interstitial inflammation in patients on high-flux hemodialysis/hemodiafiltration, as shown by our findings, may have important biological consequences in terms of an adequate performance of leukocyte functions in which the CD11b molecule plays a key role (Thylen et al. 1997; Moshfegh et al. 2002). Extravasated neutrophils and monocytes from patients on high-flux hemodialysis/hemodiafiltration showed a maintained response to fMLP as a second inflammatory stimulus after extravasation.

The mechanism behind this preserved leukocyte function in patients on high-flux biocompatible hemodialysis/hemodiafiltration could be the removal of small and middle-sized leukocyte inhibitory molecules by high-flux hemodialysis/hemodiafiltration (Vanholder et al. 1994a), but membrane compatibility could also play an important role.

2.2.2 Hydrogen peroxide formation

Results for hydrogen peroxide production in neutrophils and monocytes are displayed in Figures 3-6. The findings indicate the presence of a dose-response phenomenon in terms of leukocyte function at the site of interstitial inflammation in patients on high-flux hemodialysis/hemodiafiltration, which could be due to leukocyte refractoriness when encountered with an intense inflammatory stimulus. Refractoriness of leukocytes could be caused by previous priming, giving rise to an impaired response to a second activating stimulus.

2.2.3 Apoptosis and cell counts

There was no significant difference in the total number of leukocytes at the inflammatory sites between patients on high-flux hemodialysis/hemodiafiltration and healthy subjects.

In our study of leukocytes from patients on high-flux hemodialysis/hemodiafiltration, leukocytes were studied at their actual site of action, namely after *in vivo* extravasation. This is advantageous, since leukocyte function in patients with chronic kidney disease or on dialysis has previously almost exclusively been studied on cells collected from the peripheral circulation.

In both the neutrophil and monocyte populations, we observed no significant differences in the percentage of apoptotic cells (Annexin V+ and Annexin V+ PI+) in the peripheral circulation or at the sites of interstitial inflammation between patients on high-flux hemodialysis/hemodiafiltration and healthy subjects.

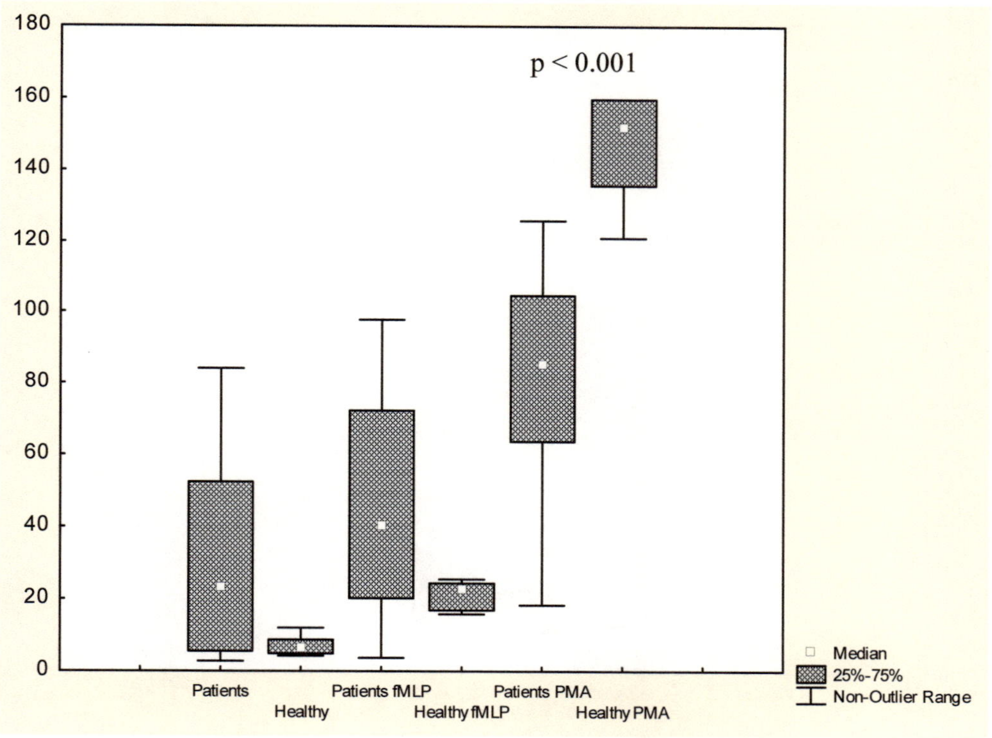

Fig. 3. Respiratory burst in neutrophils at the site of an intermediate interstitial inflammation expressed as mean fluorescence intensity (MFI). P is indicated where a significant difference is present.

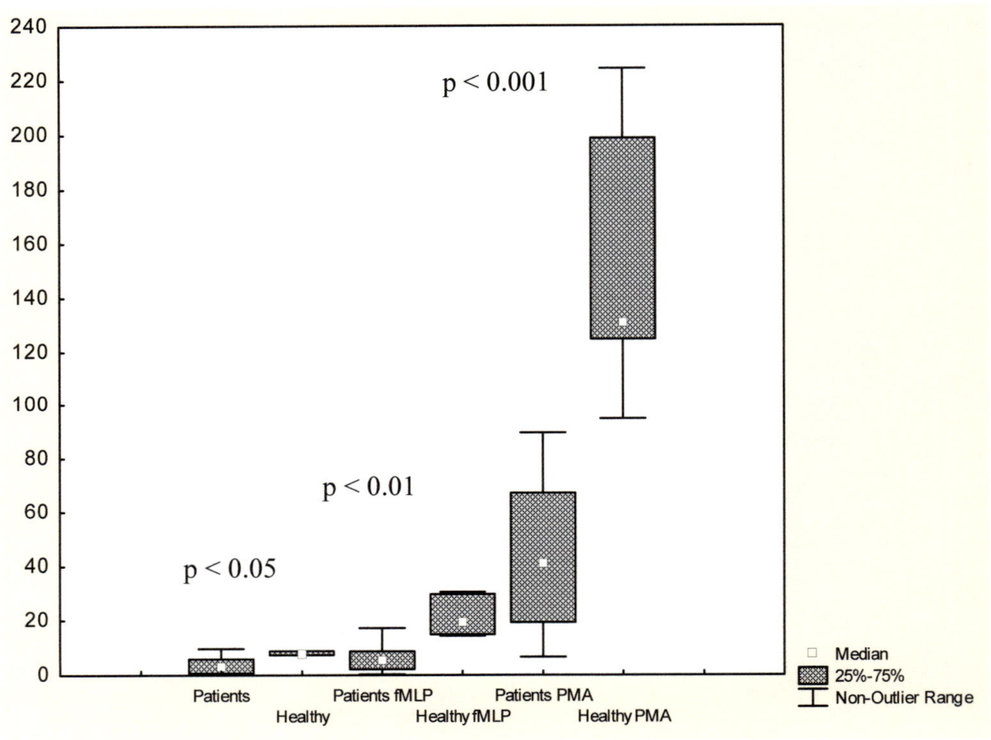

Fig. 4. Respiratory burst (MFI) in neutrophils at the site of intense interstitial inflammation.

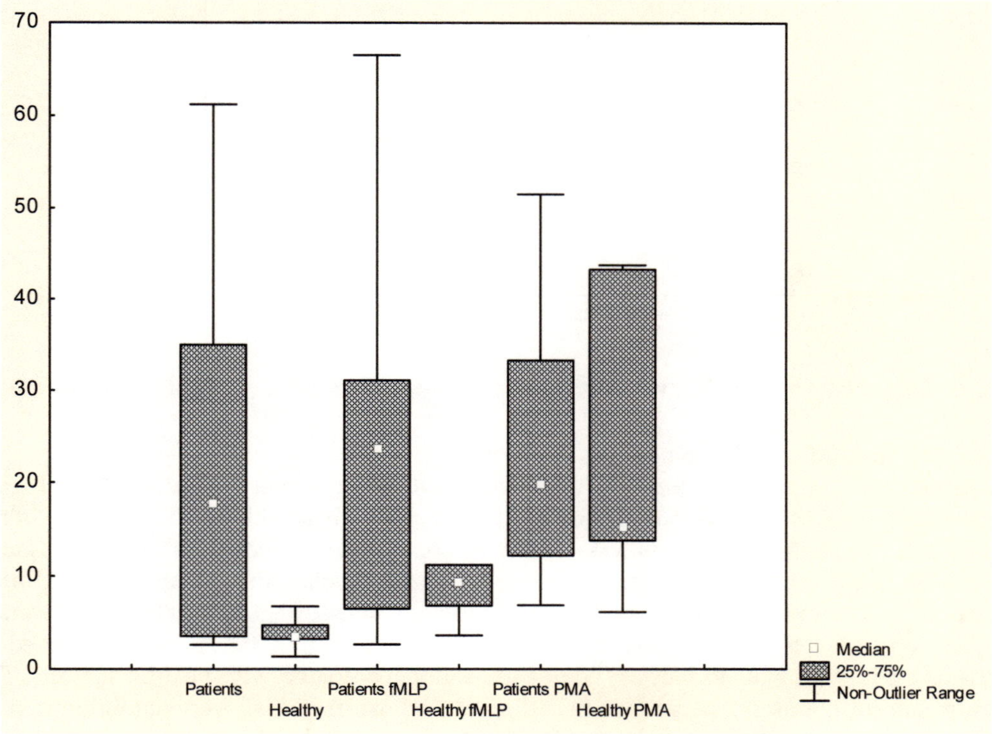

Fig. 5. Respiratory burst (MFI) in monocytes at the site of intermediate interstitial inflammation. No significant difference for any comparison.

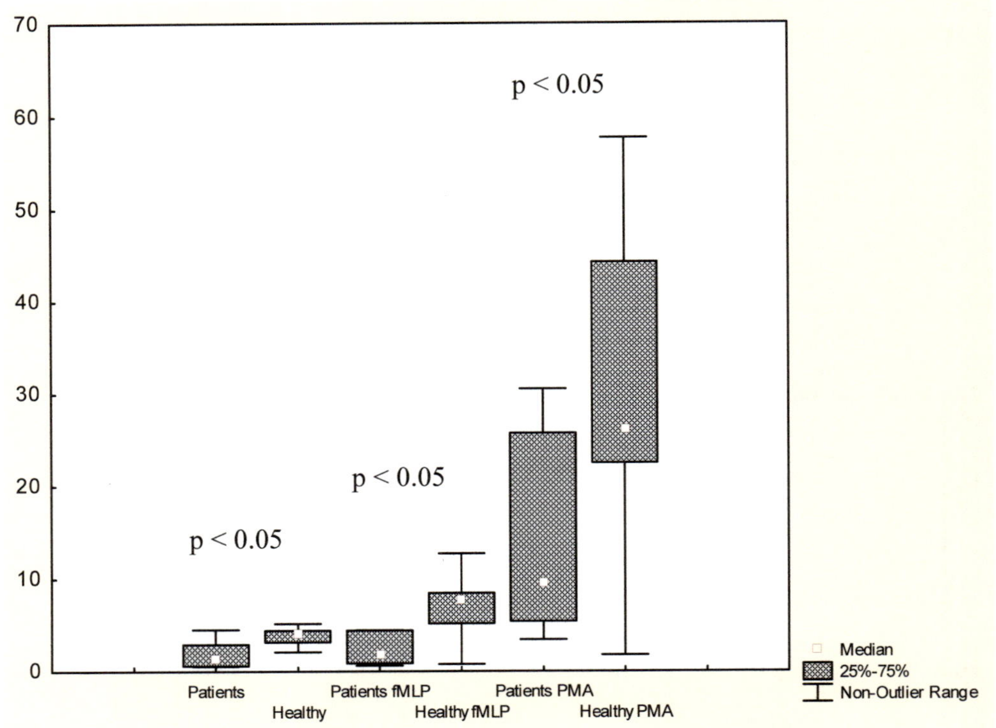

Fig. 6. Respiratory burst (MFI) in monocytes at the site of intense interstitial inflammation.

2.2.4 Concentrations of chemokines

Patients on high-flux hemodialysis/hemodiafiltration had significantly higher concentrations of MCP-1, MIP-1α, IL-6, IL-8, TNF-α and high-sensitivity CRP (hsCRP) in the peripheral circulation, prior to dialysis treatment, compared with healthy subjects (Olsson et al. 2009). MMP-9/NGAL serum concentration was similar in patients on high-flux hemodialysis/hemodiafiltration and healthy subjects (Olsson et al. 2009). Significantly higher serum levels of β2-microglobulin and serum amyloid A (SAA) were observed in patients on high-flux hemodialysis/hemodiafiltration, compared with healthy subjects. The serum concentrations of chemokines, hsCRP, SAA and oxidized LDL were not influenced by the high-flux hemodialysis/hemodiafiltration session, while the concentration of β2-microglobulin was significantly reduced (unpublished data).

The concentrations of MIP-1α, MMP-9/NGAL and IL-8 at the sites of intermediate and intense inflammation were similar in patients and healthy subjects, and the concentration of MCP-1 at the sites of intermediate and intense inflammation was significantly higher in patients on high-flux hemodialysis/hemodiafiltration, compared with healthy subjects (Olsson et al. 2009). At the site of intermediate inflammation, the concentration of IL-6 and TNF-α was significantly higher in patients compared with healthy subjects, reflecting a high inflammatory activity (unpublished data). There were no significant correlations between the concentrations of chemokines or the gradient between the concentration in the peripheral circulation and the interstitium, and the recruitment of neutrophils and monocytes and their expression of CD11b at the site of interstitial inflammation (unpublished data).

3. Conclusion

In vivo extravasated monocytes and neutrophils from patients on high-flux hemodialysis/hemodiafiltration have a preserved capacity to mobilize CD11b, compared with the corresponding cells from healthy subjects (Olsson et al. 2007). Furthermore, monocytes and neutrophils were able to respond to a second signal (fMLP) at the site of interstitial inflammation, indicating an adequate response to bacterial peptides (Olsson et al. 2007). After the most potent stimulation, both monocytes and neutrophils that had extravasated *in vivo* and been recruited to the site of intense inflammation showed a lower capacity to produce hydrogen peroxide in response to activation, compared with the corresponding cells from healthy individuals (Olsson et al. 2007). The apoptotic rates of neutrophils and monocytes were similar in patients and in healthy subjects (Olsson et al. 2007). Clearance of leukocytes from the site of infection via apoptosis is essential for the coordinated resolution of inflammation. The balance between pro-apoptotic and anti-apoptotic factors is necessary for the maintenance of an effective immune response without the harmful side effects of an excessive neutrophil activation.

The higher concentration of MCP-1 and equal concentration of IL-8, MMP-9/NGAL and MIP-1α at the sites of intermediate and intense inflammation in patients on high-flux hemodialysis/hemodiafiltration (Olsson et al. 2009) could be of importance for the maintained capacity of leukocytes to extravasate and mobilize CD11b compared with healthy subjects (Olsson et al. 2007). These data contrast with our previous studies on patients with chronic kidney disease or patients on peritoneal dialysis, in which the concentrations of MCP-1 and IL-8 are significantly lower, coupled with an impaired capacity to up-regulate CD11b on neutrophils at sites of interstitial inflammation (Dadfar et al. 2004c; Dadfar et al. 2004b, 2004a).

The results of our study support a preserved neutrophil and monocyte function in terms of extravasation and activation at the inflammatory focus. One possible explanation for the preserved capacity of monocytes and neutrophils to express CD11b in response to an interstitial inflammation in patients on high-flux hemodialysis/hemodiafiltration may be that the cells extravasate into a milieu which contains equal or higher concentrations of factors involved in transmigration and CD11b expression (MCP-1, IL-8, MIP-1α and MMP-9/NGAL) compared with healthy subjects. The maintained capacity to produce chemokines in the interstitium in patients on high-flux hemodialysis/hemodiafiltration may be due to an increased intradialytic removal of uremic substances that inhibit leukocyte function.

4. Acknowledgement

I want to thank my co-investigators and co-authors Stefan H Jacobson, Joachim Lundahl, Ali Moshfegh, Josefin Paulsson and Elham Dadfar. I also want to thank Titti Nieminen and Anette Bygdén-Nylander for skilful technical support. These studies were made possible by an unrestricted grant from Karolinska Institutet, Stockholm, Sweden and Terumo Europe N.V. *dedicated to well being*. The author also received financial support from the Swedish Society of Nephrology.

5. References

Adams DH, Shaw S (1994) Leucocyte-endothelial interactions and regulation of leucocyte migration. *Lancet* 343(8901): 831-836.

Adams DH, Lloyd AR (1997) Chemokines: leucocyte recruitment and activation cytokines. *Lancet* 349(9050): 490-495.

Albelda SM, Smith CW, Ward PA (1994) Adhesion molecules and inflammatory injury. *Faseb J* 8(8): 504-512.

Alberts, B., A. Johnson, et al. (2002) *Molecular Biology of the Cell*. New York.

Allon M, Depner TA, Radeva M, Bailey J, Beddhu S et al. (2003) Impact of dialysis dose and membrane on infection-related hospitalization and death: results of the HEMO Study. *J Am Soc Nephrol* 14(7): 1863-1870.

Babior BM (1999) NADPH oxidase: an update. *Blood* 93(5): 1464-1476.

Bainton DF, Miller LJ, Kishimoto TK, Springer TA (1987) Leukocyte adhesion receptors are stored in peroxidase-negative granules of human neutrophils. *J Exp Med* 166(6): 1641-1653.

Bloembergen WE, Port FK (1996) Epidemiological perspective on infections in chronic dialysis patients. *Adv Ren Replace Ther* 3(3): 201-207.

Bordoni V, Piroddi M, Galli F, de Cal M, Bonello M et al. (2006) Oxidant and carbonyl stress-related apoptosis in end-stage kidney disease: impact of membrane flux. *Blood Purif* 24(1): 149-156.

Borregaard N, Miller LJ, Springer TA (1987) Chemoattractant-regulated mobilization of a novel intracellular compartment in human neutrophils. *Science* 237(4819): 1204-1206.

Brogden, K. A. and J. M. Guthmiller (2002) The Host Response: A Double-edged Sword. *Polymicrobial diseases*. Herndon, VA, ASM Press.

Canaud B, Chenine L, Henriet D, Leray H (2008) Cross-membrane flux is a major factor influencing dialysis patient outcomes. *Contrib Nephrol* 161: 178-184.

Canaud B, Bragg-Gresham JL, Marshall MR, Desmeules S, Gillespie BW et al. (2006) Mortality risk for patients receiving hemodiafiltration versus hemodialysis: European results from the DOPPS. *Kidney Int* 69(11): 2087-2093.

Carracedo J, Ramirez R, Madueno JA, Soriano S, Rodriguez-Benot A et al. (2002) Cell apoptosis and hemodialysis-induced inflammation. *Kidney Int Suppl*(80): 89-93.

Carrero JJ, Yilmaz MI, Lindholm B, Stenvinkel P (2008) Cytokine dysregulation in chronic kidney disease: how can we treat it? *Blood Purif* 26(3): 291-299.

Charo IF, Ransohoff RM (2006) The many roles of chemokines and chemokine receptors in inflammation. *N Engl J Med* 354(6): 610-621.

Chauveau P, Nguyen H, Combe C, Chene G, Azar R et al. (2005) Dialyzer membrane permeability and survival in hemodialysis patients. *Am J Kidney Dis* 45(3): 565-571.

Cheung AK, Parker CJ, Wilcox L, Janatova J (1989) Activation of the alternative pathway of complement by cellulosic hemodialysis membranes. *Kidney Int* 36(2): 257-265.

Cheung AK, Greene T, Leypoldt JK, Yan G, Allon M et al. (2008) Association between serum 2-microglobulin level and infectious mortality in hemodialysis patients. *Clin J Am Soc Nephrol* 3(1): 69-77.

Cheung AK, Levin NW, Greene T, Agodoa L, Bailey J et al. (2003) Effects of high-flux hemodialysis on clinical outcomes: results of the HEMO study. *J Am Soc Nephrol* 14(12): 3251-3263.

Chuluyan HE, Issekutz AC (1993) VLA-4 integrin can mediate CD11/CD18-independent transendothelial migration of human monocytes. *J Clin Invest* 92(6): 2768-2777.

Clark WR, Hamburger RJ, Lysaght MJ (1999) Effect of membrane composition and structure on solute removal and biocompatibility in hemodialysis. *Kidney Int* 56(6): 2005-2015.

Cohen G, Horl WH (2009a) Free immunoglobulin light chains as a risk factor in renal and extrarenal complications. *Semin Dial* 22(4): 369-372.

Cohen G, Horl WH (2009b) Resistin as a cardiovascular and atherosclerotic risk factor and uremic toxin. *Semin Dial* 22(4): 373-377.

Cohen G, Haag-Weber M, Horl WH (1997) Immune dysfunction in uremia. *Kidney Int* Suppl 62: S79-82.

Cohen G, Rudnicki M, Horl WH (2001) Uremic toxins modulate the spontaneous apoptotic cell death and essential functions of neutrophils. *Kidney Int* Suppl 78: S48-52.

Cohen G, Rudnicki M, Deicher R, Horl WH (2003) Immunoglobulin light chains modulate polymorphonuclear leucocyte apoptosis. *Eur J Clin Invest* 33(8): 669-676.

Coldren CD, Nick JA, Poch KR, Woolum MD, Fouty BW et al. (2006) Functional and genomic changes induced by alveolar transmigration in human neutrophils. *Am J Physiol Lung Cell Mol Physiol* 291(6): L1267-1276.

D'Intini V, Bordoni V, Bolgan I, Bonello M, Brendolan A et al. (2004) Monocyte apoptosis in uremia is normalized with continuous blood purification modalities. *Blood Purif* 22(1): 9-12.

Dadfar E, Lundahl J, Jacobson SH (2004a) Monocyte adhesion molecule expression in interstitial inflammation in patients with renal failure. *Nephrol Dial Transplant* 19(3): 614-622.

Dadfar E, Lundahl J, Jacobson SH (2004b) Granulocyte extravasation and recruitment to sites of interstitial inflammation in patients with renal failure. *Am J Nephrol* 24(3): 330-339.

Dadfar E, Jacobson SH, Lundahl J (2007) Newly recruited human monocytes have a preserved responsiveness towards bacterial peptides in terms of CD11b up-regulation and intracellular hydrogen peroxide production. *Clin Exp Immunol* 148(3): 573-582.

Dadfar E, Lundahl J, Fernvik E, Nopp A, Hylander B et al. (2004c) Leukocyte CD11b and CD62l expression in response to interstitial inflammation in CAPD patients. *Perit Dial Int* 24(1): 28-36.

Dahlgren C, Karlsson A (1999) Respiratory burst in human neutrophils. *J Immunol Methods* 232(1-2): 3-14.

de Lemos, J. A., D. A. Morrow, et al. (2003) Association between plasma levels of monocyte chemoattractant protein-1 and long-term clinical outcomes in patients with acute coronary syndromes. *Circulation* 107(5): 690-5.

Descamps-Latscha B (1993) The immune system in end-stage renal disease. *Curr Opin Nephrol Hypertens* 2(6): 883-891.

Drost, E. M. and W. MacNee (2002) Potential role of IL-8, platelet-activating factor and TNF-alpha in the sequestration of neutrophils in the lung: effects on neutrophil deformability, adhesion receptor expression, and chemotaxis. *Eur J Immunol* 32(2): 393-403.

Eknoyan G, Beck GJ, Cheung AK, Daugirdas JT, Greene T et al. (2002) Effect of dialysis dose and membrane flux in maintenance hemodialysis. *N Engl J Med* 347(25): 2010-2019.

Follin P (1999) Skin chamber technique for study of in vivo exudated human neutrophils. *J Immunol Methods* 232(1-2): 55-65.

Gibbons RA, Martinez OM, Garovoy MR (1990) Altered monocyte function in uremia. *Clin Immunol Immunopathol* 56(1): 66-80.

Gonzalez-Amaro R, Sanchez-Madrid F (1999) Cell adhesion molecules: selectins and integrins. *Crit Rev Immunol* 19(5-6): 389-429.

Graff LR, Franklin KK, Witt L, Cohen N, Jacobs RA et al. (2002) Antimicrobial therapy of gram-negative bacteremia at two university-affiliated medical centers. *Am J Med* 112(3): 204-211.

Haag-Weber M, Horl WH (1996a) Are granulocyte inhibitory proteins contributing to enhanced susceptibility to infections in uraemia? *Nephrol Dial Transplant* 11 Suppl 2: 98-100.

Haag-Weber M, Horl WH (1996b) Dysfunction of polymorphonuclear leukocytes in uremia. *Semin Nephrol* 16(3): 192-201.

Haag-Weber M, Hable M, Fiedler G, Blum I, Schollmeyer P et al. (1991) Alterations of polymorphonuclear leukocyte glycogen metabolism and glucose uptake in dialysis patients. *Am J Kidney Dis* 17(5): 562-568.

Hermant B, Bibert S, Concord E, Dublet B, Weidenhaupt M et al. (2003) Identification of proteases involved in the proteolysis of vascular endothelium cadherin during neutrophil transmigration. *J Biol Chem* 278(16): 14002-14012.

Hernandez MR, Galan AM, Cases A, Lopez-Pedret J, Pereira A et al. (2004) Biocompatibility of cellulosic and synthetic membranes assessed by leukocyte activation. *Am J Nephrol* 24(2): 235-241.

Himmelfarb J, Lazarus JM, Hakim R (1991) Reactive oxygen species production by monocytes and polymorphonuclear leukocytes during dialysis. *Am J Kidney Dis* 17(3): 271-276.

Himmelfarb J, Ault KA, Holbrook D, Leeber DA, Hakim RM (1993) Intradialytic granulocyte reactive oxygen species production: a prospective, crossover trial. *J Am Soc Nephrol* 4(2): 178-186.

Horl WH (2001) Neutrophil function in renal failure. *Adv Nephrol Necker Hosp* 31: 173-192.

Horl WH (2002) Hemodialysis membranes: interleukins, biocompatibility, and middle molecules. *J Am Soc Nephrol* 13 Suppl 1: S62-71.

Hornberger JC, Chernew M, Petersen J, Garber AM (1992) A multivariate analysis of mortality and hospital admissions with high-flux dialysis. *J Am Soc Nephrol* 3(6): 1227-1237.

Idriss, H. T. and J. H. Naismith (2000) TNF alpha and the TNF receptor superfamily: structure-function relationship(s). *Microsc Res Tech* 50(3): 184-95.

Ikeda, U., K. Matsui, et al. (2002) Monocyte chemoattractant protein-1 and coronary artery disease. *Clin Cardiol* 25(4): 143-7.

Jacobson SH, Thylen P, Lundahl J (2000) Three monocyte-related determinants of atherosclerosis in haemodialysis. *Nephrol Dial Transplant* 15(9): 1414-1419.

Jacobson SH, Thylen P, Fernvik E, Hallden G, Gronneberg R et al. (2002) Hemodialysis-activated granulocytes at the site of interstitial inflammation. *Am J Kidney Dis* 39(4): 854-861.

Janeway C, Travers P (2005) *Immunobiology*. New York: Garland Publisher.

Jiang, Y., D. I. Beller, et al. (1992) Monocyte chemoattractant protein-1 regulates adhesion molecule expression and cytokine production in human monocytes. *J Immunol* 148(8): 2423-8.

Jiang, Y., J. F. Zhu, et al. (1994) MCP-1-stimulated monocyte attachment to laminin is mediated by beta 2-integrins. *Am J Physiol* 267(4 Pt 1): C1112-8.

Johnson-Leger C, Aurrand-Lions M, Imhof BA (2000) The parting of the endothelium: miracle, or simply a junctional affair? *J Cell Sci* 113 (Pt 6): 921-933.

Johnson F, Giulivi C (2005) Superoxide dismutases and their impact upon human health. *Mol Aspects Med* 26(4-5): 340-352.

Kaysen GA (2001) The microinflammatory state in uremia: causes and potential consequences. *J Am Soc Nephrol* 12(7): 1549-1557.

Kaysen GA, Kumar V (2003) Inflammation in ESRD: causes and potential consequences. *J Ren Nutr* 13(2): 158-160.

Kobayashi Y (2008) The role of chemokines in neutrophil biology. *Front Biosci* 13: 2400-2407.

Koller H, Hochegger K, Zlabinger GJ, Lhotta K, Mayer G et al. (2004) Apoptosis of human polymorphonuclear neutrophils accelerated by dialysis membranes via the activation of the complement system. *Nephrol Dial Transplant* 19(12): 3104-3111.

Kosch M, Levers A, Fobker M, Barenbrock M, Schaefer RM et al. (2003) Dialysis filter type determines the acute effect of haemodialysis on endothelial function and oxidative stress. *Nephrol Dial Transplant* 18(7): 1370-1375.

Ledebo I (1998) Principles and practice of hemofiltration and hemodiafiltration. *Artif Organs* 22(1): 20-25.

Liu, G., Y. J. Park, et al. (2008). Interleukin-1 receptor-associated kinase (IRAK) -1-mediated NF-kappaB activation requires cytosolic and nuclear activity. *Faseb J* 22(7): 2285-96.

Locatelli F (2003) Dose of dialysis, convection and haemodialysis patients outcome--what the HEMO study doesn't tell us: the European viewpoint. *Nephrol Dial Transplant* 18(6): 1061-1065.

Locatelli F, Martin-Malo A, Hannedouche T, Loureiro A, Papadimitriou M et al. (2009) Effect of membrane permeability on survival of hemodialysis patients. *J Am Soc Nephrol* 20(3): 645-654.

Lundberg L, Johansson G, Karlsson L, Stegmayr BG (1994) Complement activation is influenced by the membrane material, design of the dialyser, sterilizing method, and type of dialysate. *Nephrol Dial Transplant* 9(9): 1310-1314.

Malaponte G, Libra M, Bevelacqua Y, Merito P, Fatuzzo P et al. (2007) Inflammatory status in patients with chronic renal failure: the role of PTX3 and pro-inflammatory cytokines. *Int J Mol Med* 20(4): 471-481.

Martin-Malo A, Carracedo J, Ramirez R, Rodriguez-Benot A, Soriano S et al. (2000) Effect of uremia and dialysis modality on mononuclear cell apoptosis. *J Am Soc Nephrol* 11(5): 936-942.

Miller LJ, Bainton DF, Borregaard N, Springer TA (1987) Stimulated mobilization of monocyte Mac-1 and p150,95 adhesion proteins from an intracellular vesicular compartment to the cell surface. *J Clin Invest* 80(2): 535-544.

Moshfegh A, Jacobson SH, Hallden G, Thylen P, Lundahl J (2002) Impact of hemodialysis membrane and permeability on neutrophil transmigration in vitro. *Nephron* 91(4): 659-665.

Muniz-Junqueira MI, Braga Lopes C, Magalhaes CA, Schleicher CC, Veiga JP (2005) Acute and chronic influence of hemodialysis according to the membrane used on phagocytic function of neutrophils and monocytes and pro-inflammatory cytokines production in chronic renal failure patients. *Life Sci* 77(25): 3141-3155.

Olsson J, Dadfar E, Paulsson J, Lundahl J, Moshfegh A et al. (2007) Preserved leukocyte CD11b expression at the site of interstitial inflammation in patients with high-flux hemodiafiltration. *Kidney Int* 71(6): 582-588.

Olsson J, Paulsson J, Dadfar E, Lundahl J, Moshfegh A et al. (2009) Monocyte and neutrophil chemotactic activity at the site of interstitial inflammation in patients on high-flux hemodialysis or hemodiafiltration. *Blood Purif* 28(1): 47-52.

Parkin J, Cohen B (2001) An overview of the immune system. *Lancet* 357(9270): 1777-1789.

Paulsson J, Dadfar E, Held C, Jacobson SH, Lundahl J (2007) Activation of peripheral and in vivo transmigrated neutrophils in patients with stable coronary artery disease. *Atherosclerosis* 192(2): 328-334.

Panichi, V., U. Maggiore, et al. (2004) Interleukin-6 is a stronger predictor of total and cardiovascular mortality than C-reactive protein in haemodialysis patients. *Nephrol Dial Transplant* 19(5): 1154-60.

Pawlak K, Naumnik B, Brzosko S, Pawlak D, Mysliwiec M (2004) Oxidative stress - a link between endothelial injury, coagulation activation, and atherosclerosis in haemodialysis patients. *Am J Nephrol* 24(1): 154-161.

Pecoits-Filho, R., P. Barany, et al. (2002) Interleukin-6 is an independent predictor of mortality in patients starting dialysis treatment. *Nephrol Dial Transplant* 17(9): 1684-8.

Pecoits-Filho R, Lindholm B, Stenvinkel P (2002) The malnutrition, inflammation, and atherosclerosis (MIA) syndrome -- the heart of the matter. *Nephrol Dial Transplant* 17 Suppl 11: 28-31.

Powe NR, Jaar B, Furth SL, Hermann J, Briggs W (1999) Septicemia in dialysis patients: incidence, risk factors, and prognosis. *Kidney Int* 55(3): 1081-1090.

Pupim, L. B., J. Himmelfarb, et al. (2004) Influence of initiation of maintenance hemodialysis on biomarkers of inflammation and oxidative stress. *Kidney Int* 65(6): 2371-9.

Rabindranath KS, Strippoli GF, Daly C, Roderick PJ, Wallace S et al. (2006) Haemodiafiltration, haemofiltration and haemodialysis for end-stage kidney disease. *Cochrane Database Syst Rev*(4): CD006258.

Raj DS, Vincent B, Simpson K, Sato E, Jones KL et al. (2002) Hemodynamic changes during hemodialysis: role of nitric oxide and endothelin. *Kidney Int* 61(2): 697-704.

Ramos, C. D., C. Canetti, et al. (2005) MIP-1alpha[CCL3] acting on the CCR1 receptor mediates neutrophil migration in immune inflammation via sequential release of TNF-alpha and LTB4. *J Leukoc Biol* 78(1): 167-77.

Rezzonico, R., V. Imbert, et al. (2001) Ligation of CD11b and CD11c beta(2) integrins by antibodies or soluble CD23 induces macrophage inflammatory protein 1alpha (MIP-1alpha) and MIP-1beta production in primary human monocytes through a pathway dependent on nuclear factor-kappaB. *Blood* 97(10): 2932-40.

Rocco MV, Cheung AK, Greene T, Eknoyan G (2005) The HEMO Study: applicability and generalizability. *Nephrol Dial Transplant* 20(2): 278-284.

Sardenberg C, Suassuna P, Andreoli MC, Watanabe R, Dalboni MA et al. (2006) Effects of uraemia and dialysis modality on polymorphonuclear cell apoptosis and function. *Nephrol Dial Transplant* 21(1): 160-165.

Sarnak MJ, Jaber BL (2000) Mortality caused by sepsis in patients with end-stage renal disease compared with the general population. *Kidney Int* 58(4): 1758-1764.

Scheja A, Forsgren A (1985) A skin chamber technique for leukocyte migration studies; description and reproducibility. *Acta Pathol Microbiol Immunol Scand* 93: 25-30.

Schindler R, Eichert F, Lepenies J, Frei U (2001) Blood components influence cytokine induction by bacterial substances. *Blood Purif* 19(4): 380-387.

Schindler R, Ertl T, Beck W, Lepenies J, Boenisch O et al. (2006) Reduced cytokine induction and removal of complement products with synthetic hemodialysis membranes. *Blood Purif* 24(2): 203-211.

Sela S, Shurtz-Swirski R, Cohen-Mazor M, Mazor R, Chezar J et al. (2005) Primed peripheral polymorphonuclear leukocyte: a culprit underlying chronic low-grade inflammation and systemic oxidative stress in chronic kidney disease. *J Am Soc Nephrol* 16(8): 2431-2438.

Stenvinkel P, Heimburger O, Lindholm B, Kaysen GA, Bergstrom J (2000) Are there two types of malnutrition in chronic renal failure? Evidence for relationships between malnutrition, inflammation and atherosclerosis (MIA syndrome). *Nephrol Dial Transplant* 15(7): 953-960.

Swain SD, Rohn TT, Quinn MT (2002) Neutrophil priming in host defense: role of oxidants as priming agents. *Antioxid Redox Signal* 4(1): 69-83.

Theilgaard-Monch K, Porse BT, Borregaard N (2006) Systems biology of neutrophil differentiation and immune response. *Curr Opin Immunol* 18(1): 54-60.

Theilgaard-Monch K, Knudsen S, Follin P, Borregaard N (2004) The transcriptional activation program of human neutrophils in skin lesions supports their important role in wound healing. *J Immunol* 172(12): 7684-7693.

Thylen P, Fernvik E, Haegerstrand A, Lundahl J, Jacobson SH (1997) Dialysis-induced serum factors inhibit adherence of monocytes and granulocytes to adult human endothelial cells. *Am J Kidney Dis* 29(1): 78-85.

Thylen P, Lundahl J, Fernvik E, Gronneberg R, Hallden G et al. (2000) Impaired monocyte CD11b expression in interstitial inflammation in hemodialysis patients. *Kidney Int* 57(5): 2099-2106.

van Buul JD, Hordijk PL (2004) Signaling in leukocyte transendothelial migration. *Arterioscler Thromb Vasc Biol* 24(5): 824-833.

Van Den Steen, P. E., A. Wuyts, et al. (2003) Gelatinase B/MMP-9 and neutrophil collagenase/MMP-8 process the chemokines human GCP-2/CXCL6, ENA-78/CXCL5 and mouse GCP-2/LIX and modulate their physiological activities. *Eur J Biochem* 270(18): 3739-49.

Vanholder R, Van Biesen W, Ringoir S (1993a) Contributing factors to the inhibition of phagocytosis in hemodialyzed patients. *Kidney Int* 44(1): 208-214.

Vanholder R, De Smet R, Hsu C, Vogeleere P, Ringoir S (1994a) Uremic toxicity: the middle molecule hypothesis revisited. *Semin Nephrol* 14(3): 205-218.

Vanholder R, Van Loo A, Dhondt AM, De Smet R, Ringoir S (1996) Influence of uraemia and haemodialysis on host defence and infection. *Nephrol Dial Transplant* 11(4): 593-598.

Vanholder R, Baurmeister U, Brunet P, Cohen G, Glorieux G et al. (2008) A bench to bedside view of uremic toxins. *J Am Soc Nephrol* 19(5): 863-870.

Vanholder R, De Smet R, Jacobs V, Van Landschoot N, Waterloos MA et al. (1994b) Uraemic toxic retention solutes depress polymorphonuclear response to phagocytosis. *Nephrol Dial Transplant* 9(9): 1271-1278.

Vanholder R, Dell'Aquila R, Jacobs V, Dhondt A, Veys N et al. (1993b) Depressed phagocytosis in hemodialyzed patients: in vivo and in vitro mechanisms. *Nephron* 63(4): 409-415.

Vanholder R, Argiles A, Baurmeister U, Brunet P, Clark W et al. (2001) Uremic toxicity: present state of the art. *Int J Artif Organs* 24(10): 695-725.

Weber, C., K. U. Belge, et al. (2000) Differential chemokine receptor expression and function in human monocyte subpopulations. *J Leukoc Biol* 67(5): 699-704.

Woods HF, Nandakumar M (2000) Improved outcome for haemodialysis patients treated with high-flux membranes. *Nephrol Dial Transplant* 15 Suppl 1: 36-42.

Yamashiro S, Kamohara H, Wang JM, Yang D, Gong WH et al. (2001) Phenotypic and functional change of cytokine-activated neutrophils: inflammatory neutrophils are heterogeneous and enhance adaptive immune responses. *J Leukoc Biol* 69(5): 698-704.

Yan, L., N. Borregaard, et al. (2001) The high molecular weight urinary matrix metalloproteinase (MMP) activity is a complex of gelatinase B/MMP-9 and neutrophil gelatinase-associated lipocalin (NGAL). Modulation of MMP-9 activity by NGAL. *J Biol Chem* 276(40): 37258-65.

Zeilhofer, H. U. and W. Schorr (2000) Role of interleukin-8 in neutrophil signaling. *Curr Opin Hematol* 7(3): 178-82.

10

Dialysis Membrane Manipulation for Endotoxin Removal

Michael Henrie, Cheryl Ford, Eric Stroup and Chih-Hu Ho
Fresenius Medical Care North America
United States

1. Introduction

In the dialysis clinic, water is an essential vehicle to deliver life-saving treatment to patients suffering from varying degrees of kidney failure, both acute and chronic. Clean water is vital, as the key ingredient used to prepare hemodialysis fluid (dialysate solution), and on-line generation of substitution fluid for hemodiafiltration. Generally all fluids used to treat patients suffering from kidney failure may come into contact with the blood of the patient, whether directly or indirectly (across a membrane), and theoretically could transport contaminants resulting in a negative impact on patient health. Of the microbiological contaminants found in water, endotoxin is given considerable attention, given its difficulty for removal and inactivation from water and water distribution systems (Smeets et al., 2003; Perez-Garcia & Rodriguez-Benitez, 2000) and its inherent pyrogenicity (G. Lonnemann, 2000).

Endotoxins are found in all gram-negative bacteria, although slight differences in chemical structure are found between varying bacterial strains. The term endotoxin is typically used to describe a complex of protein and lipopolysaccharide (LPS) molecules found in the outer cell wall of gram-negative bacteria, that either slough off during growth, or are released upon cell lysis. Endotoxin and lipopolysaccharide are typically used interchangeably in literature, although in clinical discussion the term endotoxin is most often used, as it is the metric used to monitor water and dialysis fluid quality. Lipopolysaccharide is a vital component of the outer membrane of gram-negative bacteria, providing numerous physiological functions and comprising nearly 75% of the bacterium outer surface area (Raetz, 1991). Lipopolysaccharides consist of three components: a long heteropolysaccharide chain (O-specific chain) which represents a surface antigen; a core oligosaccharide; and a lipid component termed lipid A used as an anchor in the outer cell membrane (Rietschel et al., 1994; Gorbet & Sefton, 2005). Molecular weights of most lipopolysaccharides are 10 - 20 kDa; however, due to their amphiphilic nature, LPS molecules can form aggregates (100 - 1000 kDa) which are too large to pass through dialysis membranes. It has been shown that components of lipopolysaccharide (lipid A) are able to pass through dialysis membranes, can elicit a pyrogenic response (Naveh-Many et al., 1999), and contribute to long-term morbidity and inflammation (H. Schiffl, 2000; Raj et al., 2009).

Lipid A is the most conserved component of lipopolysaccharide throughout all gram-negative bacteria, and as such is responsible for the majority of the pyrogenic activity. Lipid A consists of a phosphorylated N-acetylglucosamine (NAG) dimmer connected to saturated fatty acid chains; variability within the composition of the fatty acids will determine the toxic property of lipid A, as well as play a role in resistance to host antimicrobial factors and avoiding recognition from specific components of the host immune system (Bland et al., 1994; Gunn, 2001; Qureshi et al., 1999). The O-specific side chain component of LPS is responsible for complement activation and contributes to fever and hypotension, as well as binding to endotoxin recognition molecules within the body (Valvano, 1992; Bailat et al., 1997). Once within the body, LPS tend to be found at higher concentrations within the spleen and liver (uptake by phagocytosis) where they are cleared from the body (Haeffner-Cavaillon et al., 1998).

Dialysis patients are typically exposed to 90 – 120 liters of dialysis fluid per treatment, which equates to an annual exposure of 20 – 30,000 liters (Weber et al., 2004; I. Ledebo, 2002). With constant exposure to large amounts of fluid, the opportunity for a dialysis patient to experience an inflammatory or pyrogenic reaction due to contamination within the dialysis fluid is increased. For hemodialysis, fluids that are used for treatments do not have to be sterile; however, the lower the microbial concentration, the lower the risk of patient reaction. Because of this risk, regional regulatory boards have implemented limits to the total microbial count that can be present in fluids that are to be used in dialysis treatments. However, even if water treatment systems are in place, contamination is still a possibility and a risk. Dialysis fluid used for clinical treatments may become contaminated from either the source water, the dialysate concentrate, or from the water distribution system. Due to the ubiquitous nature of biofilm, and its propensity to generate endotoxin, this problem affects not only hemodialysis, but all extracorporeal therapies (Kanagasundaram et al., 2009).

Regardless of the treatment processes used to create water for dialysis fluid, the final opportunity to remove microbial contaminants from the fluid path prior to patient exposure is the dialysis membrane contained within the dialyzer. Dialysis fluid comes into direct contact with this membrane, and due to transmembrane pressure differences and the permeability of the filter, especially for high-flux dialyzers, the potential for dialysis fluid to enter the blood compartment and return to the patient is significant (N. Hoenich, 2007). It is this final barrier, the dialyzer membrane, where the last opportunity resides to remove endotoxins from solution (Weber et al., 2009), by means of membrane manipulation. The aim of the following research is to achieve a more thorough understanding of how endotoxin interacts with various physical characteristics of the dialysis membrane, and how to exploit these interactions to increase endotoxin removal from dialysis fluid.

2. Membrane manipulation for endotoxin removal

The degree of contaminated dialysis fluid including bacteria, bacterial fragments and endotoxin that may enter the bloodstream of a patient during treatment depends largely upon the porosity and other physical characteristics of the membrane being utilized. Back-filtration is based upon geometrical and permeability properties of the hollow fiber membrane, and cannot be avoided in high-flux hemodialysis (Ofsthun & Leypoldt, 1995). However, both physical and chemical means can be used to prohibit endotoxin from crossing the membrane, by removing it from solution and holding it within the dialyzer membrane. Numerous studies have been performed to determine the properties of hemodialysis membranes that best manipulate the transfer of endotoxin, by removing it from the dialysis circuit (Canaud et al., 2000; Lonnemann et al., 2001). Surface treatments, polymer modifications, as well as chemical changes to the membrane composition, have been investigated to ascertain their influence on preventing or minimizing endotoxin and bacterial fragment flux across the membrane. Some studies have shown that even the choice of sterilization modality may have an impact on the membrane, and affect the ability to retain endotoxin (Gomila et al, 2006; Krieter et al., 2008). It is necessary to understand how a particular dialysis membrane interacts with endotoxin and other dialysis fluid contaminants, as the membrane is the last barrier to the patients' blood. Endotoxins (and other types of microbial contamination) are removed from dialysis fluid mainly by one of two methods: filtration and adsorption. Studies have shown that both methods of endotoxin removal occur during dialysis treatment (Osumi et al., 1995). Understanding endotoxin interactions with various membrane surfaces is imperative in order to orchestrate changes that will have a positive impact on endotoxin removal. The end goal of all endotoxin research is to limit patient exposure, in hopes of reducing the chance for pyrogenic reactions, inflammation, and shock.

2.1 Membrane geometry

Prior to synthetic membranes occupying the majority of the dialysis filter market, cellulosic membranes were the predominant choice for manufacturers. Cellulose was a material that could be modified to improve its biocompatibility; however its geometrical manipulation was limited due to the production process. As membrane materials progressed from cellulose-based to synthetic, numerous adjustments could be made to the physical characteristics of the membrane by relatively simple manufacturing process changes.

One of the most direct methods to inhibit endotoxin is to change the material structure of the membrane itself, as the physical attributes of the membrane will perhaps have the greatest effect on endotoxin removal. Typically a thin-wall membrane is not as robust as a thick-wall membrane, in terms of endotoxin adsorption, since a thicker membrane can offer more surface area for the endotoxin to come into contact with. A thicker membrane provides a longer path for the endotoxin to maneuver through, before it reaches the blood circuit. An important characteristic of this path from outer membrane surface to inner membrane lumen is tortuosity, the curving path that the endotoxin must follow in order to reach the blood compartment of the fiber membrane (Osumi et al., 1995). As tortuosity is increased, the greater the chance the membrane has at prohibiting the passage of endotoxin. Membrane geometry changes can lead to differences in the adsorptive capacity for endotoxin (Vanholder & Pedrini, 2008; Vaslaki et al., 2000) and for bacteria (Waterhouse & Hall, 1995).

Changes in membrane permeability are controlled to enhance convective transfer, which targets middle molecular removal of species such as β_2Microglobulin and vitamin B_{12}. As dialysis membranes are pushed for more convective removal ability, the opportunity for endotoxin trans-membrane flux increases due to the higher chance of back-filtration. Future membranes designed to address middle molecule removal by increasing internal filtration (Mineshima et al., 2009) will not improve on patient inflammation (Kerr et al., 2007) unless membrane geometry is modified to improve endotoxin removal.

The effect of membrane thickness and permeability on endotoxin removal was studied by testing various membrane configurations, and by observing their ability to restrict contaminant flux. Synthetic membranes for testing were manufactured with specific geometries to observe their performance relative to a control. Fiber geometries tested included low flux, high flux, thin wall, thick wall, macrovoid, and a control. Characteristics of each test membrane produced for this study are listed below in Table 1. The endotoxin challenge solution used was comprised of a 1:1 mixture of bacterial culture filtrates of Stenotrophomonas maltophilia (ATCC 13637) and Pseudomonas aeruginosa (ATCC 27853), both common water organisms. Cultures of each microorganism were ultra-sonicated to lyse the cells and release the endotoxin fragments, then filtered using a sequentially-decreasing process resulting in a final 0.2 µm filtration step.

Fiber Type	Fiber ID, µm	Fiber Wall, µm	Fiber Kuf, mL/hr*mmHg	Material, Fiber type
Control	185	35	200	Polysulfone (PS), asymmetric
Low Flux	181	39	48	PS, asymmetric
High Flux	182	37	522	PS, asymmetric
Thin Wall	187	24	231	PS, asymmetric
Thick Wall	184	44	190	PS, asymmetric
Macrovoid	212	33	130	PS, dual skin

Table 1. Fiber membrane geometries

Bacterial culture filtrates were used instead of purified LPS to produce challenge material that would closely resemble clinical experiences. Membranes were tested for their ability to restrict the passage of endotoxin across the membrane by either filtration or adsorption, by using a test setup (Figure 1) that focused on the diffusive and convective aspects of hemodialysis. The first setup focuses on diffusive testing, whereby the counter current flow mimics a typical hemodialysis treatment. The second setup in the test forces fluid to flow through the membrane, testing the filtration capacities of each fiber membrane. Initially, the test setup involved connecting the test dialyzer to a recirculating loop, where it could be connected to a peristaltic pump to control the flow of fluid on the blood loop. The dialysis fluid loop consisted of tubing that was connected to a reservoir, which allowed fluid to be recirculated through the dialysis fluid compartment, via another peristaltic pump. This reservoir held 1 liter of challenge solution, containing bacterial culture filtrate mixed into saline to produce an endotoxin concentration of 400 +/- 50 EU/mL. The blood loop

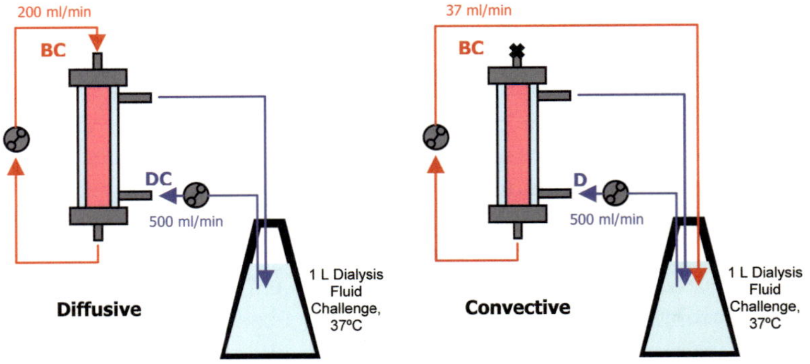

Fig. 1. Endotoxin challenge test setup, showing the blood loop and dialysis fluid loop flowrates for both diffusive and convective testing.

peristaltic pump was set at 200 mL/min to recirculate the enclosed saline, while the dialysis fluid loop pump was set at 500 mL/min to recirculate the endotoxin challenge solution from the reservoir, through the dialyzer, and back. This test setup was maintained inside an incubator set at 37 C. Prior to starting the test, the dialyzer (both blood loop and dialysis fluid loop) were primed with sterile saline, to rinse out any residual endotoxin that may be contained within the test setup. Once the pumps were initiated, a timer was started and samples were taken from both the blood loop and dialysis fluid loop at the following times: 0, 7, 15, and 60 minutes. Following the 60 minute sample, the test setup was changed according to Figure 1, so that dialysis fluid was forced across the membrane into the blood loop, and back into the challenge reservoir. Again, samples were taken following the start of the second half of the experiment at 67, 75, and 120 minutes. Samples were kept refrigerated at 4 C until ready to be analyzed for endotoxin content.
Endotoxin activity was measured using a kinetic turbidimetric Limulus Amoebocyte Lysate (LAL) assay from Charles River Labs. Each sample was measured in duplicate, along with a positive control to verify recovery within the sample. Results from these tests are shown in Figure 2, with curves to represent both blood side and dialysis fluid side endotoxin concentrations. The data were able to show that only the control and thick wall membranes were able to contain the endotoxin in the blood side below < 0.1 EU/mL; all other membrane types allowed measurable amounts of endotoxin to cross into the enclosed blood loop circuit. Also, the results indicate that some membranes perform better at prohibiting

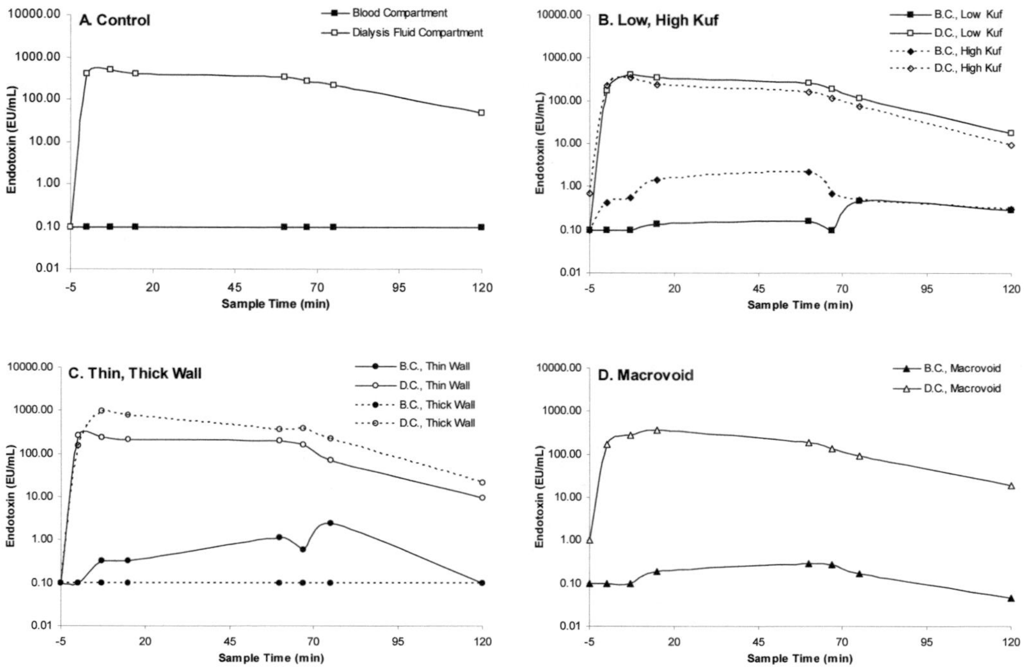

Fig. 2. Endotoxin challenge results for test simulations (all tests, n=3). a) Control membrane; b) Low and High Kuf membranes; c) Thin, Thick Wall membranes; d) Macrovoid membrane.

diffusive endotoxin flux than convective endotoxin flux, and vice versa. In particular, the high flux and thin wall membranes allowed the highest amounts of endotoxin into the blood compartment, as these membranes present the shortest tortuous path (thin wall) and the highest potential for back-diffusion along the membrane (high flux). These findings suggest that asymmetric, thick membranes are better suited at removing endotoxin from solution, as well as allowing endotoxin and other pyrogenic substances from crossing the membrane and contaminating a patient blood-flow.

Not only is a thick fiber good at preventing endotoxin contamination to the patient, but the outer or inner membrane surface of the fiber membrane are imperative at preventing trans-membrane endotoxin flux. Pore size distribution, or surface morphology, is a strictly controlled process in how to determine the flux of the dialyzer, and in allowing molecules of a certain size to either pass through the membrane surface, or be retained. Dialysis membrane pore sizes are not manufactured with endotoxin transfer in mind; however the pores play a critical role in regulating trans-membrane passage. Membrane thickness, structure, and surface morphology influence the membranes' ability in preventing endotoxin transfer through geometrical means, mostly by way of filtration. However, chemical changes within the membrane can also add benefits towards increased endotoxin performance, with respect to removal by way of adsorption.

2.2 Membrane surface changes

Similar to how membrane geometry directly affects the endotoxin sieving ability, the surface properties of membranes will govern the adsorption capacity for endotoxin by providing a suitable surface for endotoxin and endotoxin fragments to adsorb by utilizing their amphiphilic nature. The hydrophobic lipid A moiety is typically attracted to hydrophobic surfaces, however the hydrophilic polysaccharide component will also allow for adsorption to hydrophilic surfaces (Takemoto et al., 2003). Recent studies have shown this to be the case, particularly for ultrafilters which remove endotoxin by way of adsorption through ionic and hydrophobic interactions (Vaslaki et al, 2000). When adjusting the polymer ratios of dialysis fiber membrane, chemical changes as well as physical changes can be produced. The overall geometry of the fiber can be manipulated by the polymer ratio - whether the fiber is based upon a sponge structure, whether the membrane possesses macrovoids, or whether the membrane exhibits one skin or two.

Synthetic dialysis membranes from polysulfone are typically hydrophobic in nature, thus adding to their ability in being a good hemocompatible membrane for blood interaction. When manufacturing such membranes it is necessary to utilize a hydrophilic polymer that allows for the membrane to "wet"; to possess hydrophilic regions or properties. By simply adjusting the ratio of hydrophobic polymer (polysulfone) to hydrophilic polymer (polyvinylpyrrolidone or PVP), the membrane hydrophobicity composition can be changed significantly. A membrane that incorporates varying regions of hydrophobicity may be able to exploit the amphiphilic nature of endotoxin, resulting in numerous opportunities to remove it from dialysis fluid via adsorption (Maitz et al., 2009). Enhanced endotoxin removal has been shown feasible by increasing the surface polarity of the membrane (Rimmele et al, 2008). Polysulfone membranes typically exhibit a net negative surface charge, termed zeta potential, which may aid in their ability to remove endotoxin through adsorption (Mares et al, 2009; Shao et al., 2007). Similar behaviors are witnessed when endotoxin solutions are kept in glass containers; the glassware adsorbs a portion of the endotoxin, thus necessitating the glass to be cleaned or "depyrogenated."

A special consideration to not overlook is where dialysis clinics practice reuse; numerous studies have investigated the effect of reprocessing agents on dialysis membrane performance and the resulting effect on endotoxin retention (Teehan et al., 2004; Sundaram et al., 1996). For those using bleach as a disinfectant and sterilizing agent, its use has to be taken into account as repeated exposure to membranes have been shown to increase solute clearance, as well as increase the net negative charge, thus increasing hydrophilicity (Shao et al., 2007).

Polymer mixes were varied for test membranes, to study the endotoxin removal performance based upon chemical surface changes. Membranes, manufactured for this study, included those composed of high and low PVP content, a membrane consisting of a polymer mixture (polysulfone, PEG) and a membrane exposed to bleach - to determine how fiber surface differences affect the overall ability to remove endotoxin from solution. Also, membranes were tested using a fluorescent-labeled endotoxin to show the distribution of endotoxin within the membrane, modified from prior studies (Hayama et al., 2002). The experimental test setup was similar to that used to test fiber geometries - the test environment temperature, blood loop and dialysis fluid loop flow rates, endotoxin challenge concentration, and sample analysis method were all kept constant as described previously.

An additional test was performed for these membranes, using a labeled endotoxin to identify where the endotoxin molecule is removed from solution within the fiber membrane. To accomplish this, miniature dialyzers were constructed of small polycarbonate housings and T's to create a membrane dialyzer that could filter a smaller volume of fluorescent challenge solution, a mixture of Alexa Fluor 568 (Invitrogen, Carlsbad, CA) in saline to produce a concentration of 2,000 EU/mL. Membranes were challenged using a test setup similar to the diffusive setup used for the endotoxin challenge simulations, utilizing a challenge fluid flow on the dialysis fluid side of 5 mL/min, and a countercurrent fluid flow of saline on the blood side of 2 mL/min. Upon completion of the diffusive test, fibers were extracted from the miniature dialyzer housings and fixed into freezing media. A cryostat was used to slice the membrane samples into 10 um sections, which were then imaged using a microscope fit with a resorufin filter to observe the distribution of endotoxin on the membrane.

Membrane permeability tests (Figure 3) were able to show how the bleached membrane, the high PVP content membrane, as well as the polymer mixture membrane, all allowed significant amounts of endotoxin to cross into the blood loop compartment. Fluorescent imaging revealed that for all membranes the majority of the endotoxin (highest intensity) was bound at either the inner or outer lumen of the fiber; also, differences could be seen in the distribution of endotoxin inside the bulk of the membrane, with some membranes showing high intensity, while others hardly could be imaged due to the low intensity of the endotoxin (Figure 4).

These results indicate that chemical changes to the membrane can be manipulated in order to direct the preferential adsorption of endotoxin in a discreet region of the fiber, such as the outer lumen or inner lumen. These types of changes may be beneficial depending upon the intended use of the membrane, such as dialysis or ultrafiltration. Researchers have postulated that the region within the membrane where endotoxin is removed is important, as it has been shown to induce cytokine activation in blood within a dialyzer when bound adjacent to the lumen surface (Okamoto et al., 2004). These test results also provide insight into the nature of where and how endotoxin is bound or adsorbs to the membrane, furthering our understanding in how to remove it from solutions.

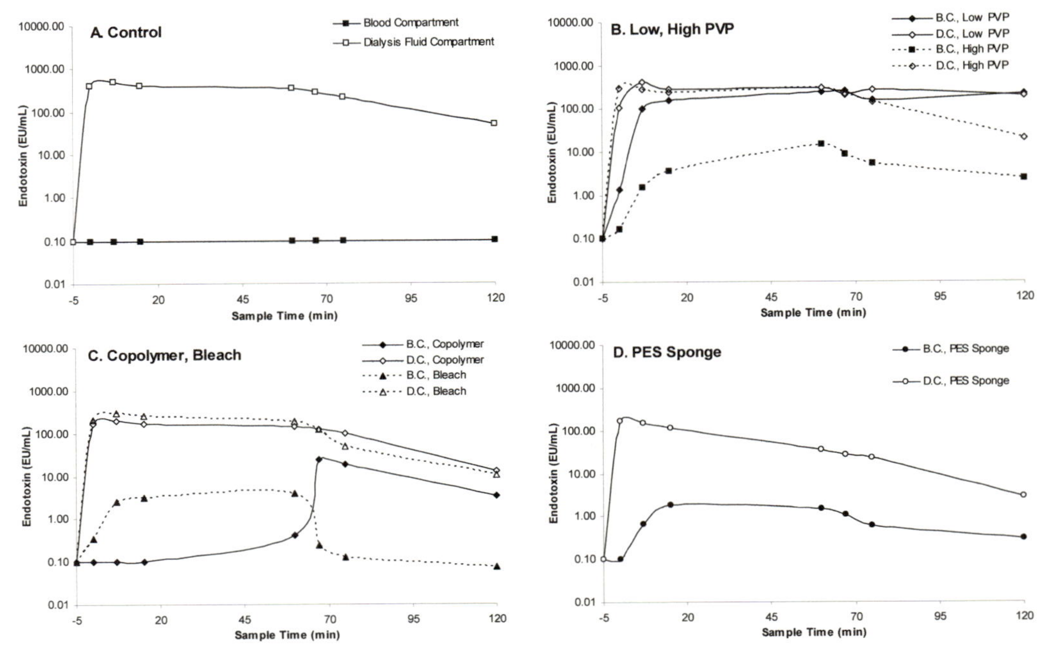

Fig. 3. Endotoxin challenge results for test simulations (all tests, n=3). a) Control membrane; b) Low, High PVP membranes; c) Copolymer, Bleach membranes; d) PES Sponge membrane.

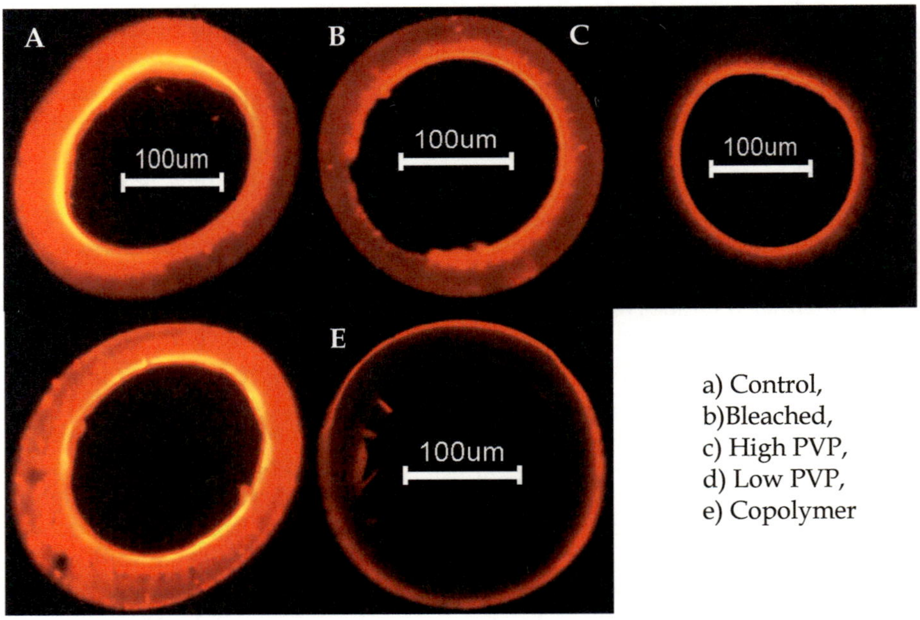

Fig. 4. Fiber membrane sections showing the distribution of fluorescent-labeled endotoxin (Alexa Fluor 568, imaged using a Resorufin filter).

2.3 Membrane material

The type of membrane structure possible, which directly relates to the endotoxin removal mechanism (filtration, adsorption), is largely governed by the material used to produce the membrane. Polysulfone is currently the most common membrane material in the chronic dialysis market, but is only one of several choices available to patients and nephrologists. Dialysis membranes may also be produced from materials such as cellulose, poly methyl methacrylate (PMMA), polyester-polymer alloy (PEPA), polyethersulfone, polyamide, and cuprophane. Use of cuprophane membranes modified with vitamin E (Girndt et al., 2000), highlight the potential for modifications of specific membrane materials. Significant research has been produced to show superior performance for endotoxin removal by synthetic membranes (Yamamoto & Kim, 1996; Nube & Grooteman, 2001); however, research has also exploited differences in the capacity for endotoxin between membranes of the same material, indicating that slight differences in the manufacturing and finishing processes may have a significant impact on the ultimate performance (Opatrny Jr. et al., 2006). On the contrary, studies have shown that in some instances it is difficult to show a clinical benefit when comparing differing membranes (Boudville et al., 2009; Urena et al., 1992).

The effect of various fiber membrane materials on endotoxin retention was studied by testing polysulfone, cellulose triacetate, and polyethersulfone dialysis membranes using endotoxin permeability studies. An endotoxin challenge of 400 ± 50 EU/mL was created by spiking sterile saline with bacterial culture filtrates of a 1:1 mixture of P. aeruginosa (ATCC 27853) and S. maltophilia (ATCC 13637). Simulation experiments were conducted to assess endotoxin transfer under both diffusive and convective conditions, with sterile saline used to model blood in the blood-side circuit. Flow rates used were similar to prior studies (Q_B = 200 mL/min, Q_D = 500 mL/min) and the experimental temperature was kept constant at 37 C. Samples were taken at times similar to prior studies, and were analyzed using a kinetic turbidimetric LAL assay with a detection limit of 0.1 EU/mL.

The results from these studies (Figure 5) show sponge-structure polysulfone performed the best at prohibiting endotoxin to cross the membrane, under diffusive and convective hydraulic conditions. Cellulose triacetate and polyethersulfone both allowed endotoxin to cross into the inner lumen space of the membrane; it is unclear if these results are indications to limits of endotoxin removal regarding the fiber lumen (pore size) or lumen surface adsorption. Material choice will dictate what type of endotoxin removal will predominate - filtration or adsorption - as certain materials will produce specific structure geometries when undergoing the manufacturing process.

Also, material choice will determine if a membrane is a good candidate for a particular coating or surface treatment to be applied; to aid in either creating a more biocompatible surface, or to enhance the endotoxin retentive properties.

2.4 Membrane coatings

Membrane coatings or surface treatments are not usually found on general use dialyzers; rather, they are used to add enhancements to dialyzers to better help a niche group of patients - whether the need is improved biocompatibility, better anticoagulation, or a reduction in circulating inflammatory cytokines. Surface treatments or coatings could be used to remove endotoxin; however, no coatings for dialyzer membranes (to date) have been produced to directly address endotoxin adsorption or removal. A coating which could produce a mixture of hydrophobic and hydrophilic regions would increase the adsorptive capacity of the membrane to retain circulating endotoxin - and at the same time may aid in filtrative endotoxin removal. Coatings applied to the membrane post-production should be designed to not decrease/impede any solute clearance performance of the membrane, or inhibit membrane performance in any way.

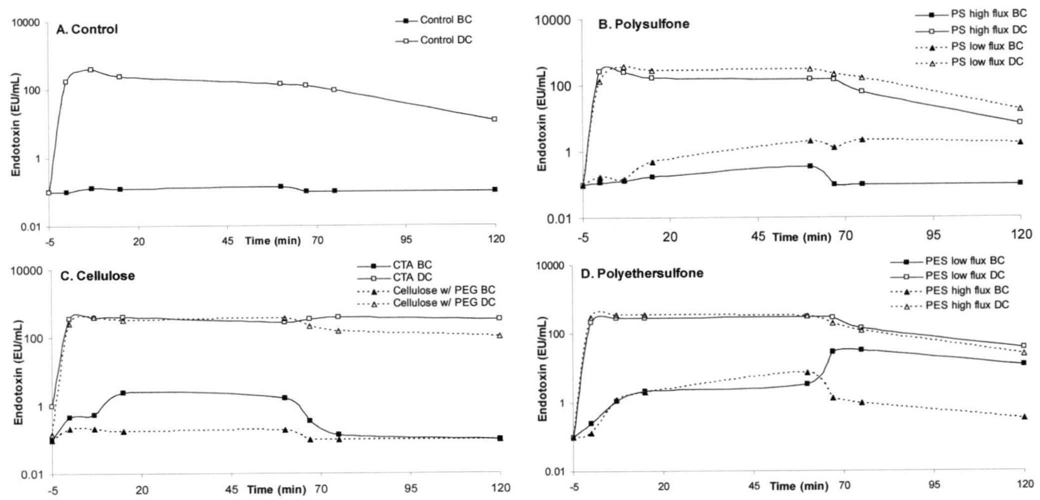

Fig. 5. Endotoxin challenge results for test simulations (all tests, n=3). a) Control membrane (PS); b) Polysulfone, low-flux and high-flux; c) Cellulose, CTA and PEG coated; d) Polyethersulfone, low-flux and high-flux.

Charcoal suspension has been tested as a potential adsorbent for diaysis, although it has been shown to induce platelet activation (Kramer et al., 2000). One significant area of research on endotoxin adsorption is for septic patients. Numerous techniques have been tested to remove circulating inflammatory cytokines from patient blood, as well as remove endotoxin. Polymyxin-B has been studied as an endotoxin binder, due to its affinity to the lipid A component and as it disrupts the permeability of cytoplasmic membranes of Gram negative bacteria (Uriu et al., 2002; Jaber & Pereira, 1997; Tani et al., 1998). Polyethylenimine has been researched as a potential endotoxin adsorbent, and may be more compatible than other types of resins in similar applications (Mitzner et al., 1993). The most prevalent treatment is to use apheresis and hemoperfusion, removing specific targets by resins or coated fibers (Ronco et al., 2000; Szathmary et al., 2004; Yaroustovsky et al., 2009; Umgelter et al., 2008). Some of these endotoxin-specific adsorbents that have been proven effective may come with deleterious side effects (Steczko et al., 1999; Tani et al., 1998).

Efficacy of a potential endotoxin-specific coating application was investigated by treating standard dialysis membranes with two specific polysaccharides (neutral and positive charged chitosan), a tri-block copolymer, and by using a bleach rinse. These modified membranes were tested for their endotoxin retention capacity by using the endotoxin simulation procedure described previously, with the same flow rates (Q_B = 200 mL/min, Q_D = 500 mL/min) and an endotoxin dialysis fluid challenge of 440 ± 55 EU/mL. However, the duration of the experiment was extended to 6 hours (3 hrs. diffusive, 3 hrs. convective) to observe if any plateau of endotoxin filtration or adsorption were to occur. Sampling from the blood and dialysis fluid circuits occurred at the following times (minutes): -5, 0, 7, 15, 30, and every 30 minutes afterwards until 3 hours had transpired. Samples were analyzed for endotoxin activity using a kinetic turbidimetric LAL assay with a detection limit of 0.1 EU/mL.

Results obtained from the test dialyzers with membrane coatings are shown in Figure 5, showing the endotoxin profile curves for the full 6 hours of testing. Samples analyzed from the chitosan and +chitosan membranes exhibited inflated spike recovery samples, indicative of false positive readings. It is likely that polysaccharide leaching out of the coating and into the recirculating saline solution in the blood compartment compromised the integrity of the samples. It is likely that the actual endotoxin crossing into the blood compartment for the chitosan and +chitosan samples is lower, however the overall endotoxin reduction in the dialysis fluid compartment did not justify repeating the tests using a buffering agent to mask the effects of the polysaccharides. The findings suggest that while all of the investigative treatments did enhance the removal of endotoxin, some were more successful than others (chitosan coatings<control<bleach treated<polymer coating).

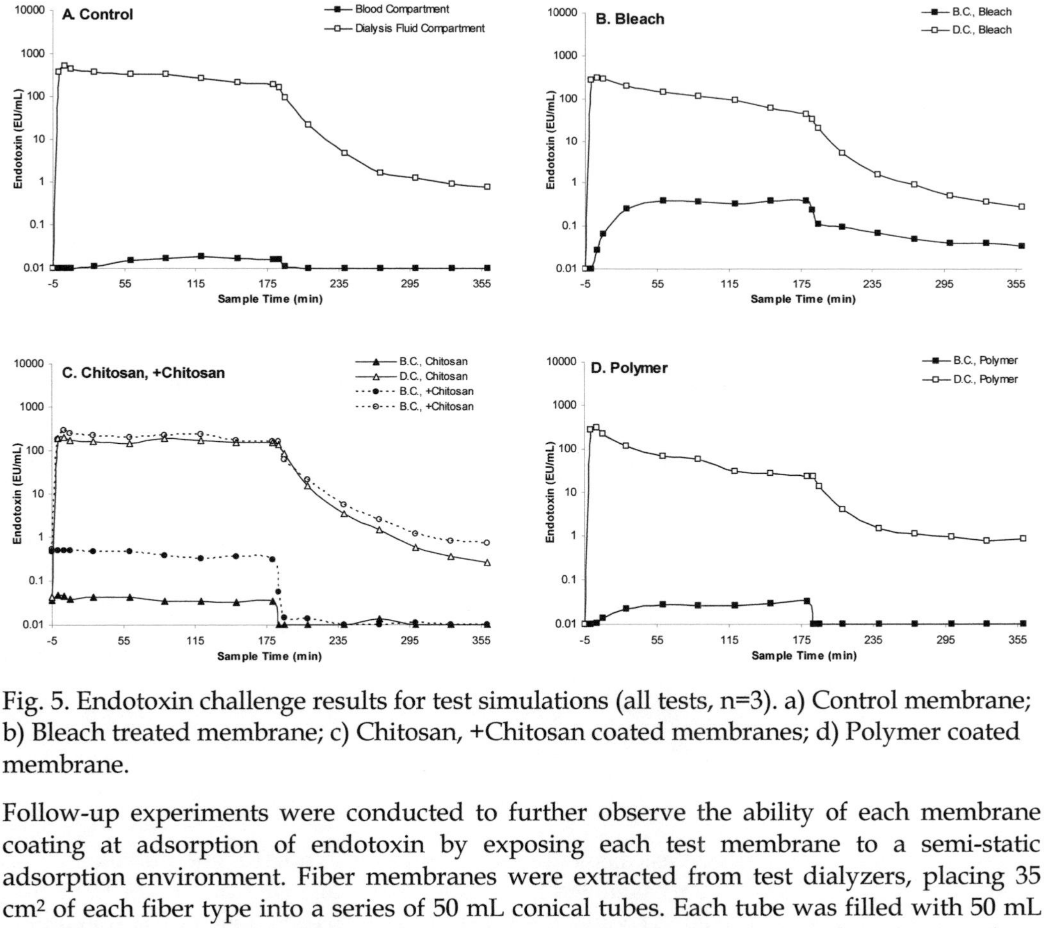

Fig. 5. Endotoxin challenge results for test simulations (all tests, n=3). a) Control membrane; b) Bleach treated membrane; c) Chitosan, +Chitosan coated membranes; d) Polymer coated membrane.

Follow-up experiments were conducted to further observe the ability of each membrane coating at adsorption of endotoxin by exposing each test membrane to a semi-static adsorption environment. Fiber membranes were extracted from test dialyzers, placing 35 cm^2 of each fiber type into a series of 50 mL conical tubes. Each tube was filled with 50 mL of sterile saline, and then spiked with varying amounts of endotoxin resulting in a gradient of concentrations for each membrane type (1, 2.5, 5, 10, 20, and 50 EU/mL). These tubes were then fixed to a rotor in a 37 C environment, which provided thorough mixing for the test duration of 72 hours. Samples were taken at set intervals, and analyzed immediately using the kinetic turbidimetric LAL assay with a detection limit of 0.01 EU/mL. Data gathered from these tests were used to generate adsorption isotherms for each membrane, shown in Figure 6. These plots indicate that the polymer coated membrane removed more endotoxin, and at a higher rate, than both the bleach treated and control membranes. For all three test membranes, adsorption rates for the 1 and 2.5 EU/mL concentrations reached a plateau at about 60 hours, although at 72 hours the 20 and 50 EU/mL concentrations were still showing measurable adsorption of endotoxin. The adsorption rates were calculated as follows: control - 0.15 ml/cm^2*hr; bleach - 0.11 ml/cm^2*hr; polymer - 0.30 mL/cm^2*hr. The results from the polymer coated membrane are promising, given that the adsorption rate of endotoxin was twice that of the control. These findings suggest that endotoxin-specific coatings for dialysis or ultra filtration membranes are a theoretical possibility, and may aid in other aspects of membrane performance.

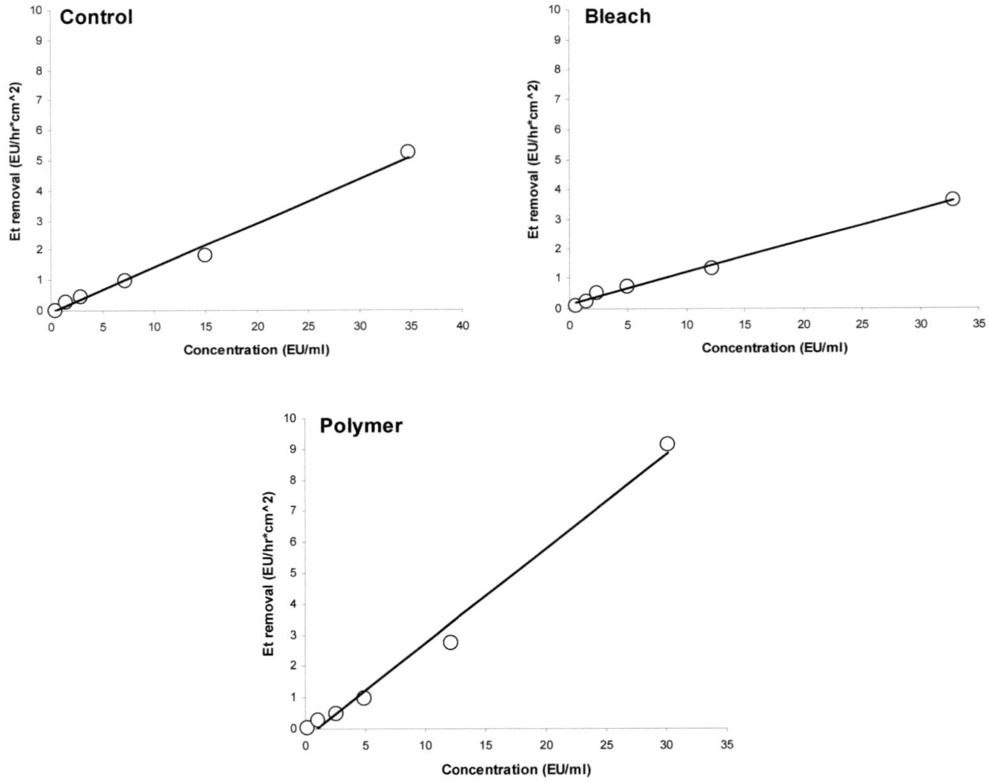

Fig. 6. Adsorption isotherm curves calculated for control, bleach treated, and polymer coated membranes. Curves were calculated from endotoxin challenge solutions of 1, 2.5, 5, 10, 20, and 50 EU/mL. Correlation coefficients for the control, bleach treated, and polymer coated membranes were $r^2 = 0.991$, $r^2 = 0.994$, and $r^2 = 0.989$, respectively.

3. Discussion

Patient health, as it relates to hemodialysis treatment, is of the utmost importance as the mortality and morbidity of ESRD patients is typically high. A strong push recently has been to move to the use of ultrapure dialysate in clinics, as studies have shown correlations between improvements in markers of inflammation and the use of dialysis fluid meeting the criteria of <0.1 CFU/mL and <0.03 EU/mL (Lonnemann & Kock, 2002; Ledebo, 2007a; Schindler, 2009; Schiffl et al., 2002). As some studies have shown that typical endotoxin concentrations are higher in dialysis fluid than RO water entering the hemodialysis machine (von Sengbusch et al., 1993), the ultrapure criteria of the dialysis fluid needs to be created just prior to the patient receiving treatment. One method to produce and ensure the production of ultrapure dialysis fluid is to place an ultrafilter in the hydraulic path between the patient and the dialysis machine, as this filter will have the greatest impact to the final dialysis fluid solution prior to entrance into the dialyzer (Oliver et al., 1992; Schindler et al., 2004).

Studies in the literature have revealed significant removal rates for ultrafilters in vitro, typically >99% for endotoxin (Oliver et al., 1992; Krautzig et al., 1996), with log reduction values >3 desirable (Tsuchida et al., 2009). Ultrafilters are commonly used in HDF, where two filters are typically used in series to guarantee sterile fluid production - manufacturers of ultrafilters state that sterility of substitution fluid is only guaranteed if the machine feed water falls within certain criteria (Penne et al., 2009). However, as ultrafilters are exposed to disinfection agents and cleaning cycles their efficacy in removing endotoxin is reduced. A desirable application would be a novel surface treatment or coating that would enhance endotoxin removal, while able to resist efficiency loss induced by age and chemical exposure. Durable membranes have been studied, with some researchers looking at ceramic or alumina membranes. As these membranes do perform well in retaining endotoxin, their expense in manufacturing seems to limit their application, as well as some membranes have been shown to leach aluminum when cleaned with NaOH (Bender et al., 2000).

The goal of endotoxin removal is ultimately to reduce patient inflammation, as contaminated dialysate has been linked to the systemic micro-inflammatory state observed in many hemodialysis patients (Ouseph et al., 2007). Other studies have reported links between inflammation and cardiovascular disease (CVD) in hemodialysis patients (Merino et al., 2008; Wang et al., 2011; Kerr et al., 2007), while some have shown association between inflammation and nutritional status (Raj et al., 2009), implicating the breadth of influence caused by repeated endotoxin exposure. As more ESRD patients are treated with high-flux dialysis membranes, the opportunity increases for bacterial contaminants in dialysis fluid to cross the membrane into the blood and activate numerous cell types, releasing pro-inflammatory cytokines which heighten the inflammatory condition (Vanholder et al., 1992; Almeida et al., 2006). This is also the case in the acute market, as membranes with increased permeabilities are being used in ARF for their higher clearances of cytokines (Haase et al., 2007; Vanholder et al., 2000); these patients will have higher risks for endotoxin contamination, based upon the membrane flux.

Aside from removal, advances in the detection of endotoxin and other pyrogenic substances at low concentrations would further propel endotoxin research forward by providing researchers tools to better distinguish bacterial contaminant changes, or by making highly sensitive endotoxin detection available to clinics to provide advanced microbiological observation of their water systems. Specific research in this field has focused on the efficacy of utilizing photometry to detect and measure endotoxin in patient plasma samples (Nakazawa et al., 2010), which would have direct impact on research clinics and for septic patients. PCR techniques have also been utilized for their application to dialysis research, by analyzing total flora in dialysis water via the 16s rDNA. As this technique guarantees a high degree of detection, it does not specify whether bacteria or live or dead, or what species are prevalent within the sample (Nystrand, 2006).

4. Future work

Studies involving endotoxin in hemodialysis have been going on for quite some time - covering how to prevent and remove biofilm from water distribution systems, how endotoxin interacts with the body, and how to increase removal efficiencies. Going forward, future work may involve identifying new bacterial contaminants that cause adverse patient reactions, but may not be identified by the LAL assay (Glorieux et al., 2009). There are a number of smaller bacterial components released during cell lysis, with bacterial DNA fragments recently receiving considerable attention in research studies (Handelman et al., 2009; Schindler et al., 2004). Some of these studies have shown a correlation between bDNA fragments present in patient blood, and higher levels of CRP and IL-6 (Bossola et al., 2009). Current limitations in endotoxin quantitative methodology, which influence how bacterial contaminant results and target values are interpreted (Ledebo, 2007b) will hopefully be improved upon and expanded to cover additional areas of focus in ESRD treatment.

The future of any therapy used to treat patients with ESRD needs to focus on the associated mortality and morbidity influencing factors. Whether ESRD therapy will focus on smaller, wearable devices (Gura et al., 2008; Ronco & Fecondini, 2007), strive for increases in home treatment (Moran, 2009), or devices utilizing living cells (Humes et al., 2006), the effect of endotoxin must be taken into account for each application - and to address the specific actions necessary to remove endotoxin thus ensuring patient safety. Future progress in endotoxin research will hopefully alleviate inflammation-related complications, and improve patient outcomes for all aspects of ESRD.

5. Conclusion

In conclusion, endotoxin contamination of fluid for dialysis therapy is an important aspect of patient safety and well-being. Regardless of the microbiological quality of the water coming into the hemodialysis machine, the dialysis membrane is the final barrier between potentially contaminated dialysis fluid, and the blood of the patient. We have examined how manipulation of specific fiber membrane parameters (geometric properties, materials, coatings, chemical modifications) can be utilized to improve the endotoxin retentive properties to limit trans-membrane flux, whether they contribute to adsorptive improvements, sieving improvements, or both. Membrane structure, surface chemistry, material, and surface coatings all have an impact on how endotoxin is filtered and adsorbed from solution. In addition to better understanding endotoxin-membrane interactions, studies of endotoxin removal by membrane modifications will result in better approaches to manufacture dialysis membranes that remove endotoxin from solution quickly and with improved efficiency.

As future hemodialysis membranes are designed to further improve upon convective removal of larger middle molecular solutes such as B2M, the opportunity for pyrogenic materials to enter the blood stream via back filtration becomes greater. An improved comprehension of how endotoxin is removed using a fiber membrane can lead to new improvements and future product designs, by streamlining concepts from development to production.

6. Acknowledgment

The authors would like to express their gratitude to Mr. Doug Olmstead and Mr. Marion Andersen for their support and guidance with the LAL analysis, and to Dr. David Britt and Dr. Ben Madsen for their assistance and work with the fluorescence assay.

7. References

Almeida, W., Maciel, T., Di Marco, G., Casarini, D., Campos, A., Schor, N. (2006). Escherichia coli lipopolysaccharide inhibits renin activity in human mesangial cells. *Kidney International*, Vol.69, No.1, pp.974-980.

Bailat, S., Heumann, D., Roy, D., Baumgartner, J., Rietschel, E., Glauser, M., Padova, F. (1997). Similarities and disparities between core-specific and O-side-chain-specific antilipopolysaccharide monoclonal antibodies in models of endotoxemia and bacteremia in mice. *Infection Immunity*, Vol.65, No.2, pp.811-814.

Bender, H., Pflanzel, A., Saunders, N., Czermak, P., Catapano, G., Vienken, J. (2000). Membranes for endotoxin removal from dialysate: Considerations on feasibility of commercial ceramic membranes. *Artificial Organs*, Vol.24, No.10, pp.826-838.

Bland, L., Oliver, J., Arduino, M., Oettinger, C., McAllister, S., Favero, M. (1994). Potency of endotoxin from bicarbonate dialysate compared with endotoxins from Escherichia coli and Shigella flexneri. *JASN*, Vol.5, No.1, pp.1634-1637.

Bossola, M., Sanguinetti, M., Scribano, D., Zuppi, C., Giungi, S., Luciani, G., Torelli, R., Posteraro, B., Fadda, G., Tazza, L. (2009). Circulating bacterial-derived DNA fragments and markers of inflammation in chronic hemodialysis patients. *Clinical JASN*, Vol.4, No.1, pp.379-385.

Boudville, N., Horner, M., McEwan, E., Lim, W., Mudge, D., Markus, H. (2009). Effect of FX dialysers on systemic inflammation and quality of life in chronic haemodialysis patients. *Blood Purification*, Vol.27, No.1, pp.187-193.

Canaud, B., Bosc, J., Leray, H., Stec, F. (2000). Microbiological purity of dialysate for on-line substitution fluid preparation. *Nephrology Dialysis Transplantation*, Vol.15, Suppl.2, pp.21-30.

Girndt, M., Lengler, S., Kaul, H., Sester, U., Sester, M., Kohler, H. (2000). Prospective crossover trial of the influence of vitamin E-coated dialyzer membranes on T-cell activation and cytokine induction. *American J Kidney Diseases*, Vol.35, No.1, pp.95-104.

Glorieux, G., Schepers, E., Schindler, R., Lemke, H., Verbeke, F., Dhondt, A., Lameire, N., Vanholder, R. (2009). A novel bio-assay increases the detection yield of microbiological impurity of dialysis fluid, in comparison to the LAL-test. *Nephrology Dialysis Transplantation*, Vol.24, No.1, pp.548-554.

Gomila, M., Gasco, J., Gil, J., Bernabeu, R., Inigo, V., Lalucat, J. (2006). A molecular microbial ecology approach to studying hemodialysis water and fluid. *Kidney International*, Vol.70, No.1, pp.1567-1576.

Gorbet, M., Sefton, M. (2005). Endotoxin: the uninvited guest. *Biomaterials*, Vol.26, No.1, (month/year of edition), pp.6811-6817.

Gunn, J. (2001). Bacterial modification of LPS and resistance to antimicrobial peptides. *J Endotoxin Res*, Vol.7, No.1, pp.57-62.

Gura, V., Ronco, C., Davenport, A. (2008). The wearable artificial kidney, why and how: from holy grail to reality. *Seminars in Dialysis*, Vol.22, No.1, pp. 13-17.

Haase, M., Bellomo, R., Baldwin, I., Haase-Fielitz, A., Fealy, N., Davenport, P., Morgera, S., Goehl, H., Storr, M., Boyce, N., Neumayer, H. (2007). Hemodialysis membrane with a high-molecular-weight cutoff and cytokine levels in sepsis complicated by acute renal failure: A phase 1 randomized trial. *American J Kidney Diseases*, Vol.50, No.1, pp.296-304.

Haeffner-Cavaillon, N., Carreno, M., Aussel, L., Caroff, M. (1998). Molecular aspects of endotoxins relevant to their biological functions. *Nephrology Dialysis Transplantation*, Vol.14, No.1, pp.853-860.

Handelman, G., Megdan, P., Handelman, S. (2009). Bacterial DNA in water and dialysate: Detection and significance for patient outcomes. *Blood Purification*, Vol.27, No.1, pp.81-85.

Hayama, M., Miyasaka, T., Mochizuki, S., Asahara, H., Tsujioka, K., Kohori, F., Sakai, K., Jinbo, Y., Yoshida, M. (2002). Visualization of distribution of endotoxin trapped in an endotoxin-blocking filtration membrane. *J Membrane Science*, Vol.210, No.1, pp.45-53.

Hoenich, Nicholas. (2007). The extracorporeal circuit: Materials, problems, and solutions. *Hemodialysis International*, Vol.11, No.1, pp.s26-s31.

Humes, H., Fissell, W., Tiranathanagul, K. (2006). The future of hemodialysis membranes. *Kidney International*, Vol.69, No.1, pp.1115-1119.

Jaber, B., Pereira, B. (1997). Extracorporeal adsorbent-based strategies in sepsis. *American J Kidney Diseases*, Vol.30, No.5, Suppl.4, pp.s44-s56.

Kanagasundaram, N., Moore, I., Hoenich, N. (2009). Biofilm in bicarbonate-based replacement fluid circuits in CVVH. *Kidney International*, Vol.76, No.1, p.682.

Kerr, P., Sutherland, W., de Jong, S., Vaithalingham, I., Williams, S., Walker, R. (2007). The impact of standard high-flux polysulfone versus novel high-flux polysulfone dialysis membranes on inflammatory markers : A randomized, single-blinded, controlled clinical trial. *American J Kidney Diseases*, Vol.49, No.1, pp.533-539.

Khan, R., Badr, K. (1999). Endotoxin and renal function: Perspectives to the understanding of septic acute renal failure and toxic shock. *Nephrology Dialysis Transplantation*, Vol.14, No.1, pp.814-818.

Kramer, L., Gendo, A., Madl, C., Ferrara, I., Funk, G., Schenk, P., Sunder-Plassmann, G., Horl, W. (2000). Biocompatibility of a cuprophane charcoal-based detoxification device in cirrhotic patients with hepatic encephalopathy. *American J Kidney Diseases*, Vol.36, No.6, pp.1193-1200.

Krautzig, S., Lonnemann, G., Shaldon, S., Koch, K. (1996). Bacterial challenge of NISSHO ultrafilter ETF 609: Results of in vitro testing. *Artificial Organs*, Vol.20, No.7, pp.798-800.

Krieter, D., Lemke, H., Wanner, C. (2008). A new synthetic dialyzer with advanced permselectivity for enhanced low-molecular weight protein removal. *Artificial Organs*, Vol.32, No.7, pp.547-554.

Ledebo, Ingrid. (2002). On-line preparation of solutions for dialysis: practical aspects versus safety and regulations. *JASN*, Vol.13, No.1, pp.78-83.

Ledebo, Ingrid. (2007a). Clinical benefits of ultrapure dialysis fluid for hemodialysis. *Hemodialysis International*, Vol.11, No.1, pp.s12-s17.

Ledebo, Ingrid. (2007b). Ultrapure dialysis fluid - how pure is it and do we need it? *Nephrology Dialysis Transplantation*, Vol.22, No.1, pp.20-23.

Lonnemann, Gerhard. (2000). Should ultra-pure dialysate be mandatory? *Nephrology Dialysis Transplantation*, Vol.15, Suppl.1, pp.55-59.

Lonnemann, G., Sereni, L., Lemke, H., Tetta, C. (2001). Pyrogen retention by highly permeable synthetic membranes during in vitro dialysis. *Artificial Organs*, Vol.25, No.12, pp.951-960.

Lonnemann, G., Kock, K. (2002). B_2-Microglobulin amyloidosis: Effects of ultrapure dialysate and type of dialyzer membrane. *JASN*, Vol.13, No.1, pp.s72-s77.

Maitz, M., Teichmann, J., Sperling, C., Werner, C. (2008). Surface endotoxin contamination and hemocompatibility evaluation of materials. *J Biomedical Materials Research Part B*, Vol.90B, No.1, pp.18-25.

Mares, J., Thongboonkerd, V., Tuma, Z., Moravec, J., Matejovic, M. (2009). Specific adsorption of some complement activation proteins to polysulfone dialysis membranes during hemodialysis. *Kidney International*, Vol.76, No.1, pp.404-413.

Merino, A., Nogueras, S., Garcia-Maceira, T., Rodriguez, M., Martin-Malo, A., Ramirez, R., Carracedo, J., Aljama, P. (2008). Bacterial DNA and endothelial damage in haemodialysis patients. *Nephrology Dialysis Transplantation*, Vol.23, No.1, pp.3635-3642.

Mineshima, M., Ishimori, I., Sakiyama, R. (2009). Validity of internal filtration-enhanced hemodialysis as a new hemodiafiltration therapy. *Blood Purification*, Vol.27, No.1, pp.33-37.

Mitzner, S., Schneidewind, J., Falkenhagen, D., Loth, F., Klinkmann, H. (1993). Extracorporeal endotoxin removal by immobilized polyethylenimine. *Artificial Organs*, Vol.17, No.9, pp.775-781.

Moran, John. (2009). Technical advances in home dialysis. *Advances in Chronic Kidney Disease*, Vol.16, No.3, pp.215-220.

Nakazawa, R., Motohashi, K., Azuma, N., Obata, T. (2010). Effectiveness of endotoxin scattering photometry (ESP) for determining endotoxin levels of dialysis fluid for haemodialysis. ?,

Nube, M., Grooteman, M. (2001). Impact of contaminated dialysate on long-term haemodialysis-related complications: Is it really that important? *Nephrology Dialysis Transplantation*, Vol.16, No.1, pp.1986-1991.

Nystrand, Rolf. (2006). Modern microbiological techniques and their use in dialysis fluid systems: What are the benefits? *Kidney International*, Vol.70, No.1, pp.1539-1540.

Ofsthun, N., Leypoldt, J. (1995). Ultrafiltration and backfiltration during hemodialysis. *Artificial Organs*, Vol.19, No.11, pp.1143-1161.

Oliver, J., Bland, L., Oettinger, C., Arduino, M., Garrard, M., Pegues, D., McAllister, S., Moone, T., Aguero, S., Favero, M. (1992). Bacteria and endotoxin removal from bicarbonate dialysis fluids for use in conventional, high-efficiency, and high-flux hemodialysis. *Artificial Organs*, Vol.16, No.2, pp.141-145.

Opatrny Jr., K., Krouzecky, A., Polanska, K., Mares, J., Tomsu, M., Bowry, S., Vienken, J. (2006). Does an alteration of dialyzer design and geometry affect biocompatibility parameters? *Hemodialysis International*, Vol.10, No.1, pp.201-208.

Osumi, M., Yamada, N., Toya, M. (1996). Bacterial retention mechanisms of membrane filters. *PDA J Pharma Sci & Tech*, Vol.50, No.1, pp.30-34.

Qureshi, N., Kutuzova, G., Takayama, K., Rice, P., Golenbock, D. (1999). Structure of lipid A and cell activation. *J Endotoxin Res*, Vol.5, No.3, pp.147-150.

Ouseph, R., Jones, S., Dhananjaya, N., Ward, R. (2007). Use of ultrafiltered dialysate is associated with improvements in haemodialysis-associated morbidity in patients treated with reused dialysers. *Nephrology Dialysis Transplantation*, Vol.22, No.1, pp.2269-2275.

Penne, E., Visser, L., van den Dorpel, M., van der Weerd, N., Mazairac, A., van jaarsveld, B., Koopman, M., Vos, P., Feith, G., Hovinga, T., van hamersvelt, H., Wauters, I., Bots, M., Nube, M., ter Wee, P., Blankestijn, P., Grooteman, M. (2009). Microbiological quality and quality control of purified water and ultrapure dialysis fluids for online hemodiafiltration in routine clinical practice. *Kidney Internatinal*, Vol.76, No.1, pp.665-672.

Perez-Garcia, R., Rodriguez-Benitez, P. (2000). Why and how to monitor bacterial contamination of dialysate? *Nephrology Dialysis Transplantation*, Vol.15, No.1, pp.760-764.

Raetz, C. (1991). Gram negative endotoxin: an extraordinary lipid with profound effets on eukaryotic signal transduction. *FASEB Journal*, Vol.5, No.1, pp. 2652-2660.

Raj, D., Carrero, J., Shah, V., Qureshi, A., Barany, P., Heimburger, O., Lindholm, B., Ferguson, J., Moseley, P., Stenvinkel, P. (2009). Soluble CD14 levels, interleukin 6, and mortality among prevalent hemodialysis patients. *American J Kidney Diseases*, Vol.54, No.1, pp.1072-1080.

Rietschel, E., Kirikae, T., Schade, F., Mamat, U., Schmidt, G., Loppnow, H., Ulmer, A., Zahringer, U., Seydel, U., Padova, F.,Schreier, M., Brade, H. (1994). Bacterial endotoxin: molecular relationships of structure to activity and function. *FASEB Journal*, Vol.8, No.1, pp. 217-225.

Rimmele, T., Assadi, A., Cattenoz, M., Desebbe, O., Lambert, C., Boselli, E., Goudable, J., Etienne, J., Chassard, D., Bricca, G., Allaouchiche, B. (2009). High-volume haemofiltration with a new haemofiltration membrane having enhanced adsorption properties in septic pigs. *Nephrology Dialysis Transplantation*, Vol.24, No.1, pp.421-427.

Ronco, C., Brendolan, A., Dan, M., Piccinni, P., Bellomo, R., De Nitti, C., Inguaggiato, P., Tetta, C. (2000). Adsorption in sepsis. *Kidney International*, Vol.58, Suppl.76, pp.148-155.

Ronco, C., Fecondini, L. (2007). The Vicenza wearable artificial kidney for peritoneal dialysis (ViWAK PD). *Blood Purification*, Vol.25, No.1, pp.383-388.

Sakamoto, Y., Mashiko, K., Obata, T., Yokota, H. (2010). Effectiveness of endotoxin scattering photometry for determining the efficacy of polymyxin B-immobilized fiber treatment in septic shock: Report of a case. *J Nippon Medical School*, Vol.77, No.2, pp.119-122.

Schiffl, H., Lang, S., Fischer, R. (2002). Ultrapure dialysis fluid slows loss of residual renal function in new dialysis patients. *Nephrology Dialysis Transplantation*, Vol.17, No.1, pp.1814-1818.

Schiffl, Helmut (2011). High-flux dialyzers, backfiltration, and dialysis fluid quality. *Seminars in Dialysis*, Vol.24, No.1, pp.1-4.

Schindler, R., Beck, W., Deppisch, R., Aussieker, M., Wilde, A., Gohl, H., Frei, U. (2004). Short bacterial DNA fragments: Detection in dialysate and induction of cytokines. *JASN*, Vol.15, No.1, pp.3207-3214.

Schindler, Ralf. (2009). Clinical effect of purification of dialysis fluids, evidence and experience. *Blood Purification*, Vol.27, Supp.1, pp.20-22.

Shao, J., Wolff, S., Zydney, A. (2007). In vitro comparison of peracetic acid and bleach cleaning of polysulfone hemodialysis membranes. *Artificial Organs*, Vol.31, No.6, pp.452-460.

von Sengbusch, G., Bowry, S., Vienken, J. (1993). Focusing on membranes. *Artificial Organs*, Vol.17, No.4, pp.244-253.

Smeets, E., Kooman, J., vander Sande, F., Stobberingh, E., Frederik, P., Claessens, P., Grave, W., Schot, A., Leunissen, K. (2003). *Kidney International*, Vol.63, No.1, pp.1574-1576.

Steczko, J., Ash, S., Blake, D., Carr, D., Bosley, R. (1999). Cytokines and endotoxin removal by sorbents and its application in push-pull sorbent-based pheresis: The biologic-DTPF system. *Artificial Organs*, Vol.23, No.4, pp.310-318.

Sundaram, S., Barrett, T., Meyer, K., Perrella, C., Neto, M., King, A., Pereira, B. (1996). Transmembrane passage of cytokine-inducing bacterial products across new and reprocessed polysulfone dialyzers. *JASN*, Vol.7, No.1, pp.2183-2191.

Szathmary, S., Hegyi, E., Amoureux, M-C., Rajapakse, N., Chicorka, L., Szalai, G., Reszegi, K., Derbyshire, Z., Paluh, J., Dodson, B., Grandics, P. (2004). Characterization of the Dialguard™ device for endotoxin removal in hemodialysis. *Blood Purification*, Vol.22, No.1, pp.409-415.

Takemoto, Y., Nakatani, T., Sugimura, K., Yoshimura, R., Tsuchida, K. (2003). Endotoxin adsorption of various dialysis membranes: In vitro study. *Artificial Organs*, Vol.27, No.12, pp.1134-1142.

Tani, T., Hanasawa, K., Endo, Y., Yoshioka, T., Kodama, M., Kaneko, M., Uchiyama, Y., Akizawa, T., Takahasi, K., Sugai, K. (1998). Theapeutic apheresis for septic patients with organ dysfunction: Hemoperfusion using a polymyxin B immobilized column. *Artificial Organs*, Vol.22, No.12, pp.1038-1044.

Teehan, G., Guo, D., Perianayagam, M., Galakrishnan, V., Pereira, B., Jaber, B. (2004). Reprocessed (high-flux) Polyflux® dialyzers resist trans-membrane endotoxin passage and attenuate inflammatory markers. *Blood Purification*, Vol.22, No.1, pp.329-337.

Tsuchida, K., Nakatani, T., Sugimura, K., Yoshimura, R., Matsuyama, M., Takemoto, Y. (2004). Biological reactions resulting from endotoxin adsorbed on dialysis membrane: An in vitro study. *Artificial Organs*, Vol.28, No.2, pp. 231-234, ISSN.

Tsuchida, K., Nakamura, M., Yoshikawa, K., Minakuchi, J., Takesawa, S. (2009). Current situation of endotoxin retentive filter. *Blood Purification*, Vol.27, Suppl.1, pp.28-35.

Umgelter, A., Reindl, W., Lutz, J., Kreymann, B., Ronco, C., Huber, W., Frank, H., Schmid, R., Heemann, U. (2008). Treatment of septic patients with an arginine-based endotoxin adsorber column improves hemodynamics and reduces oxidative stress: results of a feasibility study. *Blood Purificaiton*, Vol.26, No.1, pp.333-339.

Urena, P., Herbelin, A., Zingraff, J., Lair, M., Man, N., Descamps-Latscha, B., Drueke, T. (1992). Permeability of cellulosic and non-cellulosic membranes to endotoxin subunits and cytokine production during in-vitro haemodialysis. *Nephrology Dialysis Transplantation*, Vol.7, No.1, pp.16-28.

Uriu, K., Osajima, A., Hiroshige, K., Watanabe, H., Aibara, K., Inada, Y., Segawa, K., Anai, H., Takagi, I., Ito, A., Kamochi, M., Kaizu, K. (2002). Endotoxin removal by direct hemoperfusion with an adsorbent column using polymyxin B-immobilized fiber ameliorates systemic circulatory disturbance in patients with septic shock. *American J Kidney Diseases*, Vol.39, No.5, pp.937-947.

Valvano, Miguel. (1992). Pathogenicity and molecular genetics of O-specific side-chain lipopolysaccharides of Escherichia coli. *Canadian J Microbiology*, Vol.38, No.1, pp.711-719.

Vanholder, R., Van Haecke, E., Veys, N., Ringoir, S. (1992). Endotoxin transfer through dialysis membranes: Small- versus large-pore membranes. *Nephrology Dialysis Transplantation*, Vol.7, No.1, pp.333-339.

Vanholder, R., De Vriese, A., Lameire, N. (2000). The role of dialyzer biocompatibility in acute renal failure. *Blood Purification*, Vol.18, No.1, pp.1-12.

Vanholder, R., Pedrini, L. (2008). All high-flux membranes are equal but some high-flux membranes are less equal than others. *Nephrology Dialysis Transplantation*, Vol.23, No.1, pp.1481-1483.

Vaslaki, L., Karatson, A., Voros, P., Major, L., Petho, F., Ladanyi, E., Weber, C., Mitteregger, R., Falkenhagen, D. (2000). Can sterile and pyrogen-free on-line substitution fluid be routinely delivered? A multicentric study on the microbiological safety of on-line haemodiafiltration. *Nephrology Dialysis Transplantation*, Vol.15, Suppl.1, pp.74-78.

Wang, A., Sanderson, J. (2011). Current perspectives on diagnosis of heart failure in long-term dialysis patients. *American J Kidney Disease*, Vol. 57, No.2, pp.308-319.

Waterhouse, S., Hall, G. (1995). The validation of sterilising grade microfiltration membranes with Pseudomonas diminuta. *J Membrane Science*, Vol.104, No.1, pp.1-9.

Weber, V., Linsbetrge, I., Rossmanith, E., Weber, C., Falkenhagen, D. (2004). Pyrogen transfer across high and low-flux hemodialysis membranes. *Artificial Organs*, Vol.28, No.2, pp.210-217.

Weber, V., Linsberger, I., Falkenhagen, D. (2009). Negligible transfer of endotoxins across high-flux haemodialysis membranes designed for convective therapies. *Nephrology Dialysis Transplantation Plus*, Vol.2, Suppl.2, ii1901-.

Yamamoto, C., Kim, S. (1996). Endotoxin rejection by ultrafiltration through high-flux, hollow fiber filters. *J Biomedical Materials Research*, Vol.32, No.1, pp.467-471.

Yaroustovsky, M., Abramyan, M., Popok, Z., Nazarova, E., Stupchenko, O., Popov, D., Plushch, M., Samsonova, N. (2009). Preliminary report regarding the use of selective sorbents in complex cardiac surgery patients with extensive sepsis and prolonged intensive care stay. *Blood Purification*, Vol.28, No.1, pp.227-233.

11

Citrate Anticoagulation in Hemodialysis

Stephan Thijssen
Renal Research Institute
USA

1. Introduction

In hemodialysis, the patient's blood is flown through an extracorporeal circuit containing a hemodialyzer. This process stimulates coagulation for several reasons, most notably the blood's contact with the artificial surfaces of the tubing and dialyzer membrane and with air in the venous bubble trap, turbulent and stagnant blood flow, shear stress and hemoconcentration during the treatment [1]. Technological advances, e.g., the development of air-free blood circuits and more biocompatible materials for both tubing and dialyzer membranes, may eventually help reduce thrombogenicity of the extracorporeal circuit but are unlikely to eliminate this problem anytime soon. As a result, anticoagulation is (and will be, for the years to come) generally required for hemodialysis in the vast majority of patients.

In most cases in the United States, unfractionated heparin is the agent of choice to provide dialysis anticoagulation. While this is usually well-tolerated and relatively safe, there are significant drawbacks. The most obvious of these is that the anticoagulation is systemic in nature, which translates into an increased bleeding risk. This is certainly undesirable in end-stage renal disease patients, who are already afflicted with uremic thrombocytopathy, and it is particularly dangerous for patients with additionally increased bleeding risk, e.g., patients after surgery or trauma, and patients with active (e.g., gastro-intestinal) bleeding. Another possible complication related to heparin use, albeit rare in dialysis patients, is heparin-induced thrombocytopenia (HIT) type II [2], a potentially life-threatening condition associated with a mortality rate of 8 to 20 percent. Other possible side-effects of heparin use include osteoporosis, hair loss, and hyperlipidemia. Starting in late 2007, a series of severe anaphylactoid reactions had caused serious injuries and deaths. These reactions were later linked to heparin contaminated with oversulfated chondroitin sulfate [3, 4].

Several alternatives to heparin anticoagulation are potentially available, each of them accompanied by specific disadvantages. Intermittent saline flushes, i.e., flushing of the extracorporeal circuit with 25 to 50 mL of 0.9% sodium chloride solution every 15 to 30 minutes, is often used during acute dialysis in patients with increased bleeding risk or in patients with HIT type II. Since the procedure, surprisingly, is not automated, it is very laborious. Furthermore, its capacity to prevent clotting is rather limited, with partial clotting occurring in approximately 20 percent, and complete clotting of the extracorporeal circuit in about 7 percent of treatments [1]. Clotting of the extracorporeal system, of course, is associated with blood loss to the patient, and even with partial clotting, solute clearances will be impaired. Other agents used for systemic anticoagulation in hemodialysis are fondaparinux, danaparoid, and direct thrombin inhibitors. These have other downsides, such as long half-life, lack of an antidote, or high cost, and all of them increase the bleeding risk as they are administered systemically.

The primary purpose of anticoagulation during hemodialysis is to prevent clotting of the blood while it is traveling through the blood tubing and dialyzer. Against this background, the cornerstones of optimal anticoagulation for hemodialysis are complete suppression of the activation of the clotting cascade, strict limitation to the extracorporeal circuit, absence of serious side-effects, and low cost.

Limitation of anticoagulation to the extracorporeal circuit, also known as regional anticoagulation, is important because it eliminates the increased bleeding risk associated with systemic anticoagulation. Originally, this was accomplished by infusing heparin into the arterial line of the blood circuit and antagonizing its anticoagulant effect by infusing its antidote protamine into the venous line. Since protamine's half-life is shorter than heparin's, the anticoagulant effect may return after the dialysis procedure, increasing the bleeding risk. Also, this mode of anticoagulation is not suitable for HIT type II patients because of the heparin administration. Regional anticoagulation by infusing the arachidonic acid derivative prostacyclin into the arterial line is based on this molecule's inhibitory effect on thrombocyte aggregation and its short half-life of only a few minutes. The downsides are its vasodilatatory properties, which can cause significant hypotension during the treatment, and its prohibitive cost. Regional citrate anticoagulation is an alternative to these two methods that also confines anticoagulation to the extracorporeal circuit but does not come with the disadvantages mentioned above. In fact, it conveys a set of additional advantages that go above and beyond merely providing regional anticoagulation.

2. The principles and history of citrate anticoagulation in hemodialysis

The anticoagulant properties of citrate have been known since the late 1800s already and are based on its capacity to chelate calcium ions. Ionized calcium (iCa) is an important co-factor at several steps in the coagulation cascade and, in that role, was formerly called coagulation factor IV. Addition of citrate to whole blood leads to formation of stable calcium-citrate complexes, thereby lowering the concentration of ionized calcium. At iCa levels below 0.5 mmol/L, clotting becomes impaired; at levels below approximately 0.3 mmol/L, coagulation is virtually blocked. This principle has been applied for storage of red cells in transfusion medicine since the early 20th century and later on for blood cell apheresis and lipid apheresis. Citrate physiologically occurs in the human body. It is an intermediate metabolite in the mitochondrial Krebs cycle, and all human cells that possess mitochondria can generate and metabolize citrate, particularly those tissues that are rich in mitochondria, such as the liver.

The first mention of citrate for anticoagulation in hemodialysis dates back to 1961 [5]. Traditionally, regional citrate anticoagulation in hemodialysis involves infusion of trisodium citrate into the arterial line of the extracorporeal circuit in sufficient quantities to lower iCa levels to around 0.25 to 0.35 mmol/L in order to substantially inhibit coagulation. In the venous limb of the dialysis tubing, ideally close to the point of blood reinfusion into the patient, calcium is substituted in the form of a calcium chloride or calcium carbonate infusion. This calcium substitution primarily serves to raise the iCa concentration in the blood to safe levels before the blood re-enters the patient's circulation, but there is another aspect to it as we shall see later. Classically, a calcium-free dialysate is used in this setting so as not to compromise anticoagulation due to calcium influx from the dialysate [6]. This setup of regional citrate anticoagulation is depicted in **Figure 1**.

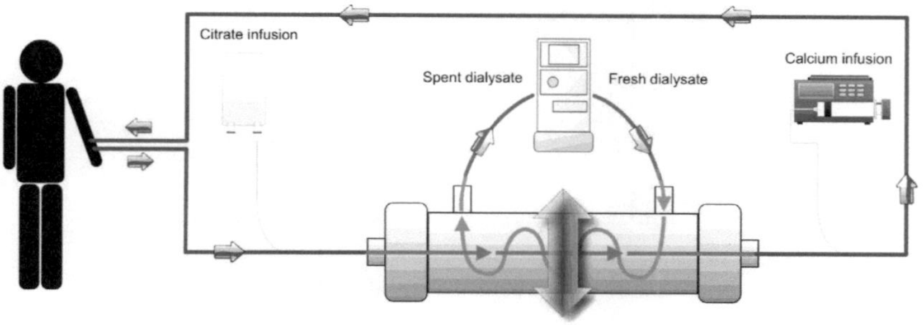

Fig. 1. Conventional setup of regional citrate anticoagulation in hemodialysis.

A question of central importance is how plasma citrate concentrations relate to iCa concentrations. We analyzed the data from 21 regional citrate anticoagulation treatments performed at Renal Research Institute facilities in New York, USA, in 10 patients, during which 4% trisodium citrate (136 mmol/L) was infused into the arterial line and iCa measured before the dialyzer. Blood flow rates were 350 mL/min in 4 treatments, 400 mL/min in 13 treatments, and 450 mL/min in 4 treatments. Hematocrit and iCa were measured 13 minutes into the treatment using an Abbott i-Stat point-of-care analyzer. Hematocrits ranged from 28% to 39% (average, 33.6%). Citrate infusion rates ranged from 140 to 480 mL/h, and iCa ranged from 0.27 to 0.68 mmol/L (average, 0.38 mmol/L). Plasma citrate concentrations were calculated based on citrate infusion rates and calculated plasma flow rates. **Figure 2** illustrates the relationship between pre-dialyzer blood iCa activity and plasma citrate concentration. As can be seen, a plasma citrate concentration of >3.5 mmol/L is typically required to bring iCa levels to below 0.3 mmol/L. The exact citrate concentration necessary depends mainly on the individual patient's plasma calcium and protein (primarily albumin) concentrations. Total calcium in the serum comprises a protein-bound and a free (ionized) fraction, and the equilibrium concentrations of each can be estimated based on the respective dissociation constant [7-10]. Likewise, free citrate reacts with free calcium to form calcium-citrate complexes, again with a known dissociation constant [11]. Strictly, the multi-ionic milieu of the plasma should be considered, but reducing the relationships to calcium, protein, and citrate is a fair approximation. In clinical practice, these relationships are, however, not calculated. Instead, the citrate infusion rate is generally based on empirical knowledge and in most cases only tailored to the patient's blood flow rate. As can be expected, this may occasionally lead to citrate concentrations that are either too low to provide sufficient anticoagulation, or unnecessarily high. To assess the individual situation, pre-dialyzer (some groups use post-dialyzer) iCa levels can be measured in the plasma to ascertain that they are within the desired target range of approximately 0.25 to 0.35 mmol/L. If they are not, adjustments to the citrate infusion rate can be implemented and the iCa levels reassessed. Likewise, the post-dialyzer iCa concentrations are not known in clinical practice, and the rate of calcium substitution is based on empirical knowledge. Routinely, systemic iCa levels are measured in the patient at multiple time points during the treatment, and the calcium substitution rate is adjusted to counter drops or rises in systemic iCa concentration. Each adjustment usually necessitates a reassessment of iCa levels after 15 to 30 minutes to monitor its effect.

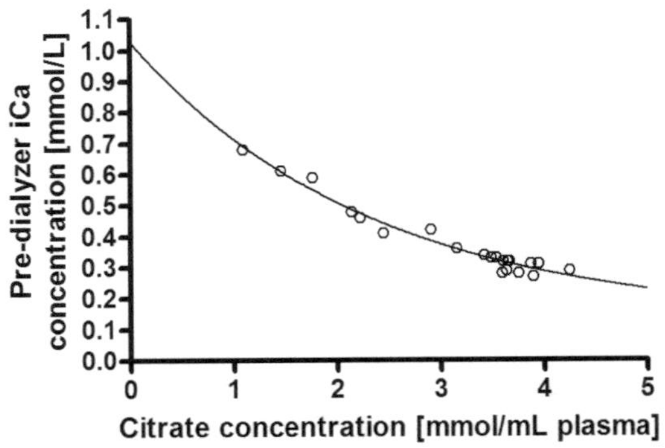

Fig. 2. Pre-dialyzer ionized calcium (iCa) concentration plotted against plasma citrate concentration.

During regional citrate anticoagulation, citrate enters the body in the form of both free citrate and calcium-citrate complexes. When this citrate is metabolized, each molecule yields three molecules of bicarbonate, which will have an impact on the acid-base status. Also, calcium is released from calcium-citrate complexes as they are metabolized, which impacts serum calcium concentration. The use of trisodium citrate or Acid Citrate Dextrose (ACD) solution further entails an additional sodium load to the patient that should be taken into account. In clinical practice, the dialysis prescriptions for regional citrate anticoagulation typically incorporate reduced sodium (by about 2 mmol/L) and bicarbonate (by about 5 mmol/L) concentrations. Magnesium concentration in the dialysate may be increased since citrate also complexes magnesium, leading to increased magnesium losses across the dialyzer.

Over the years, different algorithms for the administration of regional citrate anticoagulation have been suggested and studied, both for intermittent as well as continuous hemodialysis. These algorithms usually define blood and dialysate flow rates, the starting rates for citrate infusion and calcium substitution, rules on how these rates should be adjusted in case of iCa deviations from the specified circuit or systemic target ranges, time points for monitoring iCa, and downward adjustments for sodium and bicarbonate in the dialysate. Since citrate and calcium kinetics during dialysis depend on many factors, including the type of dialyzer used and the blood and dialysate flow rates, such algorithms generally are only applicable to the particular dialysis setting for which they have been validated. The purpose of all these algorithms is always to make the administration of regional citrate anticoagulation as safe and simple as possible, i.e. to minimize the risk for calcium or acid-base derangements, circuit clotting or other complications while requiring as little monitoring or intervention by the staff as possible.

3. The benefits of regional citrate anticoagulation

Regional citrate anticoagulation does not increase the patient's bleeding risk and is, therefore, not only an ideal mode of anticoagulation in any patient with high bleeding risk or active bleeding but also for the average hemodialysis patient. Furthermore, citrate anticoagulation avoids all the other potential side effects of heparin use noted above, which also makes it a choice mode of anticoagulation in patients with HIT type II. Aside from these obvious advantages, however, there are several additional benefits to using regional citrate anticoagulation. One of these appears to be improved biocompatibility of the dialysis procedure: comparing heparin anticoagulation with citrate anticoagulation, Böhler et al. found that citrate anticoagulation reduced complement activation, neutropenia and lactoferrin release with the use of cuprophane dialyzers, and significantly inhibited neutrophil degranulation with the use of polymethyl methacrylate membranes [12]. Likewise, Gritters and colleagues compared anticoagulation using unfractionated heparin, low molecular weight heparin and citrate in a randomized crossover trial and found that citrate anticoagulation suppressed the dialysis-associated degranulation of polymorphonuclear cells and platelets. Furthermore, pro-atherogenic oxidized low-density lipoprotein levels were reduced by a median of 26% after only one week on citrate anticoagulation [13]. In view of the heightened inflammatory state of chronic hemodialysis patients, the reduction of oxidative stress, complement and cell activation associated with citrate dialysis may be a relevant benefit with regard to reducing the high cardiovascular morbidity in these patients. Hofbauer et al. compared anticoagulation with unfractionated heparin, low molecular weight heparin and citrate during dialysis with a single-use polysulfone dialyzer and used scanning electron microscopy to quantify the degree of membrane-associated clotting [14]. The highest degree of cell adhesion and thrombus formation was observed with unfractionated heparin, and it was only slightly reduced with the use of low molecular weight heparin. With regional citrate anticoagulation, on the other hand, thrombus formation was found to be negligible, indicating a far superior anticoagulation using citrate compared to both unfractionated and fractionated heparin. Gabutti et al. employed a randomized controlled cross-over design to compare standard heparin dialysis with regional citrate anticoagulation, dosed to achieve a similar degree of coagulation activation, and study the effects on complement activation and interleukin-1 beta release. In this setting, complement activation was slightly but significantly higher in the citrate dialysis group, but at the same time, interleukin-1 beta release was markedly reduced. Citrate can, and often is, dosed higher in regional citrate anticoagulation than was done in this study, and it stands to reason that with such higher citrate concentrations, complement activation would have been lower than with standard heparin dialysis, associated perhaps with a further decrease in interleukin-1 beta secretion. In line with Hofbauer's results mentioned above, regional citrate anticoagulation appears to allow for markedly prolonged filter patency times in continuous dialysis [15-18]. Lastly, a recent study by Oudemans-van Straaten and colleagues found higher patient and kidney survival in critically ill patients on citrate versus low-molecular weight heparin [19]. On top of these benefits, citrate is a relatively inexpensive compound compared to heparin.

4. The downsides of regional citrate anticoagulation

The single biggest concern with regional citrate anticoagulation is the development of potentially life-threatening systemic calcium derangements. Acute changes in systemic iCa can develop quickly when calcium elimination across the dialyzer (in the form of free calcium and calcium-citrate complexes), calcium release from the metabolism of calcium-citrate complexes, and calcium substitution (from the calcium infusion and/or the dialysate, if a calcium-containing dialysate is used) are mismatched. From this concern springs the need to monitor, at least initially, systemic iCa levels fairly closely during regional citrate anticoagulation. This, along with the more complex setup, presents a significant strain on staff resources and, consequently, can make citrate dialysis more costly than standard heparin dialysis. The prolonged filter patency times seen with citrate anticoagulation, however, may also introduce cost savings compared to heparin dialysis in continuous dialysis therapies [20]. The administration of buffer base in the form of citrate can further lead to metabolic alkalosis [20-22]. Hypernatremia can occur secondary to the additional sodium load administered with the citrate infusion (e.g., in the form of trisodium citrate, which carries 3 moles of sodium for each mole of citrate) [5, 21]. With high citrate infusion rates and/or in patients with impaired liver function (liver failure, cirrhosis), systemic citrate accumulation may occur. Measurements of plasma citrate concentrations are not usually readily available in clinical laboratories, but citrate accumulation may be detected by looking for its effects on calcium levels: citrate accumulation traps calcium in the form of calcium-citrate complexes. The growing plasma pool of calcium-citrate complexes and the insufficient release of calcium from this pool via citrate metabolism lead to a drop in systemic iCa which is spotted in systemic iCa measurements and countered by an increase in the calcium substitution rate in order to restore systemic iCa to physiologic levels. Under such conditions, the amounts of free calcium, calcium-protein complexes and the increased amount of calcium-citrate complexes add up to an increased total calcium concentration. Therefore, citrate accumulation may be detected by an increased total calcium concentration or an increased ratio of total to ionized serum calcium concentration [23]. An increased anion gap may also point towards citrate accumulation [24].

5. The future of citrate anticoagulation in hemodialysis

The fundamental roadblocks to widespread implementation of regional citrate anticoagulation are fear of electrolyte or metabolic disturbances and the relative laboriousness of this mode of anticoagulation. These two domains are interconnected. What current citrate dialysis algorithms have in common is that they are empiric. There is some degree of individualization, but only on a relatively low level. As a consequence, while these algorithms may work for the average patient, or even a majority of patients, there will always be the concern that the characteristics of a particular patient situation are not captured adequately, leading to unexpected and possibly dangerous changes in electrolyte or acid-base parameters. And for this very reason, these algorithms will never help eliminate the intensive laboratory monitoring that, at least initially, is currently required for regional citrate anticoagulation.

Tailoring the citrate infusion rate to the blood flow rate alone is a crude oversimplification. Anticoagulation along the extracorporeal circuit depends on a myriad things, such as the hematocrit, the void volume fraction, the plasma water calcium concentration, the composition of the other ionic species in the multi-ionic milieu of the plasma, the ultrafiltration rate, the type, size and geometry of the dialyzer used and, consequently, its solute removal characteristics, the blood and dialysate flow rates, the concentration of the citrate infusion (high concentrations entail low infusion rates, which may cause mixing issues or discontinuous, pulsatile flow), the dialysate composition (e.g., in terms or calcium, magnesium and citrate concentration), the plasma protein concentration, the rates of citrate generation and metabolism, the systemic citrate levels, the degree of access recirculation, the patient's capacity to buffer changes in extracellular calcium concentration, and so on, to name but a few. Some of these have greater impact than others; some are easier to model than others. But if the kinetics of calcium and citrate are to be predicted (not on average, but for a particular patient) with any degree of reliability, then these factors must be taken into account. Needless to say, the interactions between all these factors cannot possibly be assessed (let alone integrated over an entire treatment and beyond) based on intuition or clinical experience. Computer-aided calcium and citrate kinetic modeling is the only way to simulate in detail the processes during regional citrate anticoagulation. We have recently published a comprehensive, yet versatile, mathematical model for citrate dialysis [25]. A refinement of this model (comprised of our original model combined with a statistical correction component), recently presented as a talk at the XLVII ERA-EDTA conference in Munich, Germany, showed excellent prediction quality [26]. When applied to 120 patients on pure dialysate-side citrate dialysis (dialysate containing 2.4 mEq/L citrate and 2.25 mEq/L calcium), the model overestimated end-dialysis ionized calcium levels by only 0.026 mmol/L on average. While current clinical citrate dialysis algorithms are only applicable to a rather narrow setting for which they have been developed, computer-aided calcium and citrate kinetic modeling affords much greater flexibility and could possibly even be adapted on-the-fly to different conditions.

As was mentioned above, the calcium substitution in regional citrate anticoagulation is currently dosed empirically and adjusted so as to keep systemic iCa within the physiologic range. However, it must be born in mind that this approach pays no heed to the question of calcium mass balance. This is, of course, not done deliberately but simply from necessity, because clinicians have no way of assessing intradialytic calcium mass balance reliably, let alone under such complex conditions as occur in regional citrate anticoagulation. The difference between calcium substitution and calcium loss across the dialyzer membrane determines the intradialytic calcium mass balance, and from this perspective, the calcium substitution should be chosen so as to effect the desired mass balance. The challenges with determining what calcium mass balance is required for a given patient is a related but separate issue and shall not be discussed here. With higher citrate infusion rates, and accompanying citrate accumulation and calcium "trapped" systemically in the form of calcium-citrate complexes, calcium mass balances can easily become positive. In practice, this point is often dismissed and calcium substitution rates justified with reference to the need to maintain serum ionized calcium within the normal range. What becomes clear, however, when simulating citrate dialysis is that many roads lead to Rome, and, within limits, different calcium mass balances can be achieved without compromising the extracorporeal anticoagulation by modifying parameters such as dialysate calcium and citrate concentrations and blood and dialysate flow rates. Dialysis dose issues certainly have to be considered, and the combination of calcium and citrate kinetic modeling with urea kinetic modeling would be a particularly powerful tool. Conversely, the same calcium mass balance can be achieved in different ways, potentially allowing for individualization of the citrate dialysis prescription according to particular patient characteristics, such as impaired liver function or reduced calcium buffering capacity. In view of the ever-increasing awareness of the potential importance of calcium mass balance for long-term outcomes in hemodialysis patients, calcium and citrate kinetic modeling offers a unique opportunity for actively incorporating this parameter into the dialysis prescription. This may turn out to be crucial for translating the compelling short-term benefits associated with regional citrate anticoagulation into long-term improvements in cardiovascular outcomes and ultimately survival. Currently, this mode of anticoagulation is thoroughly ignoring this aspect and is lagging behind the trend towards neutral calcium mass balance seen in standard heparin hemodialysis. Similar to calcium mass balance considerations, dialysis-related sodium

loading is another topic that has been receiving more and more attention in recent years and is another domain of solute kinetic modeling that should ultimately be integrated into citrate dialysis modeling, particularly given the additional sodium load administered with the use of regional citrate anticoagulation.
The use of dialysate-side citrate anticoagulation (i.e., the use of a citrate- and calcium-containing dialysate without arterial citrate infusion or venous calcium substitution) has sparked interest recently for its alleged heparin-sparing potential and its safety and ease of use [27-29]. At unchanged heparin doses, using citrate-containing dialysate (instead of bicarbonate dialysate acidified with acetate) appears to improve solute removal [30].
Citrate anticoagulation holds great promises for improving the outcomes of hemodialysis patients. Ultimately, kinetic modeling will be essential for taking this therapy to the next level (i.e., a high degree of individualization and increased safety through accurate prediction of electrolyte and acid-base kinetics) and to facilitate its widespread use in routine clinical practice.

6. References

[1] Suranyi M, Chow JS: Review: anticoagulation for haemodialysis. Nephrology (Carlton) 2010;15(4):386-392.
[2] Arepally GM, Ortel TL: Clinical practice. Heparin-induced thrombocytopenia. N Engl J Med 2006;355(8):809-817.
[3] Kishimoto TK, Viswanathan K, Ganguly T, Elankumaran S, Smith S, Pelzer K, Lansing JC, Sriranganathan N, Zhao G, Galcheva-Gargova Z, Al-Hakim A, Bailey GS, Fraser B, Roy S, Rogers-Cotrone T, Buhse L, Whary M, Fox J, Nasr M, Dal Pan GJ, Shriver Z, Langer RS, Venkataraman G, Austen KF, Woodcock J, Sasisekharan R: Contaminated heparin associated with adverse clinical events and activation of the contact system. N Engl J Med 2008;358(23):2457-2467.
[4] Blossom DB, Kallen AJ, Patel PR, Elward A, Robinson L, Gao G, Langer R, Perkins KM, Jaeger JL, Kurkjian KM, Jones M, Schillie SF, Shehab N, Ketterer D, Venkataraman G, Kishimoto TK, Shriver Z, McMahon AW, Austen KF, Kozlowski S, Srinivasan A, Turabelidze G, Gould CV, Arduino MJ, Sasisekharan R: Outbreak of adverse reactions associated with contaminated heparin. N Engl J Med 2008;359(25):2674-2684.
[5] Morita Y, Johnson RW, Dorn RE, Hall DS: Regional anticoagulation during hemodialysis using citrate. Am J Med Sci 1961;242:32-43.
[6] Buturovic-Ponikvar J, Cerne S, Gubensek J, Ponikvar R: Regional citrate anticoagulation for hemodialysis: calcium-free vs. calcium containing dialysate - a randomized trial. Int J Artif Organs 2008;31(5):418-424.
[7] Pedersen KO: Binding of calcium to serum albumin. I. Stoichiometry and intrinsic association constant at physiological pH, ionic strength, and temperature. Scand J Clin Lab Invest 1971;28(4):459-469.
[8] Pedersen KO: Binding of calcium to serum albumin. II. Effect of pH via competitive hydrogen and calcium ion binding to the imidazole groups of albumin. Scand J Clin Lab Invest 1972;29(1):75-83.
[9] Pedersen KO: Binding of calcium to serum albumin. IV. Effect of temperature and thermodynamics of calcium-albumin interaction. Scand J Clin Lab Invest 1972;30(1):89-94.

[10] Pedersen KO: Protein-bound calcium in human serum. Quantitative examination of binding and its variables by a molecular binding model and clinical chemical implications for measurement of ionized calcium. Scand J Clin Lab Invest 1972;30(3):321-329.
[11] Toffaletti J, Gitelman HJ, Savory J: Separation and quantitation of serum constituents associated with calcium by gel filtration. Clin Chem 1976;22(12):1968-1972.
[12] Bohler J, Schollmeyer P, Dressel B, Dobos G, Horl WH: Reduction of granulocyte activation during hemodialysis with regional citrate anticoagulation: dissociation of complement activation and neutropenia from neutrophil degranulation. J Am Soc Nephrol 1996;7(2):234-241.
[13] Gritters M, Grooteman MP, Schoorl M, Bartels PC, Scheffer PG, Teerlink T, Schalkwijk CG, Spreeuwenberg M, Nube MJ: Citrate anticoagulation abolishes degranulation of polymorphonuclear cells and platelets and reduces oxidative stress during haemodialysis. Nephrol Dial Transplant 2006;21(1):153-159.
[14] Hofbauer R, Moser D, Frass M, Oberbauer R, Kaye AD, Wagner O, Kapiotis S, Druml W: Effect of anticoagulation on blood membrane interactions during hemodialysis. Kidney Int 1999;56(4):1578-1583.
[15] Hetzel GR, Schmitz M, Wissing H, Ries W, Schott G, Heering PJ, Isgro F, Kribben A, Himmele R, Grabensee B, Rump LC: Regional citrate versus systemic heparin for anticoagulation in critically ill patients on continuous venovenous haemofiltration: a prospective randomized multicentre trial. Nephrol Dial Transplant 2011;26(1):232-239.
[16] Kutsogiannis DJ, Gibney RT, Stollery D, Gao J: Regional citrate versus systemic heparin anticoagulation for continuous renal replacement in critically ill patients. Kidney Int 2005;67(6):2361-2367.
[17] Monchi M, Berghmans D, Ledoux D, Canivet JL, Dubois B, Damas P: Citrate vs. heparin for anticoagulation in continuous venovenous hemofiltration: a prospective randomized study. Intensive Care Med 2004;30(2):260-265.
[18] Bagshaw SM, Laupland KB, Boiteau PJ, Godinez-Luna T: Is regional citrate superior to systemic heparin anticoagulation for continuous renal replacement therapy? A prospective observational study in an adult regional critical care system. J Crit Care 2005;20(2):155-161.
[19] Oudemans-van Straaten HM, Bosman RJ, Koopmans M, van der Voort PH, Wester JP, van der Spoel JI, Dijksman LM, Zandstra DF: Citrate anticoagulation for continuous venovenous hemofiltration. Crit Care Med 2009;37(2):545-552.
[20] Morgera S, Scholle C, Voss G, Haase M, Vargas-Hein O, Krausch D, Melzer C, Rosseau S, Zuckermann-Becker H, Neumayer HH: Metabolic complications during regional citrate anticoagulation in continuous venovenous hemodialysis: single-center experience. Nephron Clin Pract 2004;97(4):c131-136.
[21] Mehta RL, McDonald BR, Aguilar MM, Ward DM: Regional citrate anticoagulation for continuous arteriovenous hemodialysis in critically ill patients. Kidney Int 1990;38(5):976-981.
[22] Silverstein FJ, Oster JR, Perez GO, Materson BJ, Lopez RA, Al-Reshaid K: Metabolic alkalosis induced by regional citrate hemodialysis. ASAIO Trans 1989;35(1):22-25.

[23] Meier-Kriesche HU, Gitomer J, Finkel K, DuBose T: Increased total to ionized calcium ratio during continuous venovenous hemodialysis with regional citrate anticoagulation. Crit Care Med 2001;29(4):748-752.

[24] Cassina T, Mauri R, Engeler A, Giannini O: Continuous veno-venous hemofiltration with regional citrate anticoagulation: a four-year single-center experience. Int J Artif Organs 2008;31(11):937-943.

[25] Thijssen S, Kruse A, Raimann J, Bhalani V, Levin NW, Kotanko P: A mathematical model of regional citrate anticoagulation in hemodialysis. Blood Purif 2010;29(2):197-203.

[26] Thijssen S, Kossmann RJ, Sands JJ, Ofsthun NJ, Vienneau L, Levin NW, Kotanko P: Validation of a novel mathematical model of citrate dialysis in a large cohort of hemodialysis patients. Nephrol Dial Transplant Plus 2010;3 (Supplement 3):iii381-iii382.

[27] Hanevold C, Lu S, Yonekawa K: Utility of citrate dialysate in management of acute kidney injury in children. Hemodial Int 2010;14 Suppl 1:S2-6.

[28] Cheng YL, Yu AW, Tsang KY, Shah DH, Kjellstrand CM, Wong SM, Lau WY, Hau LM, Ing TS: Anticoagulation during haemodialysis using a citrate-enriched dialysate: a feasibility study. Nephrol Dial Transplant 2011;26(2):641-646.

[29] Sands JJ, Kotanko P, Segal JH, Ho CH, Young A, Carter M, Sergeyeva O, Korth L, Maunsell E, Zhu Y, Krishnan M, Diaz-Buxo JA: Citrasate®: Effects on Hemodialysis Adequacy and Heparin N Requirements. J Am Soc Nephrol 2010;21 (Abstract Supplement):434A.

[30] Kossmann RJ, Gonzales A, Callan R, Ahmad S: Increased efficiency of hemodialysis with citrate dialysate: a prospective controlled study. Clin J Am Soc Nephrol 2009;4(9):1459-1464.

12

Hemodialysis Principles and Controversies

Parin Makadia, Payam Benson, Filberto Kelly and Joshua Kaplan
New Jersey Medical School,
United States of America

1. Introduction

The incidence rates of End-stage renal disease (ESRD) have increased steadily internationally since 1989. The United States has the highest incident rate of ESRD, followed by Japan; Japan has the highest prevalence per million population, with the United States second (1). Of the 490,000 patients with ESRD in the United States, more than 380,000 are currently on hemodialysis (HD) (2).

ESRD on HD disproportionately affects minority populations. Whites represent the majority of the HD population (59.8%), while African Americans (33.2%), Asians (3.6%), and Native Americans (1.6%) comprise the rest of the ESRD population. However, the incidence rate of ESRD among African Americans is 4-fold higher and Native Americans 2-fold higher than that for whites. ESRD is slightly more prevalent in men than in women (male-to-female ratio, 1.2:1) and more prevalent in older adults (3).

2. Morbidity/mortality

Chronic renal failure is associated with a very high morbidity and hospitalization rate, likely due to existing comorbid conditions, such as hypertension, coronary artery disease, and peripheral vascular disease. The first-year age-adjusted mortality rate of patients on dialysis is 9.4%, the two-year mortality rate is 32.3%, and the 5-year mortality rate is 60.8% (3). ESRD patients with diabetes have a first-year mortality rate of 23% (3). In patients with ESRD, cardiovascular disease is the primary cause of death, followed by sepsis and cerebrovascular disease. The dialysis population in the United States has a 10- to 20-fold higher risk of death due to cardiovascular complications than the general population after adjusting for age, race, and sex. The relative risk with respect to the general population is much higher in younger patients, with cardiovascular event rates in ESRD patients in their 20s equivalent to the event rates in the general population in their 80s (3). Increased understanding of the disease process, new insights into pathogenic mechanisms, and new therapeutic options are emerging that may improve survival rates and quality of life for patients with ESRD.

3. The need for dialysis

Given the poor outcomes for patients on HD, every effort should be undertaken to preserve residual renal function, which is associated with improved survival (4). Early nephrology referrals, patient education, and consideration of transplant options may be helpful in decreasing the progression to ESRD. Preparation for dialysis therapy is critical for the smooth transition from CKD care to ESRD. Poor planning for initiation of dialysis is a major cause of increased morbidity and mortality. The use of temporary or tunneled dialysis catheters contributes to dialysis mortality by increasing the incidence of sepsis, acting as a stimulus for chronic inflammation, and damaging the central veins, thereby preventing or shortening the survival of more permanent vascular access once created. The chapter will discuss in detail regarding type of dialysis access.

3.1 Indications for initiation of dialysis

The appropriate time to initiate dialysis for a patient is not clearly defined. The decision to initiate dialysis in a patient with CKD involves the consideration of subjective and objective parameters by the physician and the patient. Over the past decade a trend of increasing estimated glomerular filtration rate (eGFR) at the initiation of dialysis for treatment of ESRD has been noted in the United States. In 1996, only 19% of patients began dialysis therapy with an eGFR of greater than 10 ml/min/1.73 m^2 (denoted as 'early start'), but by 2005 the fraction of early start dialysis patients had risen to 45% (5). It is not known whether early start of dialysis is beneficial, harmful or neutral with respect to the outcome of dialysis treatment for ESRD (5). The timing of initiation of dialysis for ESRD is a matter of clinical judgment guided by values of residual renal function and symptoms and signs present in the patients, including those related to comorbidity. By the time the eGFR falls below 10 ml/min/1.73 m^2, most patients require dialysis. However, many patients appear to function quite well until the eGFR approaches 5 ml/min/1.73 m^2. As a general rule, patients with diabetes require earlier intervention (eGFR<15 ml/min/1.73 m^2) than do those with other etiologies for renal failure (6). Clearly, dialysis must be initiated before the uremic symptoms of peripheral neuropathy, encephalopathy, malnutrition, or serositis (including pericarditis) become evident (See Table 1).

• Pericarditis or pleuritis (urgent indication)
• Progressive uremic encephalopathy or neuropathy, with signs such as confusion, asterixis, myoclonus, wrist or foot drop, or, in severe cases, seizures (urgent indication)
• A clinically significant bleeding diathesis attributable to uremia (urgent indication)
• Fluid overload refractory to diuretics
• Hypertension poorly responsive to antihypertensive medications
• Persistent metabolic disturbances that are refractory to medical therapy; these include hyperkalemia, metabolic acidosis, hypercalcemia, hypocalcemia, and hyperphosphatemia
• Persistent nausea and vomiting
• Evidence of malnutrition

Table 1. Clinical indications to initiate dialysis in patients with CKD. (7)

3.2 'Early' versus 'Late' dialysis

There is conflicting evidence concerning the effect of the early initiation of dialysis on survival. Some retrospective and uncontrolled prospective studies have reported no survival benefits with early dialysis while others have found that early start of dialysis may be harmful (8). After a comprehensive review of the published literature by the National

Kidney Foundation (NKF) workgroup in 1997, they recommended that initiation of dialysis be considered when the arithmetic mean of the urea and creatinine clearances fell below approximately 10.5 ml/min/1.73 m^2 except in well-nourished, asymptomatic patients (9). In 1999 Obrador *et al.*, observed that 23% of the US ESRD population, between 1995 and 1997, started dialysis at an eGFR less than 5 ml/min/1.73 m^2. They opined that this 'late start' of dialysis needed further examination, including studies of the impact on outcomes and cost of ESRD treatment (10).

In 2006, the NKF work group updated the guidelines for initiation of hemodialysis and stated that 'at CKD Stage 5, when the eGFR is < 15 ml/min/1.73 m^2, that nephrologists should evaluate the benefits, risks and disadvantages of beginning renal replacement therapy'. They also suggested that initiation of dialysis therapy before CKD Stage 5 (an eGFR of > 15 ml/min/1.73 m^2) may be appropriate in patients who have symptoms believed to be related to both their comorbidities and their level of residual kidney function (11). Only one study has reported the outcomes of patients with CKD who initiated dialysis only after the onset of symptoms due to uremia. In this prospective cohort study of 233 consecutive patients with advanced uremia, 151 were elective starters on dialysis, while 82 initially declined dialysis. Among the initial refusers, 55 percent developed a uremic emergency, while 48 percent were eventually established on maintenance dialysis. In this study, one year mortality was significantly higher among the initial refusers than the elective starters (18 versus 7 percent). However, these results are confounded by lack of randomization and by three deaths among the initial refusers resulting from treatment withdrawal (12).

Additional published studies have not been able to demonstrate any clear-cut survival benefits for early start of dialysis. The only randomized controlled trial that examined mortality and time of dialysis initiation, the IDEAL study (13), found no difference in survival between early or late initiation of dialysis. In this study, 828 patients with progressive CKD and an estimated GFR between 10.0 and 15.0 mL/min/1.73 m2 (as determined by the Cockcroft-Gault equation) were randomly assigned to dialysis initiation when the estimated GFR was either 10 to 14 mL/min/1.73 m2 or 5 to 7 mL/min/1.73 m^2. The median time to the initiation of dialysis was 1.8 and 7.4 months in the early and late start groups, respectively. At a median follow-up period of 3.6 years, the authors noted no significant difference in survival (38 and 37 percent mortality, hazard ratio of 1.05 with early initiation, 95% CI of 0.83 to 1.30) as well as no difference in cardiovascular events, infections, or dialysis complications between the late start group and early start group.

However, these results do not imply that the initiation of dialysis can be delayed until the GFR is between 5 to 7 mL/min/1.73 m^2 in all patients. The design of the IDEAL study permitted clinicians to initiate dialysis based upon the presence of symptoms due to uremia as well as on the estimated GFR. As a result, 76 percent of patients assigned to the late start arm initiated dialysis when the GFR was much greater than 5 to 7 mL/min/1.73 m^2. This resulted in a mean GFR of 9.8 mL/min/1.73 m^2 at the start of dialysis for the late start group, which was only 2.2 mL/min/1.73 m^2 less than the mean start GFR for the early group (12.0 mL/min/1.73 m^2). Thus, approximately 88 percent of all enrolled patients had initiated dialysis with an estimated GFR of approximately 10 mL/min/1.73 m^2 or more, either because of symptoms or enrollment in the early dialysis arm (13).

A recent study published in *Canadian Medical Association Journal* examined trends in initiation of hemodialysis within Canada and compared the risk of death between patients with early and late initiation of dialysis (14). Using the Canadian Organ Replacement

Registry from 2001 to 2007, the investigators identified a cohort of 25,910 patients 18 years or older who began hemodialysis. Dialysis was defined as beginning early if the eGFR exceeded 10.5 mL/minute/1.73 m^2. Mean eGFR at initiation of dialysis increased from 9.3 mL/minute/1.73 m^2 in 2001 to 10.2 mL/minute/1.73 m^2 in 2007 ($P < .001$). During the same period, the proportion of early dialysis initiations increased from 28% (95% confidence interval [CI], 27% - 30%) to 36% (95% CI, 34% - 37%). Among those starting dialysis early, mean GFR at initiation was 15.5 mL/minute/1.73 m^2 vs 7.1 mL/minute/1.73 m^2 among those who started dialysis late. For early vs late initiation of dialysis, the unadjusted hazard ratio (HR) for death was 1.48 (95% CI, 1.43 - 1.54). This suggests that early initation is associated with higher mortality. After adjustment for demographic factors, serum albumin, primary cause of end-stage renal disease, type of vascular access, comorbid conditions, late referral, and transplant status, the hazard ratio for death decreased to 1.18 (95% CI, 1.13 - 1.23). Difference in mortality per 1000 patient-years between starting dialysis early vs late decreased after 1 year of follow-up but persisted and began increasing again after 24 months of follow-up, with significant differences at 6, 12, 30, and 36 months. (14)

There may be two additional advantages to early dialysis: control of hypertension and increased dietary intake. Reversal of volume overload with dialysis often leads to a reduction in blood pressure, which is typically volume-dependent in CKD. Perhaps more important, patients on dialysis patients require at least 1 g/kg of protein per day to replace dialysis losses and maintain nitrogen balance. Thus, early institution of dialysis can allow a more liberal diet in terms of both food and fluid.

The overall conclusion of these trials largely supports current practice that dialysis initiation should be based upon clinical factors rather than the estimated GFR alone. Patients with progressive CKD require close follow up, early nephrology referral, and adequate advance dialysis planning (including the presence of a functioning peritoneal or vascular access and referral for transplantation). Among patients with progressive CKD, clinicians must be vigilant for the presence of symptoms and/or signs of uremia and dialysis should be initiated in the patient with these symptoms.

4. Dialysis modality selection

Although the life expectancy of patients with end-stage renal disease has improved since the introduction of dialysis in the 1960s, it is still far below that of the general population. As an example, the mean life span at age 49 in the United States is 33 years in the general population but only approximately seven years in patients receiving maintenance dialysis (15), in whom the overall five-year survival rate is about 30 to 50 percent in nondiabetics (depending upon the co-morbid diagnoses) and 25 percent in diabetics (15). Despite improvements in technology and patient care, the mortality rate of patients on maintenance dialysis remains alarmingly high, at approximately 15 to 20 percent per year (16).

There are two principal choices for maintenance dialysis: hemodialysis (HD) and peritoneal dialysis (PD). Selecting one of these modalities is influenced by a number of considerations such as availability and convenience, comorbid conditions, socioeconomic and dialysis center factors, the patient's home situation, method of physician reimbursement, and the ability to tolerate volume shifts (17-23). Most studies suggest a better survival rate in PD than in HD patients during the first few years after starting therapy (24). However, after 2 or 3 years, outcome on PD becomes equal to HD, or worse (25-28). This section mainly focuses on different means of receiving hemodialysis.

The European Best Practice Guidelines for Hemodialysis recommends the standard hemodialysis dose should be delivered as three times per week for 4 hours each session (29). In an attempt to improve outcomes, it was postulated that a higher dialysis dose than commonly provided during conventional dialysis may increase survival among patients undergoing renal replacement therapies (30).

However, this hypothesis was refuted in two large well-designed studies in both hemodialysis and peritoneal dialysis patients:

- The HEMO study found that increasing the dialysis dose within the general restrictions of a thrice weekly regimen failed to decrease patient mortality (31).
- In the ADEMEX study, no decrease in mortality was seen with peritoneal dialysis doses greater than a weekly Kt/V of 1.7 (32)

In light of these negative studies, significant attention has turned to alternative dialysis schedules, such as, short-daily HD (SHD), nocturnal HD (NHD), and long, intermittent hemodialysis (LHD). It is suggested that more frequent dialysis may be associated an improvement in health-related quality of life (HRQoL) and with improved survival (33-34).

The first successful use of short daily, or "quotidian" hemodialysis was first reported by DePalma in 1969 (35). This approach was based upon the premise that improved patient outcomes, compared with conventional three times per week hemodialysis, would occur with a dialysis schedule that consisted of the same number of hours of dialysis per week but delivered over twice as many sessions. More specifically, it involves five to seven treatments per week, each lasting 1.5 to 2.5 hours. The rationale for short daily hemodialysis is based upon a strategy that is proposed to enhance both dialysis efficiency and hemodynamic stability. With short daily dialysis, shortening the dialysis time while increasing the frequency of dialysis allows more time to be spent dialyzing against higher uremic solute concentration gradients. This enhances the efficiency of solute removal (36). More frequent dialysis allows for less interdialytic fluid accumulation. This is likely to improve hemodynamic stability during dialysis with increased potential for normalizing the extracellular fluid volume. This form of therapy has been associated with significant improvement in serum albumin, calcium phosphate, and volume control in small scale studies. However, no mortality data is available.

A recent study, Frequent Hemodialysis Network (FHN) Daily Trial, was a multicenter, randomized trial that included 245 patients assigned to either frequent hemodialysis (six times weekly) or conventional hemodialysis. Two primary composite outcomes were determined at one year, including death or one-year change from baseline in left ventricular (LV) mass as assessed by cardiac resonance imaging, and death or one-year change in physical health as assessed by a RAND health survey. Both composite outcomes showed significant benefit to the frequent-dialysis group compared with the conventional-dialysis group (with hazard ratios of 0.61, 95% CI, 0.46-0.82 for death or change in LV mass; and 0.70, 95% CI, 0.53-0.92, for death or change in physical health) (37). This study also demonstrated benefits in pre-determined secondary outcomes to the frequent dialysis group such as a decrease in LV mass, improved blood pressure control and phosphate balance but not on cognitive performance, depression, serum albumin concentration, or use of erythropoiesis-stimulating agents.

Nocturnal hemodialysis (e.g, long nightly home hemodialysis) was introduced as a potentially more desirable alternative to conventional dialysis, since it provides superior dialysis based upon dose, duration, and frequency (38). This can be accomplished because it is performed during nightly sleep, an otherwise unproductive time (39). The late Robert

Uldall started the first quotidian (daily) nocturnal hemodialysis program in 1994 at the Wellesley Hospital in Toronto (40). Since then, its use has been extended to more centers in Canada, the United States, Australia, and several European countries (41-44). This hemodialysis modality is performed five to seven times per week, with each treatment lasting 6 to 8 hours. Although the number of patients studied has been rather limited, but these evidence suggest signficant improvements in caloric intake and serum albumin results.

Long intermittent hemodialysis is given three times a week and a dialysis time of 6 to 8 hours. This procedure is practiced in Tassin, France, and has been associated with improvements in blood pressure control and better overall nutritional status.

Although, no data on randomized controlled trials are available on home hemodialysis, some recent well-conceived cohort studies have indicated that outcome of home (daily) HD is superior to conventional in-centre dialysis, and even equal to cadaveric transplantation, when differences in case mix are taken into account (45).

4.1 Hemofiltration and hemodiafiltration

Hemodiafiltration is a form of chronic renal replacement therapy used most in Europe, particularly Germany and Belgium, and very rarely used currently in the United States (46). Based upon relatively better clearance of larger "middle" molecules through solvent drag, some claim that replacement therapy with hemodiafiltration may be superior to that with hemodialysis, including improved hemodynamics.

For chronic renal replacement therapy, the two principal regimens used to provide substantial removal of larger MW uremic toxins via convection are intermittent hemofiltration (HF) and intermittent hemodiafiltration (HDF). Daily convective therapy has also been used.

- Hemofiltration — With HF, fluid is removed by the dialysis machine through increased transmembrane pressure and the replacement solution is infused intravenously at equal volume minus the desired fluid volume removal. The clearance of the method for a particular solute is dictated by the ultrafiltration volume and the sieving coefficient. As the sieving coefficient for low MW unbound solutes equals 1, the clearance for small molecules equals the ultrafiltrate volume. Although hemofiltration is effective in the removal of the larger MW solutes, it is less effective in the removal of small molecules as it is restricted by the ultrafiltration volume.
- Hemodiafiltration — HDF is a combination of hemodialysis and hemofiltration devised to overcome the low clearance of small solutes by hemofiltration by adding a diffusive component.

For chronic renal replacement therapy, the standard regimen for both HF and HDF includes three sessions per week for three to five hours, as with conventional intermittent hemodialysis. A typical conservative (or high dose) regimen for HDF includes a post dilution configuration with a blood flow of 300 mL/min (500 mL/min for high dose), a dialysate flow of 500 mL/min, a flow of a substitution volume of 60 mL/min (120 mL/min for high dose) and a high flux dialyzer of 1.4 m^2 (2.2 m^2 for high dose) (47).

Several small studies using daily HF/HDF have been published.

- One study that addressed the short term effects of daily HF reported that predialysis beta-2-microglobulin levels decreased by 40 percent (48).
- In one study in which 12 patients switched from HD to HF at home on a daily basis for one month, HF was associated with a lower blood pressure, higher caloric intake, and

improved quality of life, findings consistent with previous reports on short daily HD (49-50). A trend toward a decrease in serum beta-2-microglobulin could be ascribed to the HF alone. The infusion volume used was 40 percent of total body water, which offered a standard Kt/V of approximately 2.0.

- In another study of eight patients undergoing in center daily hemodiafiltration for six months, there were lower serum levels of predialysis BUN and creatinine (which were expected by the change to a daily schedule), as well as lower levels of other solutes including beta-2-microglobulin and homocysteine (51). Additional benefits included improved phosphate control, discontinuation of all antihypertensive agents, and a 30 percent regression in left ventricular mass. Although some of these results can be attributed to the daily treatment schedule, the decrease in the pretreatment levels of beta-2-microglobulin and the improvement in phosphate control are clearly attributable to both convection and the increased treatment frequency.

4.2 Adequacy of hemodialysis

For greater than 50 years hemodialysis (HD) has been performed in some form or another. Outcomes for dialysis patients expressed in terms of quality of life (QOL), mortality, and hospitalization, is reportedly similar to those seen in patients with solid organ cancer. Despite improvements in long-term outcomes demonstrated with all dialysis modalities, the adjusted annual mortality of dialysis patient remains high at 19% (52-53). There are many factors (dialysis and non-dialysis) that determines outcome. One such influential factor is "adequacy" of dialysis. Adequate dialysis was originally used to describe dialysis dosing measured by small solute removal, but is now deemed as the amount of dialysis required to keep a patient symptoms free, functional, with a life expectancy similar to that of healthy individuals. Since its inception, there have been numerous approaches to quantify the delivered dialysis dose in a reproducible manner, and to link the dialysis dose with clinical outcomes.

4.3 Importance of urea and its use as a surrogate marker of uremic toxicity

Solute removal during hemodialysis focuses on urea. Urea is produced from the anabolism, catabolism of proteins and is the principal way by which nitrogenous substances are excreted from the body. Urea is a small water soluble molecule (molecular weight 60 daltons) that is slightly toxic. Recent studies have demonstrated that urea removal does not closely parallel that of other small water-soluble compounds, protein-bound solutes, or middle molecules. (54) Despite this information, adequacy of HD dosing is predominantly evaluated by removal of urea. During the development of the uremic syndrome, losses of kidney function are accompanied by deteriorating organ function attributable to the accumulation of uremic retention solutes or uremic toxins. (54) Uremic toxins are diverse and complex, they include inorganic compounds (phosphate water, potassium, water and trace elements), as well as organic compounds that comprises small water-soluble solutes (<500 d), middle molecules (>500 d), and protein-bound solutes. These peptides can be altered by glycosylation, oxidization or carbamylation, and they can provoke inflammation, hypertrophy, oxidative stress, coagulation, constriction, thus uremia is more than the retention and accumulation of urea or water-soluble compounds alone. (54) Mortality has repeatedly been shown to be associated with the clearance of urea. Of commonly measured protein-derived substances, only the serum concentration of $ß_2$-microglobulin correlates with mortality. Recently, a higher free concentration of the protein-bound solute *p*-cresol has also been reported to be associated with mortality. (55) Current dialysis and dialysis-related treatments do not remove any significant quantity of substances larger than 10 to 15 kd. Future means of removing higher molecular weight toxins or protein-bound substances may include the use of sorbents in addition to traditional diffusive and convective dialysis strategies.

4.4 Urea kinetic modeling, URR and KT/V

The mathematical model known as urea kinetics can be used to calculate the rate of production and removal of urea. Measurement of the dialysis dose has, for the most part, relied on estimation of clearance of the small, water-soluble, and nitrogenous waste product urea, and hence the mathematical model is referred to as urea kinetic modeling (UKM). Formal (UKM) is the most accurate method for assessment of delivered dialysis dose. It assumes that urea is distributed in a single, well-mixed pool. UKM presumes that full equilibration occurs immediately between blood and tissue compartments. However, in vivo there is a delay in redistribution and it takes 30 to 60 minutes for equilibration between blood and tissue compartments post dialysis. UKM also assumes that urea is generated at a constant rate by protein metabolism and is removed at a constant rate by residual renal function, and intermittently by dialysis. Hence, in a person with negligible renal function, the extent of urea removal provides a measure of dialysis adequacy, and the rate of production correlates with dietary protein intake. (56) Thus, it's inappropriate to follows predialysis blood urea nitrogen (BUN) or serum urea only; because low serum urea could be attributed to malnutrition (insufficient protein diet) rather than adequate dialysis urea removal. UKM has formed the basis for retrospective interpretation of the National Cooperative Dialysis Study and for prescription and control of the HEMO and the Frequent Hemodialysis Network studies. (60) Due its mathematical intricacy, UKM requires advanced computer support. UKM is the most rigorous available method for prescribing and evaluating dialysis dose and is widely used in the United States. Current methods for assessment of dialysis dose are based on the predialysis and postdialysis difference in BUN and include the urea reduction ratio (URR), the single-pool *Kt/V* (*spKt/V*), the equilibrated *Kt/V* (*eKt/V*), and the weekly standard *Kt/V* (*std-Kt/V*).

Kt/V is a dimensionless ratio representing fractional urea clearance, where *K* is the dialyzer urea clearance (liters per hour), *t* is the length of HD session (hours), and *V* is the volume of distribution of urea (liters). It is the most widely used parameter to assess dialysis dose. Kt/V is derived from single-pool urea kinetics and is referred to as spKt/V. A value of spKt/V of 1 indicates that the total volume of blood completely cleared of urea during a dialysis session is equivalent to the volume of distribution of urea. Solute disequilibrium occurs when dialysis time is decreased in addition to increasing dialysis and blood flow rates. Solute disequilibrium can be corrected by adjusting the Kt/V for the rebound in urea, which happens mainly in the 30–60 minutes immediately post dialysis. The resultant Kt/V is termed equilibrated Kt/V or eKt/V. Numerous equations have been developed by Daugirdas and others to help derive the eKt/V from spKt/V.(57-59) With a conventional 4-hour HD treatment, eKt/V is usually about 0.2 units lower than spKt/V. The difference is even larger with short, high-efficiency HD or hemodiafiltration, in which urea rebound is higher. Single-pool *Kt/V* or, even better, *eKt/V* should be assessed monthly, and dialysis prescription should be adapted accordingly. In large cross-sectional studies, mortality increases when *spKt/V* falls below 1.2, and international guidelines (e.g., KDOQI) recommend a target *spKt/V* of 1.3 for a conventional dialysis schedule of three times per week.

Online clearance is the term used when the dialysis dose is calculated by measuring conductivity or ionic clearance across the dialysis membrane. Multiple ions can be tracked at the same time to minimize error, and the delivered Kt/V can be predicted in real time before the treatment is over. Although sound in theory, the practical application is limited. UKM is also used to calculate the protein catabolic rate (PCR) and the protein catabolic rate normalized to body weight (nPCR), both of which are useful measures of nutrition.

Urea reduction ratio (URR) is another way of quantifying the delivered dialysis dose. However, it's over simplified since it does not take into account intradialytic urea generation and convective urea removal by ultrafiltration. Because the relative decrease in urea concentration during dialysis is the most significant determinant of Kt/V, direct measurement of URR is an accepted method for assessment of dialysis adequacy. The URR equation is as follows: URR = (BUNpre -BUNpost)/BUNpre where BUNpre is pre-dialysis urea concentration and BUNpost is post-dialysis urea concentration. By convention, the value is multiplied by 100 and expressed as a percentage. A minimum URR of 65% to 70% is recommended for adequate HD. Kt/V and URR are mathematically linked by the following equation: Kt/V= -ln(1-URR), where ln is the natural logarithm. (60) Accordingly, *Kt/V* equals 1.0 when URR equals 0.63 or 63% of whole-body urea has been removed. (60)

4.5 Limitations of UKM

One of the criticisms of UKM is the use of urea as the reference marker for measurement. We know that it's a very small solute. Clearance of a solute is multifactorial; it is dependent on the molecular weight, charge, volume of distribution, and protein binding. Furthermore, clearance of solutes with different molecular weights from urea or bound to proteins would be different. Thus, clearance of urea cannot be extrapolated to other substances such as "uremic toxin" because they act differently. In addition UKM does not take into account residual renal function (RRF), which has a significant impact on patient outcome. (57) Also, it has been shown that V calculated by anthropometric formulas systematically overestimates volume by about 15%. (58) Kt/V underestimate that body water has an independent effect on outcomes, it is now recognized that smaller patients require higher Kt/v compared to larger patients. (61) Also, Kt/V does not confer that time (t) has an independent effect on outcome. The National Cooperative Dialysis (NCDS) was the first multicenter, randomized controlled trial of hemodialysis adequacy in which UKM was used to analyse the effect of BUN and HD time. Longer time was associated with better outcomes, however the statistical relationship between treatment time and patient outcome in was considered not to be significant (*p* value of 0.056). (61-62) Kt/V does not account for QOL, BP and volume control, clinically stability or biochemical factors. We know from the analysis of Hurricane Katrina that patients who missed three HD sessions were associated with odds ratio for hospitalization of 2.15. (61,63) Thus, Kt/V only measure the adequacy of one dialysis session, it does not incorporate missed HD sessions or shorten dialysis time.

Some of these limitations are rectifiable. One can increase HD time for intradialytic hypotension, inability to control volume, or if dialysis dosage is inadequate. HD dose can be based on body surface area (BSA), thus, smaller patients can receive more dialysis.

4.6 Hemodialysis dose

Quantifying removal of toxic uremic solutes is important to assess the adequacy of HD. The delivered dialysis dose is a function of length of the session (*t*), dialysate and blood flow rates, volume of distribution (V) of the uremic toxin studied, and the dialyzer efficiency (K_oA). Volume of distribution is very different for urea (total body water volume), than other small-molecular-weight. The minimum frequency and dosage of dialysis is three times per week, for a minimum treatment time of 3 to 4 hours, a blood flow rate of at least 250 ml/min, and a dialysate flow rate of 500 to 800 ml/min. Patients that are initiated on HD, *V* is unknown and has to be estimated (men, 58% of body weight; women, 55% of body weight). After obtaining measured *Kt/V* the dialysis prescription can be adjusted to meet the *Kt/V* goals. For patients with severe and long-standing uremia, it's recommended to provide several sessions in achieving target dose to avoid the dialysis disequilibrium syndrome.

4.7 Recommendations for dialysis dose adequacy

Current recommendations in the United States are as follows (KDOQI) (64):

- A minimum *spKt/V* of at least 1.2 for both adult and pediatric HD patients. When URR is used, the delivered dose should be equivalent to a *Kt/V* of 1.2, that is, an average URR of 65%.
- To prevent the delivered dose of HD from falling below the recommended minimum dose, the prescribed dose of HD should be *spKt/V* of 1.3, which corresponds to an average URR of 70%.
- The delivered dose of HD should be measured at least once per month in all adult and pediatric HD patients.

4.8 Factors affecting delivered Kt/V

Factors that influences delivery of Kt/V is multifactorial: hematocrit, the effective dialyzer urea clearance *Kd* depends on blood and dialysate flow rates, dialyzer K_oA, effective dialyzer surface area, anticoagulation, and recirculation. (60) Dialysis session time (*t*) is critical for reaching the *Kt/V* goal. Prescribe treatment time (PTT) and effective treatment time (ETT) may not always correlate, EET may be significantly less secondary to patient demand, clotting of dialyser, or intermittent pump stops. *V* does not substantially change during a single HD session but may change over time. Dialysis dose needs to be adjusted for an increase in *V*. However, if there is a loss in body mass (weight loss, amputation of limb), is associated with a decrease in *V*, *Kt/V* should not be reduced but rather adjusted to the higher, ideal patient *V* or BSA.

If faced with an inadequate delivered *Kt/V*, first check if that session was representative of an average session and no unusual problems may have occurred (e.g., shortened time because of patient request, needle difficulty, leaks, alarm triggering). (60) The use of commercial technologies that measure ionic dialysance can be implemented to monitor each dialysis. A frequent cause of low *Kt/V* is fistula integrity that causes a vascular access problem leading to recirculation. Blood sampling errors should be considered because delayed post-HD sampling will reduce *Kt/V*. Standardized blood sampling procedures should be implemented in each center. If, despite these checks, a low *Kt/V* remains unexplained, treatment time should be increased to 4.5 or 5 hours. Prescription of a more efficient dialyzer and higher blood and dialysate flow rates should also be considered. However, increasing treatment time, rather than increasing dialysate flow, or using two dialysers, would be more beneficial and practical to improve adequacy. Muscle exercise before or during dialysis improves *Kt/V* by increasing blood supply to poorly perfused urea rich muscle tissue and thus facilitates urea equilibration. Delivered *Kt/V* should be checked whenever the dialysis prescription has been modified substantially. Online clearance monitoring allows assessment of *Kt/V* during each single session without blood sampling.

4.9 Should volume (V) be included in Kt/V to assess target clearance?

In an attempt to address the question of optimal dialysis dose, several clinical trial have proposed that patients with small urea *V*, such as women, do worst compared to larger people. This is secondary to the notion that muscle mass closely correlate to total body water than to body weight. Thus, small urea *V* is a good indicator for low muscle mass. The Hemodialysis Study (HEMO) was performed in which 1846 patients were randomly assigned to a standard or high dose of dialysis and a low- or high-flux dialyzer (based on clearance of beta-2-microglobulin) which revealed a beneficial effect of higher *Kt/V* for women but not for men. (65) This suggests that individuals with low muscle mass may require a higher clearance in relation to *V* and therefore raises the question of whether *V* is the appropriate denominator for dialysis dose. (60) Native renal clearances, in contrast, are commonly related to body surface area (BSA), not to total body water. (60) It has been suggested to relate BSA to dialysis clearances. The ratio of BSA to urea *V* is generally higher in women than in men and decreases with an increment in *V*. Prescribing dialysis dose in relation to BSA ($K \times t/\mathrm{BSA}$) would result in more dialysis for smaller patients of either gender and for women of any size. (57,60) More work need to be done to validate this novel idea.

4.10 Other dialysis factors related to outcomes

There are many other factors that play a role in the outcome of dialysis adequacy. Such factor includes but is not restricted to middle molecule removal, hyperphosphatemia, preservation of RRF, vascular access, QOL and treatment time. In general, middle molecule removal is determined by the dialyser permeability, the presence of convection, protein binding, and dialysis duration. Given that daily dialysis results in more frequent solute level equilibration with less rebound, this technique provides higher middle molecule removal than with conventional hemodialysis. The retention of solutes of middle molecular size is proposed to play an important role in the pathogenesis of the uremic state and contribute significantly to the high mortality of dialysis patients. (60) High-flux dialyzers have the propensity to remove larger amounts of middle molecules than low-flux dialyzers due to higher membrane porosity, and this may even be further increased by the use of convective dialysis strategies, such as hemodiafiltration. Serum β_2-microglobulin, is a surrogate for other uremic middle molecules, is effectively removed by high-flux than by low-flux dialysis, and predialysis β_2-microglobulin levels were found to be related to mortality in patients treated randomly with high-flux or low-flux dialyzers. (70) Patient who has diabetes on HD, or on dialysis for longer than 3.7 years, and those with serum albumin levels below 40 g/l, may benefit most from high-flux dialysis. (69,71) The European Best Practice Guidelines have recommended maximizing the removal of middle molecules in all dialysis patients. (60,72)

Hyperphosphatemia is a major problem in HD and is managed by phosphate removal via dialysis, use of phosphate binder medication to prevent intestinal phosphate absorption

from dietary phosphate and dietary restriction. With the use of larger dialyzer surface area, hemodiafiltration, high-flux HD, removal of phosphate is significantly removal. Must monitor for hypophosphatemia with long frequent dialysis
End stage renal patients initiated on dialysis initially posess considerable residual renal function (RRF). However, most of these patients lose their RRF by the end of the first year on dialysis. By year three only 10% to 20% of patients retain their RRF. RRF of 2 to 3 ml/min urea clearance contributes significantly to the elimination of uremic toxins. (73) The retention of RRF results in lower serum β_2-microglobulin, phosphate, potassium, urea, creatinine, and uric acid levels; higher hemoglobin concentration; enhanced nutritional status; better quality of life scores; and a reduced need for dietary and fluid restrictions. (60) Left ventricular hypertrophy is associated with loss of RRF. Patient with an estimated TBW of 40 liters, a residual urea clearance of 2 to 3 ml/min is equivalent to a *std-Kt/V* of 0.5 to 0.75/week. Dialysate water impurities, nephrotoxic agents such as radiocontrast, nonsteroidal anti-inflammatory drugs, aminoglycosides and activation of the immune system by bioincompatible membranes, intradialytic hypotension are risk factors for the loss of RRF. Patients who retain urine output may enhance survival augment with the regulation of fluid and electrolyte balance.

5. Frequency of dialysis

DePalma first reported in 1969 the successful use of short daily or "quotidian" hemodialysis. (35) Short daily dialysis (SDD) was based upon the premise that patient outcomes would improved, compared with conventional three times per week hemodialysis. SDD would occur with a dialysis schedule that consisted of the same number of hours of dialysis per week but delivered over twice as many sessions. More specifically, this schedule consists of daily hemodialysis (five to seven days per week) provided for a duration of 1.5 to 3 or more hours per session. Initial attempts to popularize daily dialysis in the United States were suppressed by financial and logistical issues. This led to a decline in its use both in the home and in-center settings. However, over the last decade there has been resurgence in the use of daily dialysis, with several studies emerging from the United States and Europe showing improvements in various intermediate outcomes. Most recently, in the wake of the HEMO study, attention has turned from increasing the per-session dialytic dose, to altering variables such as treatment frequency or duration to improve outcomes (75-76) Daily dialysis has also been proposed as a rescue therapy and in the intensive care unit setting.
The mortality rate of patients undergoing maintenance hemodialysis is unacceptably high. An extremely high morbidity, relatively low quality of life (due in part to a high level of dependence and unemployment), and high cost have also been observed. Contrast this with frequent dialysis which provides a more physiological renal replacement, because it allows more gentle volume removal, reduction of hemodynamic stress and better blood pressure control. More frequent dialysis and prolonged-duration HD have the greatest effect on middle molecule clearance. (74) In addition, phosphorus removal is increased secondarily to its predominant intracellular distribution. Protein bound solutes like p-cresol are not changed, because these solutes depend on RRF. The benefits of more frequent dialysis improve BP, thus decreasing anti-hypertensive medications, decreasing intradialytic hypotension, lowering serum phosphate, raising albumin and hemoglobin with lower requirements for erythropoiesis stimulating agents. HD patients switch to nocturnal dialysis improved sleep efficiency especially in stage 3 and 4 sleep with decreased in daytime fatigue

after 6 months. (75) Nocturnal dialysis is also associated with beneficial effects on vascular smooth muscle which restore the proliferation of the apoptosis ratio, which directly associated to serum phosphorus. However, there are no published randomized trials of nocturnal hemodialysis compared to other modalities. Thus studies comparing nocturnal hemodialysis to conventional hemodialysis should be performed to better understand the benefits with nocturnal hemodialysis.

Due to the nightly schedule with nocturnal hemodialysis, the cost of consumables is higher than conventional hemodialysis and is similar to the cost of short daily hemodialysis. However, the personnel cost of nocturnal hemodialysis is lower than that with in-center hemodialysis regimens. (76)

Depending upon the consumable/personnel cost ratio in different countries, nocturnal hemodialysis can be less or more expensive than in-center conventional hemodialysis. In addition, the cost of medications, including EPO, antihypertensive agents, and phosphate binders, is lower with nocturnal hemodialysis as well as cost of hospitalization.

5.1 Vascular access

Performing hemodialysis requires the ability to access and return a patient's blood at a high rate. The optimal access would allow a high rate of blood flow, with no recirculation of dialyzed blood into the pre-dialysis blood, with maximal durability, minimal complications, and minimal gap from creation to use. Currently, no hemodialysis access approaches this goal; each available access has shortcomings.

The preferred access currently is the arteriovenous fistula (AVF). The AVF is created surgically by connecting an artery to a vein, with the subsequent increased flow and pressure causing the vein to "arterialize," with thickened wall and increased size. This arterialized vein can then be accessed for hemodialysis. The advantages to the AVF are a high rate of blood flow with minimal recirculation, minimal complications because of the absence of foreign material, and an extended functional life. The primary shortcoming of the AVF is the significant time from initial placement to maturation for use, which ranges from 25 to 98 days (81). Typically AVF is not used until 3 months after placement. However, a recent study of the practice patterns at dialysis facilities in DOPPS suggests that earlier cannulation of AVFs (even prior to 4 weeks) was not associated with increased risk of access failure (81). Other issues include a significant rate of primary failure of AVFs (82), vascular steal syndrome, inability to create AVFs because of lack of suitable vessels (82-84), and development of stenoses leading to AVF thrombosis and AVF failure (82-84).

Given the significant time for their maturation, AVFs must be placed well before initiation of hemodialysis to avoid use of other accesses, such as tunneled catheters. Currently, only 15 percent of patients starting on hemodialysis use an AVF, and only 24 percent have a maturing AVF (85). One cause is late referral to nephrologists, but even with a timely referral to nephrologists, 46% of the patients did not have a permanent access placed prior to starting HD (85). Some barriers leading to this problem include patient resistance to creation of AVFs, poor access to surgeons, and decreased rate of primary patency of AVFs (85). Possible solutions include improved patient education, often through patient support groups in CKD clinics and referral to nephrologist at earlier stage of chronic kidney disease (85).

Where creation of an AVF is impossible, insertion of an arteriovenous graft (AVG) may be feasible. The advantage of an AVG is the high primary patency rate and minimal gap between creation and first use (84,86). Because of the presence of foreign material, there is increased risk of access infection, although less than that with tunneled catheters, and there is an increased rate of stenosis, thrombosis, and graft failure compared with AVFs. One new technique in the creation of AVGs is the Hemodialysis Reliable Outflow (HeRO™) dialysis catheter, a new FDA approved device for catheter-dependent and significant vasculopathic patients. The HeRO device is an AVG that extends from the arm into the right ventricle. This may avoid problems with stenosis at the venous anastomosis leading to graft failure.

The third means of chronic hemodialysis access is the tunneled catheter. This catheter, like the standard non-tunneled dialysis catheter used for acute hemodialysis access and non-tunneled catheters used for venous access, is inserted into a central vein, usually the internal jugular vein, but the risk of infection is reduced by increasing the distance between the vein and skin entry by running the catheter through a subcutaneous tunnel. This access has the advantage of being usable immediately upon insertion, but it has the highest rate of infection, particularly catheter-related bacteremia, and is associated with higher costs, morbidity, and mortality, compared with other accesses (87-88). Other complications of the tunneled catheter include intraluminal thrombosis and fibrin sheath.

6. Management of access complications

6.1 Detection and treatment of stenosis and thrombosis of AVF and AVG

Stenosis of AVF and AVG commonly develop over time, generally resulting from response to endothelial damage. This can occur at the anastamosis between native vessels or between a graft and a native vessel, with endothelial damage caused by surgical trauma, or distal to the venous anastamosis, with endothelial damage from rapid turbulent flow. If these stenoses are not recognized and corrected, increased access pressures and decreased flow can result in thrombosis of the access. Once an access has thrombosed, even if it can be salvaged, the duration of secondary patency is relatively short, with 62% one year patency average (89). Therefore, monitoring and subsequent treatment of stenosis in AVFs and AVGs is critical to prolonging the life of these hemodialysis accesses. For an excellent review of the various methods of monitoring accesses, see reference 90. There are several ways to monitor for stenosis. Physical exam, looking for abnormalities such as change in thrill, bruit or pulse, presence of arm swelling, or prolonged bleeding after dialysis, can be quite helpful in detecting access problems (91). Another common way to detect stenosis is with dynamic venous pressure monitoring. With this technique, the pressure at the venous needle is measured with low dialysis pump rate. If the pressure is over 80, or if there is significant increase from prior pressures, there is a high likelihood of outflow stenosis (92). Measuring static access pressures (with blood pump off) is more accurate, and can also detect arterial stenoses, but this technique requires additional equipment, and is therefore not common (93). Another monitoring method growing in use is Doppler flow measurement. If the flow decreases to less than 650 mL/minute, or if there has been significant interval decrease in flow, there is a high likelihood of stenosis (94). Stenoses can be detected by Doppler ultrasound, but the gold standard for detection and treatment of access stenosis is fistulogram, or the injection of contrast into the access to demonstrate visually the stenosis. When a fistulogram demonstrates stenosis, the stenosis can be repaired with angioplasty or surgical revision. While angioplasty has a shorter secondary patency than surgical revision, angioplasty is generally the first line treatment of stenosis and thrombosis of AVF and AVG, since surgical revision can be performed after angioplasty in case of recurrent stenosis or thrombosis (95). Treatment with anticoagulant or anti-platelet therapy, e.g. aspirin, ticlopidine or warfarin, has a modest effect on reducing stenosis and increasing patency of fistulas; however, this treatment is associated with increased risk of hemorrhage (96). Antiplatelet therapy should be a part of routine care in patient with graft but not AV fistula (97). Other pharmacological approaches for prevention of stenosis and patency of vascular access including calcium channel blocker, ACE-I and fish oil have been investigated, but further research is required to determine the role of these agents in maintaining fistula patency.

Another complication of AVF and AVG is vascular access induced ischemia and is related to significant amounts of blood flow via AV fistulas. This diversion of blood via the fistula could cause decrease of blood flow to the distal tissue and cause ischemia (known as steal syndrome). It could rarely cause exacerbation of heart failure in paints with underlying disease. Elderly patients, patients with diabetics, peripheral vascular disease or coronary artery disease are at increase risk of ischemia. Pain during hemodialysis is a characteristic symptom.

Another vascular access complication is central venous obstruction occurring in patients with previously inserted venous catheter or pacemaker placement. The rate of central venous obstruction is higher in patients who had their brachial venous accessed prior to dialysis access placement compare to patient who had internal jugular vein accessed. The most common clinical presentation is pain and swelling of the ipsilateral arm usually accompanied with the superficial collateral vein around the shoulder. Other clue for diagnosis of central venous obstruction is finger ulceration, pain and inadequate dialysis. The first option for treatment is percutaneous transluminal angioplasty and stent placement (angioplasty alone has a high rate of restenosis). The second option is surgical revision with bypass grafting and placement of HERO catheter (as discussed above).

6.2 Catheter thrombosis and fibrin sheath formation

One of the most common complications of hemodialysis catheters is decrease of flow or thrombosis. Catheter thrombosis prevention is generally achieved through instillation of heparin into the catheter ports after completion of dialysis; a recent study suggests that weekly instillation of recombinant tissue plasminogen activator (tPA) may prevent thrombosis more effectively (98). Catheter thrombosis can be treated effectively by instillation of tPA into the catheter lumens or with exchange of the catheter over a guidewire; however, thrombosis frequently recurs, necessitating further procedures. One cause of frequent catheter malfunction is the formation of a fibrin sheath around the tip of the catheter. This can be treated with a 3 hour infusion of low-dose tPA or with mechanical stripping, although secondary patency rates remain low (99).

6.3 Catheter related blood stream infection (CRBSI)

The prevalence of central venous catheters in the United States is about 20-30% despite recommendations from major societies to increase the use of AV fistulas known as fistula first initiative. There is an increased risk of mortality with the use of catheters compared with the use of AV fistulas (100). This increased rate of mortality is likely related to infection. The rate of catheter related blood stream infection is 0.5 to 6.6 episodes per 1,000 catheter days (101). The source of this infection is bacterial seeding from biofilms that form on the inside and outside of the blood stream catheter. The rate of CRBSI is directly related to the species and level of virulence of the seeding bacteria. Meticulous catheter care and reeducation of personnel responsible for insertion of the catheters are the key elements in lowering the rate of catheter related infection (101). The catheter care includes but is not limited to sterile technique of catheter placement, exit –site care, sterile technique during initiation and termination of dialysis (including the use of a sterile barrier, sterile gloves, and antiseptic to clean the tubes) and the replacement of malfunctioning catheters over a guidewire (empirical administration of antibiotics does not reduce the incidence of catheter associated bacteremia) (102). Using standard antiseptic precautions the incidence of catheter related infection could drop to one episode per 1,000 catheter days which could be used to assess the quality of catheter care.

The current guidelines indicate the use of tunneled cuffed catheter for long term use (more than 3 weeks duration) in patients in need of hemodialysis based on pathophysiological considerations as well as a generally lower rate of infection of tunneled, cuffed catheters compared to nontunneled catheters (103). The location of catheters influences the risk of infection. The femoral lines carry a higher rate of infection compare with the subclavian or jugular lines. Subsequent studies, however, only confirm an increase risk of femoral catheter infection in the patients with a higher BMI (87-88,102).

Although the prophylactic use of systemic antibiotics at the time of insertion of a catheter is not currently recommended, the antimicrobial lock solutions for prevention of catheter related infection and bactremia are recommended (101). The ideal lock solution has anticoagulant and antimicrobial activity, is safe, and does not induce bacterial resistance. The antimicrobial solutions most frequently used are antibiotics or chemicals, citrate (30% concentrated since the lower concentration has little antimicrobial affect) (104). Antimicrobial lock solutions substantially reduce the risk of catheter related infection (102). The potential disadvantage of usage of antibiotics for antimicrobial lock solution is bacterial resistance and predisposition to highly resistance bacterial infection. There is also a potential adverse effect of these antibiotics including aminoglycoside-related ototoxicity. The disadvantage of usage of citrate is hypocalcemia and adverse cardiac event if the locking solution is pushed to the patient blood (105).

Application of topical antibiotics to the exit site may reduce the incidence of catheter related infection in patients on hemodialysis. The most recent CDC guideline recommends use of povidone iodine antiseptic ointment or bacitracin/gramicidin/polymyxin B at the hemodialysis catheter exit site after each dialysis session (101). A recent Cochrane review on this subject concluded that the current data support only the topical application of mupirocin alone (among antibacterial agents) for prevention of catheter related infection (106). The use of antibiotic coated catheter in hemodialysis patients has not been shown to reduce the incidence of catheter related infection (101,107).

Staphylococcus species in general and S. aureus in particular are among the most common cause of bacterial related infection. Mortality rate is high among the patient infected with S. aureus (8%). Morbidity related to S. aureus is secondary to its high propensity to colonize prosthetic materials, heart valves, bones and joints. Nasal carriage of S. aureus is common among patients on dialysis, in whom it is associated with an increased risk of S. aureus infection. Successful elimination of S. aureus nasal carriage can be achieved by a short (5-day) course of mupirocin applied daily to the anterior nares (108).

Treatment of CRBSI requires systemic antibiotics and frequently discontinuation of the catheter and placement of temporary catheter. There are four possible options for treatment of CRBSI. Intravenous antibiotics alone, prompt catheter removal with delayed placement of a new long term catheter, exchange of the infected catheter with a new one over guidewire, or use of systemic antibiotics and an antibiotic lock in the existing catheter. Antibiotic therapy for catheter-related infection is often initiated empirically. The initial choice of antibiotics will depend on the severity of the patient's clinical disease, the risk factors for infection, and the likely pathogens associated with the specific intravascular device (109). Antibiotic therapy should be administered to patients with persistent fungemia or bacteremia after catheter removal (especially if the infection is caused by S. aureus). Long-term catheters should be removed from patients with CRBSI associated with any of the following conditions: severe sepsis; suppurative thrombophlebitis; endocarditis; bloodstream infection that continues despite antimicrobial therapy to which the infecting microbes are susceptible (110). In uncomplicated CRBSI involving long-term catheters due to pathogens other than S. aureus, P. aeruginosa, fungi, because of the limited access sites in many patients who require long-term intravascular access for survival in hemodialysis patients, treatment should be attempted without catheter removal, with use of both systemic and antimicrobial lock therapy for 14 days and cultures should be repeated one week after completion of antibiotics treatment. The rate of treatment failure, however, is higher for patient treated with antibiotics alone (111). If the symptoms resolve after 2–3 days of intravenous antibiotic therapy, guidewire exchange of the catheter is associated with cure rates that are comparable to those associated with immediate removal and delayed placement of a new catheter (110). Localized Cellulites (exit site infection) should be treated with systemic antibiotics and exit site care. Tunnel track infection, however, requires catheter removal since it involves space in an area with limited vascular supply (112).

6.4 Acute vascular access

A large diameter venous catheter (a dual lumen venous catheter) usually placed in the internal jugular or femoral vein, is needed for acute or urgent hemodialysis in the absence of permanent vascular access. This catheter is used in patients with acute kidney injury who need urgent hemodialysis, in patients who need removal of a toxic agent by means of dialysis, or with chronic dialysis patients with a temporary inability to use a permanent access, as with catheter-related bacteremia. Using this type of access, one lumen of the venous catheter is allocated to draw blood (arterial side) and the other lumen is allocated to return the blood. Separation of arterial from venous lumen minimized the recirculation of blood during hemodialysis. Because of high risk of infection, non-tunneled femoral catheter should be removed within a week, while non-tunneled internal jugular catheters can be used for about 2 weeks. Hemodialysis catheters placed in the subclavian veins have a significant risk of subclavian stenosis, which can cause the arm on that side to be unsuitable for AVF or AVG placement, and so catheters are generally not placed in the subclavian veins. An indwelling cuffed catheter is tunneled under the skin and placed in the internal jugular vein by an interventional nephrologist, interventional radiologist or surgeon. It is used when acute renal failure is expected to require hemodialysis for more than 2 weeks because of the decreased rate of infection (1034).

6.5 Extracorporeal therapies in the ICU setting - continuous renal replacement therapy

Critically ill, hemodynamically unstable intensive care unit (ICU) patients are typically the most challenging to treat with conventional dialytic modalities as described above. The intermittent volume and solute fluxes may cause significant morbidity, which includes worsening of hypotension and arrhythmias. Multiple modalities of renal replacement therapy are currently available. These include intermittent hemodialysis (IHD), continuous renal replacement therapies (CRRTs), and hybrid therapies, such as sustained low-efficiency dialysis (SLED).

INDICATIONS FOR AND TIMING OF INITIATION OF DIALYSIS – Accepted indications for renal replacement therapy (RRT) in patients with Acute Kidney Injury (AKI) generally include:
Refractory fluid overload
Hyperkalemia (plasma potassium concentration >6.5 meq/L) refractory to medical therapy
Signs of uremia, such as pericarditis, neuropathy, or an otherwise unexplained decline in mental status
Metabolic acidosis (pH less than 7.1) refractory to medical therapy.
Certain alcohol and drug intoxications

CRRTs involve either dialysis (diffusion-based solute removal) or filtration (convection-based solute and water removal) treatments that operate in a continuous mode (114-117). The major advantage of continuous therapy is the slower rate of solute or fluid removal per unit of time. Thus, CRRT is generally better tolerated than conventional therapy, since many of the complications of intermittent hemodialysis are related to the rapid rate of solute and fluid loss. It must be emphasized, however, that the protection afforded by CRRT is relative, not absolute.

7. Outcomes in CRRT

Outcomes of an increased dose of CRRT have been assessed in several randomized controlled trials and two meta-analyses (78-80,116-117). Conflicting results related to survival have been reported. To address the issue of optimal dose in CRRT and IHD, the United States VA/NIH Acute Renal Failure Trial Network study (ATN), the Randomized Evaluation of Normal versus Augmented Level of RRT study (RENAL) and two meta-analyses were performed. All studies found that, compared with standard intensity dialysis, higher intensity dialysis did not result in improved survival or clinical benefits:

In the United States VA/NIH Acute Renal Failure Trial Network study (ATN), all 1124 patients were treated with IHD, CRRT, or SLED based upon hemodynamic status. Patients were randomly assigned to one of two dosing arms:

- Intensive therapy: Hemodialysis and SLED were given six times per week and a target Kt/V of 1.2 to 1.4 per treatment, while CRRT was provided with an effluent flow rate of 35 mL/kg per hour.
- Less intensive therapy: Hemodialysis and SLED were given three times per week, while CRRT was provided with a flow rate of 20 mL/kg per hour.

The death rate at day 60 was the same for both groups (53.6 percent with intensive therapy and 51.5 percent with less intensive therapy). In addition, the duration of renal replacement therapy and the rate of recovery of kidney function or nonrenal organ failure were similar for both treatment arms. The group that received intensive therapy had an increased number of hypotensive episodes. Thus, more intensive renal support beyond that obtained with a standard thrice-weekly regimen (with a target Kt/V of 1.2 to 1.4 per treatment) or standard CRRT (with an effluent flow rate of 20 mL/kg per hour) does not improve clinical outcomes.

In the RENAL study (a trial in Australia and New Zealand), 1508 patients with AKI were randomly assigned to CVVHDF at an effluent flow of either 25 or 40 mL/kg per hour (119). At 90 days, mortality was the same in each group (44.7 percent, odds ratio 1.00, 95% CI 0.31 to 1.23). In addition, the incidence of patients who continued to receive renal replacement therapy at 90 days was similar with both dialysis doses (6.8 and 4.4 percent of higher and lower-intensity groups, odds ratio 1.59, 95% CI 0.86 to 2.92).

Two meta-analyses, one consisting of 3841 patients and 8 trials and the other 3999 patients and 12 trials, found that more intense therapy did not improve survival compared with less intensive regimens (118-119). There was significant trial heterogeneity.

8. References

[1] Grassmann A, Gioberge S, Moeller S, Brown G. ESRD patients in 2004: global overview of patient numbers, treatment modalities and associated trends. Nephrol. Dial. Transplant. 2005, 20 (12): 2587-2593.

[2] United States Renal Data System. USRDS 2010 Annual Data Report: Atlas of End-Stage Renal Disease in the United States 2010; Bethesda, MD, National Institute of Health, National Institutes of Diabetes and Digestive and Kidney Diseases.

[3] Alper B, Shenava, R, Young, B, et. al. Uremia. Medscape. Batuman V. Mar 17, 2010. http://emedicine.medscape.com/article/245296-overview

[4] Termorshuizen F, Dekker FW, van Manen JG et al., Relative contribution of residual renal function and different measures of adequacy to survival in hemodialysis patients: an analysis of the Netherlands Cooperative Study on the Adequacy of Dialysis (NECOSAD)-2, J Am Soc Nephrol 2004; 15:1061-70

[5] Rosansky SJ, Clark WF, Eggers P, Glassock RJ. Initiation of dialysis at higher GFRs: is the apparent rising tide of early dialysis harmful or helpful? Kidney Int. 2009 Aug;76(3):257-61.

[6] Schrier R. Manual of Nephrology: Diagnosis and Therapy. Philadelphia: Lippincott Williams & Wilkins, 2009.

[7] Pendse, S, Singh, A, Zawada, E. Initiation of dialysis in Handbook of Dialysis, 4th ed, Daugirdas, JT, Blake, PG, Ing, TS (Eds). Lippincott Williams & Wilkins, Philadelphia 2007.

[8] Rosansky SJ, Eggers P, Jackson K, Glassock R, Clark WF. Early Start of Hemodialysis May Be Harmful. Arch Intern Med. 2011; 171(5):396-403)

[9] NKF-KDOQI Clinical Practice Guidelines. Am J Kidney Dis 1997; 30(3 Suppl 2): S67–S136.

[10] Obrador RT, Auora P, Kausz AT et al. Level of renal function at the initiation of dialysis in the US end-stage renal disease population. Kidney Int 1999; 5: 2227–2235.

[11] National Kidney Foundation. KDOQI Clinical practice guidelines and clinical practice recommendations for 2006 updates: hemodialysis adequacy, peritoneal dialysis adequacy and vascular access. Am J Kidney Dis 2006; 48(Suppl 1): S1–S322.

[12] Tang, SC, Ho, YW, Tang, AW, et al. Delaying initiation of dialysis till symptomatic uraemia--is it too late? Nephrol Dial Transplant 2007; 22:1926.

[13] Cooper, BA, Branley, P, Bulfone, L, et al. A randomized, controlled trial of early versus late initiation of dialysis. N Engl J Med 2010; 363:609.

[14] Clark, W., Na, Y., Rosansky, S., et.al. Association between estimated glomerular filtration rate at initiation of dialysis and mortality. CMAJ. 2011 Jan 11;183(1):47-53.

[15] United States Renal Data System. Excerpts from the USRDS 2009 annual data report: Atlas of end-stage renal disease in the United States. Am J Kidney Dis 2010; 1(Suppl 1):S1.

[16] USRDS: The United States Renal Data System: Overall hospitalization and mortality. Am J Kidney Dis 2010; 55(Suppl 1):S1.]

[17] Van Biesen W, Vanholder R, Lameire N. The role of peritoneal dialysis as the first-line renal replacement modality. Perit Dial Int. 2000;20(4):375

[18] Goldstein A, Kliger AS, Finkelstein FO. Recovery of renal function and the discontinuation of dialysis in patients treated with continuous peritoneal dialysis.Perit Dial Int. 2003;23(2):151

[19] Teitelbaum I, Burkart J. Peritoneal dialysis. Am J Kidney Dis. 2003;42(5):1082

[20] Wauters JP, Uehlinger D. Non-medical factors influencing peritoneal dialysis utilization: the Swiss experience. Nephrol Dial Transplant. 2004;19(6):1363

[21] Mendelssohn DC, Langlois N, Blake PG. Peritoneal dialysis in Ontario: a natural experiment in physician reimbursement methodology. Perit Dial Int. 2004;24(6):531

[22] Tonelli M, Hemmelgarn B, Culleton B, Klarenbach S, Gill JS, Wiebe N, Manns B, Alberta Kidney Disease Network. Mortality of Canadians treated by peritoneal dialysis in remote locations. Kidney Int. 2007;72(8):1023

[23] Mehrotra R, Khawar O, Duong U, Fried L, Norris K, Nissenson A, Kalantar-Zadeh K. Ownership patterns of dialysis units and peritoneal dialysis in the United States: utilization and outcomes. Am J Kidney Dis. 2009;54(2):289.

[24] Korevaar JC, Feith GW, Dekker FW, et al. Effect of starting with hemodialysis compared with peritoneal dialysis in patients new on dialysis treatment: a randomized controlled trial. Kidney Int 2003;64:2222-2228.

[25] Ganesh SK, Hulbert-Shearon T, Port FK, et al. Mortality differences by dialysis modality among incident ESRD patients with and without coronary artery disease. J Am Soc Nephrol 2003;14:415-424

[26] Stack AG, Molony DA, Rahman NS, et al. Impact of dialysis modality on survival of new ESRD patients with congestive heart failure in the United States. Kidney Int 2003;64:1071-1079

[27] Vonesh EF, Snyder JJ, Foley RN, et al. The differential impact of risk factors on mortality in hemodialysis and peritoneal dialysis. Kidney Int 2004;66:2389-2401

[28] Jaar BG, Coresh J, Plantinga LC, et al. Comparing the risk for death with peritoneal dialysis and hemodialysis in a national cohort of patients with chronic kidney disease. Ann Intern Med 2005;143:174-183.

[29] Tattersall J, Martin-Malo A, Pedrini L, Basci A, Canaud B, Fouque D, Haage P, Konner K, Kooman J, Pizzarelli F, Tordoir J, Vennegoor M, Wanner C, ter Wee P, Vanholder R: EBPG guideline on dialysis strategies. Nephrol Dial Transplant 22[Suppl 2]: ii5–ii21, 2007.

[30] Lowrie, E, Laird, NM. National Cooperative Dialysis Study. Kidney Int Suppl 1983; 23:19.

[31] Eknoyan G, Beck GJ, Cheung AK, Daugirdas JT, Greene T, Kusek JW, Allon M, Bailey J, Delmez JA, Depner TA, Dwyer JT, Levey AS, Levin NW, Milford E, Ornt DB, Rocco MV, Schulman G, Schwab SJ, Teehan BP, Toto R, Hemodialysis (HEMO) Study Group. Effect of dialysis dose and membrane flux in maintenance hemodialysis. N Engl J Med. 2002;347(25):2010.

[32] Paniagua R, Amato D, Vonesh E, Correa-Rotter R, Ramos A, Moran J, Mujais S, Mexican Nephrology Collaborative Study Group. Effects of increased peritoneal clearances on mortality rates in peritoneal dialysis: ADEMEX, a prospective, randomized, controlled trial. J Am Soc Nephrol. 2002;13(5):1307

[33] Tattersall J, Martin-Malo A, Pedrini L, Basci A, Canaud B, Fouque D, Haage P, Konner K, Kooman J, Pizzarelli F, Tordoir J, Vennegoor M, Wanner C, ter Wee P, Vanholder R: EBPG guideline on dialysis strategies. Nephrol Dial Transplant 22[Suppl 2]: ii5–ii21, 2007

[34] Kjellstrand CM, Buoncristiani U, Ting G, Traeger J, Piccoli GB, Sibai-Galland R, Young BA, Blagg CR: Short daily haemodialysis: Survival in 415 patients treated for 1006 patient-years. Nephrol Dial Transplant 23: 3283–3289, 2008.

[35] DePalma, JR, Pecker, EA, Maxwell, MH. A new automatic coil dialyser system for 'daily' dialysis. Proc EDTA 1969; 6:26....DePalma, JR, Pecker, EA, Maxwell, MH. A new automatic coil dialyser system for 'daily' dialysis. Semin Dial 1999; 12:410.

[36] Henderson LW, Leypoldt JK, Lysaght MJ, Cheung AK. Death on dialysis and the time/flux trade-off. Blood Purif. 1997;15(1):1.

[37] FHN Trial Group, Chertow GM, Levin NW, Beck GJ, Depner TA, Eggers PW, Gassman JJ, Gorodetskaya I, Greene T, James S, Larive B, Lindsay RM, Mehta RL, Miller B, Ornt DB, Rajagopalan S, Rastogi A, Rocco MV, Schiller B, Sergeyeva O, Schulman G, Ting GO, Unruh ML, Star RA, Kliger AS. In-center hemodialysis six times per week versus three times per week. N Engl J Med. 2010;363(24):2287.

[38] Kalirao P and Kaplan JM, Nocturnal Hemodialysis, Clin Exp Nephrol 2009; 13:257-62

[39] Pierratos A, Ouwendyk M, Francoeur R, Vas S, Raj DS, Ecclestone AM, Langos V, Uldall R. Nocturnal hemodialysis: three-year experience. J Am Soc Nephrol. 1998;9(5):859.

[40] Udall, PR, Francoeur, R, Ouwendyk, M. Simplified nocturnal home hemodialysis (SNHHD). A new approach to renal replacement therapy. J Am Soc Nephrol 1994; 5:428

[41] Lindsay RM, Daily/Nocturnal Dialysis Study Group. The London, Ontario, Daily/Nocturnal Hemodialysis Study. Semin Dial. 2004;17(2):85

[42] Lockridge RS Jr, Spencer M, Craft V, Pipkin M, Campbell D, McPhatter L, Albert J, Anderson H, Jennings F, Barger T. Nocturnal home hemodialysis in North America. Adv Ren Replace Ther. 2001;8(4):250.

[43] Agar JW, Somerville CA, Dwyer KM, Simmonds RE, Boddington JM, Waldron CM. Nocturnal hemodialysis in australia. Hemodial Int. 2003;7(4):278.

[44] Kooistra MP. Frequent prolonged home haemodialysis: three old concepts, one modern solution. Nephrol Dial Transplant. 2003;18(1):16.

[45] Kjellstrand CM, Buoncristiani U, Ting G, et al. Short daily haemodialysis: survival in 415 patients treated for 1006 patient-years. Nephrol Dial Transplant 2008;23:3283-3289.

[46] ERA-EDTA Registry: Annual Academic Medical Center. Amsterdam, The Netherlands, 2003.
[47] Wizemann V, Külz M, Techert F, Nederlof B. Efficacy of haemodiafiltration. Nephrol Dial Transplant. 2001;16 Suppl 4:27.
[48] Canaud B, Assounga A, Kerr P, Aznar R, Mion C. Failure of a daily haemofiltration programme using a highly permeable membrane to return beta 2-microglobulin concentrations to normal in haemodialysis patients. Nephrol Dial Transplant. 1992;7(9):924.
[49] Jaber BL, Zimmerman DL, Teehan GS, Swedko P, Burns K, Meyer KB, Leypoldt JK. Daily hemofiltration for end-stage renal disease: a feasibility and efficacy trial. Blood Purif. 2004;22(6):481.
[50] Zimmerman, DL, Swedko, P, Posen, G, Burns, K. Daily hemofiltration with a simplified method of delivery. J Am Soc Nephrol 2002; 13:61A.
[51] Maduell F, Navarro V, Torregrosa E, Rius A, Dicenta F, Cruz MC, Ferrero JA. Change from three times a week on-line hemodiafiltration to short daily on-line hemodiafiltration. Kidney Int. 2003;64(1):305.
[52] US Renal Data System: USRDS 2008 Annual Data Report: Atlas of Chronic Kidney Disease and End Stage Renal Disease in the United States, Bethesda, NIH, National Institute of Diabetes and Digestive and Kidney Disease, 2008
[53] US Renal Data System: USRDS 2008 Annual Data Report: Atlas of Chronic Kidney Disease and End Stage Renal Disease in the United States, Bethesda, NIH, National Institute of Diabetes and Digestive and Kidney Disease, 2009
[54] Vanholder R, Van Laecke S, Glorieux G: What is new in uremic toxicity?. Pediatr Nephrol 2008; 23:1211-1221.
[55] Vanholder R, De Smet R, Glorieux G, et al: Review on uremic toxins: Classification, concentration, and interindividual variability. Kidney Int 2003; 63:1934-1943.
[56] Ankit N. Mehta, MD; Andrew Z. Fenves, MD: Hemodialysis Adequacy: A Review; January 2010 Dialysis & Transplantation
[57] Daugirdas JT. Simplifi ed equations for monitoring Kt/V, PCRn, eKt/V, and ePCRn. Adv Renal Replace Ther. 1995; 2:295-304.
[58] Tattersall JE, DeTakats D, Chamney P, Greenwood RN, Farrington K. The post-hemodialysis rebound: predicting and quantifying its effect on Kt/V. Kidney Int. 1996; 50: 2094-2102.
[59] Leypoldt JK, Jaber BL, Zimmerman DL. Predicting treatment dose for novel therapies using urea standard Kt/V. Semin Dial. 2004; 17:142-145.
[60] Feehally, J, Floege, J, Johnson, R. The Comprehensive Clinical Nephrology. Chapter 90; Hemodialysis: Outcomes and Adequacy. Copyright © 2010 Elsevier
[61] Agarwal, R, Mehrotra, R, Townsend RR, Goldfarb, S. NephSap, Vol9, No. 6, November 2010;pp 366-371
[62] Powell JR, Oluwaseum O, Woo YM, Padmanabhan N, Narasingham E, Latta C, Tortolana J, Jardine AG, Geddes CC. Ten year experience of in-center thrice weekly long overnight hemodialysis. Clin J Am Soc Nephrol 4:1097-1101, 2009
[63] Anderson AH, Cohen AJ, Kutner NG, Kopp JB, Kimmel PL, Mutner P; Missed dialysis sessions and hospitalization in hemodialysis patients after Hurricane Katrina. Kidney Int 75:1202-1208, 2009

[64] National Kidney Foundation : KDOQI Clinical Practice Guidelines and Clinical Practice Recommendations for 2006 Updates: Hemodialysis Adequacy, Peritoneal Dialysis Adequacy and Vascular Access. Am J Kidney Dis 2006; 48(Suppl 1):S1-S322

[65] Eknoyan G, Beck GJ, Cheung AK, Daugirdas JT, Greene T, Kusek JW, Allon M, Bailey J, Delmez JA, Depner TA, Dwyer JT, Levey AS, Levin NW, Milford E, Ornt DB, Rocco MV, Schulman G, Schwab SJ, Teehan BP, Toto R, Effect of dialysis dose and membrane flux in maintenance hemodialysis. N Engl J Med. 2002; 347(25):2010. Hemodialysis (HEMO) Study Group

[66] DePalma, JR, Pecker, EA, Maxwell, MH. A new automatic coil dialyser system for 'daily' dialysis. Proc EDTA 1969; 6:26.

[67] DePalma, JR, Pecker, EA, Maxwell, MH. A new automatic coil dialyser system for 'daily' dialysis. Semin Dial 1999; 12:410.

[68] Uldall, PR, Francoeur, R, Ouwendyk, M. Simplified nocturnal home hemodialysis (SNHHD). A new approach to renal replacement therapy. J Am Soc Nephrol 1994; 5:428.

[69] Pierratos A, Ouwendyk M, Francoeur R, et al. Nocturnal hemodialysis: three-year experience. J Am Soc Nephrol 1998; 9:859.

[70] Cheung AK, Rocco MV, Yan G, et al: Serum β2-microglobulin levels predict mortality in dialysis patients: Results of the HEMO study. J Am Soc Nephrol 2006; 17:546-555.

[71] Locatelli F, Martin-Malo A, Hannedouche T, et al: Effect of membrane permeability on survival of hemodialysis patients. J Am Soc Nephrol 2009; 20:645-654.

[72] European Best Practice Guidelines Expert Group on Hemodialysis, European Renal Association. Nephrol Dial Transplant 2002; 17(Suppl 7):16-31.

[73] Bargman JM, Golper TA: The importance of residual renal function for patients on dialysis. Nephrol Dial Transplant 2005; 20:671-673.

[74] Kliger AS, More Intensive hemodialysis. Clin J Am Soc Nephrol 4[suppll 1] S121-S124, 2009

[75] Beecroft JM, Hoffstein V, Pierratos A, Chan Ct, McFarlane P, Hanly PJ, Nocturnal heamodialysis increases pharyngeal size in patients with sleep apnea and end stage renal disease. Nephrol Dialy Transplant 23: 673-679, 2008

[76] McFarlane PA Reducing hemodialysis costs: conventional and quotidian home hemodialysis in Canada. Semin Dial. 2004: 17(2):118.

[77] Manns M, Sigler MH, Teehan BP. Continuous renal replacement therapies: an update. Am J Kidney Dis. 1998;32(2):185.

[78] Bouman CS, Oudemans-Van Straaten HM, Tijssen JG, Zandstra DF, Kesecioglu J. Effects of early high-volume continuous venovenous hemofiltration on survival and recovery of renal function in intensive care patients with acute renal failure: a prospective, randomized trial. Crit Care Med. 2002;30(10):2205.

[79] Ronco C, Bellomo R, Homel P, Brendolan A, Dan M, Piccinni P, La Greca G. Effects of different doses in continuous veno-venous haemofiltration on outcomes of acute renal failure: a prospective randomised trial. Lancet. 2000;356(9223):26

[80] Saudan P, Niederberger M, De Seigneux S, Romand J, Pugin J, Perneger T, Martin PY. Adding a dialysis dose to continuous hemofiltration increases survival in patients with acute renal failure. Kidney Int. 2006;70(7):1312.

[81] Creation, cannulation and survival of arteriovenous fistulae: Data from the Dialysis Outcomes and Practice Patterns Study. Kidney International; Jan2003, Vol. 63 Issue 1, p323-330, 8p
[82] Schild AF: Maintaining vascular access: the management of hemodialysis arteriovenous grafts. Vasc Access. 2010 Apr-Jun;11(2):92-9.
[83] Robin M et al. Hemodialysis Arteriovenous Fistula Maturity: US Evaluation Radiology 2002, vol 221:1, 59-64
[84] Biuckians A, Scott EC, Meier GH, et al: The natural history of autologous fistulas as first-time dialysis access in the KDOQI era. J Vasc Surg 2008; 47:415-421.
[85] Ronald L Pisoni, Eric W Young, Dawn M Dykstra, Roger N Greenwood, Erwin Hecking, Brenda Gillespie, Robert A Wolfe, David A Goodkin and Philip J HeldVascular access use in Europe and the United States: Results from the DOPPS, Kidney International (2002) 61, 305–316
[86] Lazarides MK, Georgiadis GS, Papasideris CP, et al: Transposed brachial-basilic arteriovenous fistulas versus prosthetic upper limb grafts: A meta-analysis. Eur J Vasc Endovasc Surg 2008; 36:597-601.
[87] Parienti, J. J. et al. Femoral vs jugular venous catheterization and risk of nosocomial events in adults requiring acute renal replacement therapy: a randomized controlled trial. JAMA 299, 2413-2422 (2008).
[88] Hamilton, H. C. & Foxcroft, D. R. Central venous access sites for the prevention of venous thrombosis, stenosis and infection in patients requiring long-term intravenous therapy. Cochrane Database of Systematic Reviews, Issue 3. Art. No.: CD004084. doi:10.1002/14651858.CD004084.pub2 (2007).
[89] Kakkos SK, Haddad GK, Haddad JA et al., Secondary patency of thrombosed prosthethc vascular access grafts with aggressive surveillance, monitoring, and endovascular management, Eur J Endovasc Surg 2008; 36:356-65
[90] Tessitore N, Bedogna V, Melilli E et al., In search of an optimal bedside screening program for arteriovenous fistula stenosis, Clin J Am Soc Nephrol 2011; 6:819-26
[91] Beathard GA, An algorithm for the physical examination of early fistula failure, Semin Dial 2005; 18:331-335
[92] Besarab A, Asif A, Roy-Chaudury P et al., The native arteriovenous fistula in 2007. Surveillance and monitoring. J Nephrol 2007; 20:656-667
[93] Besarab A, Sullivan KL, Ross R et al., The utility of intra-access monitoring in detecting and correcting venous outlet stenoses prior to thrombosis, Kidney Int 1995; 1364-1373
[94] Tessitore N, Bedogna V, Gammaro L et al., Diagnostic accuracy of ultrasound dilution access blood flow measurement in detecting stenosis and predicting thrombosis in native forearm arteriovenous fistulae for hemodialysis, Am J Kidney Dis 2003; 42:331-341
[95] Napoli M, Prudenzano R, Russo F et al., Juxta-anastomotic stenosis of native arteriovenous fistulas: surgical treatment versus percutaneous transluminal angioplasty, J Vasc Access 2010; 11:346-351
[96] Dixon BS, Beck GJ, Vazquez MA, et al: Effect of dipyridamole plus aspirin on hemodialysis graft patency. N Engl J Med 2009; 360:2191-2201.

[97] Dember LM, Besk GJ, Allon M, et al: Effect of clopidogrel on early failure of arteriovenous fistulas for hemodialysis: A randomized controlled trial. JAMA 2008; 299:2205-2207

[98] Hemmelgarn BR, Moist LM, Lok CE et al., Prevention of dialysis catheter malfunction with recombinant tissue plasminogen activator, N Engl J Med 2011; 364:303-312

[99] Kamper L, Piroth, W, and Haage P, Endovascular treatment of dysfunctional hemodialysis catheters, J Vasc Access 2010; 11:263-268

[100] Allon M, Daugirdas J, Depner TA, et al: Effect of change in vascular access on patient mortality in hemodialysis patients. Am J Kidney Dis 2006; 47:469-477

[101] 2011 CDC Guidelines for the Prevention of Intravascular Catheter-Related Infections

[102] Rabindranath, K. S. et al. Systematic review of antimicrobials for the prevention of haemodialysis catheter-related infections. Nephrol. Dial. Transplant. 24, 3763-3774 (2009).

[103] Vanholder, R. et al. Diagnosis, prevention and treatment of haemodialysis catheter-related bloodstream infections (CRBSI): a position statement of the European Renal Best Practice (ERBP). NDTPlus 3, 234-246 (2010).

[104] Dogra GK, Herson H, Hutchison B, et al. Prevention of tunneled hemodialysis catheter-related infections using catheter-restricted filling with gentamicin and citrate: a randomized controlled study. J Am Soc Nephrol 2002; 13:2133–9

[105] Punt, C. D. & Boer, W. E. Cardiac arrest following injection of concentrated trisodium citrate. Clin. Nephrol. 69, 317-318 (2008)

[106] McCann, M. & Moore, Z. E. H. Interventions for preventing infectious complications in haemodialysis patients with central venous catheters. Cochrane Database of Systematic Reviews, Issue 1. Art. No.: CD006894. doi:10.1002/14651858.CD006894.pub2 (2010)

[107] Chatzinikolaou, I. et al. Antibiotic-coated hemodialysis catheters for the prevention of vascular catheter-related infections: a prospective, randomized study. Am. J. Med. 115, 352-357 (2003).

[108] von Eiff, C. et al. Nasal carriage as source of Stapylococcus aureus bacteremia. Study Group. N. Engl. J. Med. 344, 11-16 (2001)

[109] Wilcox MH, Tack KJ, Bouza E, et al. Complicated skin and skin structure infections and catheter-related bloodstream infections: noninferiority of linezolid in a phase 3 study. Clin Infect Dis 2009; 48: 203–12.

[110] Clinical practice guidelines for the diagnosis and management of intravascular catheter-related infection: 2009 Update by the Infectious Diseases Society of America

[111] Mokrzycki MH, Zhang M, Cohen H, Golestaneh L, Laut JM, Rosenberg SO. Tunnelled haemodialysis catheter bacteraemia: risk factors for bacteraemia recurrence, infectious complications and mortality. Nephrol Dial Transplant 2006; 21:1024–31

[112] NKF-K/DOQI Clinical Practice Guidelines for Vascular Access: update 2000. Am J Kidney Dis 2001; 37:S137-S181

[113] McCarthy JT, Moran J, Posen G, Leypoldt JK, Hull AR, Jaber BL, Correa-Rotter R. A time for rediscovery: chronic hemofiltration for end-stage renal disease. Semin Dial. 2003;16(3):199.

[114] Honore PM, Jamez J, Wauthier M, Lee PA, Dugernier T, Pirenne B, Hanique G, Matson JR. Prospective evaluation of short-term, high-volume isovolemic hemofiltration on the hemodynamic course and outcome in patients with intractable circulatory failure resulting from septic shock. Crit Care Med. 2000;28(11):3581.
[115] Palevsky PM. Dialysis modality and dosing strategy in acute renal failure. Semin Dial. 2006;19(2):165.
[116] Tolwani AJ, Campbell RC, Stofan BS, Lai KR, Oster RA, Wille KM. Standard versus high-dose CVVHDF for ICU-related acute renal failure. J Am Soc Nephrol. 2008;19(6):1233.
[117] Jun M, Heerspink HJ, Ninomiya T, Gallagher M, Bellomo R, Myburgh J, Finfer S, Palevsky PM, Kellum JA, Perkovic V, Cass A. Intensities of renal replacement therapy in acute kidney injury: a systematic review and meta-analysis. Clin J Am Soc Nephrol. 2010;5(6):956.
[118] Van Wert R, Friedrich JO, Scales DC, Wald R, Adhikari NK, University of Toronto Acute Kidney Injury Research Group. High-dose renal replacement therapy for acute kidney injury: Systematic review and meta-analysis. Crit Care Med. 2010;38(5):1360.
[119] RENAL Replacement Therapy Study Investigators, Bellomo R, Cass A, Cole L, Finfer S, Gallagher M, Lo S, McArthur C, McGuinness S, Myburgh J, Norton R, Scheinkestel C, Su S. Intensity of continuous renal-replacement therapy in critically ill patients. N Engl J Med. 2009;361(17):1627.
[120] Vesconi S, Cruz DN, Fumagalli R, Kindgen-Milles D, Monti G, Marinho A, Mariano F, Formica M, Marchesi M, René R, Livigni S, Ronco C, DOse REsponse Multicentre International collaborative Initiative (DO-RE-MI Study Group). Delivered dose of renal replacement therapy and mortality in critically ill patients with acute kidney injury. Crit Care. 2009;13(2):R57.

Part 2

Prognosis

13

Residual Renal Function in Hemodialysis Patients

Zachary Z. Brener[1], Stephan Thijssen[2], Peter Kotanko[2], James F. Winchester[1] and Michael Bergman[3]
[1]Beth Israel Medical Center, New York;
[2]Renal Research Institute, New York
[3]Rabin Medical Center – Campus Golda, Tel-Aviv University
[1,2]USA
[3]Israel

1. Introduction

The role of residual renal function (RRF) in the health and quality of life of both pre-dialysis and dialysis patients is equally important and now well established (Termorshuizen, Korevaar et al, 2003).

RRF plays an important role in maintaining fluid balance, phosphorus control, and removal of uremic toxins in dialysis patients. The importance of RRF in hemodialysis (HD) patients is less well appreciated and it is believed that RRF declined rapidly in HD patients (Morduchowicz, Winkler et al, 1994; Wang, Woo, et al, 2005). Decline of RRF also contributed significantly to anemia, inflammation, and malnutrition in end-stage renal disease (ESRD) patients (Wang, Sea et al, 2001; Pecoits-Filho, Heimburger et al, 2003; Pecoits-Filho, Heimburger et al, 2002; Wang, Wang et al, 2004). More importantly, RRF has also been shown to be a powerful predictor of mortality, especially in patients on peritoneal dialysis (PD) (Bargman, Thorpe et al, 2001; Brener, Thijssen et al, 2011; Maiorca, Brunori et al, 19951).

Glomerular filtration rate (GFR) measured by isotope clearance is considered to be the standard measure of renal function. Other tests, such as serum creatinine, creatinine clearance, urea clearance, an average of the creatinine and urea clearances, and urine volume have been used to assess RRF in chronic kidney disease (Levey, 1990). Despite its limitations, urine volume, the simplest measure of RRF, has been correlated to GFR in studies and most authors defined loss of RRF as urine volume < 200 ml/24 hours (Moist, Port et al, 2000). Urine collections (24 hours for PD, interdialytic for HD) to measure urea and/or creatinine clearance usually done at beginning of chronic dialysis and every 1-3 months in patients with RRF.

In this chapter, we will review available data that have shown a positive impact of RRF on the survival and quality of life of dialysis patients, and outline the current strategies to preserve RRF in PD and HD patients.

2. The benefits of preserved RRF (Table 1)

- Improving patients survival
- Maintaining fluid balance
- Blood pressure control
- Decrease left ventricular hypertrophy
- Anemia control
- Phosphorus control
- Potassium control
- Uric acid control
- Improving nutritional status
- Decreasing inflammatory response

Table 1. Benefits of preserved RRF

2.1 RRF and patient survival (Table 2)

In 1995, Maiorca et al noted an independent relationship between the presence of RRF and survival in dialysis patients (Maiorca, Brunori et al, 2011). In their multivariate survival analysis of 102 PD and HD dialysis patients, each 1-ml/min increase in GFR was associated with a 40% reduced risk of death in the entire cohort and a 50% reduced risk of death in PD patients. Multicenter prospective cohort Canada-USA (CANUSA) Study of 680 incident PD patients clearly demonstrated that the predictive power for mortality in PD patients was attributed to RRF and not to the dose of PD (Bargman, Thorpe et al, 2001). The impact of RRF on outcome has not been examined in large cohorts of HD patients, likely due to the more rapid rate of decrease in RRF and its smaller relative contribution to total small-molecule clearance in HD compared with PD patients. In our retrospective study of 118 incident HD patients survival time was significantly lower in patients without RRF (48 vs 55 months) (Brener, Thijssen et al, 2011). Crude mortality was 19.4% in anuric patients and 7.8% in patients with RRF, and cardiovascular disease was a leading cause of death for both groups. The presence of RRF was also associated with a strong trend toward fewer hospital days per patient-year. Shemin et al (Shemin, Bostom et al, 2001) reported that in the prospective observational study of 114 incident and prevalent HD patients, the presence of RRF was independently associated with a 65% decrease in risk of death, even after adjustment for duration of dialysis treatment, age, presence of diabetes, cardiovascular disease and serum albumin level. Netherlands Cooperative Study on the Adequacy of Dialysis (NECOSAD) (Termorshuizen, Dekkeret al, 2004) has prospectively evaluated the contribution of treatment adequacy and RRF to patients survival after 3 and 6 months of treatment in a large incident HD population (740 patients). It showed the important

- RRF is a powerful predictor of mortality
- Each 1-ml/min increase in GFR was associated with a 40% reduced risk of death
- Each 1-unit increase in renal Kt/V resulted in 66% decrease in relative risk of death
- Independent relationship between the presence of RRF and survival in dialysis patients
- Preservation of RRF is important in the survival of dialysis patients

Table 2. RRF and dialysis patient survival

contribution of RRF to the overall survival of HD patients: each 1-unit increase in renal Kt/V resulted in 66% decrease in relative risk of death. Moreover, in patients with preserved RRF, increasing dialysis dose did not result in improved patient outcomes. The international prospective observational DOPPS study has also recently reported the diuretic use and presence of RRF was associated with a better survival in prevalent HD patients (Bragg-Gresham, Fissell et al, 2007). Diuretic use declined after the start of dialysis (9.2% in Europe versus 21.3% in the United States). Patients with RRF on diuretics had almost twice the chances of retaining RRF after 1 year with 7% lower all-cause and mortality and 14% lower cardiac-specific mortality compared to patients not receiving diuretics. All these and other observational studies suggest that preservation of RRF has an important role in the survival of both HD and PD patients.

2.2 RRF, volume control and cardiac hypertrophy

RRF has been found to be important in maintaining fluid balance of dialysis patients, especially in patients on PD. Suboptimal fluid removal in PD patients is associated with greater rates of all-cause hospitalization and mortality (Ates, Nergizoglu et al, 2001). In the CANUSA Study, urine volume was a strong independent predictor of survival. Every 250 ml/imin urine output was associated with a 36% reduction in overall mortality ((Bargman, Thorpe et al, 2001). RRF may reduce or avoid the need for fluid restriction. Loss of RRF is independently associated with suboptimal blood pressure control, likely a result of chronic volume expansion (Ates, Nergizoglu et al, 2001; Konings, Kooman et al, 2003). The severity of left ventricular hypertrophy (LVH), a strong independent predictor of mortality in dialysis patients, inversely correlates with the presence of RRF Pecoits-Filho, Heimburger et al, 2002; Wang, Wang et al, 2004). In addition, loss of RRF is associated with more severe anemia, hypoalbuminemia, and higher arterial pressure (Pecoits-Filho, Heimburger et al, 2003), all of which are important risk factors for cardiac hypertrophy in dialysis patients. Extracellular fluid (ECF) volume has been also reported to be associated with hypertension and left ventricular hypertrophy in HD patients (Fagugli, Pasini et al, 2003).

2.3 RRF and metabolic control

Middle molecule clearance is one of the most widely recognized benefits of RRF. Patients with significant RRF are shown to have lower ß2-mocroglobulin (ß2M) levels (McCarthy, Williams et al, 1994; Montenegro, Martinez et al, 1992; Amici G, Virga et al, 1993) and thus are less prone to dialysis-associated amyloidosis (Copley JB, Lindberg et al, 2001). Preserved RRF is also associated with lower blood levels of uric acid, potassium (Morduchowicz, Winkler et al, 1994), and aluminium (Altmann , Butter et al, 1987), and higher levels of hemoglobin (Pecoits-Filho, Heimburger et al, 2002), presumably due to increased levels of endogenous erythropoietin.

Hyperphosphatemia is prevalent in dialysis patients (Yavuz, Ersoy et al, 2008; Wang, Woo et al, 2004) and has been linked to vascular calcification and increased cardiovascular mortality in both HD and PD patients (Block, Hulbert-Shearon et al, 1998; Wang AY, Lai et al, 2006). RRF plays a major role in improving phosphate balance in both PD and HD patients ((Morduchowicz, Winkler et al, 1994).

2.4 RRF and inflammation

Inflammation is highly prevalent in dialysis patients (Arici M, Walls et al, 2001) and established to be a strong predictor of mortality in dialysis patients. Loss of RRF was associated with an increased inflammatory response with elevated solute vascular cell adhesion molecules (VCAM-1) and C-reactive protein (CRP) levels in PD patients (Wang AY, Lam et al, 2005), possibly as a result of impaired renal elimination of proinflammatory cytokines and increased cytokine generation (Witko-Sarsat, Descamps-Latscha et al, 1997). Conversely, the presence of inflammation also accelerated the decline of RRF (Shin, Noh et al, 1999).

2.5 RRF and nutritional status

Malnutrition is a common serious problem in dialysis patients, may be result of multiple factors including impairments in protein and energy metabolism, hormonal imbalances and poor food intake because of anorexia (Ikizler, Hakim et al, 1996). Dialysis dose may affect nutritional status and low dialysis efficacy is associated with higher rates of morbidity and mortality (Gotch, Sargent, 1985; Bergstrom, Lindholm, 1993). RRF contributes significantly to the appetite and total caloric intake (Wang, Sea et al, 2001; Wang, Sea et al, 2005), and overall nutritional status assessed using subjective global assessment, handgrip strength, or lean body mass in both HD and PD patients. Nutritional status is closely related to inflammation. In our study (Brener, Thijssen et al, 2008) anuric HD patients were older with lower baseline serum albumin and showed a trend toward greater length of stay for all causes, and all cause mortality including infectious mortality. Analysis of albumin kinetics performed in HEMO Study showed that a decrease in serum albumin in adequately dialysed patients was mostly due to an increase in the level of inflammation, rather that a decrease in protein intake (Kaysen, Dubin et al, 2000).

3. Preservation of RRF (Table 3)

- PD modality
- Avoidance of ECF volume depletion
- Avoidance of nephrotoxic insults (NSAIDs, radiocontrast agents, aminoglycosides)
- Antihypertensive medications (ACE-inhibitors and calcium channel blockers)

Table 3. Preservation of RRF

3.1 Patient-related factors

Decline of RRF is an unavoidable phenomenon caused by the degenerative and fibrosis process of chronic kidney disease (CKD). However, the rate of RRF loss is different among patients and may be affected by other factors such as patient-related factors, treatment modalities and practice patterns (Jansen, Hart et al, 2002). Patient-related factors include age, causal nephropathy and comorbid conditions. Decline of RRF has been shown to be age dependent (Hung, Young, 2003). Intercurrent events such as recurrent blood pressure drop during HD, cardiac events and sepsis may precipitate loss of RRF. Diabetics on PD have been shown to have a more rapid decline in RRF than nondiabetics (Singhal, Bhaskaran et al, 2000). Comorbid conditions, including congestive heart failure, poorly controlled hypertension, and coronary artery disease, also are associated with faster rates of RRF decrease (Shin, Noh et al, 1999). Patients with CKD secondary to glomerular disease lose RRF more rapidly than those with tubulointerstitial disease (Iest, Vanholder et al, 1989). In a large multicenter study, the majority of patients with adult polycystic kidney disease were found to maintain a GFR greater than 2 ml/min for more than 4 years (Van Stone, 1995). Patients returning to dialysis therapy after kidney transplant failure have a more rapid decline in RRF than those initiating dialysis therapy with native kidney disease (Davies, 2001).

3.2 Impact of dialysis modality

Observational studies showed the advantage of PD compared to HD in preserving RRF (Moist, Port et al, 2000; Rottembourg, Issad et al, 1983; Misra, Vonesh et al, 2001) but data from prospective randomized trials are lacking. PD is associated with better hemodynamic stability that may minimize ischemic renal insults and avoidance of the extracorporeal circulation of HD that promotes systemic inflammation, oxidative stress, and subsequent kidney injury (Rottembourg, Issad et al, 1983). Treatment with ultrapure dialysate and biocompatible membranes has been shown to slow the loss of RRF in incident HD patients (Schiffl , Lang et al, 2002). It has been suggested use of PD as an initial dialysis modality in patients with RRF to maximize RRF conservation and thus survival for patients on dialysis.

3.3 Avoidance of ECF volume depletion

Observational data from NECOSAD Study suggest that episodes of volume depletion were an independent risk factor for the loss of RRF (Termorshuizen, Korevaar et al, 2003).[1] In a study by Gunal et al (Gunal AI, Duman et al, 2001) strict volume control in 47 PD patients led to 6% decrease in left ventricular hypertrophy and 28% decrease in mean urine volume in the 19 patients with RRF. Subclinical hypovolemia, even in presence of normal blood pressure, can lead to a decrease in RRF as a result of overzealous ECF volume depletion. Diuretics have been shown to increase urine volume and sodium removal, but do not affect the solute clearance (Moist, Port et al, 2000; van Olden, Guchelaar et al, 2003), and can be used, where appropriate, to provide better control of volume balance. As mentioned above, the extended use of loop diuretics may help to prolong diuresis and preserve RRF. Correction of fluid volume excess by combining dietary salt restriction and gentle ultrafiltration is a simple and effective approach to control hypertension and to reverse LVH (Konings, Kooman et al, 2003).

3.4 Avoidance of nephrotoxic insults

Avoiding the use of radiocontrast agents or nephrotoxic drugs such as non-steroidal anti-inflammatory drugs or aminoglycosides is an important approach in protecting RRF. Aminoglycoside nephrotoxicity can be decreased by once-daily dosing, avoidance of concomitant nephrotoxins, monitoring of drug levels, and choice of the least nephrotoxic aminoglycoside used (Baker, Senior et al, 2003). Recent trials that used either adequate hydration, low-osmolar radiocontrast agents (Dittrich, Puttinger et al, 2006) as well as prophylactic acetylcysteine (Tepel, van der Giet et al, 2000) did not show long-term decline after contrast exposure despite a temporary decline in GFR immediately after contrast exposure.

3.5 Antihypertensive medications

ACE-inhibitors and calcium channel blockers were associated with preservation of RRF in both PD and HD patients (Tepel, van der Giet et al, 2000). In a prospective study by Li PK et al (Li PK, Chow et al, 2003), PD patients treated with ramipril had a slower rate of RRF loss compared to the control group. Investigation of the role of combination therapy with ACE inhibitors and ARBs and direct aldosterone blockade on RRF represent promising future strategies in slowing the rate of RRF decline in dialysis patients.

4. Conclusion

RRF contributes to the clearance of both small and medium-sized solutes. It serves important metabolic and hemodynamic functions, and plays a crucial role in maintaining the cardiovascular health, nutritional status, and well-being of dialysis patients. RRF has also been shown to have a significant impact on the survival of dialysis patients, especially in PD dialysis. Health care providers need to realize that RRF is a very valuable asset to dialysis patients. Efforts to preserve RRF should continue even after patients are started on dialysis treatment, irrespective of the modality used

5. References

Altmann P, Butter KC, Plowman D, Chaput de Saintonge DM, Cunningham J & Marsh FP. Residual renal function in hemodialysis patients may protect against hyperaluminemia. *Kidney Int*, Vol.32, no.5, (November 1987), pp. 710-713

Amici G, Virga G, Da Rin G, Grandesso S, Vianello A, Gatti P & Bocci C. Serum beta-2-microglobulin level and residual renal function in peritoneal dialysis. *Nephron*, Vol.65, No.3, (March 1993), pp. 469-471

Arici M & Walls J. End-stage renal disease, atherosclerosis, and cardiovascular mortality: is C-reactive protein the missing link? *Kidney Int*, Vol.59, No.2, (February 2001), pp. 407-414

Ates K, Nergizoglu G, Keven K, Sen A, Kutlay S, Ertürk S, Duman N, Karatan O & Ertuğ AE. Effect of fluid and sodium removal on mortality in peritoneal dialysis patients. *Kidney Int*,Vol.60, No.2, (August 2001), pp.767-776

Baker RJ, Senior H, Clemenger M & Brown EA. Empirical aminoglycosides for peritonitis do not affect residual renal function. *Am J Kidney Dis*; Vol.41, No.3, (March 2003), pp. 670-675

Bargman JM, Thorpe KE & Churchill DN. Relative contribution of residual renal function and peritoneal clearance to adequacy of dialysis: a reanalysis of the CANUSA study. *J Am Soc Nephrol*; Vol.12, No.10, (October 2001), pp. 2158-2162.

Bergstrom J& Lindholm B. Nutrition and adequacy of dialysis. How do hemodialysis and CAPD compare? *Kidney Int Suppl*, Vol.43, (February 1993), pp. S39-50

Block GA, Hulbert-Shearon TE, Levin NW & Port FK. Association of serum phosphorus and calcium * phosphate product wit mortality risk in chronic hemodialysis patients: A national study. *Am J Kidney Dis*; Vol.31, No.4, (April 1998), pp. 607-617

Bragg-Gresham JL, fissell RB, Mason NA, Baille GR, Gillespie BW, Wizemann V, Cruz JM, Akiba T, Kurokawa K, Ramirez S, Young EW. Diuretic use, residual renal function, and mortality among hemodialysis patients in the Dialysis Outcomes and Practice Pattern Study (DOPPS). *Am J Kidney Dis;* Vol.49(3), (March 2007), pp. 426-431

Brener ZZ Thijssen S, Kotanko P, Kuhlmann MK, Winchester JF & Levin NW. The impact of residual renal function on infectious outcomes in incident hemodialysis patients. *J Am Soc Nephrol;* Vol.18 (2008), pp. 291

Brener ZZ, Thijssen S, Kotanko P, Kuhlmann MK, Bergman M, Winchester JF, Levin NW. The impact of residual renal function on hospitalization and mortality in incident hemodialysis patients. Blood Purif, Vol.31, No. 4, (January 2011), pp. 243-251

Copley JB & Lindberg JS. Nontransplant therapy for dialysis-related amyloidosis. *Semin Dial,* Vol.14, (2001), pp. 94-98

Davies SJ. Peritoneal dialysis in the patient with a failing renal allograft. *Perit Dial Int,* Vol. 21, (2001), pp. S280-S284

Dittrich E, Puttinger H, Schillinger M, Lang I, Stefenelli T, Hörl WH & Vychytil A. Effect of radio contrast media on residual renal function in peritoneal dialysis patients- A prospective study.

Fagugli, RM, Pasini P, Quintaliani G, Pasticci F, Ciao G, Cicconi B, Ricciardi D, Santirosi PV, Buoncristiani E, Timio F, Valente F & Buoncristiani U. Association between extracellular water, left ventricular mass and hypertension in haemodialysis patients. *Nephrol Dial Transplant,* Vol.18, No.11, (November 2003), pp. 2332-2338

Gotch F & Sargent J. A mechanistic analysis of the National Cooperative Dialysis study (NCDS). *Kidney Int,* Vol.28, No.2, (February 1985), pp. 526-534

Gunal AI, Duman S, Ozkahya M, Töz H, Asçi G, Akçiçek F & Basçi A. Strict volume control normalizes hypertension in peritoneal dialysis patients. *Am J Kidney Dis,* Vol.37, No.3, (March 2001), pp. 588-593

Hung AM, Young BS, Chertow GM. The decline in residual renal function is slow and age dependent. *Hemodial Int,* Vol. 7, (2003), pp. 17

Iest CG, Vanholder RC, Ringoir SM. Loss of residual renal function in patients on regular haemodialysis. *Int J Artif Organs,* vol. 12, (1989), pp. 159-164

Ikizler TA & Hakim RM. Nutrition in end-stage renal disease. *Kidney Int,* Vol.50, No.2, (August 1996), pp. 343-57

Jansen MA, Hart AA, Korevaar JC, Dekker FW, Boeschoten EW, Krediet RT; NECOSAD Study Group. Predictors of the rate of decline of residual renal function in incident dialysis patients. *Kidney Int,* Vol. 62, pp. 1046-1053

Kaysen GA, Dubin JA, Muller HG, Rosales LM & Levin NW. The acute-phase response varies with time and predicts serum albumin levels in hemodialysis patients. The HEMO Study Group. *Kidney Int,* Vol.8, No.1, (July 2005), pp. 346-352

Konings CJ, Kooman JP, Schonck M, Struijk DG, Gladziwa U, Hoorntje SJ, van der Wall Bake AW, van der Sande FM & Leunissen KM. Fluid status in CAPD patients is related to peritoneal transport and residual renal function: Evidence from a longitudinal study. *Nephrol Dial Transplant,*Vol.18, no.4, (April 2003), pp. 797-803

Levey AJ. Measurement of renal function in chronic renal disease. *Kidney Int* 1990; Vol. 38, No.1, (July 1990), pp. 167-184

Li PK, Chow KM, Wong TY, Leung CB & Szeto CC. Effects of an angiotensine-converting enzyme inhibitor on residual renal function in patients receiving peritoneal dialysis. A randomized, controlled study. *Ann Intern Med,* Vol.139, No.2, (July 2003), pp. 105-112

Maiorca R, Brunori G, Zubani R, Cancarini GC, Manili L, Camerini C, Movilli E, Pola A, d'Avolio G & Gelatti U. Predictive value of dialysis adequacy and nutritional indices for mortality and morbidity in CAPD and HD patients. A longitudinal study. *Nephrol Dial Transplant,* Vol.10, No.12, (December 1995), pp. 2295-2305

McCarthy JT, Williams AW & Johnson WJ. Serum beta 2-microglobulin concentration in dialysis patients: importance of intrinsic renal function. *J Lab Clin Med,* Vol.123, No.4, (April 1994), pp. 495-505

Misra M, Vonesh E, Van Stone JC, Moore HL, Prowant B & Nolph KD. Effect of cause and time of dropout on the residual GFR: a comparative analysis of the decline of GFR on dialysis. *Kidney Int*; Vol.59, No.2, (February 2001), pp. 754-763

Moist LM, Port FK, Orzol SM, Young EW, Ostbye T, Wolfe RA, Hulbert-Shearon T, Jones CA & Bloembergen WE.Predictors of loss of residual renal function among new dialysis patients. *J Am Soc Nephrol,* Vol.11, No.3, (March 2000), pp.556-564

Montenegro J, Martinez I, Sarachet & Gonzelez R. Beta 2 microglobulin in CAPD. *Adv Perit Dial,* Vol.8, (1992), pp. 369-372

Morduchowicz G, Winkler J, Zabludowski JR & Boner J. (1994). Effects of residual renal function in hemodialysis patients. *Int Urol Nephrol,* Vol.26, No.1, (1994), pp. 125-131.

Pecoits-Filho R, Heimburger M, Woo J, Law MC, Chow KM, Li PK, Lui SF & Sanderson JE. A novel association between residual renal function and left ventricular hypertrophy in peritoneal dialysis patients. *Kidney Int,* Vol.62, No.2, (August 2002), pp. 639-647.

Pecoits-Filho R, Heimburger O, Barany P, Bárány P, Suliman M, Fehrman-Ekholm I, Lindholm B & Stenvinkel P. Associations between circulating inflammatory markers and residual renal function in CRF patients. *Am J Kidney Di,s* Vol.41, No.6, (June 2003), pp. 1212-1208.

Rottembourg J, Issad B, Gallego JL, Degoulet P, Aime F, Gueffaf B & Legrain M. Evolution of residual renal function in patients undergoing maintenance haemodialysis or continuous ambulatory peritoneal dialysis. *Proc Eur Dial Transplant Assoc.,* Vol.19, (1983), pp. 397-403

Schiffl H, Lang SM & Fischer R. Ultrapure dialysis fluid slows loss of residual renal function in new dialysis patients. *Nephrol Dial Transplant* 2002; Vol.17, No.10, (October 2002), pp. 1814-1818

Shemin D, Bostom AG, Laliberty P & Dworkin LD. Residual renal function and mortality risk in hemodialysis patients. *Am J Kidney Dis,* Vol.38, No.1, (July 2001), pp. 85-90.

Shin SK, Noh H, Kang SW, Seo BJ, Lee IH, Song HY, Choi KH, Ha SK, Lee HY & Han DS. Risk factors influencing the decline of residual renal function in continuous ambulatory peritoneal dialysis patients. *Perit Dial Int,* Vol.19, No.2, (March 1999), pp. 138-142

Singhal MK, Bhaskaran S, Vidgen E, Bargman JM, Vas SI, Oreopoulos DG. Rate of decline of residual renal function in patients on continuous peritoneal dialysis and factors affecting it. *Perit Dial Int,* Vol.20, (2000), pp. 429-438

Tepel M, van der Giet M, Schwarzfeld C, Laufer U, Liermann D & Zidek W. Prevention of radiographic-contrast-agent-induced reductions in renal function by acetylcysteine. *N Engl J Med,* Vol.343, no.3, (July 2000), pp. 180-184

Termorshuizen F, Dekker FW, van Manen JG, Korevaar JC, Boeschoten EW & Krediet RT. NECOSAD Study Group: Relative contribution of residual renal function and different measures of adequacy to survival in hemodialysis patients: an analysis of the Netherlands Cooperative Study on the Adequacy of Dialysis (NECOSAD)-2. *J Am Soc Nephrol*, Vol.15, No.4, (April 2004), pp. 1061-1070.

Termorshuizen F, Korevaar JC, Dekker FW, van Manen JG, Boeschoten EW & Krediet RT. (2003). NECOSAD Study Group: The relative importance of residual renal function compared with peritoneal clearance for patient survival and quality of life: an analysis of the Netherlands Cooperative Study on the Adequacy of Dialysis (NECOSAD)-2. *Am J Kidney Dis*, Vol.41, No.6, (June 2003), pp. 1293-1302.

van Olden RW, Guchelaar HJ, Struijk DG, Krediet RT & Arisz L. Acute effects of high-dose furosemide on residual renal function in CAPD patients. *Perit Dial Int* 2003; Vol.23, No.4, (July 2003), pp. 339-347

Van Stone JC. The effect of dialysis membrane and etio9logy of kidney disease on the preservation of residual renal function in chronic hemodialysis patients. *ASAIO J*, Vol. 41, (1995), pp. M713-M716

Wang AY & Lai KN. The importance of residual renal function in dialysis patients. *Kidney Int*, Vol.69, No.10, (May 2006), pp.1726-1732

Wang AY, Lam CW, Wang M, Woo J, Chan IH, Lui SF, Sanderson JE & Li PK. Circulating soluble vascular cell adhesion molecule 1: relationships with residual renal function, cardiac hypertrophy, and outcome of peritoneal dialysis patients. *Am J Kidney Dis*,Vol.45, No.4, pp. 715-729

Wang AY, Sea MM, Ho ZS, Lui SF, Li PK & Woo J. Evaluation of handgrip strength as a nutritional marker and prognostic indicator in peritoneal dialysis patients. *Am J Clin Nutr.* Vol.81, No.1, (January 2005), pp. 79-86

Wang AY, Sea MM, Ip R, Law MC, Chow KM, Lui SF, Li PK & Woo J. Independent effects of residual renal function and dialysis adequacy on actual dietary protein, calorie, and other nutrient intake in patients on continuous ambulatory peritoneal dialysis. *J Am Soc Nephrol*, Vol.12, No.11, (Nov 2001), pp. 2450-2457.

Wang AY, Wang M, Woo J, Lam CW, Lui SF, Li PK & Sanderson JE. Inflammation, residual renal function, and cardiac hypertrophy are interrelated and combine adversely to enhance mortality and cardiovascular death risk of peritoneal dialysis patients. J Am Soc Nephrol, Vol.15, No.8, (August 2004), pp. 2186-2194.

Wang AY, Woo J, Sea MM, Lui SF & Li PK. Hyperphosphatemia in Chinese peritoneal dialysis patients with and without residual renal function: What are the implications? *Am J Kidney Dis*, Vol.43, No.4, (April 2004), pp. 712-720

Wang AY, Woo J, Wang M, See MM, Sanderson LE, Lui SF & Li PK. Important differentiation of factors that predict outcome in peritoneal dialysis patients with different degrees of residual renal function. *Nephrol Dial Transplant*, Vol.20, No.2, (Feb 2005), pp. 396-403.

Witko-Sarsat V & Descamps-Latscha B. Advanced oxidation protein products: Novel uraemic toxins and proinflammatory mediators in chronic renal failure? *Nephrol Dial Transplant*, Vol.12, no.7, (July 1997), pp. 1310-1312

Yavuz A, Ersoy FF, Passadakis PS, Tam P, Evaggelos DM, Katopodis KP, Ozener C, Akçiçek F, Camsari T, Ateş K, Ataman R, Vlachojannis GJ, Dombros NA, Utaş C, Akpolat T, Bozfakioğlu S, Wu G, Karayaylali I, Arinsoy T, Stathakis CP, Yavuz M, Tsakiris DJ, Dimitriades AC, Yilmaz ME, Gültekin M, Süleymanlar G & Oreopoulos DG. Phosphorus control in peritoneal dialysis patients. *Kidney Int Suppl*, Vol.108, (2008), pp. S152-158

14

Biomarkers in Chronic Kidney Disease - The Linkage Between Inflammation, Ventricular Dysfunction and Overhydration

Olimpia Ortega
Hospital Severo Ochoa, Leganés, Madrid
Spain

1. Introduction

Since 1970s several studies have shown a significant prevalence of cardiovascular disease (CVD) among patients with end-stage renal disease (Linder et al., 1974). Among patients treated by hemodialysis and peritoneal dialysis, the prevalence of CVD is approximately 40%. Even after stratification by age, sex, race, and diabetes, CVD mortality in chronic kidney disease (CKD) patients is 10 to 20 times higher than in the general population (Foley et al., 1998). End-stage-renal-disease patients often have a high prevalence of cardiovascular risk factors as hypertension, diabetes and dyslipemia. Nevertheless, previous studies have shown that the high prevalence of CVD in hemodialysis patients is only partly explained by traditional risk factors (Cheung et al., 2000). Non-traditional risk factors have been emerged in the last decade. One of this non-traditional risk factor is C-reactive protein (CRP).

In this chapter, it is tried to explain the results of several studies supporting an association between inflammation (measured by high levels of CRP), left-ventricular dysfunction and volume overload among patients with CKD and how volume overload, which is present at the very early stages of CKD, could be the main underlying factor contributing to the worse CV prognosis among these patients.

2. Inflammation (C-reactive protein) in patients with chronic kidney disease: prevalence and prognostic factor

CRP is considered the prototypical acute-phase reactant in man. Plasma CRP is produced by hepatocytes although other sites of local CRP synthesis have been suggested.

The plasma half-life of CRP is about 19 hours and is constant under all conditions of health and disease, so that the sole determinant of circulating CRP concentration is the synthesis rate, which thus directly reflects the intensity of the pathological process stimulating CRP production. In most disease, the circulating value of CRP reflects ongoing inflammation and/or tissue damage much more accurately than other laboratory parameters of the acute-phase response. The CRP concentration is thus a very useful nonspecific biochemical marker of inflammation, measurement of which contributes importantly to screening for organic disease, monitoring of the response to treatment of inflammation and infection and detection of intercurrent infection (Pepys et al., 2003).

Elevated CRP levels have been described in a significant proportion of end-stage-renal-disease patients on hemodialysis or peritoneal dialysis (Arici et al., 2001). About one-third of patients with chronic renal failure have serum CRP concentration > 10 mg/l (Owen et al., 1998). In healthy men, high CRP level has been identified as a risk factor for cardiovascular disease (Ridker et al., 2001). As occurs in the general population, prospective studies point to a correlation between CRP plasma levels and overall and cardio-vascular mortality also in end-stage-renal disease patients (Arici et al., 2001; Ikizler et al., 1999; Noh et al., 1998; Owen et al., 1998; Panichi et al., 2008; Wang et al., 2009; Yeun et al. 2000; Zimmermann et al., 1999).

3. Inflammation and anemia

In dialysis patients, inflammation expressed by high levels of CRP is also associated with low blood hemoglobin and/or resistance to eritropoyesis-stimulating agents (Barany et al., 1997; Bradbury et al., 2009; Gunnel et al., 1999; Owen et al., 1998). This has been attributed to the inhibition of erythropoietin secretion by pro-inflammatory cytokines. Inflammation also contributes to anemia by inducing functional iron deficiency probably blocking the delivery of iron from the reticuloendothelial cells to the hemathopoietic cells. Cytokines may also induce ferritin synthesis directly or by increasing iron uptake into hepatocytes. The increase in ferritin synthesis by hepatocytes and reticuloendothelial cells underlies in the iron storage pool during inflammation. Thus, inflammation among patients with CKD can contribute to anemia and impaired response to erythropoietin. Erythropoietin resistance by itself has been associated with higher short-term mortality in CKD patients (López-Gómez et al., 2008).

4. Inflammation and malnutrition

High concentration of acute phase protein is correlated with low serum albumin in malnourished hemodialysis patients (Kaysen et al., 1997; Qureshi et al., 1998). Low serum albumin concentrations are highly associated with increased mortality risk in patients with renal replacement therapy (Lowrie et al., 1990). Hypoalbuminemia has been traditionally been assumed to result from inadequate protein and calorie intake. However, albumin is a negative acute-phase protein. The synthesis of this protein decreases during inflammation independently of nutritional state. Albumin concentration in dialysis patients is negatively correlated with levels of positive acute-phase protein. Moreover, inflammation and malnutrition data has been associated with the presence of atherosclerotic carotid plaques (Stenvinkel et al., 1999) describing the so called MIA (malnutrition-inflammation-atherosclerosis) syndrome in patients with advanced renal failure.

In summary, inflammation is high prevalent among patients with chronic kidney disease and predicts anemia, malnutrition and CV death. An intriguing question is whether CRP is just a sensitive marker of systemic inflammation or actively contributes to the development and progression of atherosclerotic lesions and, therefore, to the CV damage. Some authors have demonstrated CRP content inside the atherosclerotic lesions, suggesting the active participation in the inflammatory process (Zhang et al., 1999) what hints that inflammation could be the cause rather than the consequence of CV damage. Based on the bad prognosis of patients with markers of inflammation, it is important to try to known the possible causes of inflammation in this population in order to prevent morbidity and mortality.

5. Possible causes of inflammation

The causes of inflammation in patients with CKD patients remained unclear over time.
Several studies have attempted to address the question as to whether some factors related to the dialysis technique by itself could induce the inflammatory response. Activation of monocytes with the subsequent enhanced release of inflammatory cytokines can be caused by membrane-induced complement activation, by direct cell-membrane interaction and by dialysis fluids containing endotoxins (Carracedo et al., 2006; Honkanen et al., 1991; Kerr et al., 2007; Schouten et al. 2000).
However, a similar prevalence of inflammation has been described in patients with advanced renal failure not yet on dialysis (Ortega et al., 2002; Panichi et al., 2002; Stenvinkel et al., 1999). An inverse correlation between CRP levels and clearance of creatinine has been observed (Panichi et al., 2002); thus, CRP levels increase as renal function declines. This finding suggests the possibility of a decreased renal clearance of CRP as a cause of an activated acute-phase response in patients with chronic kidney disease. Another possibility could be that uremia by itself could be the cause of inflammation among these patients. However, in another study performed in pre-dialysis patients with a more homogeneous clearance of creatinine (Ortega et al., 2002), a non-normal distribution of CRP levels were detected. That means that only a group of patients with advanced renal failure shows high levels of CRP, whereas other patients with the same degree of renal insufficiency have even normal CRP values. Hence, it seems that uremia by itself is not the unique cause of inflammation. Probably, inflammation could be related to some factors, frequently associated with renal failure, which can worsen with the worsening of renal function. In this study (Ortega et al., 2002), CRP levels were higher in those patients with a previous history of CVD. Comparing with patients with normal CRP levels at baseline, patients with higher levels maintained significant higher levels on follow-up. This group of inflamed patients showed during the study period persistently lower serum albumin, lower blood hemoglobin, needed higher doses of erythropoietin stimulating agents and showed higher hospitalization rate (table 1).

	Group I (CRP>6 mg/dL) n = 23	Group II (CRP<6 mg/dL) n = 43	P value
CRP (mg/L)*	21.6 (12.9 - 32.6)	2 (2 - 4.6)	0.00001
Albumin (g/dL)	3.5 ± 0.4	3.8 ± 0.4	0.017
Hemoglobin (g/dL)	11.6 ± 1.1	12.2 ± 0.8	0.045
Epo (IU/kg/week)	67 ± 32	43 ± 20	0.025
Hemoglobin/Epo	0.19 ± 0.08	0.32 ± 0.13	0.004
Hospitalization (n)	0.52 ± 0.8	0.03 ± 0.19	0.004

Table 1. Comparison of the evolution of analytical and clinical data between patients with high (Group I) or low (Group II) CRP levels at baseline. Mean ± standard deviation.
*Median (interquartile range).

In summary, at this point we know that inflammation is high prevalent among patients with CKD, that the prevalence is higher among patients with associated CVD, that inflammation tends to increase with the decline of renal function but that only about one third of patients with advance renal function shows persistently high levels of inflammatory markers. Thus, we could argue that uremia by itself is not the cause of inflammation. It seems that another factor, usually associated with uremia and which usually worsens with the decline of renal function could be the responsible of inflammation in patients with CKD. In the past decade, it has been observed that circulating inflammatory cytokines are elevated in patients with chronic heart failure (Levin et al., 1990) and it has been suggested that cytokines can be in part responsible for cardiac disease progression in these patients (Seta et al., 1996). Some authors have detected elevated plasma levels of endotoxins and cytokines during the acute phase of heart failure and that normalization of endotoxins and cytokines concentration can be achieved using intensive diuretic treatment (Niebauer et al. 1999, Peschel et al. 2003). The authors hypothesized that during acute cardiac decompensation, acute mesenteric venous congestion with subsequently altered gut permeability for endotoxins would lead to translocation of these materials into the circulation inducing the inflammatory response. Thus, the authors highlight that inflammation could be the consequence, rather than the cause of heart failure.

6. Association between inflammation, overhydratacion and cardiac disease: B-type natriuretic peptide

Cardiac disease is high prevalent among patients with CKD (Foley et al. ,1995; Hayashi et al., 2006; Levin et al., 1996; Zocali et al., 2004). The typical feature of uremic cardiomyopathy is left ventricular diastolic dysfunction related to left ventricular hypertrophy and left ventricular fibrosis (Ahmed et al., 2007; Losi et al., 2010; Mark et al., 2006). Left ventricular hypertrophy is particularly highly prevalent in end-stage renal disease patients because of hypertension, hyperparathyroidism and increased volume. However, myocardial fibrosis is a specific finding among patients with CKD comparing with patients with isolated hypertension as revealed autopsy studies (Sharer et al., 1999). Probably, volume overload could be a main cause of myocardial fibrosis among these patients as volume overload can produce mechanical stress on the ventricular wall and it has been demonstrated that mechanical factors can induce the activation of the fibroblasts of the myocardium synthesizing the extracellular matrix (MacKenna et al., 2000). Volume overload is present very early in the course of CKD and is the consequence of the inability of the insufficient kidney to eliminate the excess of water and salt. Usually, the increase in extracellular water in the very early course of CKD is modest and may easily be underestimated by clinical examination and can only be proved by accurate measurement of body water volume, as with bioimpedance. Extracellular water excess increases when glomerular filtration rate declines and has emerged as an independent factor in the structural cardiac damage, as a direct relation between extracellular water excess and left ventricular mass has been demonstrated as well as with left ventricular data of diastolic dysfunction (Essig et al., 2008). The authors also highlighted that cardiac remodeling was present at the very early stages of CKD. Over time, structural myocardial alterations progress, leading to diastolic dysfunction. The central disturbance in diastolic dysfunction involves abnormalities in myocardial relaxation and ventricular compliance (Martos et al., 2007). Thus, in order to complete ventricular filling and achieve a sufficient end-diastolic volume, which will provide adequate stroke volume, the left ventricle needs filling pressure higher than normal. Diastolic dysfunction, in fact, means that the left ventricle fills at higher pressure. Echocardiographic data of diastolic dysfunction are the most frequent findings among patients with CKD (Hayashy et al., 2006).

Based on the association between inflammation and heart failure in the general population and as myocardial dysfunction is high prevalent among patients with CKD, several authors tried to find an association between inflammation and cardiac disease also in this population. Furthermore, this hypothesis could explain why only some patients (those with more ventricular damage) show high levels of CRP, whereas other patients with similar clearance of creatinine (those with less cardiac disease) could present even normal values of CRP.

Some authors (Ates et al., 2005; Kim et al., 2005) have observed an association between CRP and left ventricular hypertrophy or dysfunction among patients with CKD. However, most authors have employed in their studies the measurement of a biochemical marker of ventricular dysfunction such as B-type natriuretic peptide.

B-type natriuretic peptide (BNP) is a cardiac neurohormone specifically secreted from cardiac ventricles in response to an increased left-ventricular wall tension (Maeda et al., 1998). When end-diastolic filling pressure is increased (related to ventricular dysfunction, hypervolemia or both conditions), the release of BNP is induced. BNP is a potent natriuretic peptide by enhancing renal sodium excretion, reducing so the intravascular volume and, therefore, the end-diastolic volume and pressure. BNP is a strong predictor of systolic and diastolic abnormalities and is a powerful marker for prognosis and risk stratification in the setting of heart failure (Tabbibizar et al., 2002). In the general population, a cut point of about 100 pg/ml can discriminate patients with heart failure from patients without it.

BNP is increased among patients with CKD and an inverse correlation between BNP levels and glomerular filtration rate has been observed (McCullough et al., 2003). This increased BNP level among these patients is in part related to the decreased renal clearance as well as the accompanying increased intravascular volume which is usually present in these patients. However, values above a cut-point reflect ventricular dysfunction and predict heart failure also among patients with CKD. In general, as CKD stage advances, a higher cut point of BNP is implied. BNP levels higher than 500 pg/ml usually predict heart failure even in patients with renal failure. Diastolic dysfunction is the most frequent cardiac disease among patients with CKD. In this setting, a small increment in end-diastolic volume lead to an exaggerated increase in diastolic pressure (Mandinov et al., 2000), inducing the release of natriuretic peptide. Probably, this pathophysiological mechanism partly explains the high levels of BNP detected among patients with CKD. In fact, several studies have observed an association between natriuretic peptide levels and echocardiographic data of left ventricular hypertrophy and dysfunction among patients with CKD (Guo et al., 2009; Paniagua et al., 2010; Zocali et al., 2001). Natriuretic peptide levels among patients with CKD predict death, as it occurs in patients with heart failure and normal renal function. Otherwise, some authors (Jacobs et al., 2010) have demonstrated a direct correlation between extracellular water, measured by bioelectrical impedance, and natriuretic peptide in CKD patients, explaining how volume overload can increase end-diastolic volume and, therefore, end-diastolic pressure favoring the release of BNP. Probably both mechanisms, volume overload and myocardial damage, both high prevalent among patients with CKD, could explained the high levels of natriuretic peptides detected in this population.

NT-proBNP is the amino-terminal peptide fragment of the precursor of BNP and shows a close correlation to BNP (Masson et al., 2002). A non-normal distribution of NT-proBNP levels was observed among patients with advanced renal failure, as previously observed with CRP (Ortega et al., 2004). Newly, it means that only a group of patients with advanced renal failure shows high levels of natriuretic peptides, whereas other patients with similar creatinine clearance show even normal values. This finding probably reflects the presence of a mixed population among patients with advanced CKD with a group of patients with more severe cardiac disease whereas other patients can achieve the end-stage disease phase with less myocardial damage. But most importantly, a strong correlation between NT-proBNP and CRP levels is found (figure 1), suggesting an association between left-ventricular filling pressure and inflammation among patients with CKD.

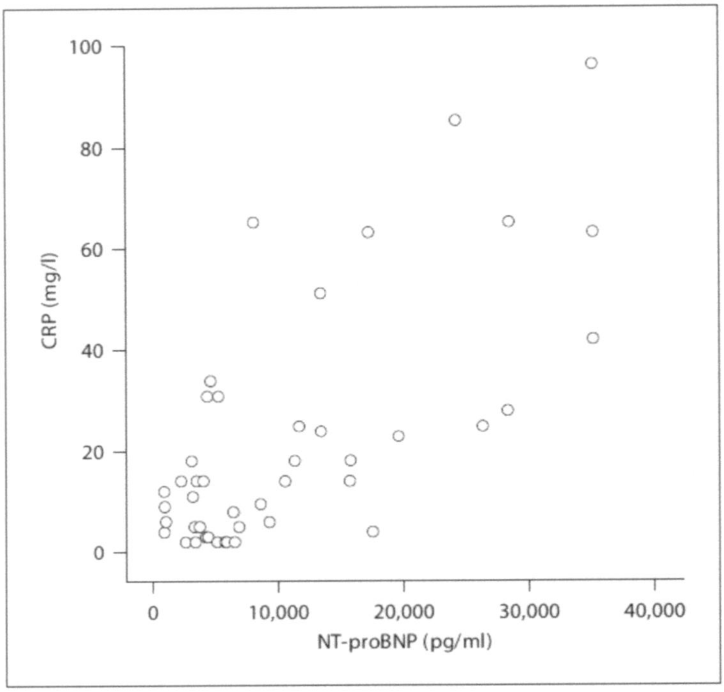

Fig. 1. Regression graph demonstrating the correlation between NT-proBNP and C-reactive protein values at baseline (r: 0.7; $p < 0.001$)

This association between left-ventricular filling pressure and inflammation among CKD patients has been confirmed in subsequent years (Guo et al., 2009; Jacobs et al., 2010; Paniagua et al., 2010). Otherwise, the same studies and other authors (Booth et al., 2010) observed a relationship between cardiac and inflammatory biomarkers and volume overload. An association between volume overload and inflammation had been previously observed among patients on peritoneal dialysis (Woodrow, 2006). Overhydration by itself has emerged as an independent predictor on mortality in chronic hemodialysis patients (Wizemann et al., 2009).

Thus, all these findings show the complex relation between overhydration, malnutrition, inflammation and cardiac biomarkers in CKD patients. Although CRP can actively participate in the atherosclerotic process inducing CV damage, it has also been suggested that inflammation among patients with CKD could be the consequence, rather than the cause, of an increased left-ventricular filling pressure, related to ventricular dysfunction, hypervolemia or both conditions (Ortega, 2005).

The complex relation between ventricular dysfunction, overhydration and inflammation highlights the importance of strict volume control in patients with CKD. Usually, ventricular dysfunction progress over time. In an interesting longitudinal study performed in hemodialysis patients, a progressive deterioration of left ventricular filling pressure (an index of diastolic dysfunction) was observed in parallel with the progression of left ventricular hypertrophy and a progressive increment in levels of NT-proBNP (Kim et al., 2011). Thus, these results suggest that diastolic dysfunction progress over time among patients with chronic kidney disease. In another longitudinal study performed in hemodialysis patients (Ortega et al., 2009), the effect of strict volume control on the evolution of cardiac biomarker levels over time was analyzed. In this study, the strategy of strict volume control permitted the stabilization of cardiac biomarker levels over time, suggesting that this strategy may prevent further progression of left ventricular hypertrophy, cardiac fibrosis and diastolic dysfunction. Patients with higher biomarker levels at baseline, probably those with more severe myocardial damage, were the most beneficed as NT-proBNP levels could even be reduced over time (figure 2). In these high risk patients, continuous prevention of fluid overload diminished the inflammatory parameters on follow-up, confirming the importance of volume control for preventing inflammation in dialysis patients (figure 3).

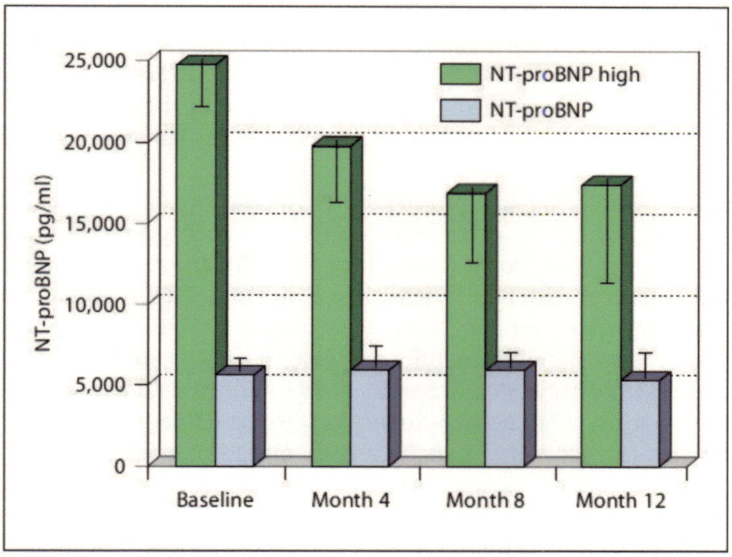

Fig. 2. Evolution over time of NT-proBNP values among patients distributed in high quartile at baseline (NT-proBNP high) and those distributed in other basal quartiles (NT-proBNP). Data expressed as mean ± standard error.

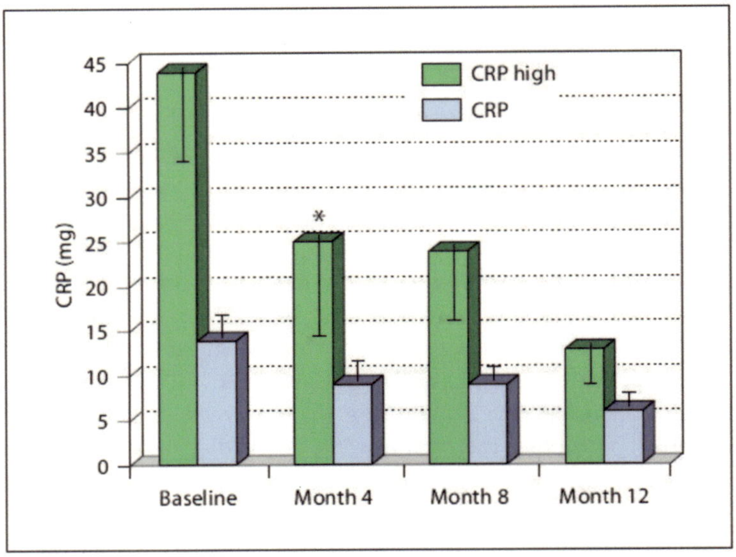

Fig. 3. Evolution over time of CRP values among patients distributed in high quartile at baseline (CRP high) and those distributed in other basal quartiles (CRP). * $p<0.05$ vs baseline levels. Data expressed as mean ± standard error.

7. Other cardiac biomarkers: Troponin T

Cardiac troponins are regulatory proteins within the myocardium that are released into the circulation when damage to the cardiomyocite has occurred. Therefore, serum troponin is an exquisitely sensitive marker of myocardial injury during the acute coronary syndrome and is necessary for establishing the diagnosis of myocardial infarction (Daubert et al., 2010).

Cardiac troponins control the calcium-mediated interaction of actin and myosin, which results in contraction and relaxation of striated muscle. The troponin complex is made up to three subunits: troponin C, troponin I and troponin T. Troponin C is expressed by cells in both cardiac and skeletal muscle. In contrast, troponin I and T are unique to cardiac muscle.

Among patients with acute coronary syndrome, cardiac troponin has not only diagnostic value, but yield prognostic information as well. It has been proven to be a potent independent indicator of recurrent ischemic events and an estimate for the risk of death among patients presenting with acute coronary syndrome (Heidenreich et al., 2001).

Persistently elevated cardiac troponin is frequently observed among asymptomatic patients with end-stage-renal-disease and is associated with increased mortality (Apple et al., 2002; de Fillipi et al., 2003; Ogi et al., 2001). There has been proposed several mechanisms for explaining the high levels of troponin among patients with CKD. Although troponin is a relative large molecule which is believed to be cleared by the reticuloendothelial system, more recent evidence suggest that troponin T is fragmented into molecules small enough to be renally excreted, which may partly explain the high prevalence of troponin T elevation in patients with renal failure (Diris et al., 2004).

Cardiac microinfarctions and arrhythmia have also been suggested as possible causes of elevations of troponin among patients with CKD.
More recently, it has been observed that CKD patients with high troponin T concentrations had clear evidence of myocardial dysfunction and raised left ventricular filling pressure (Sharma et al., 2006), supporting that volume and pressure overload can cause excessive ventricular wall tension with resultant myofibrillary damage or cardiomyocites death (Horwich TB et al., 2003). In this way, a strong association between troponin T and NT-proBNP has been observed in hemodialysis patients (figure 4) (Ortega et al., 2009) and both troponin T and NT-proBNP levels has been observed to be higher in volume-overloaded CKD patients (Sommerer et al., 2007).

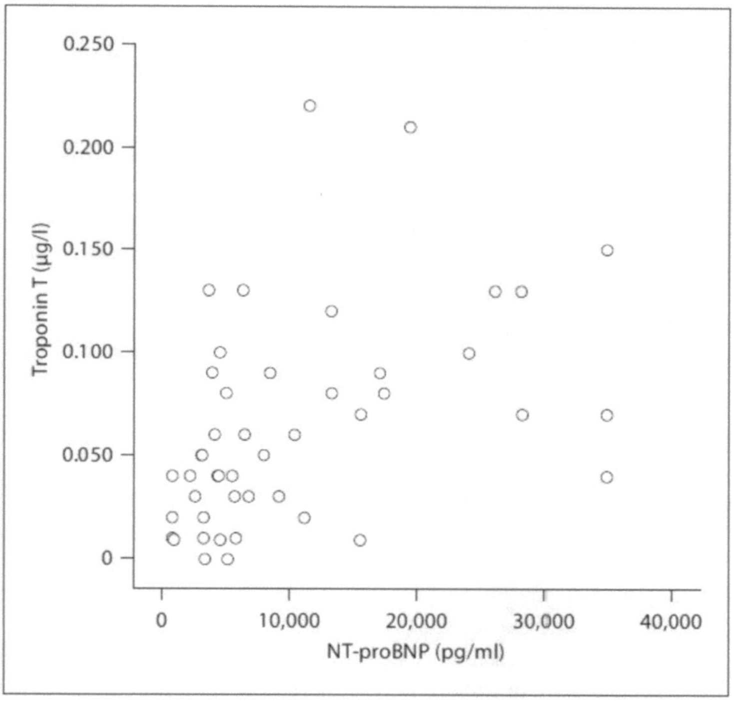

Fig. 4. Regression graph demonstrating the correlation between NT-proBNP and troponin T values at baseline (r: 0.4; p= 0.002)

Thus, it seems that the increased troponin T in a high proportion of patients with CKD could be related to myocardial injury induced by an increased left ventricular volume especially in those patients with diastolic dysfunction, in whom a small increase in end-diastolic volume produces an exaggerated increment in end-diastolic pressure with the subsequent myocardial damage. Furthermore, in hemodialysis patients, a strategy of strict volume control over time could significantly reduce the troponin T levels especially in those patients with higher biomarker levels at baseline, probably those with more severe myocardial dysfunction (figure 5) (Ortega et al., 2009).

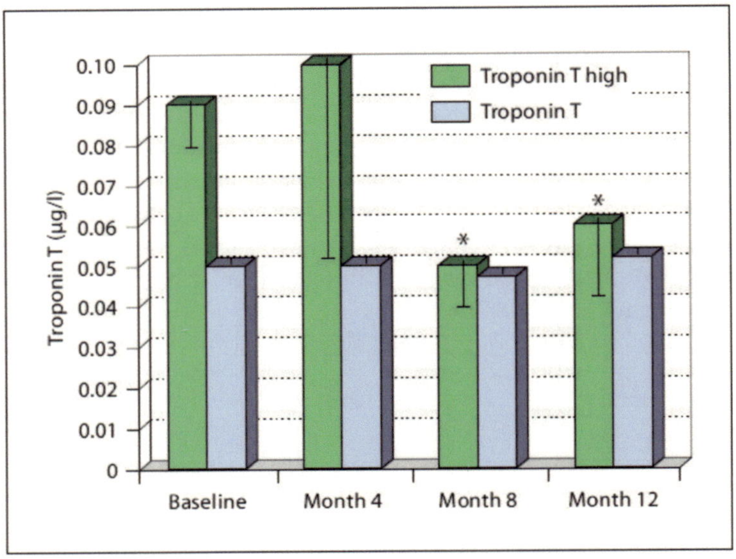

Fig. 5. Evolution over time of troponin T values among patients distributed in the high quartile at baseline (Troponin T high) vs those distributed in the other basal quartiles (Troponin T). * $p<0.05$ vs baseline levels. Data expressed as mean ± standard error.

8. Summary and future perspectives

There is a complex association between ventricular dysfunction, cardiac biomarkers, malnutrition, inflammation and overhydration among patients with CKD, which could partly explain the high CV morbidity and mortality among these patients, comparing with the general population.

Probably, these alterations begin in the very early stages of CKD and volume overload could be an important underlying factor. The inability of the insufficient kidney for excreting water and salt induces an increase in extracellular volume, which may be underestimated in the early phases of CKD. Persistently volume overload can induce an increment in blood pressure, myocardial hypertrophy and myocardial fibrosis. Over time, diastolic dysfunction develops. In this setting, further small increments in end-diastolic volume produce an exaggerated increment in end-diastolic pressure favoring the release of BNP and also, myocardial damage and cardiac remodeling. During cardiac remodeling, death of cardiomyocites is produced inducing a serum increment in troponins, and normal myocardium is progressively substituted by a fibrotic matrix, worsening so diastolic dysfunction. In this situation, systemic inflammation is produced by a yet non clear mechanism.

Thus, in this chapter, it is tried to highlight the importance of early intervention for controlling volume excess in the very early stages of CKD in order to prevent future cardiac dysfunction and inflammation, reducing so the bad CV prognosis of these patients.

It is noteworthy that at this early stage of CKD some patients can show normal plasma creatinine, especially older patients or patients with low muscle mass, but they may be subclinically overhydrated. A prescription of low sodium diet and the carefully use of diuretics at this phase of CKD could be the main tool for preventing volume overload and future CV damage.

9. References

Ahmed A, Rich MW, Sanders PW, Perry GJ, Bakris GL, Zile MR, Love TE, Aban IB, Shlipak MG (2007). Chronic kidney disease associated mortality in diastolic versus systolic heart failure; a propensity matched study. *Am J Cardiol* 99, 3 (Feb 2007): 393-398

Apple FS, Murakami MM, Pearce LA, Herzog CA (2002). Predictive value of cardiac troponin I and T for subsequent death in end-stage renal disease. *Circulation* 106, 23 (Dec 2002): 2941-2945

Arici M, Walls J (2001). End-stage renal disease, atherosclerosis and cardiovascular mortality: is C-reactive protein the missing link? *Kidney Int* 59, 2 (Feb 2001): 407-414.

Ates K, Yilmaz O, Kutlay S, Ates A, Nergizoglu G, Erturk Sl (2005). Serum C-reactive protein level is associated with renal function and it affects echocardiographic cardiovascular disease in pre-dialysis patients. *Nephron Clin Pract* 101, 14 (Aug 2005): c190-c197

Barany P, Divino Filho JC, Bergstrom J (1997). High C-reactive protein is a strong predictor of resistance to erythropoietin in hemodialysis patients. *Am J Kidney Dis* 29, 4 (Apr 1997): 565-568

Booth J, Pinney J, Davenport A. N-terminal proBNP. Marker of cardiac dysfunction, fluid overload, or malnutrition in hemodialysis patients? (2010) *Clin J Am Soc Nephrol* 5, 6 (Jun 2010): 1036-1040

Bradbury BD, Critchlow CW, Weir MR, Stewart R, Krishnan M, Hakim RH (2009). Impact of elevated C-reactive protein levels on erythropoiesis-stimulating agents (ESA) dose and responsiveness in hemodialysis patients. *Nephrol Dial Transplant*; 24, 3 (Mar 2009): 919-925

Carracedo J, Merino A, Nogueras S, Carretero D, Berdud I, Ramirez R, Tetta C, Rodriguez M, Martin-Malo A, Aljama P (2006). On-line hemodiafiltration reduces the proinflammatory CD14+CD16+monocyte-derived dendritic cells: a prospective, crossover study. *J Am Soc Nephrol* 17, 8 (Aug 2006): 2315-2321

Cheung AK, Sarnek MJ, Yan G, Dwyer JT, Heyka RJ, Rocco MV, Teehan BP, Levey AS (2000). Atherosclerotic cardiovascular disease risks in chronic hemodialysis patients. *Kidney Int* 58, 1 (Jul 2000): 407-414

Daubert MA, Jeremias A (2010). The utility of trponin measurement to detect myocardial infarction: review of the current findings. *Vasc Health Risk Manag* 6 (Sep 2010): 691-699

deFillipi C, Wasserman S, Rosanio S, Tiblier E, Sperger H, Tocchi M, Christenson R, Uretsky B, Smiley M, Gold J, Muniz H, Badalamenti J, Herzog C, Henrich W (2003). Cardiac troponin T and C-reactive protein predicting prognosis, coronary atherosclerosis, and cardyomyopathy in patients undergoing long-term hemodialysis. *JAMA* 290, 3 (Jul 2003): 353-359

Diris JH, Hackeng CM, Kooman JP, Pinto YM, Hermens WT, van Dieijen-Visser MP (2004). Impaired renal clearance explain elevated troponin T fragments in hemodialysis patients. *Circulation* 109, 1 (Jan 2004): 23-25

Essig M, Escoubet B, de Zuttere D, Blanchet F, Arnoult F, Dupuis E, Michel C, Mignon F, Mentre F, Clerici C, Vrtovsnik F (2008). Cardiovascullar remodelling and extracellular fluid excess in early stages of chronic kidney disease. *Nephrol Dial Transplant* 23, 1 (Jan 2008): 239-248

Foley RN, Parfrey PS, Harnett JD, Kent GM, Murray DC, Barré PE (1995). The prognosis of left-ventricular geometry in uremic cardiomyopathy. *J Am Soc Nephrol* 5, 12 (Jun 1995): 2024-2031

Foley RN, Parfrey PS, Sarnek MJ. Epidemiology of cardiovascular disease in chronic renal disease (1998). *J Am Soc Nephrol* 9, suppl 12 (Dec 1998): S16-S23

Gunnell J, Yeun JY, Depner TA, Kaysen GA (1999). Acute-phase response predicts erythropoietin resistance in hemodialysis and peritoneal dialysis patients. *Am J Kidney Dis* 33, 1 (Jan 1999): 63-72

Guo Q, Barany P, Qureshi AR, Snaedal S, Heimburger O, Stenvinkel P, Lindholm B, Axelsson J (2009). N-terminal pro-brain natriuretic peptide independently predicts protein energy wasting and is associated with all-cause mortality in prevalent HD patients. *Am J Nephrol* 29, 6 (2009): 516-523

Hayashi SY, Rohani M, Lindholm B, Brodin LA, Lind B, Barany P, Alvestrand A, Seeberger A (2006). Left ventricular function in patients with chronic kidney disease evaluated by colour tissue Doppler velocity imaging. *Nephrol Dial Transplant* 21, 1 (Jan 2006): 125-132

Heidenreich PA, Alloggiamento T, Melsop K, McDonald KM, Go AS, Hlatky MA (2001). The prognostic value of troponin in patients with non-ST elevation acute coronary syndromes: a meta-analysis. *J Am Coll Cardiol* 38, 2 (Aug 2001): 478-485.

Horwich TB, Patel J, MacLellan WR, Fonarow GC (2003). Cardiac troponin I is associated with impaired hemodinamics, progressive left ventricular dysfunction and increased mortality rates in advanced heart failure. *Circulation* 108, 7 (Aug 2003): 833-838

Honkanen E, Gronhagen-Riska C, Teppo AM, Maury CP, Meri S (1991). Acute-phase proteins during hemodialysis: correlations with serum interleukin-1 levels and differents dialysis membranes. *Nephron* 57, 3 (1991): 283-287

Ikizler TA, Wingard RL, Harvell J, Shyr Y, Hakim RM (1999). Association of morbidity with markers of nutrition and inflammation in chronic hemodialysis patients: a prospective study. *Kidney Int* 55, 5 (May 1999): 1945-1951.

Jacobs LH, Van de Kerkhof JJ, Mingels AM, Passos VL, Kleijnen VW, Mazairac AH, van der Sande FM, Wodzig WK, Konings CJ, Leunissen KM, van Dieijen-Visser MP, Kooman JP (2010). Inflammation, overhydration and cardiac biomarkers in hemodialysis patients: a longitudinal study. *Nephrol Dial Transplant* 25, 1 (Jan 2010): 243-248

Kaysen GA, Stevenson FT, Depner TA (1997). Determinants of albumin concentration in hemodialysis patients. *Am J Kidney Dis* 29, 5 (May 1997): 658-668

Kerr PG, Sutherland WH, de Jong S, Vaithalingham I, Williams SM, Walker RJ (2007). The impact of standard high-flux polysulfone versus novel high-flux polysulfone dialysis membranes on inflammatory biomarkers: a randomized, single-blinded, controlled clinical trial. *Am J Kidney Dis* 49, 4 (Apr 2007): 533-539

Kim BS, Jeon DS, Shin MJ, Kim YO, Song HC, Lee SH, Kim SY, Choi EJ, Chang YS, Bang BK (2005). Persistent elevation of C-reactive protein may predict cardiac hypertrophy and dysfunction in patients maintained on hemodialysis. *Am J Nephrol* 25, 3 (May-Jun 2005): 189-195

Kim YK, Shin SJ, Ihm SH, Park CS, Kim HY, Hong TY, Song HC, Yang CW, Kim YS, Choi EJ (2010). Longitudinal changes of left ventricular filling pressure and N-terminal pro-brain natriuretic peptide on chronic hemodialysis. *Clin Nephrol* 74, 3 (Sept 2010): 190-197

Levin A, Singer J, Thompson CR, Ross H, Lewis M (1996). Prevalent left-ventricular hypertrophy in the predialysis population: identifying opportunities for intervention. *Am J Kidney Dis* 27, 3 (Mar 1996): 347-354

Levine B, Kalman J, Mayer L, Fillit HM, Packer M. (1990) Elevated circulating levels of tumor necrosis factor in severe chronic heart failure. *N Eng J Med* 323, 4 (Jul 1990): 236-241

Lindner A, Charra B, Sherrard DJ, Scribner BH (1974). Accelerated atherosclerosis in prolonged maintenance hemodialysis. *N Engl J Med* 290, 13 (Mar 1974): 697-701

López-Gómez JM, Portolés JM, Aljama P (2008). Factors that condition the response to erythropoietin in patients on hemodialysis and their relation to mortality. *Kidney Int* 74, S111 (Dec 2008): S75-S81

Losi MA, Memoli B, Contaldi C, Barbati G, Del Prete M, Betocchi S, Cavallaro M, Carpinella G, Fundaliotis A, Parrella LS, Parisi V, Guida B, Chiariello M (2010). Myocardial fibrosis and diastolic dysfunction in patients on chronic hemodialysis. *Nephrol Dial Transplant* 25, 6 (Jun 2010): 1950-1954

Lowrie EG, Lew NL (1990). Death risk in hemodialysis patients: The predictive value of commonly measured variables and an evaluation of death rate differences between facilities. *Am J Kidney Dis* 15, 5 (May 1990): 458-482

Maeda K, Tsutamoto T, Wada A, Hisanaga T, Kinoshita M. Plasma brain natriuretic peptide as a biochemical marker of high left ventricular end-diastolic pressure in patients with symptomatic left ventricular dysfunction. *Am Heart J* 135, 5 (May 1998): 825-832

MacKenna D, Summerour SR, Villarreal FJ (2000). Role of mechanical factors in modulating cardiac fibroblast function and extracellular matrix synthesis. *Cardiovasc Research* 46, 2 (May 2000): 257-263

Mandinov L, Eberli FR, Seiler C, Hess OM (2000). Diastolic heart failure. *Cardiovasc Res* 45, 4 (Mar 2000): 813-825

Mark PB, Johnston N, Groenning BA, Foster JE, Blyth KG, Martin TN, Steedman T, Dargie HJ, Jardine AG (2006). Redefinition of uremic cardiomyopathy by contrast-enhanced cardiac magnetic resonance imaging. *Kidney Int* 69, 10 (May 2006): 1839-1845

Martos R, Baugh J, Ledwidge M, O'Loughlin C, Conlon C, Patle A, Donnelly SC, McDonald K (2007). Diastolic heart failure: evidence of increased myocardial collagen turnover linked to diastolic dysfunction. *Circulation* 115, 7 (Feb 2007): 888-895

Masson S, Vago T, Baldi G, Salio M, De Angelis N, Nicolis E, Maggioni AP, Latini R, Norbiato G, Bevilacqua M (2002). Comparative measurement of N-terminal pro-brain natriuretic peptide and brain natriuretic peptide in ambulatory patients with heart failure. *Clin Chem Lab Med* 40, 8 (Aug 2002): 761-763

McCullough PA, Duc P, Omland T, McCord J, Nowak RM, Hollander JE, Herrmann HC, Steg PF, Westheim A, Knudsen CW, Storrow AB, Abraham WT, Lamba S, Wu AH, Perez A, Clopton P, Krishnaswamy P, Kazanegra R, Maisel AS; Breathing Not Properly Multinantional Study Investigators (2003). B-type natriuretic peptide and renal function in the diagnosis of heart failure: an analysis from the Breathing Not Properly Multinational Study. *Am J Kidney Dis* 41, 3 (Mar 2003): 571-579

Niebauer J, Volk HD, Kemp M, Dominguez M, Schumann RR, Rauchhaus M, Poole-Wilson PA, Coats AJ, Anker SD (1999). Endotoxin and immune activation in chronic heart failure: a prospective cohort study. *Lancet* 353, 9167 (May 1999): 1838-1842

Noh H, Lee SW, Kang SW, Shin SK, Choi KH, Lee HY, Hans DS (1998). Serum C-reactive protein: a predictor of mortality in continuous ambulatory peritoneal dialysis patients. *Perit Dial Int* 18, 4 (Jul-Aug 1998): 387-394

Ooi DS, Zimmerman D, Graham J, Wells GA (2001). Cardiac troponin T predicts long-term outcomes in hemodialysis patients. *Clin Chem* 47, 3 (Mar 2001): 412-417

Ortega O, Rodriguez I, Gallar P, Carreño A, Ortiz M, Espejo B, Jimenez J, Gutierrez M, Oliet A, Vigil A (2002). Significance of high C-reactive protein levels in pre-dialysis patients. *Nephrol Dial Transplant* 17, 6 (Jun 2002): 1105-1109

Ortega O, Gallar P, Munoz M, Rodríguez I, Carreño A, Ortiz M, Molina A, Oliet A, Lozano L, Vigil A (2004). Association between C-reactive protein levels and N-terminal pro-B-type natriuretic peptide in pre-dialysis patients. *Nephron Clin Pract* 97, 4 (Aug 2004): c125-c130

Ortega O (2005). Could we reduce the prevalence of inflammation among patients with chronic kidney disease? *Nephron Clin Pract* 101, 4 (Aug 2005): c198-c199

Ortega O, Rodriguez I, Gracia C, Sanchez M, Lentisco C, Mon C, Gallar P, Ortiz M, Herrero JC, Oliet A, Vigil A (2009). Strict volume control and longitudinal changes in cardiac biomarker levels in hemodialysis patients. *Nephrol Clin Pract* 113, 2 (Jul 2009): c96-c103

Owen WF, Lowrie EG (1998). C-reactive protein as an outcome predictor for maintenance hemodialysis patients. *Kidney Int* 54, 2 (Aug 1998): 627-636

Paniagua R, Ventura MD, Avila-Diaz M, Hinojosa-Heredia H, Mendez-Duran A, Cueto-Manzano A, Cisneros A, Ramos A, Madonia-Juseino C, Belio-Caro F, Garcia-Contreras F, Trinidad-Ramos P, Vazquez R, Ilabaca B, Alcantara G, Amato D (2010). NT-proBNP, fluid overload and dialysis modality are independent predictors of mortality in ESRD patients. *Nephrol Dial Transplant* 25, 2 (Feb 2010): 551-557

Panichi V, Migliori M, de Pietro S, Taccola D, Bianchi AM, Giovannini L, Norpoth M, Metelli MR, Cristofani R, Bertelli AA, Sbragia G, Tetta C, Palla R (2002). C-reactive protein and interleukin-6 levels are related to renal function in predialytic chronic renal failure. *Nephron* 91, 4 (Aug 2002): 594-600

Panichi V, Rieza GM, Paoletti S, Bigazzi R, Aloisi M, Barsotti G, Rindi P, Donati G, Antonelli A, Panicucci E, Tripepi G, Tetta C, Palla R; RISCAVID Study Group (2008). Chronic inflammation and mortality in hemodialysis: effect of different renal replacement therapy. Results from the RISCAVID study. *Nephrol Dial Transplant* 23, 7 (Jul 2008): 2337-2343

Pepys MB, Hirschfield GM (2003). C-reactive protein: a critical update. *J Clin Invest* 111, 12 (Jun 2003): 1805-1812

Peschel T, Schonauer M, Thiele H, Anker S, Schuler G, Niebauer J (2003). Invasive assessment of bacterial endotoxin and inflammatory cytokines in patients with acute heart failure. *Europ J of Heart Fail* 5, 5 (Oct 2003): 609-614

Qureshi AR, Alvestrand A, Danielsson A, Divino-Filho JC, Gutierrez A, Lindholm B, Bergstrom J (1998). Factors influencing malnutrition in hemodialysis patients: A cross-sectional study. *Kidney Int* 53, 3 (Mar 1998): 773-782

Ridker PM (2001). High-sensitivity C-reactive protein: potential adjunt for global risk assessment in the primary prevention of cardiovascular disease. *Circulation* 103, 13 (Apr 2001): 1813-1818.

Schouten WE, Grooteman MP, van Houte AJ, Schoorl M, van Limbeck J, Nube MJ (2000). Effects of dialysers and dialysate on the acute phase reaction in clinical bicarbonate dialysis. *Nephrol Dial Trnsplant* 15, 3 (Mar 2000): 379-384

Seta Y, Shan K, Bozkurt B, Oral H, Mann DL (1996). Basic mechanism in heart failure: the cytokine hypothesis. *J Card Fail* 2,3 (Sep 1996): 243-249

Sharer K, Schmidt KG, Soergel M (1999). Cardiac function and structure in patients with chronic renal failure. *Pediatr Nephrol* 13, 9 (Nov 1999): 951-965

Sharma R, Gaze DC, Pellerin D, Mehta RL, Gregson H, Streather CP, Collinson PO, Brecker SJ (2006). Cardiac structural and functional abnormalities in end stage renal disease patients with elevated cardiac troponin T. *Heart* 92, 6 (Jun 2006): 804-809

Sommerer C, Beimler J, Schwenger V, Heckele N, Katus HA, Giannitsis E, Zeier M (2007). Cardiac biomarkers and survival in hemodialyisis patients. *Eur J Clin Invest* 37, 5 (May 2007): 350-356

Stenvinkel P, Heimburger O, Paultre F, Diczfalusy U, Wang T, Berglund L, Jogestrand T (1999). Strong association between malnutrition, inflammation and atherosclerosis in chronic renal failure. *Kidney Int* 55, 5 (May 1999): 1899-1911

Tabbibizar R, Maisel A (2002). The impact of B-type natriuretic peptide levels on the diagnoses and management of congestive heart failure. *Curr Opin Cardiol* 17, 4 (Jul 2002): 340-345.

Wang AY, Lam CW, Chan IH, Wang M, Lui SF, Sanderson JE (2009). Long-term mortality and cardiovascular risk stratification of peritoneal dialysis patients using a combination of inflammation and calcification markers. *Nephrol Dial Transplant* 24 12 (Dec 2009): 3826-3803

Wizemann V, Wabel P, Chamney P, Zaluska W, Moissl U, Rode C, Malecka-Masalska T, Marcelli D (2009). The mortality risk of overhydration in hemodialysis patients. *Nephrol Dial Transplant* 24, 5 (May 2009): 1574-1579

Woodrow G (2006). Extracellular water expansion; part of the malnutrition-inflammation-atherosclerosis syndrome? *Peri Dial Int* 26, 5 (Sep-Oct 2006):566-570

Yeun JY, Levine RA, Mantadilok V, Kaysen GA (2000). C-reacive protein predicts all-cause and cardiovascular mortality in hemodialysis patients. *Am J Kidney Dis* 35, (Mar 2000): 469-476

Zhang YX, Cliff WJ, Schoefl GI, Higgins G (1999). Coronary C-reactive protein distribution: its relation to development of atherosclerosis. *Atherosclerosis* 145, 2 (Aug 1999): 375-379

Zimmermann J, Herrlinger S, Pruy A , Metzger T, Wanner C (1999). Inflammation enhances cardiovascular risk and mortality in hemodialysis patients. *Kidney Int* 55, 2 (Feb 1999): 648-658

Zoccali C, Mallamaci F, Benedetto FA, Tripepi G, Parlongo S, Cataliotti A, Cutrupi S, Giacone G, Bellanuova I, Cottini E, Malatino LS (2001). Cardiac natriuretic peptides are related to left ventricular mass and function and predict mortality in dialysis patients. *J Am Soc Nephrol* 12, 7 (Jul 2001): 1508-1515.

Zoccali C, Benedetto FA, Mallamaci F, Tripepi G, Giacone G, Stancanelli B, Cataliotti A, Malatino LS (2004). Left ventricular mass monitoring in the follow-up of dialysis patients: prognostic value of left ventricular hypertrophy progression. *Kidney Int* 65, 4 (Apr 2004): 1492-1498.

15

Determinants of Cardiovascular Risk in Hemodialysis Patients Without Significant Comorbidities

Aysegul Zumrutdal
Baskent University,
Adana Teaching and Research Hospital
Turkey

1. Introduction

Cardiovascular (CV) disease is a major cause of morbidity and mortality in patients with end-stage renal disease. Traditional risk factors for CV disease include hypertension, smoking, diabetes, dyslipidemia, left ventricular hypertrophy, advanced age and male sex in the general population. Although hemodialysis patients have a high prevalence of many of these factors, they also have nontraditional, or uremia-related, specific factors such as anemia, altered calcium-phosphorus metabolism, inflammation, oxidative stress, nitric oxide synthase inhibitors, hypoalbuminemia, carbamylation, abnormal lipoproteins and hyperhomocysteinemia (Parfrey, 2000; London&Drüeke 1997). So the risk markers that predict CV events in hemodialysis patients may differ from those in the general population.
This increased CV risk has often been attributed to 'accelerated atherosclerosis' in end-stage renal disease (Cheung, 2000; Kasiske et al., 2000). However, CV causes of death are most prominent in the first years of dialysis and are rare in patients who have been on long term dialysis - the reverse of what would be expected if dialysis itself caused 'accelerated atherosclerosis (Mailloux et al., 1991). Because many patients with end-stage renal disease already have one or more comorbidities and clinically evident vascular disease, it is difficult to determine from clinical or epidemiological studies whether traditional or non-traditional risk factors are more responsible for the high risk of CV events.
The presence of comorbid disease is an increasingly common problem, being much more prevelant in new patients started on dialysis today than previously (Godkin et al., 2003; Mailloux et al., 1996; Merkus et al., 2000; Miskulin et al., 2009; Wallen et al., 2001). Hemodialysis patients who are under 55 years of age and without diabetes, significant comorbid diseases and obesity are very rare in the general hemodialysis population. For this reason, fewer epidemiological studies which focus on the determinants of CV risk of a relatively 'healthy' hemodialysis population are available. However, it is increasingly appreciated that chronic kidney disease alone is an independent risk factor for the development of CV disease. In this topic review of available data, an overview is presented of CV risk factors in hemodialysis patients without significant comorbidities.

2. Markers of inflammation

Chronic inflammation is one of the well-known non-traditional cardiovascular risk factors in hemodialysis patients. Chronic kidney disease results in a chronic, low-grade inflammatory process that becomes evident even in the early stages of the disease. After the start of dialysis treatment, various factors associated with the dialysis procedure may also contribute to a stronger, more active inflammatory response. All available evidence suggests that chronic inflammation in hemodialysis patients may contribute significantly to the development and progression of CV disease (Filiopoulos&Vlassopoulos, 2009; Stenvinkel, 2006; Zimmermann et al., 1999).

Although few studies are available concerning the relationship between inflammatory status and CV risk in hemodialysis patients without co-morbid diseases, the studies that do exist in this area also support the role of inflammation.

2.1 C-reactive protein (CRP)

CRP is the best studied inflammation marker associated with CV events. It is the prototypical acute phase response protein produced by the liver under the control of various proinflammatory cytokines, namely interleukin-6, interleukin-1, and tumor necrosis factor-α. Its uniquiness is due to rapid (within 6 hours) and dramatic increases (up to 1000-fold) in circulating concentrations after a cytokine-mediated response to most forms of tissue injury, infection, and inflammation. Moreover, it was shown that plasma half-life (19 hours) and fractional clearance rates of CRP were nearly constant in normal subjects, as well as in patients with infectious, inflammatory, and neoplastic conditions. This marks CRP as a 'precise objective index' of overall inflammatory activity and a surrogate of underlying cytokine stimulus (Arici& Walls, 2001; Pepys&Baltz, 1983; Vigushin et al., 1993).

Several observations have demonstrated that in a significant proportion of hemodialysis patients CRP is elevated for no apparent reason. A wide variety of factors in hemodialysis patients may be responsible for this elevation. First, the uremic state is associated with an altered immune response and uremia per se may cause a proinflammatory status with ongoing acute phase response. Also, extracorporeal circulation of blood during each hemodialysis session may act as a fresh stimulus for acute phase response. Increased cytokine release, the role of dialysis membranes, the dialysate and the patient-specific processes, such as the type of vascular access or unrecognized infections, may also play a role in inciting an inflammatory response (Arici&Walls, 2001; Stenvinkel, 2002a, 2002b).

The predictive value of CRP in CV risk and mortality in hemodialysis patients was shown in numerous studies, and evidence from experimental and clinical studies showed that CRP may contribute directly to the pathogenesis of atherosclerosis and its complications through a variety of mechanisms (Arici&Walls, 2001; Yeun&Kaysen, 2000; Zimmermann et al., 1999). So it has been suggested that this hepatic-derived protein is not only a marker, but also a mediator, of vascular disease (Lagrand et al., 1997; Torzewski et al., 1998). Although a wide variety of potential sources may be associated with elevated CRP in this patient population, underlying silent CV disease may be one of the possible links for this elevation. So the clear association between CRP and CV disease in the hemodialysis population has added CRP as a new predictive CV risk factor which may actually be in a midway position between traditional and uremia-related CV risk factors (Arici&Walls, 2001).

One of the studies investigated the associations of different risk factors with carotid artery intima-media thickness in non-diabetic hemodialysis patients who had no clinical evidence of atherosclerosis and no comorbidities (Zumrutdal et al., 2005). Seventy-two patients (43 men, 29 women; mean age 34.5 ± 10.6 years, mean time on hemodialysis 47.9 ± 40.0 months) were included in the study. Patients without history or evidence of myocardial, cerebrovascular or peripheral vascular disease, those without diabetes mellitus, and those who had been stabilized on hemodialysis therapy for more than six months and were less than 55 years old were enrolled. Patients were excluded whose chest radiograph showed calcified plaques in the aortic arch, or who had ischaemic findings on electrocardiography and/or ventricular wall motility disorders or valvular calcifications on echocardiography. Additionally, patients with conditions known to be associated with acute-phase responses were excluded. The control group consisted of 40 age-and sex-matched healthy subjects, who had been recruited from hospital staff. Body mass index, triglycerides, lipoprotein (a), fibrinogen, CRP, haematocrit-corrected erythrocyte sedimentation rate, serum cardiac troponin I, beta2 microglobulin, and homocysteine levels were found to be significantly different in patients on hemodialysis compared with control subjects. The mean value of the right and left carotid intima media thickness was 0.59 ± 0.06 mm for patients and 0.53 ± 0.07 mm for control subjects. The difference was significant (p=0.002). The carotid intima-media thickness of patients was correlated with age, body mass index, CRP, haematocrit-corrected erythrocyte sedimentation rate, beta2 microglobulin, serum cardiac troponin I, triglyceride, and fibrinogen. CRP, haematocrit-corrected erythrocyte sedimentation rate, serum cardiac troponin I, and fibrinogen were significantly correlated with each other, but not with beta2 microglobulin. The only parameter correlated with beta2 microglobulin was time on hemodialysis. The mean carotid intima-media thickness was significantly greater in patients with both left ventricular hypertrophy and a CRP level > 6.0 mg/L than it was in those with a CRP level ≤ 6.0 mg/L. In that study, multivariate regression analysis showed that age, CRP, beta2 microglobulin, and left ventricular hypertrophy were independent predictors of carotid artery intima-media thickness. The results of that study supported the hypothesis of an 'accelerated atherogenesis' in the hemodialysis population, even if those patients do not have clinical evidence of atherosclerosis. And CRP was found to be one of the independent predictors of early-onset atherosclerosis.

Most investigations of CV risk in patients on hemodialysis have been cross-sectional in nature and representative of the general hemodialysis population. In the previous study, the same subgroup of hemodialysis patients was followed up over the course of one year and the determinants of the progression of carotid artery intima-media thickness were assessed again (Zumrutdal et al., 2006). Fifty-four of the 72 patients completed the study and re-tested under the same standardized conditions after 12 months. The findings at 12 months showed that carotid artery intima-media thickness had progressed in 75.9 % patients. Age, CRP, beta2 microglobulin and left ventricular hypertrophy were independently related with baseline carotid artery intima-media thickness. At 12 months, age and CRP were found to be independent variables related with carotid artery intima-media thickness. The independent risk factors related with the change in carotid artery intima-media thickness from baseline to 12-month stage were age and male sex.

According to those results, age and male sex were related to progression of carotid artery intima-media thickness as unavoidable risk factors in this subgroup of the hemodialysis population. That agreed with the results of major clinical and epidemiological studies of the general population. The independent relation between CRP and carotid artery intima-media thickness both at baseline and 12 months supports the additional role of non-specific inflammation in hemodialysis patients without comorbidities.

2.2 Hematocrit-corrected erythrocyte sedimentation rate (Hct-corrected ESR)

Although ESR is widely used in the general population as an inflammation marker, it was judged to be of no clinical utility in chronic hemodialysis patients in the mid-1980s. So ESR has seldom been studied in patients on hemodialysis. However, in 2001, it was proposed that after correction of ESR values according to Hct levels in hemodialysis patients, Hct-corrected ESR could serve to select the inflammation-afflicted hemodialysis patients from those without this comorbid state (Borawski& Mysliwic, 2001). Supporting that study, while no relationship between ESR and carotid artery intima-media thickness was found, a relationship in hemodialysis patients without comorbidities was found between Hct-corrected ESR and carotid artery intima-media thickness, beyond other inflammatory markers, CRP, and fibrinogen. Although larger additional studies are needed to determine the potential value of Hct-corrected ESR as an inflammatory marker for early-onset atherosclerosis, this relationship may again reflect the role of non-specific inflammation in CV risk of the 'healthy' hemodialysis patients (Zumrutdal et al., 2005).

2.3 Fibrinogene

In the normal population, increased activity of procoagulant proteins including factor VII and fibrinogen is associated with coronary risk. Factor VII coagulant activity and markers of thrombin activation are elevated in patients with chronic renal failure and correlate positively with serum triglycerides and the acute phase reactants interleukin 6 and fibrinogen and negatively with serum albumin (Tomson, 2000). The presence of generalized endothelial dysfunction in uraemic patients is also suggested by higher plasma levels of fibrinogen, endothelin and other factors. The relationship between carotid artery intima-media thickness and fibrinogene in hemodialysis patients without comorbidities may reflect the role of fibrinogene in early-onset atherosclerosis as one of the best-studied inflammation markers (Zumrutdal et al., 2005).

3. Cardiac markers

3.1 Left ventricular hypertrophy

Left ventricular hypertrophy is a well-known potent predictor of CV mortality in patients on renal replacement therapy (Ma et al., 1992). This may result either from pressure overload, causing increased tensile stress, or from volume overload, causing increased shear stres (Tomson, 2000). Recently published results demonstrated that even with good control of hypertension and anaemia, conventional hemodialysis is associated with significant left ventricular hypertrophy. And high prevalence of CV disease was positively associated with left ventricular hypertrophy in hemodialysis population.

In the study assessing the predictive markers of CV risk in asymptomatic hemodialysis patients, in total, 113 hemodialysis patients were included. Demographic, anthropometric, clinical, and laboratory data were collected. Silent myocardial damage was defined by elevated cardiac troponin I values above cutoff values. Cardiac troponin I concentrations were below cutoff value in 103 (91.2%) patients (group 1), whereas 10 (8.8%) patients (group 2) had elevated concentrations. Group 1 patients had higher levels of hemoglobin and high-density lipoprotein cholesterol and lower C-reactive protein and tumor necrosis factor-alpha levels, as well as less incidence of left ventricular hypertrophy, when compared to group 2 patients. Diabetes mellitus, left ventricular hypertrophy, uncontrolled blood pressure, normalized protein equivalent of total nitrogen appearence, hemoglobin and tumor necrosis factor-alpha were found to be independently associated with silent myocardial damage (Afsar et al., 2009).

In hemodialysis patients without comorbidities, mean carotid intima-media thickness, which reflects generalized atherosclerosis and CV risk, was significantly greater in patients with left ventricular hypertrophy, than it was in patients without left ventricular hypertrophy. Mean carotid intima-media thickness in subjects in the heathy control group was significantly lower than it was in hemodialysis patients both with and without left ventricular hypertrophy. The mean serum cardiac troponin I level in the control group was significantly lower than it was in patients both with and without left ventricular hypertrophy. The mean serum cardiac troponin I level was significantly higher in patients with left ventricular hypertrophy than it was in those without left ventricular hypertrophy (Zumrutdal et al., 2005). The relationship between carotid artery intima-media thickness, serum cardiac troponin I levels and left ventricular hypertrophy may demonstrate that subclinical atherosclerotic changes and/or adaptation may occur along with cardiac alterations. So it may be reasonable to apply early strategies for prevention and treatment of left ventricular hypertrophy in hemodialysis patients before clinically evident CV disease.

3.2 Cardiac troponins

Cardiac troponins are the most specific biomarkers for myocardial damage, although they may be elevated in situations other than acute coronary syndrome. Hemodialysis patients often have raised cardiac troponin I and T levels in the absence of acute ischaemic symptoms. The source of this increase has been a point of confusion over the past decade. At the beginning, some authors suggested that this might be related to the cardiac expression of troponins, while others argued for the skeletal muscle as a possible extracardiac source of abnormally elevated cardiac troponins in hemodialysis patients (Bodor et al., 1997; Kals et al., 2011; McLaurin et al., 1997).

In initial experience with two troponin subunits, serum troponin T was elevated more frequently than troponin I in patients with renal failure, and that led the clinicians to question its specificity for the diagnosis of myocardial infarction. Additionally, the poorer specificity of troponin T was attributed to subclinical myocardial injury in the setting of left ventricular hypertrophy or to uremia-induced skeletal muscle expression of the cardiac isoform of troponin T, while cardiac troponin I has been exclusively of cardiac origin and does not express in the skeletal muscle at any developmental stage. Thus, troponin I was proposed to be a better marker of myocardial injury in renal failure than T (Yeun&Kaysen, 2000). However, subsequent studies reported the absence of extracardiac cardiac troponin T expression in truncal skeletal muscle biopsy specimens from patients with end-stage renal failure at the RNA and protein levels (Haller et al., 1998). Another study, based on the electromyographic evaluation of 50 chronic hemodialysis patients, investigated the relationship between increased cardiac troponin T levels and uremic myopathy. Proximal-extremity muscles-deltoid, biceps, vastus laterali-, which were the most common targets of uremic myopathy, were studied. Five of 50 patients (10%) had a positive troponin T test, but only 1 of those patients had characteristic electromyographic findings. Totally, 4 of 50 patients (8%) had electromyographic findings characteristic of uremic myopathy. Positive troponin test results were not associated with calcium, phosphate, parathormone levels. There was no association between serum cardiac troponin T levels and uremic myopathy (Zumrutdal AO et al., 2000).

Subsequent studies showed that frequently positive T test results in hemodialysis patients were likely due to use of the older and less specific troponin T assay with some cross-reactivity to skeletal muscle (Yeun&Kaysen, 2000). And with the use of the latest generation assays, accumulated data from groups of renal failure patients have suggested that elevated levels of both troponin T and I in asymptomatic hemodialysis patients could be associated with added CV risk, including general mortality. Most of the recent studies supported the troponin tests as predictive markers of asymptomatic atherosclerosis and silent myocardial damage in hemodialysis patients (Kanderian& Francis, 2006; Kanwar et al., 2006).

The carotid artery intima-media thickness measurement has been proposed as a method for establishing risk stratification for CV events. To the best of our knowledge, we were the first to examine the relationship between serum cardiac troponin I level and early onset atherosclerosis in a selected subgroup of hemodialysis patients without any clinical evidence of either atherosclerosis or comorbidities. Based on those results, the increased serum cardiac troponin I level was positively correlated with the carotid intima-media thickness and seemed to be a valuable predictive marker for the assessment of CV risk in asymptomatic hemodialysis patients (Zumrutdal et al., 2005). Also, a possible association was found between elevated serum cardiac troponins and inflammatory markers such as CRP, fibrinogen and Hct-corrected ESR. The association between carotid intima-media thickness, serum cardiac troponin I levels and inflammatory parameters needs to be clarified with further studies. Although the underlying pathophysiology of elevated cardiac troponins is still not clearly understood, it may reflect ongoing, often subclinical, myocardial damage or microinfarctions that are partially independent of acute ischaemic injury. So serum cardiac troponin elevations might be very effective in elucidating cardiac risks of hemodialysis patients without any clinical evidence of atherosclerosis and comorbidities.

In conclusion, in addition to traditional risk factors such as age and male sex, non-specific inflammation may play a key role in the progression of atherosclerosis in patients on hemodialysis without comorbidities. Although it is well-established that end-stage renal failure is a state of chronic systemic inflammation, both nondialysis-related factors and the dialysis procedure per se may be responsible for this high risk. Beta2 microglobulin and serum cardiac troponins may be the potential new additions for CV risk in this group of patients. Further studies are needed to determine whether there is a causal relationship.

4. Metabolic markers

4.1 Beta 2 microglobulin

Elevated plasma beta2 microglobulin is a well-known characteristic of chronic renal failure, and among uremic toxins in the middle molecule range, it is certainly one of the most studied compounds. Beta 2 microglobulin is a key component in the genesis of dialysis-associated amyloidosis. The source of the elevated serum beta2 microglobulin has not been explained absolutely in hemodialysis patients. There is controversy as to whether elevated levels are caused predominantly by increased synthesis of beta2 microglobulin, the use of membranes in hemodialysis with different clearance capacities, or diminished renal elimination (Drüeke et al., 2009). Use of middle and high-flux biocompatible membranes was shown to be associated with a notable reduction in beta2 microglobulin and, in some other studies, the systemic inflammatory response, in the general hemodialysis population. However, the role of proinflammatory monocytic cytokines, such as interleukin-1 and interleukin-6, in the pathogenesis of elevated beta2 microglobulin, and its role as a potential initiator of the inflammatory response were discussed (Vraetz et al., 1999; Xie & Yi, 2003). Recently, a study comparatively evaluated the effect of hemodialysis and peritoneal dialysis on oxidative stress and inflammatory biomarkers and the associated factors. It found similar degrees of inflammaton and oxidative stress activation in both groups. In that study, beta2 microglobulin was one of the parameters which correlated to oxidative stress and inflammatory biomarkers. It was negatively correlated both with total antioxidant capacity in hemodialysis patients and with superoxide dismutase in peritoneal dialysis patients (Filiopoulos et al., 2009).

Previously, for what was probably the first time in the available literature, we provided data about the association between beta2 microglobulin and early-onset atherosclerosis in hemodialysis patients without comorbidities (Zumrutdal et al., 2005). In our study, the only parameter correlated with beta2 microglobulin was time on hemodialysis therapy. At that time, we speculated that the relationship we found might be casual (inflammatory) or just an epiphenomenon, and added that further follow up studies were needed to elucidate the importance of beta2 microglobulin as a new nontraditional cardiovascular risk factor in hemodialysis patients. Subsequently, few studies have evaluated the association of beta 2 microglobulin levels with clinical outcome in dialyzed patients. The patients were divided into two groups according to their serum beta2 microglobulin levels (lower beta2 microglobulin group, n=245 and higher beta2 microglobulin group, n=245) and followed-up. During the follow-up period of 40±15 months, there were 91 all-cause deaths, and out of them, 36 were from CV disease. All cause mortality in the higher beta2 microglobulin group was significantly higher compared to that in the lower beta2 microglobulin group. And serum beta2 microglobulin level was a significant predictor of mortality in hemodialysis patients, independent of hemodialysis duration, diabetes, malnutrition and chronic inflammation (Okuno et al., 2009).

A few studies also supported the correlation between serum beta2 microglobulin levels and various cardiovascular risk factors, including CRP, in hemodialysis patients (Kuragano et al., 2010). And recently, beta2 microglobulin has been suggested to be a novel biomarker of peripheral arterial disease and an independent predictor of aortic stiffness in atherosclerosis, in the general population (Wilson et al., 2007). Additionally, higher serum beta2 microglobulin levels were proposed to be a novel marker to distinguish levels of risk in acute heart failure patients with creatinine ≤ 3mg/dl (Kawai et al., 2010).

All of those findings strongly support the role of beta2 microglobulin in CV risk of hemodialysis patients, and it seems it will be a potential new CV risk marker in the future. Further studies are needed to clarify the importance of beta2 microglobulin as a CV risk factor in hemodialysis patients without comorbidities.

5. Determinants of cardiovascular risk in nondiabetic hemodialysis patients

Diabetes is not only a traditional risk factor for CV disease, but also one of the most common causes of end-stage renal disease. While a decline in CV deaths has occurred in the general population, a similar trend has not been observed in dialysis patients. This discrepancy is in part due to the demographics of patients about to be started on dialysis: about 40 percent are diabetic. Also, the average age of hemodialysis patients is approximately 60 years and about 20 percent are over 75 years, and many patients have underlying cardiac disease

(Mailloux, 2010). Thus, epidemiologic studies concerning the predictive factors of CV disease in nondiabetic hemodialysis patients are less available.

5.1 Association with traditional and nontraditional risk factors

In a study of the CV assessment of 75 nondiabetic hemodialysis patients, the main cause of renal failure was hypertension. Compared with normal controls, the patients were found to have increased inflammatory cytokines such as interleukin- 6, tumor necrosis factor alpha, and intercelluler adhesion molecule, as well as a high frequency of carotid intima media thickening, left ventricular hypertrophy, and aortic calcifications (Kunstmann et al., 2009).

Mortality predictors among 84 diabetic and 161 nondiabetic patients undergoing hemodialysis were investigated for two years. Forty-three diabetic patients and 30 nondiabetic patients died. Among diabetic patients, oliguria, elevated CRP, and elevated D-dimer levels predicted all-cause mortality. Oliguria was the most important predictor, particularly for infectious disease-related death. Among nondiabetic patients elevated cardiac troponin T levels, elevated D-dimer levels, and low cholesterol levels predicted all-cause mortality rates. Subdivision of the causes of death among nondiabetic patients revealed that cardiac troponin T levels predicted CV mortality rates. According to those results, mortality predictors among hemodialysis patients differed between diabetic and nondiabetic patients (Hocher et al., 2003).

In one comparison, two groups of nondiabetic hemodialysis patients (both groups n=30) matched for age and sex, were selected according to the absence or presence of symptomatic atherothrombotic vascular disease affecting the coronary, cerebral, or peripheral arteries. The two groups were identical regarding primary renal disease, duration of hemodialysis, and Epo treatment. The presence of hypertension, lipoprotein (a), and fibronectin levels were independent predictors for the presence of atherothrombotic CV disease which may contribute to the high prevalence of CV risk. Smoking was not a predictor. (Tzanatos et al., 2009).

Left ventricular hypertrophy: Left ventricular hypertrophy is one of the strongest predictors of CV mortality in the general dialysis population. It is an independent predictor of survival in patients with chronic renal failure and it is present in a large number of patients on hemodialysis. In 30 nondiabetic hemodialysis patients, predictive factors associated with left ventricular hypertrophy at baseline and in the follow-up period (at 0, 12, and 24 months) were studied. Systolic blood pressure, residual glomerular filtration rate and serum albumin levels were the predictive factors for left ventricular mass index at initiation of hemodialysis. Systolic blood pressure, human atrial natriuretic peptide, and hemoglobin levels were independent risk factors for left ventricular mass index, after 24 months. Systolic blood pressure, human atrial natriuretic peptide, and hemoglobin levels were also predictive factors for left ventricular mass index after initiation of hemodialysis (Io et al., 2010). Better management of hypertension and anaemia may be priorities for preventing or improving CV risk in these patients.

Carotid intima-media thickness: Carotid intima-media thickness is a strong predictor of CV events in the general population. The predictive value of carotid intima-media thickness in 99 nondiabetic hemodialysis patients was investigated. During a follow-up of 42.4±19.5 months, 33 patients died, 19 (57.6%) of them of CV causes. In those 19 patients carotid thickness was significantly higher than in those who survived. So carotid intima-media thickness was an independent predictor of CV death in nondiabetic hemodialysis patients (Ekart et al., 2005).

Asymptomatic atherosclerosis and major risk factors in 104 nondiabetic patients with different stages of chronic kidney disease (stage 1-5) were also investigated. Carotid intima-media thickness and plaque occurrence were compared with 40 healthy control subjects. Nondiabetic patients with chronic kidney disease showed advanced atherosclerosis, intima-media thickness, and plaque occurrence, and their numbers increased directly with the level of renal dysfunction. Another important risk factor was hypertension (Ekart et al., 2008).

Vascular calcification: The uremic state is associated with numeous metabolic abnormalities and endocrine disturbances primarily involving calcium and phosphorus metabolism. Vascular calcification is highly prevelant in dialysis patients and increases CV mortality. The presence and progression of vascular calcification in hemodialysis patients have been significantly associated with chronic inflammation, malnutrition, and disorders of mineral metabolism. Through a review of the literature examining vascular calcification in end stage renal failure patients, hyperphosphatemia is significantly associated with vascular calcification in nondiabetic patients, while it may not be a significant risk factor for vascular calcification in diabetic patients. In diabetic patients vascular calcification occurs long before the initiation of dialysis therapy and and the factors associated with vascular calcification in non-uremic diabetics appear to be hyperglycemia and related metabolic disorders, such as increased glycation and oxidative stress. In diabetic end stage renal failure patients, hyperglycemia is also suggested to be a significant factor associated with the progression of vascular calcification. Thus, the importance of glycemic control in diabetic and phosphate control in nondiabetic end stage renal failure patients is suggested (Ishimura et al., 2008).

The accumulating data demonstrate the role of abnormalities of calcium, phosphorus, vitamin D, and parathyroid hormone in CV disease and the importance of phosphate control is suggested for preventing vascular calcification and CV risk (Andress, 2008; London et al., 2000).

Diabetes mellitus and ethnicity are known factors that affect the extent of CV calcifications. The extent of CV calcifications was assessed in non-diabetic Caucasian hemodialysis patients by a novel composite calcification score. Body mass index, cholesterol, triglycerides, intact PTH, and serum levels of fetuin-A and uncarboxylated matrix Gla protein were not associated with CV calcifications. Age, male gender, dialysis vintage, smoking, calcium-phosphate product, CRP, and lower Kt/V were independent risk factors for CV calcifications (Schlieper et al., 2009). Increasing dialysis efficiency and lowering calcium-phosphate product can reduce CV calcifications. Generally, a calcium X phosphate product of less than 55 is the therapeutic optimum and it is possible that even lower levels offer further survival advantage. However, no prospective randomized studies have demonstrated a CV benefit and/or a survival advantage with any of the current therapeutic options. But observational studies have shown improved survival in hemodialysis patients treated with active vitamin D analogues (Levin&Li, 2005).

Metabolic abnormalities: Chronic kidney disease is associated with complex metabolic changes including insulin resistance, and insulin resistance is associated with increased CV risk (O'Sullivian&Kelly, 2007). In contrast to the general population, a higher body mass index is associated with better survival among hemodialysis patients. Theoretically, high energy supplementation in nondiabetic hemodialysis patients might adversely affect insulin resistance, and with this goal in mind, the effects of high energy supplementation on nondiabetic hemodialysis patients was investigated. According to the results, body fat mass and CRP were the primary determinants of insulin resistance in nondiabetic hemodialysis patients. High energy supplementation, increased adiposity, and inflammation exacerbated insulin resistance. However, long term metabolic effects of this strategy were unclear (Hung & Tang, 2009).

Another study on nondiabetic hemodialysis patients showed that liver fat, visceral adiposity, and sleep disturbances contributed to the development of insulin resistance and glucose intolerance. However, further studies in the long term are still needed to clarify whether interventions that improve insulin sensitivity improve clinical outcomes and CV risk in nondiabetic hemodialysis patients (Sakkas et al., 2008). The study comparing fasting glucose levels and impaired fasting glucose levels with malnutrition and inflammatory parameters in nondiabetic hemodialysis patients demonstrated that fasting glucose levels predict one-year all-cause mortality in non-diabetic hemodialysis patients. And they also showed that basal fasting glucose levels, or the presence of impaired fasting glucose, plays an important role in inflammation, malnutrition and short term mortality (Lin-Tan, 2007).

Diabetes mellitus and deficiency in n-3 long-chain polyunsaturated fatty acids are known to increase the incidence of CV disease. The study investigated the relationship between n-3 long-chain polyunsaturated fatty acids and the pulse wave velocity from the brachium to the ankle, which was measured as a marker of atherosclerosis in 54 diabetic and 93 nondiabetic hemodialysis patients. The mean pulse wave velocity in diabetic patients was significantly higher than that of nondiabetic patients. There was a significant inverse association between pulse wave velocity and docasahexaenoic acid levels and docasahexaenoic acid/aracidonic acid ratios in nondiabetic patients. It was concluded that n-3 long-chain polyunsaturated fatty acids may be a negative risk factor for CV disease in nondiabetic hemodialysis patients (Hamazaki et al., 2009).

Numerous abnormalities of lipid and lipoprotein metabolism are described in renal disease. These abnormalities are caused by complex alterations in several pathways of lipoprotein metabolism. In addition, nonenzymatic modification of lipoprotein particles enhances their atherogenicity without affecting the measured levels of cholesterol, triglycerides, or the HDL, LDL and very-low-density lipoprotein fractions (Tomson, 2000). Dyslipidemia may be present in more than 90 % of hemodialysis patients and has been reported to correlate with CV disease in some, but not all, cross sectional studies of nondiabetic patients on hemodialysis. Among other lipid parameters, low HDL cholesterol was one of the independent determinants of coronary artery disease in nondiabetic hemodialysis patients (Zumrutdal et al., 2007). However there are limited data concerning the effectiveness of lipid lowering with statins in decreasing CV outcomes in patients on hemodialysis.

Coagulation defects: In 68 nondiabetic hemodialysis patients, the probable association of circulating levels of plasminogen activator inhibitor type-1 and the expression of plasminogen activator inhibitor type-1 in internal iliac artery walls with atherosclerotic disease was investigated. Fifty age- and sex-matched healthy normotensive controls participated in the study. Atherosclerotic disease in both groups was assessed by measuring carotid intima-media thickness. Compared with control subjects, hemodialysis patients had significantly increased carotid thickness. Atherosclerotic plaques were detected in 61.7% of hemodialysis patients and 4% of controls. Carotid intima-media thickness was correlated with age, systolic blood pressure, low-density lipoprotein, CRP, and interleukin-6. In hemodialysis patients, a close correlation was found between serum plasminogen activator inhibitor type-1 level, CRP, and interleukin-6 level. Also, carotid intima-media thickness and plaque score were correlated with circulating levels of plasminogen activator inhibitor type-1 and with the expression of it in internal iliac artery walls. The circulating levels of plasminogen activator inhibitor type-1 and the expression of plasminogen activator inhibitor type-1 in internal iliac rtery walls were statistically associated with CRP, interleukin-6, and low density lipoprotein cholesterol. With all of those correlations, authors have suggested that increased circulating plasminogen activator inhibitor type-1 and an upregulated expression of plasminogen activator inhibitor type- 1 in the vasculature could indicate a chronic endothelium activated state and that may identify the risk of atherothrombosis related with inflammation in nondiabetic hemodialysis patients (Peng et al., 2008). Among nondiabetic patients, generalized endothelial dysfunction is associated with an increase in CV risk.

Gene polymorphisms: Cytokine gene polymorphisms have been implicated as potential genetic risk factors for CV disease. The study assessed the role of cytokine gene polymorphisms in carotid intima-media thickness and left ventricular mass index, as surrogate markers for CV risk, in nondiabetic hemodialysis patents. Carotid intima-media thickness and left ventricular mass index progression for 2 years were detected at higher levels in patients with high-producer genotypes than in the patients with the low-producer genotype during the study period. The TNF-alpha-308 G/A polymorphism was closely associated with CRP. So polymorphisms in inflammatory genes could be additional factors affecting inflammation and CV risk in non diabetic hemodialysis patients (Yilmaz et al., 2010).

Synthesis of nitric oxide by endothelial nitric oxide synthase plays a key role in the atherosclerotic process. Several polymorphisms of the gene encoding endothelial nitric oxide synthase are known and have been investigated with respect to their influence on CV disease risk in the general population. The association between endothelial nitric oxide synthase gene polymorphism and CV events in nondiabetic Japanese hemodialysis patients was also investigated. Three endothelial nitric oxide synthase polymorphisms were genotyped for the patients and two endothelial nitric oxide synthase polymorphisms were found to be associated with major cardiac, cerebrovascular, or peripheral vascular events (Asakimori et al., 2004).

5.2 Coronary artery disease in nondiabetic hemodialysis patients

It is increasingly appreciated that chronic renal failure alone is an independent risk factor for the development of coronary artery disease. For evaluating the determinants of coronary artery disease in nondiabetic hemodialysis patients, among 312 consecutive patients on regular hemodialysis, 26 nondiabetic patients with angiographically defined coronary artery disease were compared with a subject group of nondiabetic hemodialysis patients of the same gender, smoking status, and hypertension with similar ages and body mass indexes, who had normal electrocardiography and myocardial perfusion scintigraphy. Demographics, CRP, ESR, Hct-corrected ESR, beta 2 microglobulin, cardiac troponin I, parathyroid hormone, albumin, calcium X phosphorus, and lipid profiles were compared between the groups. The nondiabetic patients with coronary artery disease had higher CRP, higher cardiac troponin I, and lower HDL-cholesterol levels than the patients without coronary artery disease. Backwards stepwise logistic regression analysis revealed that high CRP and troponin I levels and low HDL cholesterol levels were independently related with coronary artery disease in nondiabetic hemodialysis patients (Zumrutdal et al., 2007).

The predictive value of CRP in CV risk and mortality in hemodialysis patients was previously shown in numerious studies, and underlying coronary artery disease may be one of the possible links for this elevation. Additionally, even small elevations of serum cardiac troponin I concentration, at levels lower than those traditionally used for the diagnosis of acute events, were independently associated with the presence of coronary artery disease in asymptomatic hemodialysis patients. Thus, small and non-specific increases in cardiac troponin I levels may reflect underlying coronary artery disease in nondiabetic hemodialysis patients.

6. Conclusion

All hemodialysis patients, diabetic or nondiabetic, are at markedly increased CV risk, with chronic renal disease alone currently considered a coronary heart disease risk equivalent. A large number of risk factors for CV disease and decreased survival that are related or unrelated to the dialysis procedure have been identified. Since no data are available about the outcome comparing hemodialysis patients with comorbidities with those without, it is not possible to suggest increased benefits for survival for hemodialysis patients without comorbidities. Cardiovascular risk factor modification should be undertaken for all dialysis patients with or without comorbidities, given that they are considered a coronary heart disease equivalent.

7. References

Afsar, B., Elsurer, R., Akgul, A., Sezer, S., & Ozdemir, FN. (2009). Factors related to silent myocardial damage in hemodialysis patients. *Renal Failure*. Vol.31, No:10, pp.933-941, ISSN 0886-022X

Andress, DL. (2008). Bone and mineral guidelines for patients with kidney disease: a call for revision. *Clinical Journal of the American Society of Nephrology*. Vol.3, No:1, pp.179-183, ISSN1555-9041

Arici, M., Walls, J. (2001). End stage renal disease, atherosclerosis, and cardiovascular mortality: Is C- reactive protein the missing link? *Kidney International*. Vol.59, No:2, pp. 407-414, ISSN0085-2538

Asakimori, Y., Yorioka, N., Tanaka, J., Takasugi, N., Harada, S., Shigemoto, K., Yamashita, K. et al. (2004). Association between ENOS gene polymorphism and cardiovascular events in nondiabetic hemodialysis patients: a prospective study. *American Journal of Kidney Disease*. Vol.44, No:1, pp.112-120,0272-6386.

Bodor, GS., Survant, L., Voss, EM., Smith, S., Porterfield, D., & Apple, FS. (1997). Cardiac troponin T composition in normal and regenerating human skeletal muscle. *Clinical Chemistry*. Vol. 43, No:3, pp.476-484, ISSN0009-9147

Borawski, J., Mysliwic, M. The hematocrit corrected erythrocyte sedimentation rate can be useful in diagnosing inflammation in hemodialysis patients. (2001). *Nephron*. Vol.89, No:4, pp.381-383, 0028-2766

Cheung, AK.,Sarnak, MJ., Yan, G., Dwyer, JT., Heyka, RJ., Rocco, MV., Teehan, BP. et al.(2000). Atherosclerotic cardiovascular disease risks in chronic hemodialysis patients. *Kidney International*. Vol.58, No:1, pp.353-362, ISSN0085-2538

Cianciolo, G., Cli, L., La Mana, G., Donati, G., D'Addio, F. Comai, G., Ricci, D., et al. (2007). Is beta 2 microglobulin- related amyloidosis of hemodialysis patients a multifactorial disease? A new pathogenetic approach. *The Internal Journal of Artificial Organs*. Vol 30, No: 10, pp. 864-878, ISSN0391-3988

Drüeke, TB., Massy, ZA. (2009). Beta 2 microglobulin. *Seminars in Dialysis*. Vol.22, No: 4, pp. 378-380, 0894-0959

Ekart, R., Hojs, R., Hojs-Fabjan, T., & Balon, BP.(2005). Predictive value of carotid intima media thickness in hemodialysis patients. *Artificial Organs*. Vol. 29, No: 8, pp. 615-619, ISSN0160-564X

Ekart, R., Hojs, R., Bevc, S., & Balon, BP. (2008). Asymptomatic atherosclerosis and hypertension in nondiabetic patients with chronic kidney disease. *Artificial Organs*. Vol. 32, No: 3, pp.220-225, ISSN0160-564X

Filiopoulos, V., Hadjiyannakos, D., Takouli, L., Metaxaki, P., Sideris, V., & Vlassopoulos, D. (2009). Inflammation and oxidative stres in end stage renal disease patients treated with hemodialysis or peritoneal dialysis. *The International Journal of Artificial Organs.* Vol. 32, No: 12, pp. 872-882, ISSN 0391-3988

Filiopoulos, V., Vlassopoulos, D. (2009). İnflammatory syndrome in chronic kidney disease: pathogenesis and influence on outcomes. *İnflammation& Allergy Drug Targets.* Vol. 8, No:5, pp. 369-382. ISSN 1871-5281

Goodkin, Da., Bragg-Gresham, JL., Koenig, KG., Wolfe, RA., Akiba, T., Andreucci, VE., & Saito, A et al. (2003). Association of comorbid conditions and mortality in hemodialysis patients in Europe, Japan, and the United States: the dialysis Outcomes and Practice Patterns Study (DOPPS). *Journal of American Society of Nephrology*. Vol.14, No:12, pp. 3270-3277, ISSN 1046-6673

Haller, C., Zehelein, J., Remppis, A., Müler-Bardorff, M., & Katus, HA. (1998). Cardiac Troponin T in patients with end stage renal disease. Absence of expression in truncal skeletal muscle. *Clinical Chemistry*. Vol.44, No:5, pp. 930-938, ISSN0009-9147

Hamazaki, K., Terashima, Y., Itomura, M., Sawazaki, S., Inagaki, H., Kuroda, M., Tomita, S. et al. (2009). The relationship between n-3 long-chain polyunsaturated fatty acids and pulse wave velocity in diabetic and non-diabetic patients under long-term hemodialysis. *Clinical Nephrology*. Vol.71, No: 5, pp. 508-513, ISSN0301-0430

Hocher, B., Ziebig, R., Altermann, C., Krause, R., Asmus, G., Richter, CM., Slowinski, et al. Different impact of biomarkers as mortality predictors among diabetic and nondiabetic patients undergoing hemodialysis. (2003). *Journal of American Society of Nephrology*. Vol.14, No: 9, pp. 2329-2337, ISSN1046-6673

Hung, SC., Tarng, DC. (2009). Adiposity and insulin resistance in nondiabetic hemodialysis patients: effects of high energy supplementation. *The American Journal of the Clinical Nutrition*. Vol.90, No:1, pp.64-69,0002-9165

Io, H., Matsumoto, M., Okumura, K., Sato, M., Masuda, A., Furukawa, M., Nohara N, et al. (2010). Predictive factors associated with left ventricular hypertrophy at baseline and in the follow-up period in non-diabetic hemodialysis patients. *Seminars in Dialysis*. Epub ahead of print.Augst.13., ISSN0894-0959

Ishimura, E., Okuno, S., Taniwaki, H., Kizu, A., Tsuchida, T., Shioi A, Shoji T, et al. (2008). Different risk factors for vascular calcification in end-stage renal disease between diabetics and non-diabetics: the respective importance of glycemic and phosphate control. *Kidney Blood Pressure Research*. Vol. 31, No: 1, pp.10-15, ISSN1420-4096

Kals, J., Zagura, M., Serg, M., Kampus, P., Zilmer, K., Unt, E., Lieberg, et al. (2011). Beta 2 microglobulin, a novel biomarker of peripheral arterial disease, idependently predicts aortic stifness in these patients. *Scandinavian Journal of Clinical and Laboratory Investigation*. Epub ahead of print. 2011 Feb.14. ISSN 0085-591X

Kanderian, AS., Francis, GS. (2006). Cardiac troponins and chronic kidney disease. *Kidney International*. Vol. 69, No:7, pp.1112-1114, ISSN0085-2538

Kanwar, M., Hashem, M., Romsan, H., Kamalakannan, D., Cheema, A., Ali, A., Gadrin, J., & Maciejko, JJ. (2006). Usefulness of clinical evaluation, troponins, and C-reactive protein in predicting mortality among stable hemodialysis patients. *American Journal of Cardiology*. Vol.98, No: 9, pp.1283-1287, ISSN 0002-9149

Kasiske, BL.,Chakkera, HA., Roel, J. (2000). Explained and unexplained ischemic herat disease risk after renal transplantation. *Journal of the American Society of Nephrology*. Vol.11, No:9, pp. 1735-1743, ISSN1046-6673

Kawai, K., Kawashima, S., Miyazaki, T., Tajiri, E., Mori, M., Kitazaki, K., Shirotani, T. et al. (2010). Serum Beta 2 microglobulin concentration as a novel marker to distinguish levels of risk in acute heart failure patients. *Journal of Cardiology*. Vol.55, No:1, pp.99-107, ISSN0914-5087

Kaysen, GA., Eiserich, JP. (2004). The role of oxidative stres-altered lipoprotein structure and function and microinflammation on cardiovascular risk in patients with minor renal dysfunction. *Journal of American Society of Nephrology*. Vol:15, No:3, pp. 538-548,ISSN 1046-6673

Kumar, J., Shah, SV. (2005). Kidney disease as an independent risk factor for cardiovascular events. *Journal of Renal Nutrition*. Vol. 15, No:1, pp. 99-104. ISSN 1051-2276

Kunstmann, S., Vukusich, A., Michea, L., Varela, C., Allende, I., Bravo S, Gainza D, et al. (2009). Cardiovascular assessment of non diabetic patients on hemodialysis. *Revista Medica de Chile*. Vol. 137, No:3, pp: 351-360, ISSN0034-9887

Kuragano, T., Kida, A., Furuta, M., Nanami, M., Otaki, Y., Hasuike, Y., Nonoguchi, H., & Nakanishi, T. (2010). The impact of beta 2microglobulin clearence on the risk factors of cardiovascular disease in hemodialysis patients. *American Society for Artificial Internal Organs*. Vol. 56, No:4, pp. 326-332, ISSN1058-2916

Lagrand, WK., Niessen, HWM., Wolbink, GJ., Jaspars, LH., Visser, CA., Verheugt, FW., Meijer, CJ,. et al. (1997). C-reactive protein colocalizes with complement in human hearts during acute myocardial infarction. *Circulation*. Vol.95, No:1, pp. 97-103, ISSN0009-7322

Levin, A., Li, YC. (2005). Vitamin D and its analogues: do they protect against cardiovascular disease in patients with kidney disease? *Kidney International*. Vol.68, No: 5, pp.1973-1981, ISSN0085-2538

Lin-Tan, DT., Lin, JL., Wang, LH., Wang, LM., Huang, LM., Liu, L., Huang, JY., & Huang, YL. (2007). Fasting glucose levels in predicting 1-year mortality in patients who do not have diabetes and are on maintenance hemodialysis. *Journal of the American Society of Nephrology*. Vol. 18, No: 8, pp. 2385-2391, ISSN1046-6673

London, GM; Drüeke, TB. (1997). Atherosclerosis and arteriosclerosis in chronic renal failure. *Kidney International*. Vol.51, No. 6, pp. 1678-1695, ISSN0085-2538

London, GM., Marchais, SJ., Metivier, F., & Guerin, AP. (2000). Cardiovascular risk in end stage renal disease: vascular aspects. *Nephrology Dialysis Transplantation*. Vol.15, Suppl 5, pp.97-101, ISSN0931-0509

Ma, KW., Grene, EL., Raij, L. Cardiovascular risk factors in chronic renal failure and hemodialysis populations. (1992). *American Journal of Kidney Disease*. Vol. 19, No:6, pp.505-513, 0272-6386

Mailloux, LU., Bellluci, AG., Wilkes, BM.,Napolitano, B., Mosset, RT., Lesser, M., & Bluestone, PA. (1991). Mortality in dialysis patients: analyses of the causes of death. *American Journal of Kidney Diseases*. Vol.18, No:3, pp. 326-335, ISSN0272-6386

Mailloux, LU., Napolitano, B., Bellucci, AG., Mossey, RT., Vernace, MA., & Wilkes, BM. (1996). The impact of co-morbid risk factors at the start of dialysis upon the survival of ESRD patients. *American Society for Artificial Internal Organs*. Vol 42, No:3, pp.164-169, ISSN 1058-2916

Mailloux, LU., Henrich, WL. (2010). Patient survival and maintenence dialysis. wwwUpToDatecom, Editors; Berns JS& Post WT, pp.1-27

McLaurin, MD., Apple, FS., Voss, EM., Herzog, CA., & Sharkey, SW. (1997). Cardiac troponin I, cardiac troponin T, and creatinine kinase MB in dialysis patients without ischemic heart disease: Evidence of cardiac troponin T expression in skeletal muscle. *Clinical Chemistry*. Vol.43, No:6, pp.976-982, ISSN 0009-9147

Merkus, MP., Jager, KJ., Dekker, FW., de Haan, RJ., Boeschoten, EW., & Kredit, RT. (2000). Predictors of poor outcome in chronic dialysis patients: The Netherlands Cooperative Study on the Adequacy of Dialysis. The NECOSAD Study Group. *American Journal Of Kidney Disease*. Vol.35, No:1, pp. 69-79, ISSN 0272-6386

Miskulin, D., Bragg-Gresham, J., Gillespie, BW., Tentori, F., Pisoni, RL., Tiqhiouart, H., Levey, AS. et al. (2009). Key comorbid conditions that are predictive of survival among hemodialysis patients. *Clinical Journal of the American Society of Nephrology*. Vol. 4, no:11, pp.1818-1826, 1555-9041

O' Sullivan, AJ., Kelly, JJ. (2007). Insulin resistance and protein catabolism in non diabetic hemodialysis patients. *Kidney International*. Vol.71, No:2, pp.98-100, ISSN0085-2538

Okuno, S., Ishimura, E., Kohno, K., Fujino-Katoh, Y., Maeno, Y., Yamakawa, T., Inaba, M., & Nishizawa, Y. (2009). *Nephrology Dialysis Transplantation*. Vol.24, No: 2, pp.571-577, ISSN0931-0509

Parfrey, PS. (2000). Cardiac disease in dialysis patients: diagnosis, burden of disease, prognosis, risk factors and management. *Nephrology Dialysis and Transplantation*, Vol.15, Suppl.5, pp. L58-68, ISSN0931-0509

Peng, Y., Liu, H., Liu, F., Ouyang, L., Cheng M, Gao L, Pan F. et al. (2008). Atherosclerosis is associated with plasminogen activator inhibitor type-1 in chronic hemodialysis patients. *Nephrology (Carlton)*. Vol.13, No: 7, pp. 579-586, ISSN1320-5358

Pepys, MB., Baltz, ML.(1983). Acute phase proteins with special reference to C-reactive protein and related proteins (pentaxins) and serum amyloid a protein. *Advances in Immunology*. Vol: 34, pp. 141-212, ISSN 0065-2776

Sakkas, GK., Karatzaferi, C., Zintzaras, E., Giannaki, CD., Liakopoulos, V., Lavdas, E., Damani, E. et al. (2008). Liver fat, visceral adiposity, and sleep disturbances contribute to the development of insulin resistance and glucose intolerance in nondiabetic dialysis patients. *American Journal of Physiology: Regulatory, Integrative and Comparative Physiology*. Vol. 295, No: 6, pp.1721-1729, ISSN0363-6119

Sarnak, MJ., Levey, AS., Scoolwerth, AC., Coresh, J., Culleton B, Hamm, LL., McCullough, PA. et al. (2003). Kidney disease as a risk factor for development of cardiovascular disease: a statement from the American Heart Association Councils on Kidney in Cardiovascular Disease, High Blood Pressure Research, Clinical Cardiology, and Epidemiology and Prevention. *Circulation*. Vol. 108, No:17, pp. 2154-2169, ISSN 0009-7322

Schlieper, G., Brandenburg, V., Djuric, Z., Damjanovic, T., Markovic, N., Schurgers, L., Kruger, T. et al. (2009). Risk factors for cardiovascular calcifications in-diabetic Caucasian Hemodialysis patients. *Kidney Blood Pressure Research*.. Vol.32, No: 3, pp161-168, ISSN1420-4096

Stenvinkel, P. (2002). İnflammation in end-stage renal failure: could it be treated? *Nephrology Dialysis Transplantation*. Vol.17, suppl.8, pp. 33-38, ISSN0931-0509

Stenvinkel, P., Alvestrand, A. (2002). Inflammation in end-stage renal disease: sources, consequences, and therapy. *Seminars in Dialysis*. Vol.15, No:5, pp. 329-337, ISSN 0894-0959

Stenvinkel, P. (2006). İnflammation in end-stage renal disease: the hidden enemy. *Nephrology* (Carlton). Vol. 11, No:1, pp.36-41, ISSN 1320-5358

Tomson, CRV. (2000). Cardiovascular disease in chronic renal failure. In: *Comprehensive Clinical Nephrology (2nd edition)*. Johnson RJ & Feehally J, pp. 887-904, Mosby-Elsevier, ISBN 07234 32589, Philadelphia

Torzewski, J., Torzewski, M., Bowyer, DE., Fröhlich, M., Koenig, W., Waltenberger, J., Fitzsimmons, C. et al. (1998). C-reactive protein frequently colocalizes with the terminal complement complex in the intima of early atherosclerotic lesions of human coronary arteries. *Arteriosclerosis, Thrombosis, and Vascular Biology*. Vol. 18, No:9, pp.1386-1392,ISSN 1079-5642

Tzanatos, HA., Tseke, PP., Pipili, C., Retsa, K., Skoutelis, G., & Grapsa, E. (2009). Cardiovascular risk factors in non-diabetic hemodialysis patients: a comparative study. *Renal Failure*. Vol. 31, No:2, pp.91-97, ISSN0886-022X

Vigushin, DM., Pepys, MB., Hawkins, PN.(1993). Metabolic and scintigraphic studies of radioiodinated human C- reactive protein in health and disease. *The Journal of Clinical Investigation*. Vol. 91, No:4, pp. 1351-1357, ISSN 0021-9738

Vraetz, T., Ittel, TH., Mackelenbergh, MG., Heinrich, PC., Sieberth, HG., & Graeve, L. (1999). Regulation of beta 2 microglobulin expression in different human cell lines by proinflammatory cytokines. *Nephrology Dialysis and Transplantation*. Vol.14, no:9, pp.2137-2143, 0931-0509

Wallen, MD., Radhakrishnan, J., Appel, G., Hodgson, ME., & Pablos-Mendez, A. (2001). An analysis of cardiac mortality in patients with new-onset end stage renal disease in New York state. *Clinical Nephrology*. Vol. 55, No.2, pp.101-108, ISSN0301-0430

Wilson, AM., Kimura, E., Harada, RK., Nair, N., Narasimhan, B, Meng, XY., Zhang, F., et al. (2007). Beta 2 microglobulin as a biomarker in peripheral arterial disease: proteomic profiling and clinical studies. *Circulation*. Vol.116, No: 12, pp.1396-1403, ISSN0009-7322

Xie, J., Yi Q. (2003). Beta 2 microglobulin as a potential initiator of inflammatory responses. *Trends in Immunology*. Vol. 24, No:5, pp. 228-229, ISSN1471-4906

Yeun, JY., Kaysen GA. (2000). C-reactive protein, oxidative stres, homocysteine, and troponin as inflammatory and metabolic predictors of atherosclerosis in ESRD. *Current Opinion in Nephrology and Hypertension*. Vol. 9, No:6, pp.621-630, ISSN1062-4821

Yılmaz, R. Altun, B., Ozer, N., Hazirolan, T.,& Turgan, C. (2010). Impact of cytokine genotype on cardiovascular surrogate markers in hemodialysis patients. *Renal Failure*. Vol.32, No:7, pp.806-816, ISSN0886-022X.

Zimmermann, J., Herrlinger, S., Pruy, A., Metzger, T., & Wanner, C. (1999). İnflammation enhances cardiovascular risk and mortality in hemodialysis patients. *Kidney International Suppl*. Vol. 55, No:2, pp. 648-658, ISSN 0098-6577

Zumrutdal, AO., Bakıner, O., Ucan, H., Atalay, HV., & Bodur, H. (2000). Relationship between uremic myopathy and false-positive cardiac troponin T test. *Nephron*. Vol. 86, No:4, pp. 522-523, ISSN0028-2766

Zumrutdal, A., Sezer, S., Demircan. S., Seydaoglu. G., Ozdemir, FN, & Haberal, M. (2005). Cardiac troponin I and beta 2 microglobulin as risk factors for early- onset atherosclerosis in patients on haemodialysis. *Nephrology*. Vol. 10, No:5, pp. 453-458, ISSN 1320-5358

Zumrutdal, A., Demircan, S., Seydaoglu, G., Singan, M., Sezer, S., Ozdemir, FN., & Haberal, M. (2006). Atherosclerosis in haemodialysis patients without significant comorbidities: Determinants of progression. *Nephrology*. Vol. 11, No:6, pp 489-493, ISSN 1320-5358

Zumrutdal, A., Baltali, M., Micozkadioglu, H., Torun, D., Sezer, S., Ozdemir, FN. & Haberal M. (2007). Determinants of coronary artery disease in nondiabetic hemodialysis patients: A matched case-control study. *Renal Failure*. Vol. 29, No:1, pp.67-71, ISSN0886-022X

16

Malnutrition, Inflammation and Reverse Epidemiology in Hemodialysis Patients

Rodney G. Bowden, Neil A. Schwarz and Brian D. Shelmadine
Baylor University , Waco, TX
USA

1. Introduction

Reverse epidemiology, or risk factor paradox, has been used to describe the observed effect that traditional risk factors for cardiovascular disease may not necessarily signify the same risk for hemodialysis patients (HP) as for healthy populations. In fact, recent published findings have suggested counter-intuitive outcomes (Chavalitdhamrong, Danovitch, & Bunnapradist, 2007; Tsirpanlis et al., 2009) regarding the role cholesterol may play in disease progression in HP with chronic inflammation and malnutrition comorbidities (Dungan, Guster, DeWalt, & Buse, 2007). However, contemporary experimental studies regarding reverse epidemiology are lacking. The few published findings on this topic suggest chronic inflammation, as measured by C-reactive protein (CRP), and malnutrition, as measured by albumin, is associated with normal cholesterol levels yet higher levels of mortality (Chavalitdhamrong, et al., 2007; Chmielewski, Carrero, Nordfors, Lindholm, & Stenvinkel, 2008).

In contrast, traditional risk factors such dyslipidemia, hyperhomocysteinemia, obesity, or hypertension may provide protective effects in HP, at least in the short term (Kalantar-Zadeh, Block, Humphreys, & Kopple, 2003). Important predictors of clinical outcomes in HP are protein-energy wasting (malnutrition) (PEM) and inflammation (Fleischmann, Bower, & Salahudeen, 2001; Kalantar-Zadeh & Kopple, 2001; Kopple, 1997; Kopple, Zhu, Lew, & Lowrie, 1999; Lowrie & Lew, 1990; Nishizawa, Shoji, Ishimura, Inaba, & Morii, 2001). Because inflammation and PEM are interconnected and similarly affect markers of nutritional status both are considered part of a malnutrition inflammation complex (MIC) (Kalantar-Zadeh, et al., 2003; Kalantar-Zadeh & Kopple, 2001; Kalantar-Zadeh, Kopple, Block, & Humphreys, 2001). Thus, this chapter will address inflammation, malnutrition, cholesterol, and the overall concept of reverse epidemiology in HP relative to MIC as well as the implications of this information on short- and long-term treatment.

2. Inflammation in hemodialysis patients

2.1 Acute vs. chronic inflammation

Initially, the inflammatory response is a defense mechanism to cellular injury or pathogenic invasion. The acute response includes vasodilatation, hyperemia and vascular permeability and can be detected within a relatively short amount of time (minutes to days) via an increase in neutrophils and the presence of fluid protein exudates (Sprague & Khalil, 2009).

Additional responders involved in the inflammatory response are cytokines (Sprague & Khalil, 2009) and acute phase proteins, which reach peak circulating levels within two days in the acute setting (Ceciliani, Giordano, & Spagnolo, 2002). Typically, the inflammatory process ceases when the mechanism responsible for cellular injury is removed, subsequent cellular intermediaries are inhibited, and healing takes place (Sprague & Khalil, 2009). However, in some instances that inflammatory process is not resolved. Thus, the response remains active and proceeds into a chronic process, which can result in necrosis and/or loss of functional tissue.

2.2 Markers of inflammation in hemodialysis patients

In HP the inflammatory response and markers of inflammation, namely CRP and the inflammatory cytokine interleukin-6 (IL-6), are predictive of mortality (Barreto et al., 2009; Pecoits-Filho, Barany, Lindholm, Heimburger, & Stenvinkel, 2002; Stenvinkel, Barany, Heimburger, Pecoits-Filho, & Lindholm, 2002; Yeun, Levine, Mantadilok, & Kaysen, 2000; Zimmermann, Herrlinger, Pruy, Metzger, & Wanner, 1999). In addition to CRP and IL-6, albumin and the inflammatory cytokine tumor necrosis factor-alpha (TNF-α) are markers of inflammation commonly found in the literature. Each marker can provide evidence regarding the inflammatory state of HP, but there is debate as to which marker should be used and even debate as to the role in the inflammatory process of certain markers, namely CRP. For example, IL-6 and TNF-α are known pro-inflammatory cytokines and are also associated with declining kidney function. Various cells including, macrophages and mast cells, produce TNF-α and IL-6 (Sprague & Khalil, 2009). Among the numerous effects of TNF-α are the stimulation of a febrile response, up-regulation of other cytokines, such as IL-6, and stimulation of acute phase reactants (Sprague & Khalil, 2009). IL-6, in turn, has pleiotropic effects that include antibody secretion, the acute phase response and has also been shown to be pro-atherogenic, to name a few. However, TNF-α and IL-6 are not typically used in clinical medicine and are more often found in research; therefore other means of assessing inflammation are used as these tests can become costly. Conversely, albumin and CRP are measurements of inflammation readily available to physicians. Interestingly, albumin levels are also commonly used to assess nutritional status as both nutrition and inflammation can affect albumin (more on this topic will be presented later in the chapter).

CRP, however, is frequently used to confirm the presence of inflammation, as it is an acute phase protein produced by the liver and greatly regulated by IL-6. Additionally CRP is associated with reduction in nitric oxide production, induces monocyte recruitment and plays a strong role in foam cell formation. However, the causal role of CRP in cardiovascular events is still being debated (Genest, 2010; Lippi, Favaloro, Montagnana, & Franchini, 2010; Sattar & Lowe, 2006) and the use of CRP must be justified as it incurs added cost (Kaysen, 2009). Regardless, it is a marker of inflammation that in the native form consists of five noncovalently bonded subunits and is termed pentameric CRP or pCRP. This is typically the CRP measured in plasma or serum, and is also known as high sensitivity CRP (hsCRP). High sensitivity CRP can dissociate into monomeric CRP (mCRP) after binding with activated platelets (Eisenhardt et al., 2009). New evidence suggests that mCRP, through the interaction of hsCRP with activated platelets, may play a more dominant role in the inflammatory process than hsCRP as mCRP was found to colocalize with macrophages and platelets (Eisenhardt, Habersberger, Murphy, et al., 2009). High sensitivity CRP has also been found in atherosclerotic lesions (Sun et al., 2005), but the antibodies used to detect CRP in this study detected both pCRP and mCRP (Eisenhardt, Habersberger, & Peter, 2009). It has been reported that once pCRP dissociates into mCRP, mCRP stimulates monocytes to a greater extent than pCRP, leads to increased monocyte adhesion, and exerts proinflammatory properties (Eisenhardt, Habersberger, Murphy, et al., 2009). Additionally, mCRP may be more effective at regulating LDL metabolism than pCRP (Ji, Wu, Potempa, Qiu, & Zhao, 2006).

2.3 Causes of inflammation in hemodialysis patients

Aside from the primary reason for the patient being placed on hemodialysis, often a disease associated with inflammation, dialysis and the integral pieces of hemodialysis can be sources of inflammation. Kaysen (2009) indicates that the type of vascular access used in dialysis, the insertion of the catheters, biofilm on catheters, bacterial components present in dialysate, and water supply can all be sources of inflammation (Kaysen, 2009). Markers of inflammation associated with vascular access alone include albumin (Chand, Teo, Fatica, & Brier, 2008; Wystrychowski et al., 2009), CRP (Costa et al., 2008; Movilli et al., 2006; Sachdeva, Kovalchuk, Bitzer, & Mokrzycki, 2009), and IL-6 (Costa, et al., 2008; Sachdeva, et al., 2009). As Kaysen (2009) points out, the type of vascular access in HP is associated with mortality (Xue, Dahl, Ebben, & Collins, 2003). Acutely, initial insertion of vascular access, especially catheter or arteriovenous graft (AVG), resulted in transient elevations of CRP and IL-6 whereas arteriovenous fistulas (AVF) did not demonstrate a transient rise in inflammatory markers (Sachdeva, et al., 2009). In regards to chronic inflammation, changing vascular access type from a catheter to AVG was shown to cause an increase in albumin, where as a change from AVG to catheter caused a decrease in albumin (Wystrychowski, et al., 2009). Similarly, catheter and AVG use have been demonstrated to result in elevated levels of CRP and IL-6 and lower levels of albumin than AVF (Costa, et al., 2008; Movilli, et al., 2006). Thus, the type of vascular access has an impact on inflammation levels. An additional impact on inflammation levels is adipose tissue as adipocytes produce IL-6 (Fasshauer, Klein, Lossner, & Paschke, 2003), which is also a strong predictor of mortality in HP (Barreto, et al., 2009; Pecoits-Filho, et al., 2002; Stenvinkel, et al., 2002).

3. Malnutrition in hemodialysis patients

3.1 Albumin as a marker of nutritional status

Albumin is the most abundant plasma protein with a half-life of about twenty-one days. It is a negative acute-phase protein that functions to maintain oncotic pressure and act as a transport protein (Carlson, 2004). Normal serum albumin concentration is between 3.5 and 5.2 g/dL, and this reference range is often utilized as a marker of nutritional status in healthy older populations (Carlson, 2004; Covinsky, Covinsky, Palmer, & Sehgal, 2002). The cutoff point for low serum albumin concentration (hypoalbuminemia) has been proposed to be even higher at about 3.9 g/dL in HP (Trivedi, Xiang, & Klein, 2009). However, it must be noted that conclusions derived from measures of serum albumin concentration are not always in agreement with the conclusions derived from clinical assessments regarding nutritional status (Covinsky, et al., 2002). Forty HP with CRP levels below 0.80 mg/dL were evaluated for malnutrition by measuring serum albumin and through the use of the Subjective Global Assessment (SGA) described by Detsky, McLaughlin, and Baker et al. (1987). The SGA was used to determine whether a patient was classified as well-nourished or malnourished. Using 3.5 g/dL as the cutoff point for hypoalbuminemia resulted in a sensitivity of just 14.3% compared to the results of the SGA. Raising the hypoalbuminemia cutoff point to 4.1 g/dL increased the sensitivity of the measurement to 64%. Furthermore, the mean albumin concentrations for the well-nourished and malnourished groups were 4.3 g/dL and 4.0 g/dL, respectively, with considerable overlap between the two groups. These data suggest that serum albumin alone may not be a sensitive marker of malnutrition in the absence of inflammation in HP (Santos et al., 2003). Regardless, serum albumin is a very important marker of mortality risk in HP (Iseki, Kawazoe, & Fukiyama, 1993). Despite the lack of total agreement with clinical assessments of nutritional status, hypoalbuminemia has been demonstrated to be an independent risk factor for all-cause mortality in older persons especially when combined with measures of physical disability (Corti, Guralnik, Salive, & Sorkin, 1994). Additionally, hypoalbuminemia is associated with mortality in various disease populations including cardiovascular, cancer, and HP (Iseki, et al., 1993; Phillips, Shaper, & Whincup, 1989). A 1 g/dL reduction in serum albumin has been associated with a 47% greater risk of mortality in HP, with the serum albumin concentration in these particular HP being linked to inflammation more so than the presence of malnutrition (de Mutsert et al., 2009).

3.2 Regulation of serum albumin: malnutrition and inflammation

Serum albumin concentration is controlled by the rate of its synthesis, fractional catabolic rate (FCR), and distribution between intra and extravascular compartments. These three variables controlling albumin concentration are heavily influenced by both nutritional status and inflammation (Kaysen, 2003). In healthy individuals and HP without inflammation that are malnourished, albumin levels usually stay within a normal range until the degree of starvation is preterminal (Kaysen, 2009). Renal disease is associated with anorexia and PEM due to the build-up of uremic toxins. Additionally, hemodialysis for the removal of these toxins is also associated with anorexia and PEM because of the resulting nausea and post-dialysis fatigue (Bergstrom, 1996). PEM leads to a decreased rate of albumin synthesis. In normal individuals, the FCR of albumin and resting energy expenditure are also down-regulated in order to compensate for its decreased synthesis during periods of PEM. For HP that are in an inflammatory state, normal down-regulation of FCR is blunted leading to an imbalance between albumin synthesis and catabolism that result in hypoalbuminemia (Kaysen, 2009). Even in the absence of malnutrition, positive acute phase proteins that result from the production of pro-inflammatory cytokines are associated with decreased albumin synthesis. Additionally, inflammation leads to a greater than normal albumin FCR for a given serum albumin level (Kaysen, 2003). On top of the challenges presented by malnutrition and inflammation in HP, amino acid loss from hemodialysis itself may contribute further to nitrogen restriction and hypoalbuminemia (Kaysen, 2009).

3.3 Nutritional supplementation and hemodialysis patients

Recently, studies have investigated the effects of protein and amino acid supplements on serum albumin levels in HP (Bolasco, Caria, Cupisti, Secci, & Saverio Dioguardi, 2011; Moretti, Johnson, & Keeling-Hathaway, 2009; Taylor et al., 2011). When selecting an appropriate nutritional supplement for HP, phosphorus levels must be taken into consideration as it has been demonstrated that high-protein intake with concurrent low-phosphorus ingestion and normal serum phosphorus levels is associated with the lowest mortality rate among HP (Kalantar-Zadeh et al., 2010). Supplementation with 15 grams of liquid hydrolyzed collagen protein three times per week after each hemodialysis treatment in one crossover group increased serum albumin by month 3 of supplementation. However, this change was small (+0.03 g/dL) and was not sustained throughout the remaining 3 months of treatment (Moretti, et al., 2009). Conversely, two pilot studies have shown promising effects of nutritional supplementation on serum albumin. In one study, maintenance HP consumed eight ounces of egg whites (egg whites are low in phosphorus) once per day for six weeks (Taylor, et al., 2011). Mean serum albumin concentrations increased by 0.19 g/dL along with a fall in mean serum phosphorus of 0.94 mg/dL. In the other pilot study, four grams of oral amino acid supplementation three times daily increased mean serum albumin concentration by 0.50 g/dL after 3 months of treatment (Covinsky, et al., 2002). Also, inflammation was attenuated in the study group as demonstrated by a decrease in CRP levels. Based on these pilot studies, protein and amino acid supplementation may benefit HP, but more research including larger sample sizes with controlled trials is needed before a definite conclusion or treatment protocol can be formulated.

4. Cardiovascular disease and hemodialysis patients

The number of HP patients in the United States is approximately 350,000 with an expectation of reaching 1.5 million by 2016. Most HP have a significant decline in quality of life with two-thirds dying within 5 years of dialysis initiation; a survival rate worse than most cancers (Kilpatrick et al., 2007). Cardiovascular disease (CVD) is a leading cause of death in HP with rates higher than the general population and risk primarily associated with elevated lipids, inflammation, malnutrition, hypertension, hyperhomocysteinemia, obesity, and insulin resistance (Third Report of the National Cholesterol Education Program Expert Panel on Detection, Evaluation, and Treatment of High Blood Cholesterol in Adults (Adult Treatment Panel III) Final Report, 2002). Most HP patients' elevated lipid profiles are associated with a higher incidence of CVD morbidity and mortality (Vaziri, 2009) and all-cause mortality (Tsirpanlis, et al., 2009). Additionally, non-fatal CVD is 10-30 times higher in HP suggesting this population is more prone to heart disease (Nanayakkara & Gaillard, 2010). Though traditional treatment of CVD in HP has demonstrated promise, many large randomized trials in HP have not demonstrated a survival benefit from traditional treatment strategies (Nanayakkara & Gaillard, 2010). The challenge becomes understanding why traditional risk factors are less predictive and whether the progression of disease is so advanced in HP that risk factor management should be different in this patient population. It should be noted however, that traditional and non-traditional risk factors for CVD in HP do have some crossover, complicating our understanding of how risk factor management may assist in disease causation and association. Though this chapter focuses on HP, chronic kidney disease patients who are predialysis share some of the same counter-intuitive findings. Therefore it should be noted that progression of CVD begins well before HP begin dialysis and could be detected as early as stage I CKD. Finally, it has been suggested that plaque accumulation may occur differently in HP. In the general population arterial plaque is more associated with lipid accumulation, but with HP it is more likely to be associated with calcified plaques and increased arterial stenosis (Diepeveen, Wetzels, Bilo, van Tits, & Stalenhoef, 2008). Various research groups, including the National Cholesterol Education Program (NCEP) (Third Report of the National Cholesterol Education Program Expert Panel on Detection,

Evaluation, and Treatment of High Blood Cholesterol in Adults (Adult Treatment Panel III) Final Report, 2002) have established that lipids play a significant role in the progression of CVD and with reductions in cholesterol levels there is a similar and graded reduction in risk (Kalantar-Zadeh, et al., 2003). Dyslipidemia characterized in HP is primarily associated with hypertriglyceridemia, low HDL concentrations, elevated levels of LDL, elevated LDL particle numbers, a higher propensity of smaller and denser LDL particles which contain high levels of residual triglycerides, and elevated levels of lipoprotein (a) (Vaziri, 2009).
Cholesterol metabolism in HP can be significantly altered by dialysis protocol, lipid controlling medication, malnutrition, and inflammation (Montazerifar, Hashemi, Karajibani, & Dikshit, 2010). HDL can be significantly reduced in HP due to a reduced plasma concentration of ApoA-I and ApoA-II (Bowden, Hebert, Wilson, Gentile, & Lanning, 2007; Vaziri, 2009), reduced transporter proteins such as ABCA-1 (Vaziri, 2009), and the down-regulation of enzymatic process associated with HDL maturation (Malgorzewicz et al., 2010). Down-regulation also occurs with HDL paraoxonase which is associated with impaired protection against oxidative stress. Hypertriglyceridemia also occurs in HP, is normally associated with impaired VLDL and is the most prominent dyslipidemic abmormality reported in 70% of HP (Eisenhardt, Habersberger, & Peter, 2009). Additionally, hypertriglyceridemia is associated with increases in IDL, chylomicrons, and chylomicron remnants postprandial (Chmielewski, et al., 2008). Primarily a reduction in lipoprotein lipase, an enzyme associated with binding to VLDL and the release of the corresponding triglycerides, is associated with changes that cause a concomitant increase in plasma triglycerides that seems to correspond with a decrease in VLDL receptors. Finally, LDL in HP is normally more atherogenic as particles are usually smaller, denser and are more likely to be oxidized and engulfed by macrophages leading to more unstable arterial plaques (Kaysen, 2009). Oxidation can further cause LDL to no longer be recognizable to LDL receptors on the cell causing less deposition of LDL in intracellular pools. Less deposition can lead to the same amount of circulating LDL cholesterol being associated with smaller and denser LDL particles which can carry more risk for CVD. Excess LDL cholesterol is then removed from circulation primarily by being engulfed by macrophages which lead to more atherogenic foam cells leading to risk acceleration. Lipoprotein (a) is a LDL-like lipid with higher levels associated with increased risk of CVD and is associated with overproduction of apolipoproteins, specifically apoB. Apolipoprotein B is bound with LDL and is associated with increased numbers of LDL particles.

4.1 Reverse epidemiology

Though cholesterol metabolism in HP is associated with dyslipidemia and many CVD related deaths are associated with elevated levels of lipoproteins, recent evidence suggests that many HP have normal or reduced plasma cholesterol levels that are associated with a higher rate of mortality (Bowden & Wilson, 2010). CVD related mortality accounts for 40-45% of all-cause mortality in HP suggesting factors other than lipids may be associated with CVD in this patient population (Dungan, et al., 2007; Tsirpanlis, et al., 2009). Counter-intuitive outcomes regarding the role cholesterol may play in disease progression in HP may be affected by chronic inflammation and malnutrition with much of the published literature concerned with MIC (Bowden & Wilson, 2010; Chavalitdhamrong, et al., 2007). The term, though controversial, that has been used in the literature associated with this counter-intuitive finding is reverse epidemiology (Dungan, et al., 2007). Experimental studies are deficient, but the few published on this topic have suggested that HP with chronically elevated levels of inflammation, as measured by C-reactive protein (CRP) or interleukin-6 (IL-6), and malnutrition, as measured by albumin, are associated with normal cholesterol values but higher levels of mortality (Chavalitdhamrong, et al., 2007; Chmielewski, et al., 2008).

5. Malnutrition-inflammation complex

Cano et al. (2009) has reported that between 20-60% of HP may have MIC and that patients also have lower body weights, lower BMI, lower albumin levels, lower blood pressure and elevated CRP (Diepeveen, et al., 2008). Albumin has been specifically mentioned as a marker of nutritional status and identified as one of the criteria used to measure PEM which is associated with MIC. The association between hypoalbuminemia (< 3.9 mg/dL) and mortality has been well-established and albumin has been identified as a strong predictor of cardiovascular disease (Kaysen, 2009). Supporting this theory is the fact that most studies reporting on reverse epidemiology report no counter-intuitive findings with HDL. The cholesterol esters in HDL are primarily received from albumin (Vaziri, 2009) and therefore hypoalbuminemia would be associated with low HDL. This is also one possible explanation for why other lipoproteins would be low, yet still associated with a significantly higher mortality rate in HP. Challenging our understanding of how this might impact mortality and cholesterol is that albumin is also used as a measure of inflammation and may not necessarily be related a nutritional etiology (Trivedi, et al., 2009). Finally, CRP along with IL-6 are inflammatory markers that have been associated with higher rates of mortality as well (Bowden & Wilson, 2010).

5.1 Reverse epidemiology and cholesterol

In a subset of HP a decrease in baseline cholesterol levels, excluding HDL, has been associated with decreases in CVD mortality and all-cause mortality when patients have chronic levels of inflammation and poor nutritional status (Krane et al., 2009). Recent study authors have suggested the need to consider both malnutrition and inflammation simultaneously as albumin has been shown to be affected by inflammation levels. Inflammatory cytokines and acute phase reactants have been reported to decrease appetite, reduced albumin, increase catabolism (Liu et al., 2004) and quite possibly cause lower levels of cholesterol suggesting that low albumin levels may simply be a reflection of inflammation rather than malnutrition. Specifically most lipoproteins seem to be affected by MIC with the exception of HDL. In most studies where HDL was either low or unaffected most patients experience hypoalbuminemia and low protein intake in the diet (Kilpatrick, et al., 2007). Krane et al. (2009) in a study of 1,229 Type II diabetics who were HP reported that high levels of CRP strongly predicted all-cause mortality, sudden death and myocardial infarction when cholesterol levels were both low and high. Yet, when CRP levels were high and cholesterol levels were low, relative risks for CVD related deaths were even greater. It was further reported that CRP level and not LDL level was the variable more likely to predict risk for mortality and cardiovascular events. Another study confirmed the existence of reverse epidemiology in the presence of high inflammation suggesting the inflammation better predicted both morbidity and mortality (Tsirpanlis, et al., 2009). The study authors also reported that nutritional cachexia along with low cholesterol were good nutritional indices for malnutrition and may be the reason low cholesterol levels are associated with higher levels of mortality in HP. A more recent study reported on the cross-sectional association with MIC and the effects on cholesterol in HP (Bowden & Wilson, 2010). When comparing cholesterol levels, those classified as having hypoalbuminemia had a reverse epidemiological effect with LDL particle number. In the same study when HP were classified as having high inflammation, based on CRP, LDL, VLDL, and LDL particle number reported counter-intuitive findings. But, in patients classified as having both hypoalbuminemia and high inflammation, all lipid variables, with the exception of HDL, reported a reverse epidemiological effect. This suggests that though inflammation may play a more prominent role with reverse epidemiology, both inflammation and malnutrition can have a pronounced effect on lipids causing low cholesterol levels to be associated with more mortality. Additionally, other study authors have reported inverse associations with cholesterol and all-cause mortality, but also a U-shaped relationship with cholesterol in the presence of malnutrition and inflammation (Liu, et al., 2004). When malnutrition and inflammation were controlled for in the analysis, a strong, graded and positive association existed between high cholesterol levels and mortality further supporting the thought that reverse epidemiological associations with cholesterol in HP is associated with MIC. An additional review paper has suggested that previous studies that have controlled statistically for factors associated with MIC in HP, risk associated with cholesterol was the same as the general population and further speculates that cholesterol may be an additional marker of malnutrition (Chmielewski, et al., 2008). It should be noted that not all studies agree with these findings.

Another theory behind why low cholesterol in HP patients can be associated with high mortality has been called survival selection. It is well-established that most chronic kidney disease patients will not survive to kidney failure and End-Stage Renal Disease. Presently, it is suggested that only 10% (Trivedi, et al., 2009) of patients will live long enough to initiate dialysis. Therefore, since so few survive it is thought that only those who have a strong genetic predisposition for survival may be more likely to live but may also have a poorer risk profile. Additionally, simply stated, HP may not live long enough to die of the consequences of traditional CVD risk factors. Though this theory is not very new, it has yet to be confirmed with well controlled studies that take into consideration the age of the patients. Kalantar-Zadeh et al. (2003) also suggests that reverse epidemiology may be normal and that over-nutrition is primarily a 20th and 21st century phenomenon and that our understanding of traditional Framingham risk factors may in fact be new and the exception. Though over-nutrition is a problem in many countries it has been associated with longer living populations in Western nations. As one would expect this idea is highly controversial among scientist and nephrologists.

Additional study authors (Nanayakkara & Gaillard, 2010) have reported reverse epidemiology in HP concerning lipids could possibly be due oxidative stress. Reactive oxygen species (ROS) production that is not balanced by antioxidant control is associated with oxidative stress. Furthermore, oxidative injury has been reported to alter lipids in both the general population and HP and is involved in CVD acceleration (Diepeveen, et al., 2008). Though HP are normally supplemented with B vitamins and folic acid, many still have deficiencies in antioxidants with many patients shifting to a more pro-oxidative stress profile. High oxidized LDL is a well established comorbidity in both HP and CKD patients and is associated with small, dense LDL particles. Moreover, modification of LDL through oxidation is thought to be the first step in the development of CVD and specifically atherosclerosis. Oxidative stress occurs routinely in HP, especially in patients with a long-term dialysis vintage, making LDL smaller and denser and is associated with more endothelial dysfunction, inflammation, stenosis and intima media thickness. Therefore, the oxidative stress hypothesis may help to further explain reverse epidemiology. Oxidative stress in combination with MIC could cause lower levels of LDL and LDL particle numbers, but more atherogenic particles that can accelerate mortality and morbidity. Yet, those associations do exist, a causal relationship between oxidative stress, CVD, and reverse epidemiology has yet to be established suggesting the need for further study.

Chmielewski (2008) reports on an endotoxinlipoprotein hypothesis that suggests higher levels of cholesterol may be beneficial in HP. The theory suggests that higher levels of lipoproteins more readily bind bacterial lipopolysaccharide or endotoxins and modulate inflammatory immune responses. The authors continues to state that cholesterol levels and their ability to predict CVD fall on a continuum with lower and higher levels associated with mortality (Kalantar-Zadeh, 2007). Liu, et al. (2004) may help support this theory as they have reported a U-shaped curve regarding cholesterol levels and moratlity in HP. This theory is highly speculative and needs further study.

Finally, as mentioned previously, HP patients have been reported to have smaller, dense LDL particles that are more oxidized which may play a stronger role than LDL. Small LDL particle size has been identified as an emerging risk factor for CVD (*Third Report of the National Cholesterol Education Program Expert Panel on Detection, Evaluation, and Treatment of High Blood Cholesterol in Adults (Adult Treatment Panel III) Final Report*, 2002). A previous study (Bowden, Griggs, Wilson, & Gentile, 2009) has demonstrated that LDL particle number and LDL size can classify more HP at risk when compared to LDL and triglycerides. Since more HP have small, dense LDL particles there may be mortality associated with smaller LDL particles even when LDL particle number is lower. Therefore, though HP may have less LDL cholesterol and less of the smaller LDL particles, because smaller LDL particles are more atherogenic, more patients have increased morality with decrease levels of cholesterol.

6. Treatment

Reverse epidemiology has been associated with cholesterol but also body mass index (BMI), systolic and diastolic blood pressure, homocysteine, and creatinine levels (Balakrishnan & Rao, 2007) in HP suggesting the need for novel treatments. Since the counter-intuitive findings are prevalent in HP additional approaches are necessary to help identify novel treatments and to discover if new therapies are warranted. Though counter-intuitive findings are present in HP as well as advanced age, congestive heart failure, malignancies, and AIDS little data exists to support changes in non-traditional risk factors as a means to control CVD. To help increase albumin levels it has been proposed to increase protein content in the diet. But levels of protein augmentation with HP patients on chronic hemodialysis has not been sufficiently elucidated simply because dietary protein can be a significant source of uremic toxins and increase phosphate levels which can have deleterious effects on the health of HP patients (Stolic, 2010). It should be noted that hypercaloric consumption may take several years and even decades for serious health effects to occur, yet hypocaloric consumption, measured by albumin levels in HP patients, normally causes a more rapid deterioration in health. Combined with high inflammation levels, a decreased appetite and hypocaloric levels may cause a significant decrease in cholesterol but accelerated risk for mortality (Kalantar-Zadeh, et al., 2001). This short-term effect of malnutrition enhanced by inflammation may overcome the long-term impact of traditional risk factors for CVD and may cause the HP patients to not live long enough to develop elevated levels of cholesterol causing them die sooner than is expected. Also, evidence suggests that lipid levels become more elevated and more strongly associated with CVD the longer the HP receives dialysis and suggests that even though counter-intuitive cholesterol findings are evident in early dialysis traditional therapies such as statins, fibrates and niacin are necessary even with cholesterol levels are low (Chavalitdhamrong, et al., 2007). Therefore, treatment for HP patients with MIC needs to focus short-term on inflammation and malnutrition through dietary counseling and medication. Once MIC is controlled, a more long-term therapy may need to look at controlling lipids associated with CVD risk.

7. Conclusions

Reverse epidemiology in cholesterol levels associated with HP introduces a number of questions concerning our understanding of CVD and findings from the Framingham study. The questions becomes whether nephrologists should recommend the same cut-points for HP as is normally used in general populations. Should nephrologists attempt to control malnutrition and inflammation first and focus on lipids once HP have MIC under control? Though statins can help control lipids they may also help control inflammation which in turn may help to regulate appetite and increase albumin levels suggestions that statin therapy may still need to be used in most HP. Finally, more clinical trials are needed to discover if reverse epidemiology is "normal" in HP or simply a new understanding of traditional risk factors.

Author	Year	Sample	Population	Study Design	Study Findings
Bowden, et al	In Press	438	HP	Prospective ~ 3 years	Reverse epidemiological effects for total cholesterol, LDL, LDL particle number, LDL, triglycerides, and VLDL
Bowden, et al	2010	105	HP	Cross-sectional	Reverse epidemiology in number in hypoalbuminemia group; LDL, VLDL, and LDL particle number in inflamed group; total cholesterol, VLDL, large VLDL, triglycerides, Lp(a), LDL, and LDL particle number in hypoalbuminemia and inflamed group
Bowden, et al	2009	117	HP	Cross-sectional	Reverse epidemiology effect existed for LDL, large LDL, LDL particle size, and HDL
Krane, et al	2009	1255	HP with Type II Diabetes	Prospective ~ 4 years	Patients with low cholesterol and high inflammation had an

					adjusted relative risk equivalent to patients with high cholesterol and low inflammation in CVD death and all-cause mortality
Tsirpanlis, et al	2009	136	HP	Prospective ~ 2 years	Low cholesterol levels together with selected inflammatory markers predict CVD and all-cause mortality and morbidity
Kilpatrick, et al	2007	15,859	HP	Prospective ~ 3 years	Inverse associations between hyperlipidemia and survival, however, black HP with high LDL show almost two-fold increase in cardiovascular death risk
Liu, et al	2004	823	HP	Prospective ~ 3 years	Inverse association of cholesterol levels with all-cause mortality and a U-shaped relationship with CVD mortality in the presence of inflammation/malnutrition
Iseki, et al	2002	1167	HP	Prospective ~ 10 years	Hypercholesterolemia was an independent predictor on survival but was only evident in a sub-group of patients whose serum albumin was more than 4.5 g/dl

Table 1. Studies reporting a reverse epidemiology affect regarding cholesterol and HP (2002-Present).

8. References

Balakrishnan, V. S., & Rao, M. (2007). Genetics and reverse epidemiology among patients on chronic hemodialysis. *Seminars in Dialysis, 20*(6), 570-576.

Barreto, D. V., Barreto, F. C., Liabeuf, S., Temmar, M., Lemke, H. D., Tribouilloy, C., et al. (2009). Plasma interleukin-6 is independently associated with mortality in both hemodialysis and pre-dialysis patients with chronic kidney disease. *Kidney International, 77*(6), 550-556.

Bergstrom, J. (1996). Anorexia in dialysis patients. *Seminars in Nephrology, 16*(3), 222-229.

Bolasco, P., Caria, S., Cupisti, A., Secci, R., & Saverio Dioguardi, F. (2011). A novel amino acids oral supplementation in hemodialysis patients: a pilot study. *Renal Failure, 33*(1), 1-5.

Bowden, R. G., Griggs, J., Wilson, R. L., & Gentile, M. (2009). Cholesterol values are poor markers of disease risk in a chronic disease population. *Clinical Lipidology, 4*(5), 545-551.

Bowden, R. G., Hebert, S., Wilson, R., Gentile, M., & Lanning, B. A. (2007). Comparison of lipid measures and risk stratification among end-stage renal disease patients. *J Nephrol, 20*(2), 212-218.

Bowden, R. G., & Wilson, R. L. (2010). Malnutrition, inflammation, and lipids in a cohort of dialysis patients. *Postgraduate Medicine, 122*(3), 196-202.

Cano, N. J., Miolane-Debouit, M., Leger, J., & Heng, A. E. (2009). Assessment of body protein: energy status in chronic kidney disease. *Seminars in nephrology, 29*(1), 59-66.

Carlson, T. H. (2004). Laboratory Data in Nutrition Assessment. In L. K. Mahan & S. Escott-Stump (Eds.), *Krause's Food, Nutrition, & Diet Therapy* (11th ed., pp. 436-454). Philadelphia, PA: Saunders.

Ceciliani, F., Giordano, A., & Spagnolo, V. (2002). The systemic reaction during inflammation: the acute-phase proteins. *Protein and Peptide Letters, 9*(3), 211-223.

Chand, D. H., Teo, B. W., Fatica, R. A., & Brier, M. (2008). Influence of vascular access type on outcome measures in patients on maintenance hemodialysis. *Nephron Clinical Practice 108*(2), c91-98.

Chavalitdhamrong, D., Danovitch, G. M., & Bunnapradist, S. (2007). Is there a reversal of reverse epidemiology in renal transplant recipients? *Seminars in Dialysis, 20*(6), 544-548.

Chmielewski, M., Carrero, J. J., Nordfors, L., Lindholm, B., & Stenvinkel, P. (2008). Lipid disorders in chronic kidney disease: reverse epidemiology and therapeutic approach. *Journal of Nephrology, 21*(5), 635-644.

Corti, M. C., Guralnik, J. M., Salive, M. E., & Sorkin, J. D. (1994). Serum albumin level and physical disability as predictors of mortality in older persons. *The Journal of the American Medical Association, 272*(13), 1036-1042.

Costa, E., Rocha, S., Rocha-Pereira, P., Castro, E., Reis, F., Teixeira, F., et al. (2008). Cross-talk between inflammation,coagulation/fibrinolysis and vascular access in hemodialysis patients. *The Journal of Vascular Access, 9*(4), 248-253.

Covinsky, K. E., Covinsky, M. H., Palmer, R. M., & Sehgal, A. R. (2002). Serum albumin concentration and clinical assessments of nutritional status in hospitalized older people: different sides of different coins? *Journal of the American Geriatrics Society, 50*(4), 631-637.

de Mutsert, R., Grootendorst, D. C., Indemans, F., Boeschoten, E. W., Krediet, R. T., & Dekker, F. W. (2009). Association between serum albumin and mortality in dialysis patients is partly explained by inflammation, and not by malnutrition. *Journal of Renal Nutrition 19*(2), 127-135.

Detsky, A. S., McLaughlin, J. R., Baker, J. P., Johnston, N., Whittaker, S., Mendelson, R. A., et al. (1987). What is subjective global assessment of nutritional status? *Journal of Parenteral and Enteral nutrition, 11*(1), 8-13.

Diepeveen, S. H., Wetzels, J. F., Bilo, H. J., van Tits, L. J., & Stalenhoef, A. F. (2008). Cholesterol in end-stage renal disease: the good, the bad or the ugly? [Review]. *The Netherlands journal of medicine, 66*(2), 53-61.

Dungan, K. M., Guster, T., DeWalt, D. A., & Buse, J. B. (2007). A comparison of lipid and lipoprotein measurements in the fasting and nonfasting states in patients with type 2 diabetes. *Current Medical Research and Opinion, 23*(11), 2689-2695.

Eisenhardt, S. U., Habersberger, J., Murphy, A., Chen, Y. C., Woollard, K. J., Bassler, N., et al. (2009). Dissociation of pentameric to monomeric C-reactive protein on activated platelets localizes inflammation to atherosclerotic plaques. *Circulation Research, 105*(2), 128-137.

Eisenhardt, S. U., Habersberger, J., & Peter, K. (2009). Monomeric C-reactive protein generation on activated platelets: the missing link between inflammation and atherothrombotic risk. *Trends in Cardiovascular Medicine 19*(7), 232-237.

Fasshauer, M., Klein, J., Lossner, U., & Paschke, R. (2003). Interleukin (IL)-6 mRNA expression is stimulated by insulin, isoproterenol, tumour necrosis factor alpha, growth hormone, and IL-6 in 3T3-L1 adipocytes. *Hormone and Metabolic Research, 35*(3), 147-152.

Fleischmann, E. H., Bower, J. D., & Salahudeen, A. K. (2001). Risk factor paradox in hemodialysis: better nutrition as a partial explanation. *Asaio Journal, 47*(1), 74-81.

Genest, J. (2010). C-reactive protein: risk factor, biomarker and/or therapeutic target? *The Canadian Journal of Cardiology, 26 Suppl A*, 41A-44A.

Iseki, K., Kawazoe, N., & Fukiyama, K. (1993). Serum albumin is a strong predictor of death in chronic dialysis patients. *Kidney International, 44*, 115-119.

Ji, S. R., Wu, Y., Potempa, L. A., Qiu, Q., & Zhao, J. (2006). Interactions of C-reactive protein with low-density lipoproteins: implications for an active role of modified C-reactive protein in atherosclerosis. *The International Journal of Biochemistry & Cell Biology, 38*(4), 648-661.

Kalantar-Zadeh, K. (2007). What is so bad about reverse epidemiology anyway? *Seminars in Dialysis, 20*(6), 593-601.

Kalantar-Zadeh, K., Block, G., Humphreys, M. H., & Kopple, J. D. (2003). Reverse epidemiology of cardiovascular risk factors in maintenance dialysis patients. *Kidney International, 63*(3), 793-808.

Kalantar-Zadeh, K., Gutekunst, L., Mehrotra, R., Kovesdy, C. P., Bross, R., Shinaberger, C. S., et al. (2010). Understanding sources of dietary phosphorus in the treatment of patients with chronic kidney disease. *Clinical journal of the American Society of Nephrology : CJASN, 5*(3), 519-530.

Kalantar-Zadeh, K., & Kopple, J. D. (2001). Relative contributions of nutrition and inflammation to clinical outcome in dialysis patients. *American Journal of Kidney Diseases, 38*(6), 1343-1350.

Kalantar-Zadeh, K., Kopple, J. D., Block, G., & Humphreys, M. H. (2001). A malnutrition-inflammation score is correlated with morbidity and mortality in maintenance hemodialysis patients. *American Journal of Kidney Diseases, 38*(6), 1251-1263.

Kaysen, G. A. (2003). Serum albumin concentration in dialysis patients: why does it remain resistant to therapy? *Kidney international. Supplement*(87), S92-98.

Kaysen, G. A. (2009). Biochemistry and biomarkers of inflamed patients: why look, what to assess. *Clinical Journal of the American Society of Nephrology : CJASN, 4 Suppl 1*, S56-63.

Kilpatrick, R. D., McAllister, C. J., Kovesdy, C. P., Derose, S. F., Kopple, J. D., & Kalantar-Zadeh, K. (2007). Association between serum lipids and survival in hemodialysis patients and impact of race. *Journal of the American Society of Nephrology 18*(1), 293-303.

Kopple, J. D. (1997). Nutritional status as a predictor of morbidity and mortality in maintenance dialysis patients. *Asaio Journal, 43*(3), 246-250.

Kopple, J. D., Zhu, X., Lew, N. L., & Lowrie, E. G. (1999). Body weight-for-height relationships predict mortality in maintenance hemodialysis patients. *Kidney Int, 56*(3), 1136-1148.

Krane, V., Winkler, K., Drechsler, C., Lilienthal, J., Marz, W., & Wanner, C. (2009). Association of LDL cholesterol and inflammation with cardiovascular events and mortality in hemodialysis patients with type 2 diabetes mellitus. *American Journal of Kidney Diseases, 54*(5), 902-911.

Lippi, G., Favaloro, E. J., Montagnana, M., & Franchini, M. (2010). C-reactive protein and venous thromboembolism: causal or casual association? *Clinical Chemistry and Laboratory Medicine 48*(12), 1693-1701.

Liu, Y., Coresh, J., Eustace, J. A., Longenecker, J. C., Jaar, B., Fink, N. E., et al. (2004). Association between cholesterol level and mortality in dialysis patients: role of inflammation and malnutrition. *The Journal of the American Medical Association, 291*(4), 451-459.

Lowrie, E. G., & Lew, N. L. (1990). Death risk in hemodialysis patients: the predictive value of commonly measured variables and an evaluation of death rate differences between facilities. *American Journal of Kidney Diseases, 15*(5), 458-482.

Malgorzewicz, S., Aleksandrowicz-Wrona, E., Owczarzak, A., Debska-Slizien, A., Rutkowski, B., & Lysiak-Szydlowska, W. (2010). Adipokines and nutritional status for patients on maintenance hemodialysis. *Journal of Renal Nutrition, 20*(5), 303-308.

Montazerifar, F., Hashemi, M., Karajibani, M., & Dikshit, M. (2010). Hemodialysis alters lipid profiles, total antioxidant capacity, and vitamins A, E, and C concentrations in humans. *Journal of Medicinal Food, 13*(6), 1490-1493.

Moretti, H. D., Johnson, A. M., & Keeling-Hathaway, T. J. (2009). Effects of protein supplementation in chronic hemodialysis and peritoneal dialysis patients. *Journal of Renal Nutrition, 19*(4), 298-303.

Movilli, E., Brunori, G., Camerini, C., Vizzardi, V., Gaggia, P., Cassamali, S., et al. (2006). The kind of vascular access influences the baseline inflammatory status and epoetin response in chronic hemodialysis patients. *Blood Purification, 24*(4), 387-393.

Nanayakkara, P. W., & Gaillard, C. A. (2010). Vascular disease and chronic renal failure: new insights. [Review]. *The Netherlands Journal of Medicine, 68*(1), 5-14.

Nishizawa, Y., Shoji, T., Ishimura, E., Inaba, M., & Morii, H. (2001). Paradox of risk factors for cardiovascular mortality in uremia: is a higher cholesterol level better for atherosclerosis in uremia? *American Journal of Kidney Diseases, 38*(4 Suppl 1), S4-7.

Pecoits-Filho, R., Barany, P., Lindholm, B., Heimburger, O., & Stenvinkel, P. (2002). Interleukin-6 is an independent predictor of mortality in patients starting dialysis treatment. *Nephrology Dialysis Transplantation, 17*(9), 1684-1688.

Phillips, A., Shaper, A. G., & Whincup, P. H. (1989). Association between serum albumin and mortality from cardiovascular disease, cancer, and other causes. *The Lancet, 334*(8677), 1434-1436.

Sachdeva, M., Kovalchuk, O., Bitzer, M., & Mokrzycki, M. H. (2009). Vascular access type and changes in inflammatory markers in incident dialysis patients: a pilot study. *The Journal of Vascular Access, 10*(3), 174-179.

Santos, N. S., Draibe, S. A., Kamimura, M. A., Canziani, M. E., Cendoroglo, M., Junior, A. G., et al. (2003). Is serum albumin a marker of nutritional status in hemodialysis patients without evidence of inflammation? *Artificial Organs, 27*(8), 681-686.

Sattar, N., & Lowe, G. D. (2006). High sensitivity C-reactive protein and cardiovascular disease: an association built on unstable foundations? *Annals of Clinical Biochemistry, 43*(Pt 4), 252-256.

Sprague, A. H., & Khalil, R. A. (2009). Inflammatory cytokines in vascular dysfunction and vascular disease. *Biochemical Pharmacology, 78*(6), 539-552.

Stenvinkel, P., Barany, P., Heimburger, O., Pecoits-Filho, R., & Lindholm, B. (2002). Mortality, malnutrition, and atherosclerosis in ESRD: what is the role of interleukin-6? *Kidney International Supplement*(80), 103-108.

Stolic, R. (2010). Obesity in renal failure--health or disease? *Medical Hypotheses, 75*(6), 497-500.

Sun, H., Koike, T., Ichikawa, T., Hatakeyama, K., Shiomi, M., Zhang, B., et al. (2005). C-reactive protein in atherosclerotic lesions: its origin and pathophysiological significance. *American Journal of Pathology, 167*(4), 1139-1148.

Taylor, L. M., Kalantar-Zadeh, K., Markewich, T., Colman, S., Benner, D., Sim, J. J., et al. (2011). Dietary egg whites for phosphorus control in maintenance haemodialysis patients: a pilot study. *Journal of Renal Care, 37*(1), 16-24.

Third Report of the National Cholesterol Education Program Expert Panel on Detection, Evaluation, and Treatment of High Blood Cholesterol in Adults (Adult Treatment Panel III) Final Report. (2002).

Trivedi, H., Xiang, Q., & Klein, J. P. (2009). Risk factors for non-fatal myocardial infarction and cardiac death in incident dialysis patients. *Nephrology, Dialysis, Transplantation : Official Publication of the European Dialysis and Transplant Association - European Renal Association, 24*(1), 258-266.

Tsirpanlis, G., Boufidou, F., Zoga, M., Triantafyllis, G., Fatourou, A., Stamatelou, K., et al. (2009). Low cholesterol along with inflammation predicts morbidity and mortality in hemodialysis patients. *Hemodialysis International, 13*(2), 197-204.

Vaziri, N. D. (2009). Causes of dysregulation of lipid metabolism in chronic renal failure. *Seminars in Dialysis, 22*(6), 644-651.

Wystrychowski, G., Kitzler, T. M., Thijssen, S., Usvyat, L., Kotanko, P., & Levin, N. W. (2009). Impact of switch of vascular access type on key clinical and laboratory parameters in chronic haemodialysis patients. *Nephrology Dialysis Transplantation, 24*(7), 2194-2200.

Xue, J. L., Dahl, D., Ebben, J. P., & Collins, A. J. (2003). The association of initial hemodialysis access type with mortality outcomes in elderly Medicare ESRD patients. *American Journal of Kidney Diseases, 42*(5), 1013-1019.

Yeun, J. Y., Levine, R. A., Mantadilok, V., & Kaysen, G. A. (2000). C-Reactive protein predicts all-cause and cardiovascular mortality in hemodialysis patients. *American Journal of Kidney Diseases, 35*(3), 469-476.

Zimmermann, J., Herrlinger, S., Pruy, A., Metzger, T., & Wanner, C. (1999). Inflammation enhances cardiovascular risk and mortality in hemodialysis patients. *Kidney International, 55*(2), 648-658.

Part 3

Complications

17

Complications and Managements of Hyperphosphatemia in Dialysis

Eiji Takeda, Hironori Yamamoto, Hisami Yamanaka-Okumura and Yutaka Taketani
University of Tokushima Graduate School
Japan

1. Introduction

1.1 High mortality in dialysis patients

Dialysis patients have extraordinarily high mortality rates. Cardiac disease is the major cause of death accounting for 43% of all-cause mortality among patients receiving hemodialysis and peritoneal dialysis [Henry et al., 2002; US Renal Data System Annual Data Report Bethesta, 2005]. In previous report, patients with end-stage kidney disease (chronic kidney disease (CKD) stage 5) on dialysis, in comparison with the general population, also have a 3- to 30-fold increase in mortality, depending on the age group examined, and cardiovascular disease accounts for more than half of all deaths, with myocardial infarction, ischaemic cardiomyopathy, stroke and peripheral vascular disease making up the bulk of deaths (Foley et al., 1998). The marked excess in cardiovascular mortality in CKD, compared with the general population, is not explained by the presence of traditional Framingham risk factors, such as diabetes, smoking, hypertension and elevated cholesterol levels (Zoccali, 2000; Longenecker et al., 2002). With vascular calcification and arterial stiffness being observed in young and middle-aged dialysis patients without conventional cardiovascular risk factors (London et al., 2003), the search for non-traditional risk factors has led to increasing evidence of a multitude of factors that contribute to ectopic calcification in CKD.

1.2 High mortality rate and hyperphosphatemia

Inorganic phosphate (phosphate) retention, or hyperphosphatemia, has been identified as playing a major role in the progression of renal failure and in the generation of secondary hyperparathyroidism and uremic bone disease (Slatopolsky et al., 2002). Further observational data have also shown a significant association of hyperphosphatemia with increased mortality among patients who have end-stage kidney disease and are on hemodialysis (Block et al., 1998; Owen & Lowrie, 1998; Ganesh et al., 2001). Moreover, elevated serum phosphorus has been associated with an increased risk for cardiovascular mortality and hospitalization (all-cause, cardiovascular, and fracture) among dialysis patients (Block et al., 2004). Elevated phosphorus and Ca × P are also independent risk factors for all-cause and cardiovascular mortality in CKD stage 5, and increased levels of parathyroid hormone may be associated with both cardiovascular disease and increased vascular calcification (Braun et al., 1996; Block et al., 1998; Ganesh et al., 2001; Wang et al., 2003; Young et al., 2005). Thus, phosphorus has the potential to induce vascular calcification and may be cardiotoxic (Achinger & Ayus, 2006). Hyperphosphatemia is sometimes regarded as a distinct syndrome (Hruska et al., 2008), and its treatment should be considered preferentially and even independently of other laboratory values (Fig. 1).

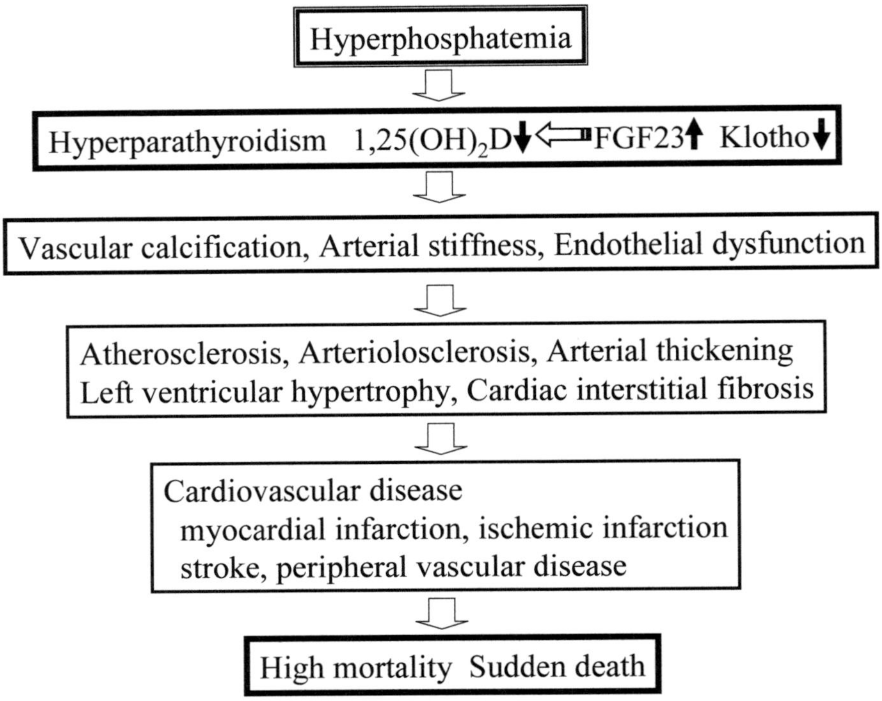

Fig. 1. Hyperphosphatemia in hemodialysis

2. Phosphate metabolism in human

2.1 Phosphate metabolism in normal physiology

Phosphorus is essential for multiple and diverse biological functions, including cellular signal transduction, mineral metabolism, and energy exchange. Although more than 80% of total body phosphorus is stored in bone and teeth, intracellular phosphorus exists in the form of organic compounds such as adenosine triphosphate and as free anions like $H_2PO_4^-$, which are commonly referred to as phosphate. Serum phosphorus primarily occurs in the form of inorganic phosphate, which is maintained within the physiological range by regulation of dietary absorption, bone formation, and renal excretion, as well as equilibration with intracellular stores (Takeda et al., 2000; Bringhurst et al., 2004; Fukagawa et al., 2004; Blumsohn, 2004).

Phosphate absorption in the renal proximal tubule and the small intestine is important for phosphate homeostasis. This is a major regulator of phosphate homeostasis and has the phosphate reabsorptive capacity to accommodate physiologic phosphate requirement. Up to 70% of filtered phosphate is reabsorbed in the proximal tubule where sodium-dependent

phosphate transport systems in the brush-border membrane mediate the rate limiting step in the overall phosphate reabsorptive process (Murer et al, 2000; Takeda et al, 2000; Miyamoto et al, 2007; Tenenhouse, 2005; Biber et al, 2009). Three different types of sodium-dependent phosphate transporters have been identified till now, types I, II and III. The sodium-dependent phosphate transport system includes the type IIa and type IIc Na-dependent phosphate cotransporters, which are localized in the apical membrane of the renal proximal tubular cells, and the type IIb Na-dependent phosphate cotransporter, which is localized in the apical membrane of the intestinal epithelial cells. The type IIa Na-dependent phosphate transporter is the major determinant of plasma phosphate level and urinary phosphate excretion (Murer et al, 2000; Takeda et al, 2000; Miyamoto et al, 2007; Tenenhouse, 2005; Biber et al, 2009). This transporter is regulated by physiological stimuli, for example, type IIa transporter levels in the apical membrane are increased in response to dietary restriction of phosphate and 1,25-dihydroxy-vitamin D_3 [$1,25(OH)_2D_3$] and decreased in response to parathyroid hormone, or a high- phosphate diet. In addition, intestinal phosphate transport activity and type IIb Na-dependent phosphate transporter levels are upregulated by $1,25(OH)_2D_3$ (Xu et al., 2002; Segawa et al., 2004).
In addition, fibroblast growth factor 23 (FGF23), a recently identified member of the FGF family, is involved in renal phosphate homeostasis (Yu X & White, 2005; Yu & White, 2005). FGF23 induces urinary phosphate excretion by suppressing the expression of type IIa and IIc Na-dependent phosphate cotransporters in the brush border of renal proximal tubules (Shimada et al., 2004; Shimada et al., 2005). It also suppresses $1,25(OH)_2D$ production by inhibiting 1a-hydroxylase (CYP27B1), which converts 25-hydroxyvitamin D [25(OH)D] to $1,25(OH)_2D$, and by stimulating 24-hydroxylase (CYP24), which converts $1,25(OH)_2D$ to inactive metabolites in the proximal tubule of the kidney (Shimada et al., 2004; Shimada et al., 2005). Given the fact that FGF23 promotes renal phosphaturia, its secretion should be regulated by serum phosphate levels. Experimental and clinical studies showed that several days of dietary phosphate loading lead to an increase in serum FGF23 in humans (Ferrari et al, 2005; Perwad et al., 2005; Nishida et al., 2006).

2.2 Phosphate metabolism in hemodialysis patients

Several studies have measured circulating FGF23 levels in predialysis and dialysis patients and reported progressively elevated FGF23 levels as serum creatinine or phosphate levels increase (Larsson et al., 2003; Imanishi et al., 2004). Thus, it appears that in patients with CKD, FGF23 production increases to counteract chronic phosphate retention by promoting urinary phosphate excretion in the face of reduced nephron mass. Notably, in this setting, a previous study showed that FGF23 was a strong independent predictor of diminished $1,25(OH)_2D$ levels, even after adjustment for renal function, serum phosphorus levels and 25(OH)D levels (Gutierrez et al., 2005). This finding suggests that in patients with CKD, increases in FGF23 intended to maintain neutral phosphate balance result in suppression of renal $1,25(OH)_2D$ production, thereby triggering the early development of secondary hyperparathyroidism (Fig. 1).

3. Cardiovascular disease in hemodyalysis

3.1 Hyperphosphatemia and cardiovascular disease

Cardiomyopathy and ischemic heart disease including acute myocardial infarctions, which are both common conditions in dialysis patients, likely play a role in the development of sudden death. After percutaneous and surgical coronary revascularization, dialysis patients are still remaining at a high risk for sudden cardiac death (Furgeson, 2008). Hyperphosphatemia is a known factor contributing to the increased risk of cardiac death both in patients with end-stage renal disease and in those under renal replacement treatment with dialysis (Goodman et al., 2000). In patients with renal disease, in fact, the well-known relationship between hyperphosphataemia, secondary hyperparathyroidism, bone turnover and extra osseous calcifications has recently been followed by the recognition of a major role played by elevated serum phosphorus levels in the induction of vascular calcification, cardiac interstitial fibrosis and arterial thickening which highly increase the risk of cardiac death (Goodman et al., 2000; Block & Port, 2000; Amann et al., 2003; Goldsmith et al., 2004; Floege & Ketteler, 2004).

3.2 Vascular calcification

Phosphate is probably the predominant inducer of vascular calcification, and elevated serum levels are strongly associated with increased vascular calcification and mortality (Goodman et al., 2000). Elevated phosphate triggers a concentration-dependent precipitation of calcium in vascular smooth muscle cells, and phosphate is also a potent stimulus for the differentiation of vascular smooth muscle cells. In vitro studies demonstrate that high phosphate levels in incubation media enhance calcification with associated extracellular matrix synthesis(Jono et al., 2000). Phosphate and sodium dependent phosphate transporter seem to play a very important role in vascular smooth muscle cells mineralization. Type III sodium-dependent phosphate transporter presents two discrete subtypes, Pit-1 and Pit-2. In human vascular smooth muscle cells, Pit-1 is mainly expressed (London et al., 2000). Apatite formation by smooth muscle cells, as a response to increased phosphate levels, is fully inhibited by phosphonoformic acid (PFA), a sodium dependent phosphate transporter inhibitor, a finding supporting the notion that vascular calcification is an active rather than passive cellular process (Giachelli et al., 2001; Ketteler et al., 2003).

Hyperphosphataemia induces osteocalcin and Cbfa-1 in vascular smooth muscle cells and promotes vascular calcification. Animals deficient in Cbfa-1 fail to mineralize bone(Komori et al., 1997), and there is also increased expression of Cbfa-1 when vascular smooth muscle cells are incubated in uremic serum compared with pooled human serum (Moe et al., 2003). There is now considerable evidence that hyperphosphataemia regulates several signalling pathways of cell functions. Of great interest is the recent identification of a novel phosphate-regulating gene, klotho (Kuro-o et al., 1997; Yoshida et al., 2002), which in mice is involved in the development of a syndrome resembling human ageing. The klotho mutant mice show abnormal calcium phosphate vitamin D metabolism and develop hyperphosphataemia and vascular calcification (Kuro-o et al., 1997; Yoshida et al., 2002). Hyperphosphataemia also down-regulates klotho gene expression (Fig. 1).

3.3 Endothelial dysfunction

Endothelial dysfunction is the principal cause of atherosclerosis resulting in cardio vascular disease (Ross, 1999). High phosphate loading on endothelial cells inhibited nitrogen oxide (NO) production through increased reactive oxygen species (ROS) production and endothelial NO syntase (eNOS) inactivation via conventional protein kinase C, resulting in impaired endothelium-dependent vasodilation (Shuto et al., 2009). Furthermore, dietary phosphate loading can deteriorate flow-mediated vasodilation in healthy men, suggesting that dietary phosphate loading or elevation of serum phosphorus level may be a risk factor for cardiovascular disease in healthy persons as well as CKD patients (Takeda et al., 2006; Shuto et al., 2009). Di Marco et al. also reported that high phosphate loading increased ROS production via phosphate influx and induced apoptosis in endothelial cells (Di Marco et al., 2008). Association of serum phosphorus level and vascular dysfunction has been well investigated, because fasting serum phosphorus level could not increase in healthy persons, even if dietary phosphate was overloaded. However, postprandial phosphorus elevation was associated with %FMD in young healthy men (Shuto et al., 2009). Thus, dietary phosphate loading can cause endothelial dysfunction within a short time. Oxidative stress and decreased NO production in endothelial cells are possible mechanisms for the impaired endothelial function mediated by phosphate loading (Fig. 2).

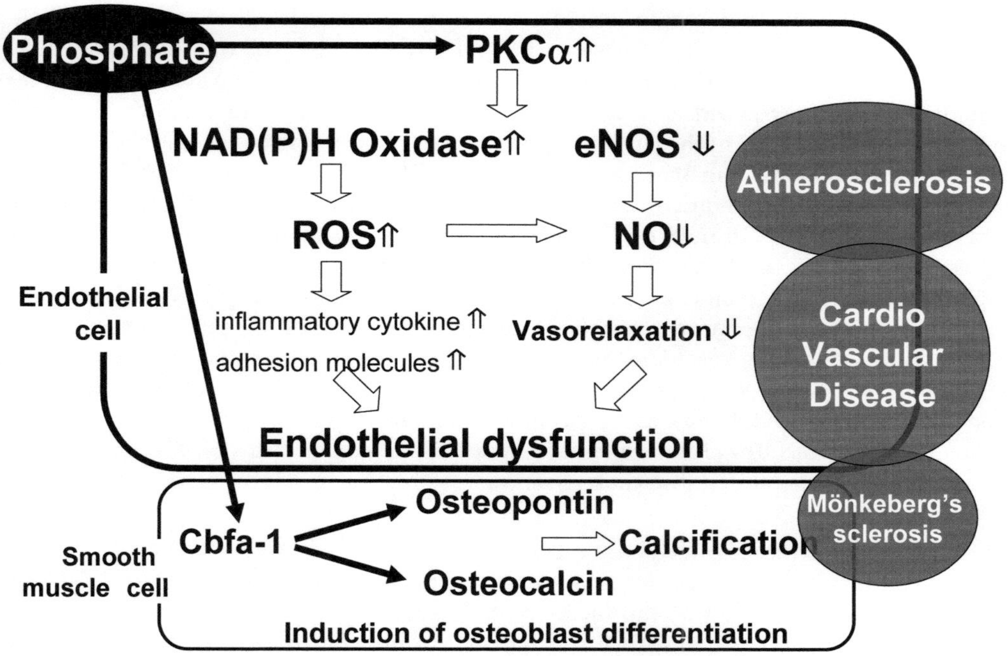

Fig. 2. Dual pathways for vascular dysfunction caused by hyperphosphatemia

3.4 Arterial stiffness

Arterial disease observed in end-stage kidney disease patients is characterized by extensive intimal as well as medial calcification. Histological changes in coronary arteries from dialysis patients, compared with age matched controls, reveal a similar magnitude of atherosclerotic plaque burden and intimal thickness but markedly increased medial calcification (arteriolosclerosis) (Schwarz et al., 2000). Medial calcification has been shown to affect vascular elasticity and leads to increased arterial wall stiffness of large capacity, elastic-type arteries like the aorta and the common carotid artery, increased pulse pressure and decreased perfusion of coronary arteries during diastole (Blacher et al., 1998; London, 2003; Speer & Giachelli, 2004). Recent studies also demonstrated that elevated FGF23 levels were associated with arterial stiffness, increased left ventricular mass index and increased prevalence of left ventricular hypertrophy in patients with CKD (Hsu & Wu, 2009; Mirza et al., 2009; Gutierrez et al., 2009).

4. Management of hyperphosphatemia in hemodialysis patients

4.1 Target of management

As elevated serum phosphorus and calcium levels are associated with vascular calcification and cardiovascular mortality in CKD, priority should be given to normalization of these parameters. It is generally accepted that adequate control of serum phosphorus remains a cornerstone in the clinical management of patients with CKD not only to attenuate the progression of secondary hyperparathyroidism but also possibly to reduce the risk for vascular calcification and cardiovascular mortality. A Ca x P more tan 72 mg^2/dl^2 is associated with a significant increase in the relative risk (RR) of mortality (RR = 1.34) compared with Ca x P less than 50 mg^2/dl^2 (Cozzolino et al., 2001). In a study in patients on hemodialysis, those who did not experience valvular calcification had maintained Ca x P at an average of 51 mg^2/dl^2 in the 6 months prior to the study, while those who did experience valvular calcification had an average Ca x P of 60 mg^2/dl^2 (Ribeiro et al., 1998). The target of treatment should be to maintain serum phosphorus level less than 5 mg/dl with serum calcium level less than 10 mg/dl to prevent cardio vascular consequences. This will allow the maintenance of Ca x P less than 50 mg^2/dl^2, a level which available evidence has so far shown not to promote calcification or increase mortality (Ribeiro et al., 1998).

High FGF23 levels are more strongly associated with kidney disease progression, left ventricular hypertrophy, vascular disease, and mortality than serum phosphorus levels, and were most predictive of adverse events in patients with normal serum phosphorus (Thadhani et al., 2008; Oliveira et al., 2010). Dietary phosphate binders can lower FGF23 in CKD (Oliveira et al., 2010). Management of hyperphosphatemia relies on dietary restriction, the use of phosphate binders and dialysis.

4.2 Dietary restriction of phosphate intake

The average diet in North America and Europe contains approximately 1,000 to 1,500 mg of phosphorus per day (Willett & Buzzard, 1998). Dietary approach to phosphate retention in advanced renal failure patients, dietary approach to phosphate reduction is an important step in the treatment of hyperphosphatemia. The level of expression of klotho mRNA was greatly reduced in the kidneys of all chronic renal failure patients. Dietary phosphate restriction induced klotho expression, which enhances the beneficial effect of phosphate restriction in patients with chronic renal failure and or on hemodialysis. However, dietary restriction cannot considerably reduce the level of phosphate retention. As dialysis patients tend to need higher levels of protein due to the losses via dialysis, tight restriction on phosphate is difficult without compromising a patient's nutritional status. Because most dietary phosphate is contained in protein-rich foods, there is some concern about excessive protein restriction. In fact, the minimum amount of protein of 1.2 g/kg body weight/day, recommended to prevent malnutrition makes planning a diet with less than 1 g of phosphorus impossible (Kopple, 2001; Eknoyan et al., 2003). Recommendations that call for 1.0 to 1.2 g/kg/day protein will usually obligate a phosphorus intake of 800 to 1,400

mg/day. Net phosphorus absorption averages 60% to 70% of intake (Delmez & Slatopolsky, 1992; Sheikh et al., 1989), however, this percentage can rise as high as 86% of ingested phosphate with calcitriol use and decrease to 30% to 40% of ingested phosphate with optimal binder usage.(Sheikh et al., 1989; Delmez & Slatopolsky, 1992).
Other foods that are high in phosphate are processed foods such as processed meats which have phosphate based additives to improve the consistency and appearance of the food. Since 1990, intake of phosphate from additives has doubled and has been 1,000 mg in USA (Calvo & Park, 1996). This is the amount that some renal patients are advised for the whole day from all food groups (James & Jackson, 2002). As people are becoming more reliant on processed and packaged meals due to convenience, phosphate from these sources needs to be considered when advising on diet. Fresh meat is considered suitable for someone following a phosphate restriction, however processed foods may in fact be providing much more phosphate than realised (Sullivan et al., 2007). Beverages such as sodas, juices and sport drinks also contain phosphate additives (Murphy-Gutekunst, 2007). It has been estimated that for a person on hemodialysis the average phosphate removal per day is 300 mg (Vaithilingham et al., 2004). This leaves the patient with a positive balance for phosphate.

4.3 Hemodialysis

The clearance of phosphate varies among the different modalities of dialysis. Ideally, adequate dialysis in any form would remove adequate amounts of all uremic toxins, including phosphate. Unfortunately, conventional thrice-weekly hemodialysis (4 h duration) removes approximately 900 mg of phosphorus each treatment (an average of only 300 mg/day) (Gotch et al., 2003). Increasing the dosage of dialysis, preferably to lengthy three times per week dialysis, hemodiafiltration, or, even better, daily/nightly dialysis may prevent phosphorus retention and even require no dietary phosphate restriction or the withdrawal of phosphate binders (Maduell et al., 2003; Benaroia et al., 2008). However, regular dialysis treatment is not able to remove all the phosphorus ingested with a diet containing protein of 1.0 - 1.2 g/kg/day (Mallick & Gokal, 1999).

4.4 Phosphate binders

Isakova et al analyzed a prospective cohort study of 10,044 incident hemodialysis patients at Fresenius Medical Care facilities in 2004 and 2005 comparing 1-year all-cause mortality among patients who were treated with phosphate binders (Isakova et al., 2009). In an intention-to-treat analysis, they compared patients who began treatment with any phosphate binder during the first 90 days after initiating hemodialysis, with those who remained untreated during that period. Treatment with phosphate binders was independently associated with decreased mortality compared with no treatment. In the unmatched cohort, the phosphate binder-treated group had a relative risk reduction of 42%, while in the intention-to-treat and as-treated analyses, the magnitude of the survival benefit ranged between 18% and 30% in multivariate models. The association between use of phosphorus binders and survival was observed within each quartile of baseline serum phosphorus except the lowest. Results from human data suggest that lowering of phosphorus levels by intake of phosphate binders will substantially reduce serum FGF-23 levels (Koiwa et al., 2005; Pande et al., 2006). In this prospective observational study, treatment with phosphate binders was associated with a reduced 1-year mortality among incident hemodialysis patients (Isakova et al., 2009).

Sevelamer hydrochloride and lanthanum carbonate are a phosphate binders containing neither calcium nor aluminium, and are useful in those being administered concurrent vitamin D to reduce the potential for hypercalcemia. Attenuation in the progression of coronary artery calcification, after 6 and 12 months, was shown in hemodialysis patients treated with sevelamer, with reduced serum calcium, compared with patients on calcium carbonate (Chertow et al., 2002). A more recent randomized study of 114 incident hemodialysis patients demonstrated a survival advantage for patients on sevelamer compared with calcium carbonate after 18-month follow up (Block et al., 2007). A further beneficial effect of sevelamer has been proved on markers of coronary artery and aortic calcification compared with calcium based phosphate binders (Chertow et al., 2002). The attenuation of vascular and, in particular, coronary calcifications compared with calcium-based phosphate binders in end-stage kidney disease patients under dialysis has been studied by electron beam computed tomography (Raggi, 2002; Raggi, 2004). High doses of sevelamer (3.2–8 g/day) are necessary to bring hyperphosphatemia back to target level, and the number of pills per day (about 8 x 800 mg tablets) may certainly be a conditioning factor for the patient's compliance (Chertow et al., 2002).
Patients with end-stage kidney disease treated with lanthanum carbonate up to 2.5–3.8 g/day for up to 2 years have been reported to obtain effective reduction of serum phosphorus level (Finn, 2006). Lanthanum-carbonate-treated patients have, also been shown to reach a significantly reduced calcium/phosphate product and parathyroid hormone level compared with the placebo (Joy & Finn, 2009). Lanthanum carbonate, therefore, is an effective, at least as effective as calcium carbonate, well-tolerated phosphate binder (Hutchison, 2004; Hutchison et al., 2006). However, despite the very encouraging results, further studies involving larger numbers of patients are needed to definitively establish the long-term safety of lanthanum regarding tissue deposition, as well as its efficacy on vascular calcifications or outcomes in treated patients, which also need to be confirmed in the long term.

4.5 Combination in treatment

A multiple-factor approach can be used to reduce serum phosphate including reduced phosphorus intake in the diet, using phosphate binders efficiently and avoidance of under- dialysis. The patient's diet should be high in nutrition but with the lowest possible phosphorus content. Since dietary control of phosphorus intake and dialysis removal are usually not sufficient, phosphate binders are usually needed as adjuvants to increase fecal excretion (Bover et al; 2005). For an optimal protein diet of 1-1.2 g/kg/day, the phosphorus intake was 778-1,444 mg/day and 5,500-10,000 mg/week. Dialysis has limited ability for phosphate control, although phosphate removal by hemodialysis is very much a time-dependent process. The amount of phosphorus removed by hemodialysis, extrapolated to an average week, is 250-300 mg/day. The introduction of non-calcium-based phosphate binders has enabled a reduction in the total phosphate load and provides a useful tool in the prevention of vascular calcification in CKD. The use of phosphate binders may decrease the phosphorus absorbed from the diet to 40% (Llach & Bover, 2000). In these circumstances, 320 mg of phosphorus and 21g of protein (0.3-0.35g of protein/kg/day) intake should be the critical value above which a positive balance of phosphate may occur (Fig. 3).

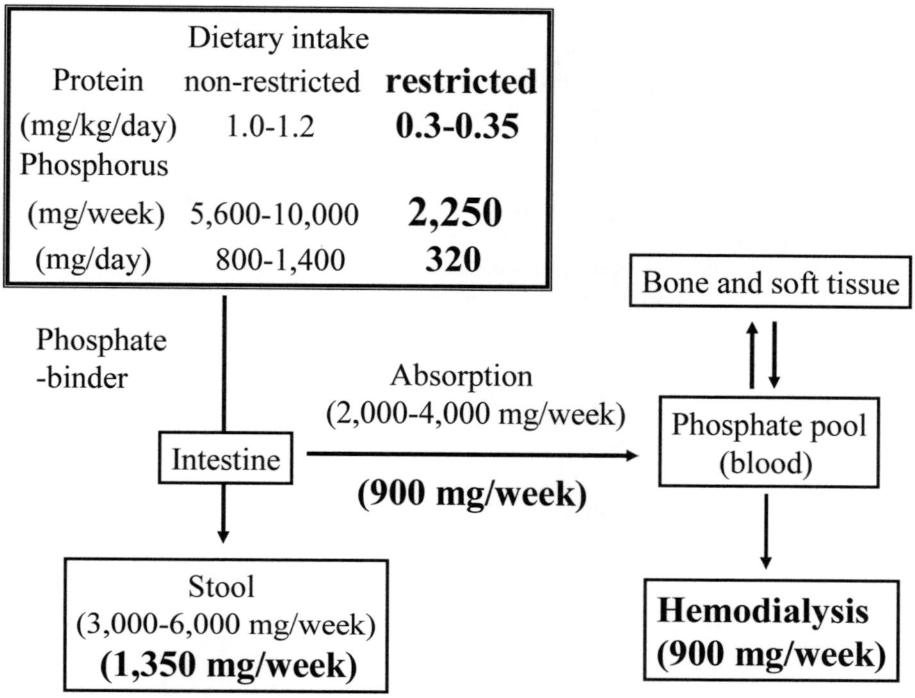

Fig. 3. Phosphate balance in hemodialysis patient
Those in restricted protein and phosphate intake are shown in bold.

Successful control of phosphate is one of the key aspects in the management of dialysis patients (Rodriguez-Benot et al., 2005; Young et al., 2004, Young et al., 2005), However, numerous studies have revealed the difficulty in achieving phosphorus targets less than 5.5 mg/dl (Arenas et al., 2006; Lorenzo et al., 2006: Wei et al., 2006), despite the wide variety of drugs available for its treatment (Joy & Finn, 2003; Sprague, 2007; Arenas et al., 2008). Both endothelial dysfunction and medial calcification are closely associated with development of cardiovascular disease. It is well known that long-term exposure to phosphate, generally observed in end-stage renal failure patients, can mediate vascular calcification (Jono et al., 2000; Giachelli, 2003). Dietary high phosphate loading can be involved in the postprandial elevation of serum phosphorus level, and this short-term exposure to phosphate was enough to decrease endothelium-dependent vasodilation.

5. Conclusion

The goals of therapy have been to reduce phosphorus intake with low protein diet and phosphate binders. Since low protein diet is thought to be induce malnutrition, it is thought that strict adherence to a low protein diet is not practical. A diet rich in proteins is usually also rich in phosphorus. However, proteins with very different phosphorus contents can provide equivalent nutritional value, as can be seen from the difference in phosphorus content between meat, cheese, and eggs. Egg white is an excellent example of food with a high level of protein but low phosphorus content. Moe et al. demonstrates the importance of the protein source of phosphate in overall mineral metabolism after only 7 days of controlled diets. Despite equivalent protein and phosphorus concentrations in the diets, subjects had lower serum phosphorus levels, a trend toward decreased urine 24-hour phosphorus excretion, and significantly decreased FGF23 levels in the vegetarian diet compared with the meat-based diet (Moe et al., 2011).

Lafage et al. (Lafage et al., 1992) used a very low protein diet (0.3 g/kg/d) supplemented with amino acids and ketoanalogues and with only 1 g of calcium carbonate and 1,000 IU of vitamin D_2 in 17 patients with advanced renal failure. They have shown not only a beneficial effect related to the control of hyperphosphatemia on the biologic and histologic parameters of hyperparathyroidism but also a correction of acidosis, which resulted in the disappearance of the osteomalacic component. Thus, dietary control often considered to be of minor importance, is actually one of the major keys to success in the management of hyperphosphataemia.

6. Acknowledgements

The work described in this publication was supported by Grants-in-Aid for Scientific Research from the Ministry of Education, Culture, Sports, Science and Technology in Japan (to ET, HY, and YT).

7. References

Achinger SG, Ayus JC. (2006) Left ventricular hypertrophy: is hyperphosphatemia among dialysis patients a risk factor? *J Am Soc Nephrol* 17(12 suppl 3): S255-S261.

Amann K, Törnig J, Kugel B, Gross ML, Tyralla K, El-Shakmak A, Szabo A, Ritz E. (2003) Hyperphosphatemia aggravates cardiac fibrosis and microvascular disease in experimental uremia. *Kidney Int* 63: 1296–1301.

Arenas MD, Alvarez-Ude F, Gil MT, Soriano A, Egea JJ, Millán I, Amoedo ML, Muray S, Carretón MA. (2006) Application of NKFK/DOQI clinical practice guidelines for bone metabolism and disease: changes of clinical practices and their effects on outcomes and quality standards in three haemodialysis units. *Nephrol Dial Transplant.* 21: 1663-1668.

Arenas MD, Malek T, Gil MT, Moledous A, Nunez C, Alvarez-Ude F. (2008) Use of aluminum-based phosphate-chelators in hemodialysis in the era of ultrapure water. *Nefrologia.* 28: 168-173.

Benaroia M, Pierratos A, Nesrallah GE. (2008) A primer for the prescription of short-daily and nocturnal hemodialysis. *Hemodial Int* 12: 23-29.

Biber J, Hernando N, Forster I, Murer H. (2009) Regulation of phosphate transport in proximal tubules. *Pflu¨gers Arch* 458: 39–52.

Blacher J, Demuth K, Guerin AP, Safar ME, Moatti N, London GM, (1998) Influence of biochemical alterations on arterial stiffness in patients with end-stage renal disease. *Arterioscler Thromb Vasc Biol* 18: 535-541.

Block GA, Hulbert-Shearon TE, Levin NW, Port FK. (1998) Association of serum phosphorus and calcium x phosphate product with mortality risk in chronic hemodialysis patients: A national study. *Am J Kidney Dis* 31: 607–617.

Block GA, Port FK. (2000) Re-evaluation of risks associated with hyperphosphatemia and hyperparathyroidism in dialysis patients: recommendations for a change in management. *Am J Kidney Dis* 35: 1226–1237.

Block GA, Klassen PS, Lazarus JM, Ofsthun N, Lowrie EG, Chertow GM. (2004) Mineral metabolism, mortality, and morbidity in maintenance hemodialysis. *J Am Soc Nephrol* 15: 2208–2218.

Block GA, Raggi P, Bellasi A, Kooienga L, Spiegel DM. (2007) Mortality effect of coronary calcification and phosphate binder choice in incident hemodialysis patients. *Kidney Int.* 71: 438–441.

Blumsohn A. (2004) What have we learnt about the regulation of phosphate metabolism? *Curr Opin Nephrol Hypertens.* 13: 397- 401.

Bover J, Ortiz-Herbener F, Ballarín J, Andrés E, Barceló P. (2005) New therapy strategies in secondary hyperparathyroidism on dialysis (I): new concepts, new treatments. *Nefrologia.* 25 Suppl 2: 100-108.

Braun J, Oldendorf M, Moshage W, Heidler R, Zeitler E, Luft FC. (1996) Electron beam computed tomography in the evaluation of cardiac calcification in chronic dialysis patients. *Am. J. Kidney Dis.* 27: 394–401.

Bringhurst FR, Demay BM, Krane SM, Kronenberg HM. (2004) Bone and mineral metabolism in health and disease. In: Kasper DL, Braunwald E, Fauci AS, Hauser SL, Longo DL, Jameson L, Isselbacher KJ, eds. *Harrison's Principles of Internal Medicine.* New York, NY: McGraw-Hill.

Calvo & Park 1996. Calvo MS, Park YK. (1996).Changing phosphorus content of the U.S. diet: potential for adverse effects on bone. *J Nutr.* 126(4 Suppl):1168S-1180S.

Chertow GM, Burke SK, Raggi P. (2002) Sevelamer attenuates the progression of coronary and aortic calcification in hemodialysis patients. *Kidney Int.* 62: 245–52.

Cozzolino M, Dusso AS, Slatopolsky D. (2001) Role of calciumphosphate product and bone-associated proteins on vascular calcification in renal failure. *J Am Soc Nephrol* 12: 2511–2516.

Delmez JA, Slatopolsky E. (1992) Hyperphosphatemia: its consequences and treatment in patients with chronic renal disease. *Am J Kidney Dis.* 19(4):303-317.

Di Marco GS, Hausberg M, Hillebrand U, Rustemeyer P, Wittkowski W, Lang D, Pavensta¨dt H. (2008) Increased inorganic phosphate induces human endothelial cell apoptosis in vitro. *Am J Physiol Renal Physiol* 294: F1381–1387.

Eknoyan G, Levin A, Levin NW. National Kidney Foundation. (2003) Bone metabolism and disease in chronic kidney disease. *Am J Kidney Dis* 42 [Suppl 3]: S1–S201

Ferrari SL, Bonjour JP, Rizzoli R. (2005) Fibroblast growth factor-23 relationship to dietary phosphate and renal phosphate handling in healthy young men. *J Clin Endocrinol Metab.* 90: 1519-1524.

Finn WF. SPD 405–307 Lanthanum Study Group. (2006) Lanthanum carbonate versus standard therapy for the treatment of hyperphosphatemia: safety and efficacy in chronic maintenance hemodialysis patients. *Clin Nephrol* 65(3): 191-202.

Floege J, Ketteler M. (2004) Vascular calcification in patients with endstage renal disease. *Nephrol Dial Transplant.* 19 [Suppl 5]: V59–V66.

Foley RN, Parfrey PS, Sarnak MJ. (1998) Clinical epidemiology of cardiovascular disease in chronic renal disease. *Am. J. Kidney Dis.* 32: S112–19.

Fukagawa M, Kurokawa K, Papadakis MA. (2004) Fluid and electrolyte disorders. In: Tierney LM, McPhee SJ, Papadakis MA, eds. *Current Medical Diagnosis and Treatment 2005*. New York, NY: McGraw-Hill/Appleton & Lange; 837–867.

Furgeson SB. (2008) Chonchol: Beta-blockade in chronic dialysis patients. *Semin Dial* 21: 43–48.

Ganesh SK, Stack AG, Levin NW, Hulbert-Shearon T, Port FK. (2001) Association of elevated serum PO(4), Ca x PO(4) product, and parathyroid hormone with cardiac mortality risk in chronic hemodialysis patients. *J Am Soc Nephrol* 12: 2131–2138.

Giachelli SM, Jono S, Mori K, Morii H, (2001) Vascular calcification and inorganic phosphate. *Am J Kidney Dis* 38: S34-37.

Giachelli CM. (2003) Vascular calcification: In vitro evidence for the role of inorganic phosphate. *J Am Soc Nephrol* 14: S300–S304.

Goldsmith D, Ritz E, Covic A. (2004) Vascular calcification: a stiff challenge for the nephrologist. *Kidney Int* 66: 1315–1333

Goodman WG, Goldin J, Kuizon BD, Yoon C, Gales B, Sider D, Wang Y, Chung J, Emerick A, Greaser L, Elashoff RM, Salusky IB. (2000) Coronary-artery calcification in young adults with end-stage renal disease who are undergoing dialysis. *N Engl J Med* 342: 1478–1483

Gotch FA, Panlilio F, Sergeyeva O, Rosales L, Folden T, Kaysen G, Levin NW. (2003) A kinetic model of inorganic phosphorus mass balance in hemodialysis therapy. *Blood Purif* 21: 51–57.

Gutierrez O, Isakova T, Rhee E, Shah A, Holmes J, Collerone G, Jüppner H, Wolf M. (2005) Fibroblast growth factor-23 mitigates hyperphosphatemia but accentuates calcitriol deficiency in chronic kidney disease. *J Am Soc Nephrol.* 16: 2205-2215.

Gutiérrez OM, Mannstadt M, Isakova T, Rauh-Hain JA, Tamez H, Shah A, Smith K, Lee H, Thadhani R, Jüppner H, Wolf M. (2008) Fibroblast growth factor 23 and mortality among patients undergoing hemodialysis. *N Engl J Med.* 359(6): 584-592.

Gutiérrez OM, Januzzi JL, Isakova T, Laliberte K, Smith K, Collerone G, Sarwar A, Hoffmann U, Coglianese E, Christenson R, Wang TJ, deFilippi C, Wolf M. (2009) Fibroblast growth factor-23 and left ventricular hypertrophy in chronic kidney disease. *Circulation.* 119: 2545-2552.

Henry RM, Kostense PJ, Bos G, Dekker JM, Nijpels G, Heine RJ, Bouter LM, Stehouwer CD: (2002) Mild renal insufficiency is associated with increased cardiovascular mortality: the Hoorn Study. *Kidney Int* 62: 1402–1407.

Hruska KA, Mathew S, Lund R, Qiu P, Pratt R. (2008) Hyperphosphatemia of chronic kidney disease. *Kidney Int* 74: 148-157.

Hsu HJ, Wu MS. (2009) Fibroblast growth factor 23: a possible cause of left ventricular hypertrophy in hemodialysis patients. *Am J Med Sci.* 337:116-122.

Hutchison AJ. (2004) Improving phosphate-binder therapy as a way forward. *Nephrol Dial Transplant* 19 [Suppl 1]: i19–i24.

Hutchison AJ, Maes B, Vanwalleghem J, Asmus G, Mohamed E, Schmieder R, Backs W, Jamar R, Vosskühler A. (2006) Long-term efficacy and tolerability of lanthanum carbonate: results from a 3-year study. *Nephron Clin Pract* 102: c61–c71.

Imanishi Y, Inaba M, Nakatsuka K, Nagasue K, Okuno S, Yoshihara A, Miura M, Miyauchi A, Kobayashi K, Miki T, Shoji T, Ishimura E, Nishizawa Y. (2004) FGF-23 in patients with end-stage renal disease on hemodialysis. *Kidney Int.* 65: 1943-1946.

Isakova T, Gutiérrez OM, Chang Y, Shah A, Tamez H, Smith K, Thadhani R, Wolf M. (2009) Phosphorus binders and survival on hemodialysis. *J Am Soc Nephrol.* 20: 388-396.

James G, Jackson H: European guidelines for the nutritional care of adult renal patients. (2002) *EDTNA/ERCA*, pp1-52.

Jono S, McKee MD, Murry CE, Shioi A, Nishizawa Y, Mori K, Morii H, Giachelli CM. (2000) Phosphate regulation of vascular smooth muscle cell calcification. *Circ. Res.* 87: E10–17.

Joy MS, Finn WF. (2003) Randomized, double-blind, placebocontrolled, dose-titration, Phase III study assessing the efficacy and tolerability of lanthanum carbonate: a new phosphate binder for the treatment of hyperphosphatemia. *Am J Kidney Dis* 42: 96–107.

Ketteler M, Bongartz P, Westenfeld R, Wildberger JE, Mahnken AH, Böhm R, Metzger T, Wanner C, Jahnen-Dechent W, Floege J. (2003) Association of low fetuin-A (AHSG) concentrations in serum with cardiovascular mortality in patients on dialysis: a cross-sectional study. *Lancet* 361: 827–833.

Koiwa F, Kazama JJ, Tokumoto A, Onoda N, Kato H, Okada T, Nii-Kono T, Fukagawa M, Shigematsu T; ROD21 Clinical Research Group. (2005) Sevelamer hydrochloride and calcium bicarbonate reduce serum fibroblast growth factor 23 levels in dialysis patients. *Ther Apher Dial* 9: 336–339.

Komori T, Yagi H, Nomura S, Yamaguchi A, Sasaki K, Deguchi K, Shimizu Y, Bronson RT, Gao YH, Inada M, Sato M, Okamoto R, Kitamura Y, Yoshiki S, Kishimoto T. (1997) Targeted disruption of Cbfa1 results in a complete lack of bone formation owing to maturational arrest of osteoblasts. *Cell.* 89(5):755-764.

Kopple JD. (2001) National Kidney Foundation K/DOQI clinical practice guidelines for nutrition in chronic renal failure. *Am J Kidney Dis* 37 [Suppl 2]: S66–S70.

Kuro-o M, Matsumura Y, Aizawa H, Kawaguchi H, Suga T, Utsugi T, Ohyama Y, Kurabayashi M, Kaname T, Kume E, Iwasaki H, Iida A, Shiraki-Iida T, Nishikawa S, Nagai R, Nabeshima YI. (1997) Mutation of the mouse klotho gene leads to a syndrome resembling ageing. *Nature* 390: 45–51.

Lafage MH, Combe C, Fournier A, Aparicio M. (1992) Ketodiet, physiological calcium intake and native vitamin D improve renal osteodystrophy. *Kidney Int.* 42(5): 1217-1225.

Larsson T, Nisbeth U, Ljunggren O, Jüppner H, Jonsson KB. (2003) Circulating concentration of FGF-23 increases as renal function declines in patients with chronic kidney disease, but does not change in response to variation in phosphate intake in healthy volunteers. *Kidney Int.* 64: 2272-2279.

Llach L, Bover J. (2000) Renal osteodystriphies; in Brenner BM (ed): *The Kidney.* Philadelphia, Saunders, pp2103-2186.

London GM. (2000) Alterations of arterial function in end-stage renal disease. *Nephron* 84: 111-118.

London GM. (2003) Cardiovascular Calcifications in Uremic Patients: Clinical Impact on Cardiovascular Function. *J Am Soc Nephrol* 14: S305–S309.

London GM, Guérin AP, Marchais SJ, Métivier F, Pannier B, Adda H. (2003) Arterial media calcification in end-stage renal disease: Impact on all-cause and cardiovascular mortality. *Nephrol. Dial. Transplant* 18: 1731–1740.

Longenecker JC, Coresh J, Powe NR Levey AS, Fink NE, Martin A, Klag MJ. (2002) Traditional cardiovascular disease risk factors in dialysis patients compared with the general population: The CHOICE Study. *J. Am. Soc. Nephrol.* 13: 1918–1927.

Lorenzo V, Martin-Malo A, Perez-Garcia R, Torregrosa JV, Vega N, de Francisco AL, Cases A. (2006) Prevalence, clinical correlates and therapy cost of mineral abnormalities among haemodialysis patients: a cross-sectional multicentre study. *Nephrol Dial Transplant.* 21: 459-465.

Maduell F, Navarro V, Torregrosa E, Rius A, Dicenta F, Cruz MC, Ferrero JA. (2003) Change from three times a week on-line hemodiafiltration to short daily on-line hemodiafiltration. *Kidney Int* 64: 305-313.

Mallick NP, Gokal R. (1999) Haemodialysis. *Lancet* 353: 737–742

Mirza MA, Larsson A, Lind L, Larsson TE. (2009) Circulating fibroblast growth factor-23 is associated with vascular dysfunction in the community. *Atherosclerosis.* 205: 385-390.

Miyamoto K, Ito M, Tatsumi S, Kuwahata M, Segawa H. (2007) New aspect of renal phosphate reabsorption: the type IIc sodium-dependent phosphate transporter. *Am J Nephrol* 27: 503–515.

Miyamoto K, Segawa H, Ito M, Kuwahata M. (2004) Physiological regulation of renal sodium-dependent phosphate cotransporters. *Jpn J Physiol* 54: 93–102.

Moe SM, Duan D, Doehle BP, O'Neill KD, Chen NX. (2003) Uremia induces the osteoblast differentiation factor Cbfa1 in human blood vessels. *Kidney Int.* 63: 1003–1011.

Moe SM, Zidehsarai MP, Chambers MA, Jackman LA, Radcliffe JS, Trevino LL, Donahue SE, Asplin JR. (2010) Vegetarian compared with meat dietary protein source and phosphorus homeostasis in chronic kidney disease. *Clin J Am Soc Nephrol.* 6(2): 257-264.

Murer H, Hernando N, Forster I, Biber J. (2000) Proximal tubular phosphate reabsorption: molecular mechanisms. *Physiol Rev* 80: 1373–1409.

Murphy-Gutekunst L. (2007) Hidden phosphorus: where do we go from here ? *J Ren Nutr* 4: e31-e36.

Nishida Y, Taketani Y, Yamanaka-Okumura H, Imamura F, Taniguchi A, Sato T, Shuto E, Nashiki K, Arai H, Yamamoto H, Takeda E. (2006) Acute effect of oral phosphate loading on serum fibroblast growth factor 23 levels in healthy men. *Kidney Int.* 70: 2141-2147.

Oliveira RB, Cancela AL, Graciolli FG, Dos Reis LM, Draibe SA, Cuppari L, Carvalho AB, Jorgetti V, Canziani ME, Moysés RM.. (2010) Early control of PTH and FGF23 in normophosphatemic CKD patients: a new target in CKD-MBD therapy? *Clin J Am Soc Nephrol.* 5(2): 286-291.

Owen WF, Lowrie EG: (1998) C-reactive protein as an outcome predictor for maintenance hemodialysis patients. *Kidney Int* 54: 607–617.

Pande S, Ritter CS, Rothstein M, Wiesen K, Vassiliadis J, Kumar R, Schiavi SC, Slatapolsky E, Brown AJ. (2006) FGF-23 and sFRP-4 in chronic kidney disease and post-renal transplantation. *Nephron Physiol* 104: 23–32.

Perwad F, Azam N, Zhang MY, Yamashita T, Tenenhouse HS, Portale AA. (2005) Dietary and serum phosphorus regulate fibroblast growth factor 23 expression and 1,25-dihydroxyvitamin D metabolism in mice. *Endocrinology.* 146: 5358-5364.

Raggi P. (2000) Detection and quantification of cardiovascular calcifications with electron beam tomography to estimate risk in hemodialysis patients. *Clin Nephrol* 54: 325–333.

Raggi P. (2002) Effects of excess calcium load on the cardiovascular system measured with electron beam tomography in end-stage renal disease. *Nephrol Dial Transplant* 17: 332–335.

Ribeiro S, Ramos A, Brandão A, Rebelo JR, Guerra A, Resina C, Vila-Lobos A, Carvalho F, Remédio F, Ribeiro F. (1998) Cardiac valve calcification in haemodialysis patients: role of calcium-phosphate metabolism. *Nephrol Dial Transplant* 13: 2037–2040.

Rodriguez-Benot A, Martin-Malo A, Alvarez-Lara MA, Rodriguez M, Aljama P. (2005) Mild hyperphosphatemia and mortality in hemodialysis patients. *Am J Kidney Dis.* 46: 68-77.

Ross R. (1999) Atherosclerosis-an inflammatory disease. *N Engl J Med* 340: 115–126.

Schwarz U, Buzello M, Ritz E, Stein G, Raabe G, Wiest G, Mall G, Amann K. (2000) Morphology of coronary atherosclerotic lesions in patients with end-stage renal failure. *Nephrol. Dial. Transplant.* 15: 218–223.

Segawa H, Kaneko I, Setsuko Y, Ito M, Kuwahata M, Inoue Y, Kato S, Miyamoto K. (2004) Intestinal Na-Pi cotransporter adaptation to dietary Pi content in vitamin D receptor null mice. *Am J Physiol Renal Physiol* 287: F39–F47.

Seiler S, Reichart B, Roth D, Seibert E, Fliser D, Heine GH. (2010) FGF-23 and future cardiovascular events in patients with chronic kidney disease before initiation of dialysis treatment. *Nephrol Dial Transplant.* 25(12): 3983-3989.

Sheikh MS, Maguire JA, Emmett M, Santa Ana CA, Nicar MJ, Schiller LR, Fordtran JS. (1989) Reduction of dietary phosphorus absorption by phosphorus binders. A theoretical, in vitro, and in vivo study. *J Clin Invest.* 83(1): 66-73.

Shimada T, Hasegawa H, Yamazaki Y, Muto T, Hino R, Takeuchi Y, Fujita T, Nakahara K, Fukumoto S, Yamashita T. (2004) FGF-23 is a potent regulator of vitamin D metabolism and phosphate homeostasis. *J Bone Miner Res.* 19: 429-435.

Shimada T, Yamazaki Y, Takahashi M, Hasegawa H, Urakawa I, Oshima T, Ono K, Kakitani M, Tomizuka K, Fujita T, Fukumoto S, Yamashita T. (2005) Vitamin D receptor-independent FGF23 actions in regulating phosphate and vitamin D metabolism. *Am J Physiol Renal Physiol.* 289: F1088-F1095.

Shuto E, Taketani Y, Tanaka R, Harada N, Isshiki M, Sato M, Nashiki K, Amo K, Yamamoto H, Higashi Y, Nakaya Y, Takeda E. (2009) Dietary phosphorus acutely impairs endothelial function. *J Am Soc Nephrol.* 20(7): 1504-1512.

Slatopolsky E, Brown A, Dusso A. (2002) Role of phosphorus in the pathogenesis of secondary hyperparathyroidism. *Am J Kidney Dis* 37: S54–S57.

Speer MY, Giachelli CM, (2004) Regulation of cardiovascular calcification. *Cardiovascular Pathology* 13: 63-70.

Sprague SM. (2007) A comparative review of the efficacy and safety of established phosphate binders: calcium, sevelamer, and lanthanum carbonate. *Curr Med Res Opin.* 23: 3167-3175.

Sullivan CM, Leon JB, Sehgal AR. (2007) Phosphorus-containing food additives and the accuracy of nutrient databases: implications for renal patients. *J Ren Nutr.* 17(5): 350-354.

Takeda E, Taketani Y, Morita K, Tatsumi S, Katai K, Nii T, Yamamoto H, Miyamoto K. (2000) Molecular mechanisms of mammalian inorganic phosphate homeostasis. *Adv Enzyme Regul* 40: 285-302.

Takeda E, Taketani Y, Nashiki K, Nomoto M, Shuto E, Sawada N, Yamamoto H, Isshiki M. (2006) A novel function of phosphate-mediated intracellular signal transduction pathways. *Adv Enzyme Regul* 46: 154–161.

Tenenhouse HS. (2006) Regulation of phosphorus homeostasis by the type IIa Na/phosphate cotransporter. *Annu Rev Nutr* 25: 197–214.

US Renal Data System Annual Data Report Bethesta (2005) *National Institutes of Health National Institute of Diabetes and Digestive and Kidney Diseases.*

Vaithilingam I, Polkinghorne KR, Atkins RC, Kerr PG. (2004) Time and exercise improve phosphate removal in hemodialysis patients. *Am J Kidney Dis.* 43(1): 85-89.

Wang AY, Wang M, Woo J, Lam CW, Li PK, Lui SF, Sanderson JE. (2003) Cardiac valve calcification as an important predictor for all-cause mortality and cardiovascular mortality in long-term peritoneal dialysis patients: A prospective study. *J. Am. Soc. Nephrol.* 14: 159–168.

Wei M, Taskapan H, Esbaei K, Jassal SV, Bargman JM, Oreopoulos DG. (2006) K/DOQI guideline requirements for calcium, phosphate, calcium phosphate product, and parathyroid hormone control in dialysis patients: can we achieve them? *Int Urol Nephrol.* 38: 739-743.

Willett WC, Buzzard M. (1998) *Nature of Variation in Diet in Nutritional Epidemiology,* 2nd Ed., edited by Willett WC, New York, Oxford University Press, pp33-49.

Xu H, Bai L, Collins JF, Ghishan FK. (2002) Age-dependent regulation of rat intestinal type IIb sodium-phosphate cotransporter by 1,25-(OH2) vitamin D3. *Am J Physiol Cell Physiol* 282: C487–C493.

Yoshida T, Fujimori T, Nabeshima Y. (2002) Mediation of unusually high concentrations of 1,25-dihydroxyvitamin D in homozygous klotho mutant mice by increased expression of renal 1 alpha-hydroxylase gene. Endocrinology 143: 683–689.

Young EW, Akiba T, Albert JM, McCarthy JT, Kerr PG, Mendelssohn DC, Jadoul M. (2004) Magnitude and impact of abnormal mineral metabolism in hemodialysis patients in the Dialysis Outcomes and Practice Patterns Study (DOPPS). *Am J Kidney Dis.* 44(Suppl 2): 34-38.

Young EW, Albert JM, Satayathum S, Goodkin DA, Pisoni RL, Akiba T, Akizawa T, Kurokawa K, Bommer J, Piera L, Port FK. (2005) Predictors and consequences of altered mineral metabolism: The Dialysis Outcomes and Practice Patterns Study. *Kidney Int.* 67: 1179–1187.

Yu X, White KE. (2005) Fibroblast growth factor 23 and its receptors. *Ther Apher Dial* 9: 308–312.

Yu X, White KE. (2005) FGF23 and disorders of phosphate homeostasis. Cytokine Growth Factor Rev 16: 221–232.

Zoccali C. (2000) Cardiovascular risk in uraemic patients - Is it fully explained by classical risk factors? *Nephrol. Dial. Transplant.* 15: 454–457.

18

Management of Secondary Hyperparathyroidism in Hemodialysis Patients

Emanuel Zitt[1,2] and Ulrich Neyer[2]
[1]*Department of Nephrology and Dialysis, Academic Teaching Hospital Feldkirch,*
[2]*Vorarlberg Institute for Vascular Investigation and Treatment (VIVIT), Feldkirch, Austria*

1. Introduction

Secondary hyperparathyroidism (sHPT) represents the adaptive and very often finally maladaptive response of the organism to control the disturbed homeostasis of calcium, phosphorus and vitamin D metabolism caused by declining renal function. Dysregulation of calcium and phosphorus homeostasis leads to elevated levels of the phosphatonin fibroblast growth factor 23 (FGF23), decreased renal phosphorus excretion, increased serum phosphorus, and diminished synthesis of calcitriol (1,25$(OH)_2D_3$), the active form of vitamin D. These alterations result in increased secretion and synthesis of parathyroid hormone (PTH) and parathyroid cell hyperplasia (Cunningham et al., 2011).

Evidence is available that these disturbances in mineral metabolism lead to vascular (Goodman et al., 2000; Raggi et al., 2002) and valvular (Ribeiro et al., 1998) calcifications and are directly linked to an increased risk of cardiovascular morbidity and mortality as well as excess all-cause mortality (Covic et al., 2009). In accordance to a recent systematic review, the risk of cardiovascular and all-cause mortality is greatest with elevated serum phosphorus followed by increased serum calcium and PTH (Covic et al., 2009). Apart from extra-skeletal side effects, sHPT also leads to profound alterations in bone metabolism which become obvious in the different forms of renal osteodystrophy (Malluche & Faugere, 1990; Moe et al., 2006). This clinical syndrome encompassing mineral, bone and cardiovascular abnormalities has been termed CKD-related Mineral and Bone Disorder (CKD-MBD) (Moe et al., 2006). Furthermore, sHPT is thought to play a role in various other complications of end-stage renal disease as bone pain, bone fractures, muscle dysfunction, sexual dysfunction, disturbed hematopoiesis, immune dysfunction, pruritus and calcific uremic arteriolopathy (calciphylaxis) (Rodriguez & Lorenzo, 2009). An overview of the current understanding of the pathogenesis of sHPT is given in Figure 1.

In an attempt to improve clinical care, the National Kidney Foundation's Kidney Disease Outcomes Quality Initiative (NKF-K/DOQI™ [KDOQI]) has recommended target ranges for serum intact PTH, serum phosphorus and total corrected serum calcium (KDOQI, 2003). More recently, the Kidney Disease Improving Global Outcomes (KDIGO) guidelines for diagnosis, evaluation, prevention and treatment of CKD-MBD have been published (KDIGO, 2009) and endorsed by the US KDOQI (Uhlig et al., 2010) and European Renal Best Practice (Goldsmith et al., 2010) groups. These latter guidelines have tried to provide evidence-based recommendations, but due to the very limited availability of high quality

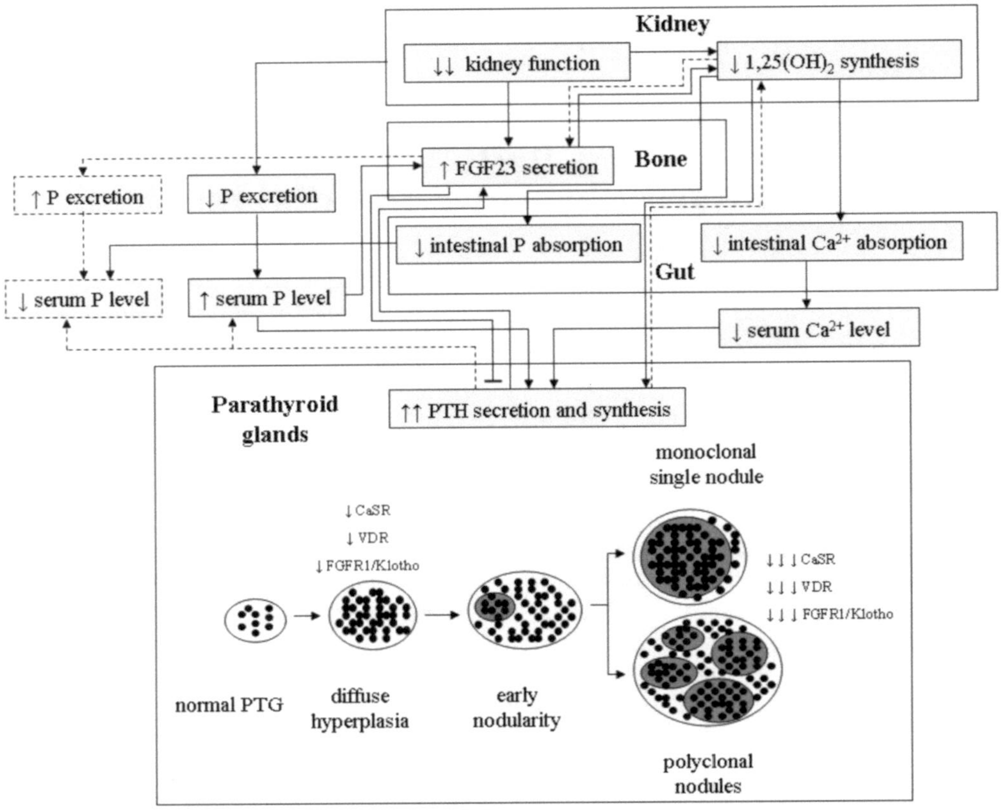

Fig. 1. Pathogenesis of secondary hyperparathyroidism. Declining kidney function causes reduced renal conversion of 25(OH)D to $1,25(OH)_2D$ by CYP27B1 (25(OH)D-1α-hydroxylase) and elevated serum phosphorus levels due to diminished phosphorus excretion. Increased phosphorus concentration, decreased calcium concentration and markedly reduced serum calcitriol levels lead to increased PTH synthesis and secretion in the parathyroid glands. Elevated FGF23 expression, to counteract the reduced phosphorus excretion, downregulates residual renal 25(OH)D-1α-hydroxylase, additionally promoting the development of sHPT. These metabolic changes are accompanied by a variable downregulation and underexpression of the calcium-sensing receptor and vitamin D receptor on parathyroidal cells, rendering the parathyroid gland unable to respond appropriately to calcium and calcitriol. Dashed lines indicate counter-regulatory pathways. Abbreviations: FGF23, fibroblast growth factor 23; P, phosphorus; Ca^{2+}, calcium; CaSR, calcium-sensing receptor; VDR, vitamin D receptor; FGFR1, fibroblast growth factor receptor 1, PTG, parathyroid gland.

clinical interventional trials with skeletal, cardiovascular or mortality end-points in this field, fewer and less mandatory recommendations are given compared to the older KDOQI guidelines.

The achievement of these target ranges set by the KDOQI or KDIGO guidelines is quite challenging (Young et al., 2004) and failure to reach these targets has been shown to be associated with increased risk for death compared to simultaneously achieving the targets for all three biochemical parameters PTH, calcium and phosphorus (Danese et al., 2008).

The 84-amino-acid peptide hormone PTH has a very short half-life of two to four minutes after parathyroid secretion. It is metabolized to shorter fragments in the liver which are then excreted by the kidneys. With increasing renal failure and progressive CKD the proportion of these fragments with a 5 to 10 times longer half-life raises due to decreased renal clearance. Although the exact composition and possible function of the various PTH fragments are not yet fully elucidated, experimental data clearly found a clinically relevant biological activity of some of these fragments. Routinely used second-generation PTH assays, globally called "intact" PTH assays because they were thought to measure the full-length PTH 1-84 molecule only, recognize with various cross-reactivities (from approximately 50 to 100%) a PTH fragment, which co-elutes in high-performance liquid chromatography with a synthetic PTH 7–84 fragment. With progressive renal failure the amount of this and related PTH fragments gradually increases from about 20% in healthy individuals to about 50% in hemodialysis patients (Brossard et al., 2000). Therefore, at least in part, the progressive increase in measured PTH with decreasing renal function is also linked to the decreased renal metabolism and clearance of PTH 1-84 and its fragments. The different commercially available second-generation PTH assays have variable cross-reactivity with the PTH 7-84 fragment, therefore PTH measurements with different assays are not fully comparable and due to lacking standardization of PTH measurement sHPT patients might be classified differently according to KDOQI or KDIGO guidelines, resulting in different and due to misclassification potentially disadvantageous therapeutic interventions (Koller et al., 2004). Newer third-generation PTH assays, which show no cross-reactivity with the PTH 7-84 and related fragments, have been developed. Unfortunately, in all bone biopsy studies, which were later used to establish the KDOQI and KDIGO PTH target ranges, the first available second-generation PTH assay was used, but this assay is no longer commercially available. In an attempt to provide some kind of comparability of PTH measurements and consistent classification, correcting factors for the different second-generation PTH assays were proposed (Souberbielle et al., 2010).
Current therapeutic strategies include the modification of calcium and phosphorus balance through restricted dietary calcium and phosphorus intake and removal during hemodialysis, administration of phosphate binders, vitamin D receptor activators (calcitriol and newer vitamin D analogues) and the calcimimetic cinacalcet, and ultimately parathyroidectomy in very severe sHPT. These interventions have been shown to improve the biochemical parameters (PTH, calcium, phosphorus), bone histology or histomorphometry and cardiovascular calcification, but still there is lacking evidence that improvements in these surrogate parameters translate into better patient outcomes. Traditionally interventions to treat sHPT primarily aimed at bone health, but over the years new experimental insights into cardiovascular calcification and epidemiological data about associated cardiovascular morbidity and mortality risk switched the emphasis from bone to cardiovascular health.

2. Treatment of hyperphosphatemia

Declining renal function inevitably causes phosphorus retention due to decreased renal phosphorus clearance. This mechanism starts early in chronic kidney disease. However, hyperphosphatemia is prevented until the late stages of chronic kidney disease by an increase in FGF23 and PTH which control phosphorus homeostasis for a definite time. Initially, phosphorus retention stimulates FGF23 and PTH secretion, which in turn suppress renal phosphorus reabsorption and increase renal phosphorus excretion. FGF23 also suppresses calcitriol ($1,25(OH)_2D_3$) production, which diminishes intestinal phosphorus absorption but allows increases in PTH levels. Whereas FGF23 suppresses PTH secretion in normal parathyroid glands, resistance to its effect occurs with further loss of kidney function because of decreased Klotho and FGF receptor 1 expression in the parathyroid glands and the kidney. Thus, as chronic kidney disease progresses to late stages, these homeostatic mechanisms are inevitably overwhelmed, hyperphosphatemia ensues, and the levels of PTH and FGF23 increase progressively (Cunningham et al., 2011).

Robust observational data show a clear association of higher serum phosphorus levels with cardiovascular events and mortality (Block et al., 1998, 2004). The exact threshold above which risk significantly increases is not definitely known and varies across the studies from 5.0 to 7.0 mg/dL (1.6 to 2.3 mmol/L) (Covic et al., 2009). However, it has never been determined in randomized placebo-controlled trials whether treating hyperphosphatemia to specific target ranges improves clinical patient outcomes. The KDIGO guidelines therefore suggest to decrease serum phosphorus levels toward the reference range in patients with chronic kidney disease 5D (KDIGO, 2009).

Therapeutic interventions to treat hyperphosphatemia include restriction of dietary phosphorus intake, administration of phosphate binders and increasing the frequency or length of dialysis sessions.

2.1 Dietary phosphorus restriction

Dietary phosphorus assessment and restriction is the cornerstone of the treatment of hyperphosphatemia. Educational support and dietary guidelines should be offered to the patients by a skilled dietician. Restriction of dietary phosphorus intake, however, requires a reduction in oral protein intake, as protein-rich foods are the main source of dietary phosphorus (Shinaberger et al., 2008). Lowering protein intake can lead to malnutrition and protein-energy wasting and thereby increasing mortality in dialysis patients (Lacson et al., 2007). It is very important to avoid concomitant malnutrition by forced dietary protein restriction, as protein restriction as means to lower dietary phosphorus intake may outweigh the benefit of controlled phosphorus and may lead to greater mortality (Shinaberger et al., 2008). One possibility for overcoming the problem of concordant overall protein restriction and the risk of malnutrition with reduced dietary phosphorus intake would be to avoid phosphorus-rich ingredients that are added to processed foods and beverages (Sherman & Mehta, 2009a, 2009b). Contrary to natural sources of organic phosphorus, such as meat or dairy products, such phosphorus sources are dissociated from protein intake. Reducing the consumption of such phosphorus additives might help to decrease phosphorus intake without the risk of protein-energy wasting (Sullivan et al., 2009). Additionally, the intake of protein sources with low phosphorus to protein ratios might further help to limit phosphorus intake (Noori et al., 2010). Nutritional guidelines recommend a maximum of 800 to 1000 mg (25 to 35 mmol) daily dietary phosphorus intake (Fouque et al., 2007). Nevertheless, dietary modifications alone are generally not sufficient to reduce phosphorus intake sufficiently in most patients, but help to save phosphate binders and probably reduce the high pill burden.

2.2 Phosphate binders

The use of oral phosphate binders to block intestinal phosphorus absorption has been shown to effectively reduce serum phosphorus levels irrespective of the phosphate binder class. Although no placebo-controlled randomized trial has been done so far to prove that reduction in serum phosphorus by the use of phosphate binders improves patient outcomes, a recent prospective observational study in a large number of incident dialysis patients has shown that the use of any phosphate binder (versus none) offers a clear survival benefit independent of absolute serum phosphorus concentration and co-medication (Isakova et al., 2009).

Available phosphate binders include the calcium salts calcium acetate and calcium carbonate, aluminium hydroxide, the polymeric anion-exchange resins sevelamer hydrochloride and sevelamer carbonate, lanthanum carbonate and the newer so far not well studied compounds ferric citrate, SBR759 (iron-based), magnesium/calcium carbonate and magnesium carbonate/calcium acetate. They differ in composition, phosphate-binding capacity, form and have specific potential advantages and disadvantages, which are summarized in Table 1.

Considering the different agents there are no data at present to favour one phosphate binder, because there is no proven superiority of any phosphate binder or binder class for relevant clinical outcomes. According to a recent systematic review and meta-analysis of available randomized controlled trials all phosphate binders decrease serum phosphorus levels compared with placebo. The newer drugs sevelamer hydrochloride and lanthanum carbonate do not result in superior control of biochemical parameters compared with calcium salts. In contrast, in head-to-head studies calcium salts enable a greater reduction of serum phosphorus than sevelamer hydrochloride. Whereas both calcium salts (calcium acetate and carbonate) do not differ with regard to serum calcium levels, sevelamer hydrochloride and lanthanum carbonate are associated with significantly lower rates of treatment-related hypercalcemia, which may result in decreased cardiovascular calcification. However, the finding of slower or less progression of cardiovascular calcification in sevelamer-treated patients is inconsistent across the studies. Studies revealed no difference in PTH suppression when comparing calcium acetate with calcium carbonate or lanthanum

Binder source	**Form**	**Content (mineral/metal/element)**	**Phosphate-binding capacity**	**Daily dose**	**Advantages**	**Disadvantages**
Calcium carbonate	tablet, capsule, chewable, gum, liquid	200 mg elemental Ca^{2+} per 500 mg carbonate (40% elemental Ca^{2+})	39 mg phosphate per 1 gramm calcium carbonate	1500 to 3500 mg (3–7 tablets)	effective phosphate-binding, inexpensive, readily available, long-term experience	potential for hypercalcemia and hypercalcemia-associated risks, gastrointestinal side effects
Calcium acetate	capsule, tablet	126.7 mg elemental Ca^{2+} per 500 mg tablet, 169 mg elemental Ca^{2+} per 667 mg capsule (25% elemental Ca^{2+})	45 mg phosphate per 1 gramm calcium acetate	3000 to 6000 mg (6 to 12 tablets)	effective phosphate-binding, potentially higher binding capacity and lower Ca^{2+} absorption than carbonate, inexpensive, long-term experience	potential for hypercalcemia and hypercalcemia-associated risks, gastrointestinal side effects, more costly than carbonate

Aluminium hydroxide	tablet, capsule, liquid	Varying with 100 to 600 mg aluminium per tablet	22.3 mg phosphate per 5 ml, 18.8 mg phosphate per 1000 mg	600 to 1800 mg (pill burden dependent on content per tablet)	very effective phosphate-binding capacity	potential for aluminium toxicity, gastrointestinal side effects
Sevelamer-HCl	tablet	none	64 mg phosphate per 800 mg sevelamer-HCl	2400 to 9600 mg (3 to 12 tablets)	effective phosphate-binding capacity, no Ca^{2+} and metal content, reduces LDL-cholesterol, possible potential for reduced calcification	costs, potential for decrease in bicarbonate levels, in presence of hypocalcemia need for Ca^{2+} supplement, higher risk of gastrointestinal side effects compared to Ca^{2+} salts
Sevelamer carbonate	tablet, powder	none	same as sevelamer-HCl	2400 to 9600 mg (3 to 12 tablets, 1 to 4 packets)	same as sevelamer-HCl, but lower risk of metabolic acidosis	assumed to have same disadvantages as sevelamer-HCl except decrease in bicarbonate levels, less well studied
Lanthanum carbonate	chewable tablet	250, 500, 750 or 1000 mg elemental lanthanum per tablet	NA	750 to 3750 mg (3 to 5 chewable tablets)	effective phosphate-binding capacity, no Ca^{2+}, chewable, reduced pill burden	costs, gastrointestinal side effects, potential for accumulation
Magnesium carbonate/calcium acetate	tablet	60 mg Mg per 235 mg $MgCO_3$, 110 mg elemental Ca^{2+} per 435 mg Ca^{2+} acetate	NA	705/1305 mg to 2820/5220 mg (3 to 12 tablets)	effective, potential for lower Ca^{2+} load than pure Ca^{2+}-based binders	potential for hypermagnesemia, gastrointestinal side effect, not well studied
Ferric citrate	capsule	176 mg elemental iron per 1g ferric citrate				potential for iron accumulation, not well studied, gastrointestinal side effects, less effective than Ca^{2+} salts
SBR759 (polymeric complex of starch with ferric iron)	powder	1.25 g per sachet			powder form	potential for iron accumulation, not well studied (1 phase I trial), gastrointestinal side effects, hypocalcemia

Table 1. Overview of available phosphate binders (adapted from KDOQI, 2003; KDIGO, 2009; Tonelli et al., 2010; Uhlig et al., 2010). Abbrevations: Ca^{2+}, calcium; HCl, hydrochloride; Mg, magnesium; CO_3, carbonate; NA, not available.

carbonate with calcium carbonate, but found a significantly lower PTH reduction with sevelamer hydrochloride in comparison to calcium salts. When all studies were pooled, gastrointestinal side effects occurred more often with sevelamer hydrochloride than with calcium salts. With the use of sevelamer hydrochloride significantly lower serum bicarbonate is found, aggravating already existing metabolic acidosis. The new formula of sevelamer carbonate does not negatively influence acid-base status. A possible advantage of sevelamer is its significant reduction of LDL-cholesterol. However, no difference in all-cause mortality could be found comparing calcium acetate and carbonate, or sevelamer with calcium salts. All-cause mortality as endpoint has not been studied with all other phosphate binders (Navaneethan et al., 2009).

Hypercalcemia is a known side effect of calcium salts, especially when combined with vitamin D receptor activators. Persistent hypercalcemia necessitates a dose reduction or cessation of calcium salts as phosphate binders. The KDOQI guidelines suggest limiting the daily calcium intake from calcium-containing phosphate binders to 1500 mg per day for elemental calcium and 2000 mg per day for total intake of elemental calcium including the dietary calcium content (KDOQI, 2003). Nevertheless, there is no data available to recommend a specific upper limit of a safe amount of calcium intake. Restrictive use of calcium-based phosphate binders may be considered in the following situations (Cozzolino et al., 2011; Goldsmith et al., 2010):

- presence of cardiovascular disease
- presence of vascular or valvular calcification
- older age (>65 years)
- diabetes mellitus
- evidence of adynamic bone disease
- hypercalcemia

Although very effective, a prolonged (>3 months continuously, or >6 months cumulative) use of aluminium hydroxide should be avoided because of the potential toxicity of accumulated aluminium leading to encephalopathy, osteomalacia and anemia (Goldsmith et al., 2010).

Irrespective of the phosphate binder class the successful practical management of hyperphosphatemia with phosphate binders includes:

- concomitant dietary phosphorus restriction (especially phosphorus-rich additives)
- administration of phosphate binders with the meal
- individual dosing with respect to eating habits and serum phosphorus level

A new and promising concept for the management of hyperphosphatemia was recently developed to enable patients to self-adjust the phosphate binder dose in relation to the phosphorus content of each individual meal: "Phosphate Education Program" (PEP) (Ahlenstiel et al., 2010). Patients are taught to eye-estimate the meal phosphorus content based on "phosphate units" (PU; 1 PU is defined per 100 mg of phosphorus per serving size of the meal) and then phosphate binders are prescribed dependent on an individual phosphate binder/PU ratio. This concept is similar to the individualized adjustments of insulin dose to carbohydrate intake in the treatment of diabetes mellitus.

Novel agents under development for the treatment of hyperphosphatemia are MCI-196 (colestilan) (Locatelli et al., 2010), a non-metallic anion-exchange resin, and niacin and nicotinamid, which probably directly inhibit the sodium-dependent phosphate cotransporter Na-Pi-2b in the gastrointestinal tract (Muller et al., 2007).

2.3 Dialytic methods for phosphorus removal

Dialytic methods to improve phosphorus removal include prolonged (nocturnal) hemodialysis (Culleton et al. 2007; Walsh et al., 2010) and convective strategies (Tonelli et al., 2009).

3. Vitamin D therapy

3.1 Correction of vitamin D deficiency and insufficiency

Neither the normal nor the desirable target ranges for 25-hydroxyvitamin D (25(OH)D) levels are known in patients on hemodialysis. In accordance with patients without chronic kidney disease, 25(OH)D levels <12.5 ng/mL (<30 nmol/L) are defined as vitamin D deficiency, values <30 ng/mL (<75 nmol/L) as vitamin D insufficiency. Observational studies have shown an association between low 25(OH)D levels and adverse clinical outcomes (Holick, 2005; Wolf et al., 2007; Giovannucci, 2008). Although data from clinical trials are missing to show a survival benefit after increasing 25(OH)D levels in insufficient or deficient hemodialysis patients, current guidelines suggest to replete 25(OH)D stores in these patients on grounds of low costs, relative safety of repletion and potential therapeutic impact (KDIGO, 2009). After initial measurement and diagnosis of vitamin D deficiency, a supplementation using cholecalciferol or ergocalciferol may be initiated with remeasurement after 3 months of supplementation. There are no data regarding the choice of vitamin D product or the administration route. Altogether, oral repletion seems to be more favourable compared to intramuscular route in hemodialysis patients. In accordance with the general population a daily dose of 1000 to 2000 IU of cholecalciferol or a corresponding weekly dose are given (KDOQI, 2003; KDIGO, 2009; Uhlig et al., 2010). In a recent study in 107 hemodialysis patients, 91% of the patients had a serum 25(OH)D level higher than the target level of 75 nmol/L (30 ng/mL) after 3 months of monthly oral substitution of 100,000 IU (at first dialysis session of the month) (Jean et al., 2009). This approach seems to be safe and guarantee patient compliance. If hypercalcemia or hyperphosphatemia occurs, vitamin D repletion should be temporarily discontinued or abandoned. Table 2 gives an overview of the key differences between 25(OH)D and its "active" form 1,25(OH)$_2$D.

	25(OH)D	**1,25(OH)$_2$D**
Total plasma concentration (recommended normal values)	30 to 50 ng/mL (75 to 125 nmol/L)	30 to 50 pg/mL (75 to 125 pmol/L)
Total plasma concentration (relative values)	1000	1
Binding affinity to vitamin D-binding protein (relative values)	1000	1
Free concentration (relative values)	1	1
Half-life	25 to 30 days	4 to 8 hours
VDR affinity (relative values)	1	500 to 1000

Table 2. Characteristics and differences of 25(OH)D and 1,25(OH)$_2$D. Abbrevations: VDR, vitamin D receptor.

3.2 Vitamin D receptor activators

Treatment of sHPT with active vitamin D receptor activators (VDRA) is a well established therapeutic modality, and current practice guidelines recommend to treat patients with elevated and/or increasing PTH levels with a VDRA (KDIGO, 2009). Observational studies are indicating a survival benefit of VDRA in hemodialysis patients in comparison with patients without VDRA treatment (Teng et al., 2003, 2005; Tentori et al., 2006; Naves-Diaz et al., 2008). Again, prospective controlled randomised clinical trials indicating a benefit on patient-level clinical outcomes with VDRA therapy are missing but strongly awaited. Calcitriol, the physiological VDRA, is the natural regulator of parathyroid gland function and growth and exerts its effect on PTH secretion by inhibiting mRNA synthesis through its action on the vitamin D receptor (VDR), a highly specific receptor that acts as a transcription factor. In addition, calcitriol is able to inhibit PTH secretion by increasing calcium absorption in the intestine, while also increasing bone resorption and, consequently, calcium release from bone. Moreover, calcitriol regulates the expression of its own receptor, stimulating its synthesis. The deficit of calcitriol observed in hemodialysis patients as well as a transformation into nodular hyperplasia with progressive sHPT is associated with a decrease in VDR levels in the parathyroid gland. Decreased VDR expression may than cause resistance to VDRA. VDRA generally control sHPT well in patients with moderately increased hypertrophic glands and less well in patients with enlarged hyperplastic glands and should therefore be started early in the development of sHPT (Cunningham et al., 2011). Beyond the classical endocrine effects on parathyroid gland, bone and intestine, the pleiotropic paracrine and autocrine effects of vitamin D have been associated with improvement of cardiovascular risk factors, including increased renin activity, hypertension, inflammation, insulin resistance, diabetes, albuminuria and an improved immune response.

Besides the native active hormone calcitriol ($1{,}25(OH)_2D_3$), the two prodrugs alfacalcidol ($1(OH)D_3$) and doxercalciferol ($1(OH)D_2$) and the two vitamin D analogues paricalcitol (19-nor-$1{,}25(OH)_2D_2$) and maxacalcitol (22-oxa-$1{,}25(OH)_2D_3$) can be used. Paricalcitol and maxacalcitol (oxacalcitriol) bind directly to the VDR, whereas doxercalciferol and alfacalcidol need an enzymatic 25-hydroxylation activation step in the liver. So far no prospective, placebo-controlled and blinded clinical trial involving 22-oxacalcitriol, paricalcitol, or doxercalciferol has yet demonstrated additional clinical benefits when compared with calcitriol, nor have any studies been published showing that either calcitriol or alfacalcidol has an advantage over the other with respect to biochemical or clinical end points (Cunningham & Zehnder, 2011). Therefore, low dose therapy with calcitriol (e.g. 0.25 µg/d orally or 0.25 µg thrice weekly orally or intravenously as a starting dose) is recommended with elevated or increasing PTH levels (KDIGO, 2009). Characteristics and oral calcitriol equivalent doses of various available VDRA are presented in Table 3.

According to current practice guidelines, the target range for PTH is now 2-9 times the upper limit of the normal range (KDIGO, 2009; Uhlig et al., 2010; Goldsmith et al., 2010). This wide range takes into account a significant interassay variability of values obtained with different commercial PTH assays (Koller et al., 2004; Souberbielle et al., 2010), inability to uniformly predict bone histologic and histomorphometric states by means of PTH within this range and the epidemiological observation of increased all-cause mortality starting from PTH values >400 to 600 pg/mL (Uhlig et al., 2010). If there is no successful response with PTH reduction into the suggested target range, or dose-limiting side effects occur, especially hypercalcemia and hyperphosphatemia, a calcimimetic can be initiated instead or combined with a low dose of VDRA.

VDRA	Chemical structure	Oral calcitriol equivalent dose (thrice weekly)
Calcitriol	$1{,}25(OH)_2D_3$; natural hormone	oral 0.25 µg intravenous 0.5 µg
Alfacalcidol	$1(OH)D_3$; synthetic prohormone	oral 0.5 µg intravenous 1 µg
Doxercalciferol	$1(OH)D_2$, synthetic prohormone	oral 2.5 µg intravenous 5 µg
Paricalcitol	19nor-$1{,}25(OH)_2D_2$; synthetic analogue	oral 1 µg intravenous 2 µg
Maxacalcitol (Oxacalcitriol)	22oxa-$1{,}25(OH)_2D_3$; synthetic analogue	NA

Table 3. Characteristics and oral calcitriol equivalent doses of vitamin D receptor activators (VDRA). Abbreviation: NA, not available.

4. Calcimimetics

Calcimimetics are allosteric modulators of the calcium sensing receptor that sensitize the receptor to extracellular calcium. This results in reduced PTH secretion and inhibited parathyroid cell proliferation (Nemeth et al., 1998; Chin et al., 2000). This decrease in serum PTH is accompanied by control of serum calcium and phosphorus levels in patients with sHPT as well as a halt or regression of parathyroid gland hyperplasia (Meola et al., 2009). Initial phase III trials and various observational studies have shown that cinacalcet enables more patients to reach the recommended biochemical targets (Block et al., 2004; Lindberg et al., 2005; Urena et al., 2009) and allows sustained biochemical control for long term up to 3 years (Sprague et al., 2009). At present cinacalcet hydrochloride is the only calcimimetic available for clinical use. In contrast to VDRA, cinacalcet decreases all three important biochemical parameters of CKD-MBD (PTH, phosphorus, calcium) (Urena et al., 2009). In addition to excellent results on laboratory parameters, cinacalcet has also shown favourable effects on cardiovascular hospitalization, bone fracture rate, parathyroidectomy rate and quality of life (Cunningham et al., 2005). In a prospectively designed observational study use of cinacalcet on top of standard sHPT therapy with VDRA and phosphate binders resulted in a 26% lower all-cause mortality and a 24% lower cardiovascular mortality than in patients without cinacalcet, with the largest survival benefit for patients with most severe sHPT (PTH >600 pg/mL) (Block et al., 2010). The ongoing double-blind, randomised placebo-controlled EVOLVE trial (Evaluation of cinacalcet HCl therapy to lower cardiovascular events) currently determines whether cinacalcet reduces all-cause mortality or non-fatal cardiovascular events (Chertow et al., 2007).

Generally, initial therapy starts with a daily dose of 30 mg followed by dose-titration every 2 to 4 weeks if necessary. Serum calcium levels must be monitored regularly because of its known hypocalcemic effect.

Whereas VDRA reduce PTH gene transcription and hormone synthesis over a period of several hours or even days, cinacalcet inhibits PTH secretion within minutes, with a maximal decrease occurring within 2 to 4 hours after administration. Besides gastrointestinal side effects, hypocalcemia is one of the most common adverse events seen with cinacalcet. It is thought to occur after decreased mobilization of calcium from bone caused by lowered PTH levels. In most patients, this hypocalcemia can be successfully managed with dose adjustments or a combination with low doses of VDRA in patients with moderate to severe sHPT. Clinical trials have demonstrated the superior suppression of PTH production and control of calcium and phosphorus in hemodialysis patients who use cinacalcet, both as adjunctive therapy to VDRA and as primary therapy with reduced doses of VDRA , compared with sHPT therapy with VDRA and phosphate binders only (Chertow et al., 2006; Block et al., 2008; Fishbane et al., 2008; Messa et al., 2008).

5. Parathyroidectomy

Persistently increased serum PTH levels >800 pg/mL (88.0 pmol/L) in presence of hypercalcemia or hyperphosphatemia refractory to medical therapy and calcific uremic arteriolopathy (calciphylaxis) with concomitantly elevated PTH levels are an indication for surgery (KDOQI, 2003; KDIGO, 2009). Subtotal and total parathyroidectomy (PTX) with or without forearm autograft arose as a treatment option in the 1990s (Tominaga et al., 1997) and PTX continues to be a primary therapeutic option for refractory sHPT in both Europe and the US. Rates of PTX increased for US patients on hemodialysis from 1998 to 2002 despite an increase in therapeutic options (Foley et al., 2005). The frequency of PTX across Europe has remained relatively stable since the mid-1980s (Malberti et al., 2001) and is lower in older patients (Pelletier et al., 2010).

PTX effectively decreases PTH, calcium and phosphorus and offers the highest percentage cure for sHPT, compared to all other medical and surgical treatments. However, recurrent hyperparathyroidism can be observed in 10 - 70% of patients dependent on follow-up time (Johnson et al., 1988; Gagne et al., 1992; Gasparri et al., 2001). For total parathyroidectomy with autotransplantation an intra-operative selection of parathyroid tissue with diffuse hyperplasia but low proliferative potential (and exclusion of nodular tissue) is feasible and minimizes the risk of graft-dependent recurrent hyperparathyroidism (Neyer et al., 2002). Alternatively to surgery, ultrasound-guided percutaneous fine-needle ethanol injection into nodular hyperplastic parathyroid glands is very common in Japan (Giangrande et al., 1992; Kitaoka et al., 1994; Fukagawa et al., 1999). Apart from ethanol, also calcitriol or novel VDRA can be directly placed into enlarged parathyroid glands using the same technique (Shiizaki et al., 2003).

To date no specific guidelines considering sHPT treatment in hemodialysis patients on kidney transplant waiting list have been established. After successful kidney transplantation persistent HPT can be observed in up to 25% of patients one year after transplantation despite adequate renal graft function. Severity of sHPT at time of transplantation was found to be a significant indicator of persistent HPT (Evenepoel et al., 2004). If indicated, therapy for persistent HPT should be initiated about three months after renal transplantation because further spontaneous improvement thereafter is rare. Because this special situation of persistent HPT after transplantation is usually accompanied by hypercalcemia and hypophosphatemia, conventional therapy with phosphate binders, VDRA or calcium supplements is not indicated in most patients. Therefore, PTX is the preferred treatment option in this situation and has been shown to be effective, safe, though associated with a mild deterioration of graft function in the early postoperative phase but similar graft survival in the long-term compared to kidney transplant patients without PTX and linked to a blood pressure and lipid lowering effect (Triponez et al., 2008). Recently, also cinacalcet has been proposed to offer an alternative therapeutic option to PTX, although not approved

for the use in this situation and cost-intensive if used for many years (Kruse et al., 2005; Serra et al., 2005; Srinivas et al., 2006; Zitt et al., 2007).
Therefore, we believe that a good and early control of sHPT prior to kidney transplantation is mandatory. This should be initially done using all medical options including cinacalcet, but if unsuccessful in control of severe sHPT proceeding straight to PTX for an optimal and cost-effective treatment. Randomized clinical trials directly comparing medical with surgical therapy of sHPT are lacking.
To avoid severe postoperative hypocalcemia ("hungry bone syndrome), pre-/peri- and postoperative calcium and calcitriol supplementation (e.g. 1 to 2 g elemental calcium thrice a day, 1 to 4 μg calcitriol per day; parenteral calcium substitution if symptomatic hypocalcemia is present with 1 to 2 mg elemental calcium/kg/h) must be guaranteed along with frequent controls of serum calcium levels. In case of recurrent or persistent hyperparathyroidism after parathyroidectomy, cinacalcet has been shown to be a viable and safe treatment option (Zitt et al., 2010).

6. Dialysate calcium concentration

A near-neutral calcium flux could be expected in patients with a dialysate calcium concentration of 1.25 mmol/L (2.5 mEq/L), although there is considerable interindividual variability among patients (Hou et al., 1991; Argiles et al., 1993). Based on calcium kinetic modelling even lower dialysate calcium concentrations of 1.0 mmol/L (2.0 mEq/L) might be needed to avoid net positive calcium balance (Gotch et al., 2010). The risks of hemodynamic instability and cardiac rhythm disturbances with a very low dialysate calcium concentration must be kept in mind (Drueke & Touam, 2009). Overall calcium balance is influenced by dietary calcium intake, vitamin D level, calcium-containing phosphate binders, use of VDRA and calcimimetics and dialysate calcium concentration. Therefore, selecting an individual dialysate calcium concentration is based on various parameters and must always be a compromise between the need to guarantee cardiovascular stability during the hemodialysis session and the goal to maintain normal bone turnover and mineralization in order to avoid bone pain and fractures but avoid extraskeletal calcification.

7. Summary

Whereas there are insufficient high-quality randomized controlled trials in the field, this shortcoming should not lead to a nihilistic approach to the relevant clinical problems of hemodialysis patients with sHPT. Nevertheless, because of insufficient clinical data, a single treatment modality, be it phosphorus binders, vitamin D substitution with inactive forms or vitamin D receptor activators, calcimimetics or parathyroidectomy may not claim to be uniformly superior to the others, and a wider therapeutic window often prompts the use of a combination of these options and individualization of sHPT management. The ultimate goal is to improve the very poor survival of hemodialysis patients, so any suggested approach for the management of sHPT should be tested.

8. References

Ahlenstiel, T., Pape, L., Ehrich, J. H., & Kuhlmann, M. K. (2010). Self-adjustment of phosphate binder dose to meal phosphorus content improves management of hyperphosphataemia in children with chronic kidney disease. *Nephrol Dial Transplant* 25(10): pp. 3241-3249

Argiles, A., Kerr, P. G., Canaud, B., Flavier, J. L., & Mion, C. (1993). Calcium kinetics and the long-term effects of lowering dialysate calcium concentration. *Kidney Int* 43(3): pp. 630-640

Block, G. A., Hulbert-Shearon, T. E., Levin, N. W., & Port, F. K. (1998). Association of serum phosphorus and calcium x phosphate product with mortality risk in chronic hemodialysis patients: a national study. *Am J Kidney Dis* 31(4): pp. 607-617

Block, G. A., Klassen, P. S., Lazarus, J. M., Ofsthun, N., Lowrie, E. G., & Chertow, G. M. (2004). Mineral metabolism, mortality, and morbidity in maintenance hemodialysis. *J Am Soc Nephrol* 15(8): pp. 2208-2218

Block, G. A., Martin, K. J., de Francisco, A. L., Turner, S. A., Avram, M. M., Suranyi, M. G., Hercz, G., Cunningham, J., Abu-Alfa, A. K., Messa, P., Coyne, D. W., Locatelli, F., Cohen, R. M., Evenepoel, P., Moe, S. M., Fournier, A., Braun, J., McCary, L. C., Zani, V. J., Olson, K. A., Drueke, T. B., & Goodman, W. G. (2004). Cinacalcet for secondary hyperparathyroidism in patients receiving hemodialysis. *N Engl J Med* 350(15): pp. 1516-1525

Block, G. A., Zaun, D. Smits, G., Persky, M., Brillhart, S., Nieman, K., Liu, J., & St Peter, W. L. (2010). Cinacalcet hydrochloride treatment significantly improves all-cause and cardiovascular survival in a large cohort of hemodialysis patients. *Kidney Int* 78(6): pp. 578-589

Block, G. A., Zeig, S., Sugihara, J., Chertow, G. M., Chi, E. M., Turner, S. A., & Bushinsky, D. A. (2008). Combined therapy with cinacalcet and low doses of vitamin D sterols in patients with moderate to severe secondary hyperparathyroidism. *Nephrol Dial Transplant* 23(7): pp. 2311-2318

Brossard, J.H., Lepage, R., Cardinal, H., Roy, L., Rousseau, L., Dorais, C., & D'Amour, P. (2000). Influence of glomerular filtration rate on non-(1-84) parathyroid hormone (PTH) detected by intact PTH assays. *Clin Chem* 46(5): pp. 697-703

Chertow, G. M., Blumenthal, S., Turner, S., Roppolo, M., Stern, L., Chi, E. M., & Reed, J. (2006). Cinacalcet hydrochloride (Sensipar) in hemodialysis patients on active vitamin D derivatives with controlled PTH and elevated calcium x phosphate. *Clin J Am Soc Nephrol* 1(2): pp. 305-312

Chertow, G. M., Pupim, L. B., Block, G. A., Correa-Rotter, R., Drueke, T. B., Floege, J., Goodman, W. G., London, G. M., Mahaffey, K. W., Moe, S. M., Wheeler, D. C., Albizem, M., Olson, K., Klassen, P., & Parfrey, P. (2007). Evaluation of Cinacalcet Therapy to Lower Cardiovascular Events (EVOLVE): rationale and design overview. *Clin J Am Soc Nephrol* 2(5): pp. 898-905

Chin, J., Miller, S. C., Wada, M., Nagano, N., Nemeth, E. F., & Fox, J. (2000). Activation of the calcium receptor by a calcimimetic compound halts the progression of secondary hyperparathyroidism in uremic rats. *J Am Soc Nephrol* 11(5): pp. 903-11

Covic, A., Kothawala, P., Bernal, M., Robbins, S., Chalian, A., & Goldsmith, D. (2009). Systematic review of the evidence underlying the association between mineral metabolism disturbances and risk of all-cause mortality, cardiovascular mortality and cardiovascular events in chronic kidney disease. *Nephrol Dial Transplant* 24(5): pp. 1506-1523

Cozzolino, M., Mazzaferro, S., & Brandenburg, V. (2011). The treatment of hyperphosphataemia in CKD: calcium-based or calcium-free phosphate binders? *Nephrol Dial Transplant* 26(2): pp. 402-407

Culleton, B. F., Walsh, M., Klarenbach, S. W., Mortis, G., Scott-Douglas, N., Quinn, R. R., Tonelli, M., Donnelly, S., Friedrich, M. G., Kumar, A., Mahallati, H., Hemmelgarn, B. R., & Manns, B. J. (2007). Effect of frequent nocturnal hemodialysis vs conventional hemodialysis on left ventricular mass and quality of life: a randomized controlled trial. *JAMA* 298(11): pp. 1291-1299

Cunningham, J., Danese, M., Olson, K., Klassen, P., & Chertow, G. M. (2005). Effects of the calcimimetic cinacalcet HCl on cardiovascular disease, fracture, and health-related quality of life in secondary hyperparathyroidism. *Kidney Int* 68(4): pp. 1793-1800

Cunningham, J., Locatelli, F., & Rodriguez, M. (2011). Secondary hyperparathyroidism: pathogenesis, disease progression, and therapeutic options. *Clin J Am Soc Nephrol* 6(4): pp. 913-921

Cunningham, J. & Zehnder D. (2011). New Vitamin D analogs and changing therapeutic paradigms. *Kidney Int* 79(7): 702-707

Danese, M. D., Belozeroff, V., Smirnakis, K., & Rothman, K. J. (2008). Consistent control of mineral and bone disorder in incident hemodialysis patients. *Clin J Am Soc Nephrol* 3(5): pp. 1423-9

Drueke, T. B. & Touam M. (2009). Calcium balance in haemodialysis--do not lower the dialysate calcium concentration too much (con part). *Nephrol Dial Transplant* 24(10): pp. 2990-2993

Evenepoel, P., Claes, K., Kuypers, D., Maes, B., Bammens, B., & Vanrenterghem Y. (2004). Natural history of parathyroid function and calcium metabolism after kidney transplantation: a single-centre study. *Nephrol Dial Transplant* 19: pp. 1281-1287

Fishbane, S., Shapiro, W. B., Corry, D. B., Vicks, S. L., Roppolo, M., Rappaport, K., Ling, X., Goodman, W. G., Turner, S., & Charytan, C. (2008). Cinacalcet HCl and concurrent low-dose vitamin D improves treatment of secondary hyperparathyroidism in dialysis patients compared with vitamin D alone: the ACHIEVE study results. *Clin J Am Soc Nephrol* 3(6): pp. 1718-1725

Foley, R. N., Li, S., Liu, J., Gilbertson, D. T., Chen, S. C., & Collins, A. J. (2005). The fall and rise of parathyroidectomy in U.S. hemodialysis patients, 1992 to 2002. *J Am Soc Nephrol* 16(1): pp. 210-218

Fouque, D., Vennegoor, M.,ter Wee, P., Wanner, C., Basci, A., Canaud, B., Haage, P., Konner, K., Kooman, J., Martin-Malo, A., Pedrini, L., Pizzarelli, F., Tattersall, J., Tordoir, J., & Vanholder, R. (2007). EBPG guideline on nutrition. *Nephrol Dial Transplant* 22 Suppl 2: pp. 45-87

Fukagawa, M., Tominaga, Y., Kitaoka, M., Kakuta, T., & Kurokawa, K. (1999). Medical and surgical aspects of parathyroidectomy. *Kidney Int Suppl* 73: pp. 65-69

Gagne, E. R., Urena, P., Leite-Silva, S., Zingraff, J., Chevalier, A., Sarfati, E., Dubost, C., & Drueke, T. B. (1992). Short- and long-term efficacy of total parathyroidectomy with immediate autografting compared with subtotal parathyroidectomy in hemodialysis patients. *J Am Soc Nephrol* 3(4): pp. 1008-1017

Gasparri, G., Camandona, M., & Dei Poli, M. (2001). Secondary and tertiary hyperparathyroidism: causes of recurrent disease after 446 parathyroidectomies. *Ann Surg* 233(1): pp. 65-69

Giangrande, A., Castiglioni, A., Solbiati, L., & Allaria, P. (1992). Ultrasound-guided percutaneous fine-needle ethanol injection into parathyroid glands in secondary hyperparathyroidism. *Nephrol Dial Transplant* 7(5): pp. 412-421

Giovannucci, E. (2008). Vitamin D status and cancer incidence and mortality. *Adv Exp Med Biol* 624: pp. 31-42

Goldsmith, D. J., Covic, A., Fouque, D., Locatelli, F., Olgaard, K., Rodriguez, M., Spasovski, G., Urena, P., Zoccali, C., London, G. M., & Vanholder, R. (2010). Endorsement of the Kidney Disease Improving Global Outcomes (KDIGO) Chronic Kidney Disease-Mineral and Bone Disorder (CKD-MBD) Guidelines: a European Renal Best Practice (ERBP) commentary statement. *Nephrol Dial Transplant* 25(12): pp. 3823-3831

Goodman, W. G., Goldin, J., Kuizon, B. D., Yoon, C., Gales, B., Sider, D., Wang, Y., Chung, J., Emerick, A., Greaser, L., Elashoff, R. M., & Salusky, I. B. (2000). Coronary-artery calcification in young adults with end-stage renal disease who are undergoing dialysis. *N Engl J Med* 342(20): pp. 1478-1483

Gotch, F. A., Kotanko, P., Thijssen, S., & Levin, N. W.. (2010). The KDIGO guideline for dialysate calcium will result in an increased incidence of calcium accumulation in hemodialysis patients. *Kidney Int* 78(4): pp. 343-350

Holick, M. F. (2005). Vitamin D for health and in chronic kidney disease. *Semin Dial* 18(4): pp. 266-275

Hou, S. H., Zhao, J., Ellman, C. F., Hu, J., Griffin, Z., Spiegel, D. M., & Bourdeau, J. E. (1991). Calcium and phosphorus fluxes during hemodialysis with low calcium dialysate. *Am J Kidney Dis* 18(2): pp. 217-224

Isakova, T., Gutierrez, O. M., Chang, Y., Shah, A., Tamez, H., Smith, K., Thadhani, R., & Wolf, M. (2009). Phosphorus binders and survival on hemodialysis. *J Am Soc Nephrol* 20(2): pp. 388-396

Jean, G., Souberbielle, J. C., & Chazot, C. (2009). Monthly cholecalciferol administration in haemodialysis patients: a simple and efficient strategy for vitamin D supplementation. *Nephrol Dial Transplant* 24(12): pp. 3799-3805

Johnson, W. J., McCarthy, J. T., van Heerden, J. A., Sterioff, S., Grant, C. S., & Kao, P. C. (1988). Results of subtotal parathyroidectomy in hemodialysis patients. *Am J Med* 84(1): pp. 23-32

K/DOQI (2003). K/DOQI clinical practice guidelines for bone metabolism and disease in chronic kidney disease. *Am J Kidney Dis* 42(4 Suppl 3): pp. S1-201

KDIGO (2009). KDIGO clinical practice guideline for the diagnosis, evaluation, prevention, and treatment of Chronic Kidney Disease-Mineral and Bone Disorder (CKD-MBD). *Kidney Int Suppl*(113): pp. S1-130

Kitaoka, M., Fukagawa, M., Ogata, E., & Kurokawa, K. (1994). Reduction of functioning parathyroid cell mass by ethanol injection in chronic dialysis patients. *Kidney Int* 46(4): pp. 1110-1117

Koller, H., Zitt, E., Staudacher, G., Neyer, U., Mayer, G.,& Rosenkranz, A. R. (2004). Variable parathyroid hormone(1-84)/carboxylterminal PTH ratios detected by 4 novel parathyroid hormone assays. *Clin Nephrol* 61(5): pp. 337-343

Kruse, A. E., Eisenberger, U., Frey, F. J., & Mohaupt, M. G. (2005). The calcimimetic cinacalcet normalizes serum calcium in renal transplant patients with persistent hyperparathyroidism. *Nephrol Dial Transplant* 20: pp. 1311-1314

Lacson, E., Jr., Ikizler, T. A., Lazarus, J. M., Teng, M., & Hakim, R. M. (2007). Potential impact of nutritional intervention on end-stage renal disease hospitalization, death, and treatment costs. *J Ren Nutr* 17(6): pp. 363-371

Lindberg, J. S., Culleton, B., Wong, G., Borah, M. F., Clark, R. V., Shapiro, W. B., Roger, S. D., Husserl, F. E., Klassen, P. S., Guo, M. D., Albizem, M. B., & Coburn, J. W. (2005). Cinacalcet HCl, an oral calcimimetic agent for the treatment of secondary hyperparathyroidism in hemodialysis and peritoneal dialysis: a randomized, double-blind, multicenter study. *J Am Soc Nephrol* 16(3): pp. 800-807

Locatelli, F., Dimkovic, N., Pontoriero, G., Spasovski, G., Pljesa, S., Kostic, S., Manning, A., Sano, H., & Nakajima, S. (2010). Effect of MCI-196 on serum phosphate and cholesterol levels in haemodialysis patients with hyperphosphataemia: a double-blind, randomized, placebo-controlled study. *Nephrol Dial Transplant* 25(2): pp. 574-581

Malberti, F., Marcelli, D., Conte, F., Limido, A., Spotti, D., & Locatelli, F. (2001). Parathyroidectomy in patients on renal replacement therapy: an epidemiologic study. *J Am Soc Nephrol* 12(6): pp. 1242-1248

Malluche, H. & Faugere M. C. (1990). Renal bone disease 1990: an unmet challenge for the nephrologist. *Kidney Int* 38(2): pp. 193-211

Meola, M., Petrucci, I., & Barsotti, G. (2009). Long-term treatment with cinacalcet and conventional therapy reduces parathyroid hyperplasia in severe secondary hyperparathyroidism. *Nephrol Dial Transplant* 24(3): pp. 982-989

Messa, P., Macario, F., Yaqoob, M., Bouman, K., Braun, J., von Albertini, B., Brink, H., Maduell, F., Graf, H., Frazao, J. M., Bos, W. J., Torregrosa, V., Saha, H., Reichel, H., Wilkie, M., Zani, V. J., Molemans, B., Carter, D., & Locatelli, F. (2008). The OPTIMA study: assessing a new cinacalcet (Sensipar/Mimpara) treatment algorithm for secondary hyperparathyroidism. *Clin J Am Soc Nephrol* 3(1): pp. 36-45

Moe, S., Drueke, T., Cunningham, J., Goodman, W., Martin, K., Olgaard, K., Ott, S., Sprague, S., Lameire, N., & Eknoyan, G. (2006). Definition, evaluation, and classification of renal osteodystrophy: a position statement from Kidney Disease: Improving Global Outcomes (KDIGO). *Kidney Int* 69(11): pp. 1945-1953

Muller, D., Mehling, H., Otto, B., Bergmann-Lips, R., Luft, F., Jordan, J., Kettritz, R. (2007). Niacin lowers serum phosphate and increases HDL cholesterol in dialysis patients. *Clin J Am Soc Nephrol* 2(6): pp. 1249-1254

Navaneethan, S. D., Palmer, S. C., Craig, J. C., Elder, G. J., & Strippoli, G. F. (2009). Benefits and harms of phosphate binders in CKD: a systematic review of randomized controlled trials. *Am J Kidney Dis* 54(4): pp. 619-637

Naves-Diaz, M., Alvarez-Hernandez, D., Passlick-Deetjen, J., Guinsburg, A., Marelli, C., Rodriguez-Puyol, D., & Cannata-Andia, J. B. (2008). Oral active vitamin D is associated with improved survival in hemodialysis patients. *Kidney Int* 74(8): pp. 1070-1078

Nemeth, E. F., Steffey, M. E., Hammerland, L. G., Hung, B. C., Van Wagenen, B. C., DelMar, E. G., & Balandrin, M. F. (1998). Calcimimetics with potent and selective activity on the parathyroid calcium receptor. *Proc Natl Acad Sci U S A* 95(7): pp. 4040-4045

Neyer, U., Hoerandner, H., Haid, A., Zimmermann, G., & Niederle, B. (2002). Total parathyroidectomy with autotransplantation in renal hyperparathyroidism: low recurrence after intra-operative tissue selection. *Nephrol Dial Transplant* 17(4): pp. 625-629

Noori, N., Kalantar-Zadeh, K., Kovesdy, C. P., Bross, R., Benner, D., & Kopple, J. D. (2010). Association of dietary phosphorus intake and phosphorus to protein ratio with mortality in hemodialysis patients. *Clin J Am Soc Nephrol* 5(4): pp. 683-692

Pelletier, S., Roth, H., Bouchet, J. L., Drueke, T., London, G., & Fouque, D. (2010). Mineral and bone disease pattern in elderly haemodialysis patients. *Nephrol Dial Transplant* 25(9): pp. 3062-3070

Raggi, P., Boulay, A., Chasan-Taber, S., Amin, N., Dillon, M., Burke, S. K., & Chertow, G. M. (2002). Cardiac calcification in adult hemodialysis patients. A link between end-stage renal disease and cardiovascular disease? *J Am Coll Cardiol* 39(4): pp. 695-701

Ribeiro, S., Ramos, A., Brandao, A., Rebelo, J. R., Guerra, A., Resina, C., Vila-Lobos, A., Carvalho, F., Remedio, F., & Ribeiro, F. (1998). Cardiac valve calcification in haemodialysis patients: role of calcium-phosphate metabolism. *Nephrol Dial Transplant* 13(8): pp. 2037-2040

Rodriguez, M. & Lorenzo V. (2009). Parathyroid hormone, a uremic toxin. *Semin Dial* 22(4): pp. 363-836

Serra, A. L., Schwarz, A. A., Wick, F. H., Marti, H.P., & Wuthrich, R. P. (2005). Successful treatment of hypercalcemia with cinacalcet in renal transplant recipients with persistent hyperparathyroidism. *Nephrol Dial Transplant* 20: pp. 1315-1319

Sherman, R. A. & Mehta O. (2009). Dietary phosphorus restriction in dialysis patients: potential impact of processed meat, poultry, and fish products as protein sources. *Am J Kidney Dis* 54(1): pp. 18-23

Sherman, R. A. & Mehta O. (2009). Phosphorus and potassium content of enhanced meat and poultry products: implications for patients who receive dialysis. *Clin J Am Soc Nephrol* 4(8): pp. 1370-1373

Shiizaki, K., Hatamura, I., Negi, S., Narukawa, N., Mizobuchi, M., Sakaguchi, T., Ooshima, A., & Akizawa, T. (2003). Percutaneous maxacalcitol injection therapy regresses hyperplasia of parathyroid and induces apoptosis in uremia. *Kidney Int* 64(3): pp. 992-1003

Shinaberger, C. S., Greenland, S., Kopple, J. D., Van Wyck, D., Mehrotra, R., Kovesdy, C. P., & Kalantar-Zadeh, K. (2008). Is controlling phosphorus by decreasing dietary protein intake beneficial or harmful in persons with chronic kidney disease? *Am J Clin Nutr* 88(6): pp. 1511-1518.

Souberbielle, J. C., Roth, H., & Fouque, D. P. (2010). Parathyroid hormone measurement in CKD. *Kidney Int* 77(2): pp. 93-100

Sprague, S. M., Evenepoel, P., Curzi, M. P., Gonzalez, M. T., Husserl, F. E., Kopyt, N., Sterling, L. R., Mix, C., & Wong, G. (2009). Simultaneous control of PTH and CaxP Is sustained over three years of treatment with cinacalcet HCl. *Clin J Am Soc Nephrol* 4(9): pp. 1465-1476

Srinivas, T. R., Schold, J. D., Womer, K.L., Kaplan, B., Howard, R. J., Bucci, C. M., & Meier-Kriesche, H. U. (2006). Improvement in hypercalcemia with cinacalcet after kidney transplantation. *Clin J Am Soc Nephro* 1: pp. 323-326.

Sullivan, C., Sayre, S. S., Leon, J. B., Machekano, R., Love, T. E., Porter, D., Marbury, M., & Sehgal, A. R. (2009). Effect of food additives on hyperphosphatemia among patients with end-stage renal disease: a randomized controlled trial. *JAMA* 301(6): pp. 629-635

Teng, M., Wolf, M., Lowrie, E., Ofsthun, N., Lazarus, J. M. ,& Thadhani, R. (2003). Survival of patients undergoing hemodialysis with paricalcitol or calcitriol therapy. *N Engl J Med* 349(5): pp. 446-456

Teng, M., Wolf, M., Ofsthun, M. N., Lazarus, J. M., Hernan, M. A., Camargo, C. A., Jr., & Thadhani, R. (2005). Activated injectable vitamin D and hemodialysis survival: a historical cohort study. *J Am Soc Nephrol* 16(4): pp. 1115-1125

Tentori, F., Hunt, W. C., Stidley, C. A., Rohrscheib, M. R., Bedrick, E. J., Meyer, K. B., Johnson, H. K., & Zager, P. G. (2006). Mortality risk among hemodialysis patients receiving different vitamin D analogs. *Kidney Int* 70(10): pp. 1858-1865

Tominaga, Y., Tanaka, Y., Sato, K., Nagasaka, T., & Takagi, H. (1997). Histopathology, pathophysiology, and indications for surgical treatment of renal hyperparathyroidism. *Semin Surg Oncol* 13(2): pp. 78-86

Tonelli, M., Pannu, N., & Manns, B. (2010). Oral phosphate binders in patients with kidney failure. *N Engl J Med* 362(14): pp. 1312-1324

Tonelli, M., Wang, W., Hemmelgarn, B., Lloyd, A., & Manns, B. (2009). Phosphate removal with several thrice-weekly dialysis methods in overweight hemodialysis patients. *Am J Kidney Dis* 54(6): pp. 1108-1115

Triponez, F., Clark, O.H., Vanrenterghem Y., & Evenepoel, P. (2008). Surgical Treatment of Persistent Hyperparathyroidism After Renal Transplantation. *Ann Surg* 248: pp. 18-30

Uhlig, K., Berns, J. S., Kestenbaum, B., Kumar, R., Leonard, M. B., Martin, K. J., Sprague, S. M., & Goldfarb, S. (2010). KDOQI US commentary on the 2009 KDIGO Clinical Practice Guideline for the Diagnosis, Evaluation, and Treatment of CKD-Mineral and Bone Disorder (CKD-MBD). *Am J Kidney Dis* 55(5): pp. 773-799

Urena, P., Jacobson, S. H., Zitt, E., Vervloet, M., Malberti, F., Ashman, N., Leavey, S., Rix, M., Os, I., Saha, H., Ryba, M., Bencova, V., Banos, A., Zani, V., & Fouque, D. (2009). Cinacalcet and achievement of the NKF/K-DOQI recommended target values for bone and mineral metabolism in real-world clinical practice--the ECHO observational study. *Nephrol Dial Transplant* 24(9): pp. 2852-2859

Walsh, M., B. J. Manns, et al. (2010). "The effects of nocturnal compared with conventional hemodialysis on mineral metabolism: A randomized-controlled trial." *Hemodial Int* 14(2): 174-81.

Wolf, M., Manns, B. J., Klarenbach, S., Tonelli, M., Hemmelgarn, B., & Culleton, B. (2007). Vitamin D levels and early mortality among incident hemodialysis patients. *Kidney Int* 72(8): pp. 1004-1013

Young, E. W., Young, E. W., Akiba, T., Albert, J. M., McCarthy, J. T., Kerr, P. G., Mendelssohn, D. C., & Jadoul, M. (2004). Magnitude and impact of abnormal mineral metabolism in hemodialysis patients in the Dialysis Outcomes and Practice Patterns Study (DOPPS). *Am J Kidney Dis* 44(5 Suppl 2): pp. 34-38

Zitt, E., Haid, A., Köberle-Wührer, R., Sprenger-Mähr, H., Hörandner, H., Zimmermann, G., & Neyer, U. (2007). Long-term observation after parathyroidectomy with autotransplantation of selected parathyroid tissue in chronic dialysis patients. *Nieren-Hochdruckkrkh* 36(3): pp. 87-95

Zitt, E., Rix, M., Urena Torres, P., Fouque, D., Jacobson, S. H., Petavy, F., Dehmel, B., & Ryba, M. (2010). Effectiveness of cinacalcet in patients with recurrent/persistent secondary hyperparathyroidism following parathyroidectomy: results of the ECHO study. *Nephrol Dial Transplant* Oct 28. [Epub ahead of print]

19

Lipid and Lipoprotein Abnormalities in Chronic Renal Insufficiency: Review

Oliver Rácz[1], Rudolf Gaško[2] and Eleonóra Klímová[3]
[1]*Šafárik University, Medical School, Košice*
[2]*Railway Hospital, Košice*
[3]*University of Prešov,*
Faculty of Health Care, Prešov
Slovak Republic

1. Introduction

1.1 Kidney disease and cardiovascular mortality

Cardiovascular disease is a leading case of mortality not only in the whole population but also in groups with different, noncardiovascular chronic conditions. Kidney disease is one of these and many patients with kidney disease paradoxically do not die from end stage kidney failure but from cardiovascular causes. Already mild or moderate renal impairment represents a considerable excess risk of cardiovascular mortality. The probability of premature death is even more striking in some subgroups of kidney patients - e.g. the cardiovascular mortality rate of young end stage renal disease (ESRD) patients is 500 times higher as compared with an age-matched control group. The situation is moreover complicated by the fact that traditional risk factors (the "Framingham factors") are of lesser predictive value in kidney disease than in general population (Foley et al, 1998, Magnus and Beaglehole, 2001, Go et al, 2004).

To explain this dismal picture it is not sufficient to disclose that chronic kidney disease (CKD) and chronic renal insufficiency (CRI) is associated with accelerated atherosclerosis and abnormal lipid/lipoprotein metabolism (Felström et al., 2003, Lacquaniti, 2010). One should keep in mind that "CKD", "CRI" and "ESRD" are collective terms and the actual diseases and conditions behind them are manifold (Table 1). Some of them (e.g. diabetes mellitus and hypertension) have a profound effect on lipid metabolism and atherosclerosis independently from kidney function already before the manifestation of renal impairment. From the data in Table 1 is evident that diabetes and hypertension is behind ESRD in one quarter (Great Britain) or even two thirds (USA) of cases.

The natural history of each underlying disease is dependent on a wide range of factors and although the K/DOQI classification based on glomerulal filtration rate is a very useful one from practical point of view it does not reveal anything about the pathogenesis of the particular condition.

Etiology of ESRD	Great Britain	Australia	USA	Japan
Chronic glomerulonephritis	30%	30%	9%	47%
Diabetic nephropathy	16%	22%	43%	31%
Hypertension	12%	14%	26%	10%
Chronic interstitial nephritis	8%	10%	2%	2%
Polycystic degeneration	6%	6%	2%	2%
Other/unkown	28%	18%	13%	8%

Table 1. Etiology of end stage renal disease in different regions of word. (According to Viklický, 2006)

1.2 Accelerated atherosclerosis in CKD

Despite all above mentioned uncertanities concerning the causal association between renal disease and accelerated atherosclerosis there is a considerable amount of knowledge in the field of pathophysiology and pathobiochemistry of this topic (Felström et al, 2003, Vaziri, 2006, Kwan et al, 2007, Saland &t Ginsberg, 2007, Tsimihodimos et al. 2008 and 2011, Basnakian at al, 2010; Karumanchi & Thadhani, 2010). An overview of different factors influencing the rate of atherosclerosis in CKD, CRI and ESRD is summarized in Table 2. These factors however do not act independently but in the frame of a complicated and not yet fully understood network (Fig 1.). They are present already in the early phases of kidney diseases and in many cases other pathological conditions associated with accelerated atherosclerosis (obesity, diabetes, hypertension, etc.) are present, too.

Dyslipidemia (increased triglycerides and LDL-cholesterol, decreased HDL-cholesterol)
Atherogenic lipid fractions (oxidized and carbamylated LDL, small dense LDL, triglyceride rich particles)
Abnormal values and forms of apolipoproteins (apoB, apoAI, $Lp_{(a)}$)
Uremic toxins
Alterations of calcium and phosphorus metabolism
Oxidative stress (increased formation of reactive oxygen species and advanced glycation endproducts, decreased acitivty of antioxidants)
Immunodeficiency
Inflammation
Malnutrition, hypalbuminemia and proteinuria
Anaemia
Physical inactivity
Ethnicity and genetic polymorphism
Drug treatment
Hemodialysis modalities
Peritoneal dialysis

Table 2. Factors influencing atherosclerosis development in CKD, CRI and ESRD

1.3 The aim of this chapter

In this chapter the authors try to answer some question conserning accelerated atherosclerosis and its assessment in CRI patients. In the subsequent parts they:

1. Describe and analyze the lipid and lipoprotein abnormalities in CRI, ESRD and HD.
2. Show the results of a metaanalysis dealing with methodological problems measuring LDL-cholesterol in CRI, ESRD and HD patients and results from a study on analytical quality of LDL-cholesterol assessment in real word laboratories.
3. Give simple advice how to assess cardiovascular risk in CRI, ESRD and HD patients in everyday clinical practice.

Therapeutic attempts and possibilities to normalize the lipid abnormalities and decrease the high risk of cardiovascular events in CRI, ESRD and HD patients are not the topics of this chapter.

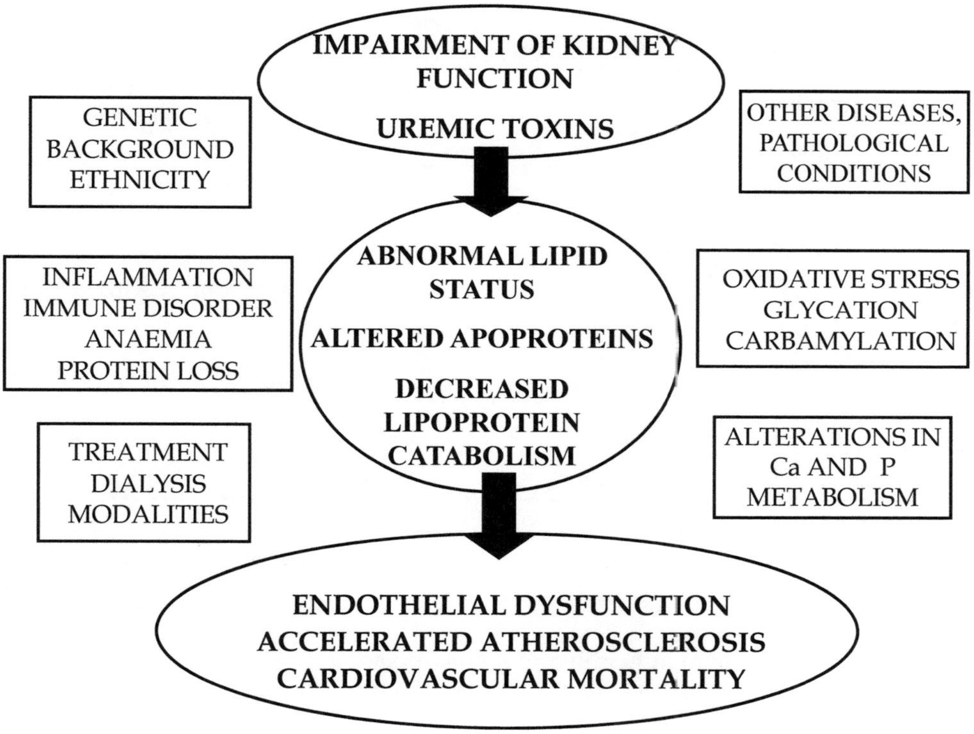

Fig. 1. Factors responsible for abnormal lipid metabolism and accelerated atherosclerosis in kidney disease form a complicated and intertwined network

2. Lipid and lipoprotein abnormalities in kidney disease

2.1 Changes of routinely measured lipid parameters in CRI and HD

The changes of two basic lipid parameters - the concentration of triglycerides (TG) and total cholesterol (TC) in different forms of renal disease are in Table 3. Increased triglyceride concentration is a general feature of kidney disease whereas increased cholesterol is not. Assesment the risk of atherosclerosis related morbidity from these two parameters is of course not possible because they do not reflect the real metabolic situation sufficiently. Lipids are insoluble in blood plasma and therefore they can circulate only in the form of lipoproteins. On the other side increased TG alone is an important warning sign of the presence of highly atherogenic triglyceride rich lipoprotein particles (TRL). The concentration of total cholesterol on the other side does not provide a valuable information because its carriers can be less and more atherogenic or even antiatherogenic. In table 4 data on changes of HDL-cholesterol, non-HDL-cholesterol and the highly atherogenhic $Lp_{(a)}$ in CRI are shown. LDL-cholesterol is not involved in this table for reasons of its analytical uncertainity which is further analyzed in part 3 of this chapter. From data in Table 3 and 4 the shift towards accelerated atherosclerosis is evident - high amount of triglycerides in the lipoproteins and a low level of antiatherogenic HDL particles regardless on the form and stage of kidney disease (Vazari, 2006, Saland et Ginsberg, 2007, Tsimihodimos et al., 2008, Attman et al., 2010).

Condition	Triglycerides	Total cholesterol
Minimal proteinuria	Increased	No change or decrease
Heavy proteinuria	Increased	Highly increased in nephrotic syndrome
Chronic renal insufficiency	Increased	No change
Hemodialysis	Increased	Controversial data - mostly no change
Peritoneal dialysis	Increased	Increased

Table 3. Triglycerides and total cholesterol in different conditions associated with kidney disease

Condition	Non-HDL cholesterol	HDL-cholesterol	$Lp_{(a)}$
Chronic renal insufficiency	Increased	Decreased	Increased
Hemodialysis	Increased	Decreased	Increased
Peritoneal dialysis	Increased	Decreased	Increased

Table 4. Non-HDL cholesterol, HDL cholesterol and $lipoprotein_{(a)}$ in chronic renal insufficiency, hemodialysis and peritoneal dialysis

2.2 Lipoprotein metabolism in health and kidney disease

Lipoproteins are complex particles consisting from lipids transferred from and to the tissues and a phospholipid envelope containing different proteins. They are not passive containers of TG and cholesterol but dynamic particles with variable composition. Both lipoprotein turnover and composition is altered in kidney diseases and therefore basic knowledge about it is essential for the proper assessment of cardiovascular risk in this special case. Lipoprotens are divided int three families: Chylomicrons and their remnants, the VLDL-IDL-LDL family and the HDL family. Their composition and apoprotein content is in Tables 5 and 6.

Chylomicrons produced in enterocytes are carriers of lipids from guts to liver. There are much bigger than the other lipoproteins and during ultracentrifugation they do not sediment at all. Chylomicrons contain one molecule of apoprotein is B48 and some apoprotein molecules A I, A II and A IV. During their life span they acquire apo E and apo C from HDL particles. In contact with muscle and fat tissue capillary endothelial cells they release fatty acids through triglyceride lipolysis catalyzed by endothelium-bound lipoprotein lipase. Remnants of chylomicrons are removed by the liver.

Lipoprotein	Size, nm	Density, g/l	Lipid content, %		
			TG	CH	PL
Chylomicrons Chylomicron remnants	80 – 500 > 50	< 0,940	80 – 95	2-7	3-9
VLDL IDL LDL	30 – 80 25 – 35 18 – 25	0,950 – 1,005 1,000 – 1,019 1,019 – 1,063	55 – 80 20 – 50 5 – 15	5 – 15 20 – 40 40 – 50	10 – 20 15 -25 20 – 25
HDL_2 HDL_3	9 – 12 5 - 9	1,063 – 1,125 1,125 – 1,210	5 – 10	15 – 25	20 – 30

Table 5. Basic characteristics of lipoproteins (According to Žák, 2002, modified; PL = phospholipids)

Apoprotein, function	Gene	Finding
A I – activator of LCAT	11q23-qter	HDL, CHY
A II – activator of liver lipase, Inhibitor of LCAT	11q21-q23	HDL, CHY
A IV – activator of LCAT	11q23-qter	HDL, CHY
B 100 - key protein for assembly and receptor binding	2p23-24	LDL, IDL, VLDL
B 48 - short form of B 100	The same as B100	CHY
C I -Cofactor of LCAT	19q12-q13.2	CHY, VLDL
C II – activator of lipoprotein lipase	19q12-q13.2	CHY, VLDL, HDL
C III – inhibitor of VLDL transfer into liver	11q23-qter	CHY, VLDL, IDL
D – regulator of cholesterol ester transfer	3q14.2-qter	HDL
E – Transfer of CHY remnants into liver	19q12-q13.2	CHY, VLDL, IDL

Table 6. Apoprotein function and their occurence in lipoproteins

After a meal rich in fat the peak value of chylomicrons occurs approximately in 3 hours and they disappear in 8 – 9 hours. Visible plasma turbidity is a clear sign of chylomicron presence (mostly caused when blood sampling is not realized in fasting state). Chylomicrons are not involved singificantly in atherogenesis but in the case of their decreased catabolism (which is a case in kidney disease) the accumulated remnants can be atherogenic (Chan et al, 2009).

Endogenous lipid carrier particles are formed in the liver as VLDL. They contain a bigger variant of apoB (apoB100) but the function of this protein is the same as in chylomicrons. Apoproteins B are of key importance during the assembly of lipoprotein particles and also serve as a docking structure when the lipoprotein binds to the LDL-receptor. The interaction of VLDL with HDL and with the tissues is similar to that of chylomicrons and during their circulation they became smaller – known as IDL and LDL. LDL particles during their relatively long life span ($t_{1/2}$ = 2 – 4 hours and in CRI probably even more) can undergo oxidation, glycation and carbamylation. These random postsynthetic events alter the quality of liporoteins with a profound effect on their cellular metabolism – e.g. the uptake of damaged LDL particles through the scavenger receptor and not through the LDL-receptor. Another important topic important for the rate of atherosclerosis (not only) in CRI patients is the presence of small dense LDL particles and (Table 7) and increased levels of abnormal particles as $Lp_{(a)}$ - Tables 4 and 8. All these features render the interpretation of basic laboratory parameters of lipid/lipoprotein metabolism in regard to the assessment of atherosclerosis difficult (Table 9).

Despite the complicated and sometimes contradictory data on LDL metabolism in CRI, ESDR and HD it is possible to summarize the underlying picture in a relatively simple way. According to Ikerwaka et al (2005) and Chan et al (2009) all lipid and lipoprotein alterations associated with LDL particles have a common soil - their decreased catabolism. Increased synthesis can play an additonal role in the case of massive proteinuria.

Class	Density, g/ml	Size, nm	% of LDL
I	1.026	27.5 - 26.0	3
II	1.028	26.0 - 25.5	16
III	1.034	25.5 - 24.2	50
IV	1.048	24.2 - 21.8	22
V	> 1.048	< 21.8	9

Table 7. Normal density distribution of LDL particles

Lipoprotein $Lp_{(a)}$	has a similar structure and composition as LDL particles
Density:	1,050 - 1,100
Size:	25 - 35 nm
Proteins:	ApoB 100 and an abnormal protein, $Apo_{(a)}$ attached to the B 100 $Apo_{(a)}$ has a variable molecular weight between 300 – 800 kDa, its structure is similar to the plasminogen (involved in fibrinolysis).
Subtypes:	6 different forms – F, B and S1 – S4
Concentration:	0 - 1200 mg/l with abnormal distribution of values. As atherogenic are considered concentrations above 200 - 300 mg/l
Lp(a) in CRI:	Increased but the cause of increase is not clear. The basic level of $Apo_{(a)}$ is probably associated with gene polymorphisms and the kidney disease is a provocative factor for further increase (Danesh et al, 2000)

Table 8. Structure of $Lp_{(a)}$

The basic function of HDL is the reverse transport of surplus cholesterol from the tissues to liver. HDL particles are synthetized as discoid particles poor in lipids. Nascent HDL (or HDL_3) particles contain a lot of different apoproteins (70 % of total protein is Apo A-I and 20 % Apo A-II) crucial in TG and cholesterol metabolism which they exchange with chylomicrons and VLDL. Cholesterol bound to the surface of HDL is esterified by the enzyme LCAT and the esters are internalized. The cholesterol-ester loaded HDL_2 particles unload their content through a specific receptor into the liver. The low number and decreased function of LDL particles (manifest as "low HDL-C") is probably a consequence of the enzyme LCAT and the apoprotein A-I. Recently Rosenson et al (2011) highlighted the topic of HDL heterogeneity and its possible role in the pathophysiology of accelerated atherosclerosis in kidney disease. According to this concept not the low level of "good cholesterol" but rather the altered constellation of HDL structure and function is of importance in atherogenesis.

Tiacylglycerols and cholesterol are insoluble in water. They circulate in the blood exclusively as lipoproteins.
Lipoproteins are complex particles; their cholesterol content (measured or calculated as HDL-C and LDL-C) does not reflect their real composition and structure.
Lipoproteins are dynamic, changing their lipid and protein composition during their life span in the circulation.
Lipoproteins are heterogeneous and their different density is not a simple biological variation but it has profound effect on their metabolism. Small dense lipoproteins are more atherogenic than those with low density.
In some people and in some pathological conditions there are also abnormal lipoproteins in the blood. One of them is $lipoprotein_{(a)}$ which is highly aterogenic and its concentration is increased in renal disease.
Some of the assay methods for lipids and lipoproteins are not bulletproof from analytical point of view – see part 3 of this chapter

Table 9. Pitfalls in interpretation of basic lipid parameters from clinical point of view

3. Methods for measurement and lipids, lipoproteins with special attention to LDL-cholesterol measurement

3.1 Basic lipid assays and the short history of lipid and lipoprotein measurement

The first cumbersome but at that time reliable colorimetric methods for cholesterol and triglyceride assays were developed in the first half of the last century. From today's point of view obsolete methods were crucial for understanding the association between lipid metabolism and cardiovascular disease. Later there were replaced with enzymatic assays and adjusted for the use in automatic analyzers. Isolation of lipoproteins by ultracentrifugation giving basis for the today lipoprotein terminology was introduced in the 40's of the last century. Analytical and preparative ultracentrifugation is also today the gold standard method for quantification, separation and research on lipoproteins. About the same time paper electrophoresis (later replaced by agarose and polyacrylamide gel) gave the rise not only to an alternative nomenclature (alpha, pre-beta and beta lipoproteins) but also to the epoch-making phenotypic classification of dyslipoproteinemias by Fredrickson & Lees in 1965 and a better understanding of the pathobiochemistry of atherosclerosis. This methodology is currently reserved only for specialized applications. (For an excellent review on this topic see Mcnamara et al., 2006).

Triglyceride and total cholesterol assays are the starting points of lipid status assessment also today but their information value is different. Strictly speaking both are "artefacts" but whereas total triglycerides provide an important information about the presence of TRLs, total cholesterol itself has a limited diagnostic value.

3.2 Estimation of LDL-cholesterol

Lipoproteins are prone to differential precipitation in arteficial conditions (e.g. heparin-manganese or dextran-magnesium solutions) and this allowed to develop methods to separate them without ultracentrifugation or electrophoresis. Based on this procedure in 70's first the direct measurement of HDL-C was developed and introduced into clinical chemistry. On the other side direct measurement of LDL-C was not possible until the end of the century. In the 25 year long interim period there was only one possibility to estimate the

concentration of LDL-C in everyday practice. It was the calculation according to Friedewald formula (Friedewald et al, 1972). The formula was based on the analysis of a large LDL database created in research laboratories using ultracentrifugation. It was however clear that a calculation from three (TC, TG, HDL-C) measured values with their own analytical uncertainity is only a recourse from necessity.
The uncertainity of the currently employed 3rd generation methods is much lower than that of the Friedewald formula or the older methods but from strictly analytical point of view they are also not sufficient to obtain accurate results (Bairaktari et al., 2005). Another unsolved problem is that the assay methods from different providers are not yet harmonized at all (Fuentes-Arderiu et al, 2009, Miller et al, 2010).

3.3 Apoprotein measurements

The discovery of immunochemical methodology in 70's made apoprotein assays possible. In the same time their function and their role in lipid metabolism was identified. According to recent view some of them belong to parameters providing important information when assessing cardiovascular disease risk (Ritz & Wanner, 2004, Batista et al, 2005) There are three apoproteins which should be measured in each patiens with elevated risk of cardiovascular disease: Apoprotein B100, apoprotein A-I and lipoprotein$_{(a)}$.
Only one molecule of ApoB100 is present in each LDL-type particle (Fig 2). ApoB100 is a big molecule (m.w. 550 kDa) crucial already in the synthesis of VLDL and playing an essential role in the removal of LDL from the circulation. Measurement of ApoB100 in routine clinical practice is possible and in contrast to dynamic and heterogenous entities as "HDL-cholesterol" and "LDL-cholesterol" is an unambiguously defined analyte. The concentration of ApoB100 therefore provides the best information about the presence of LDL-type particles circulating in the blood (Olofsson et al, 2007). Elevated concentration apoB100 and normal or slightly elevated LDL-C or nonHDL-C is an indirect but valuable marker of small dense LDL particles
Apoprotein A-I is a small molecule (28 kDa) and HDL particles contain several of them. They are activators of LCAT, that means the concentration of Apo A-I is a marker of HDL particle function and the metabolic activity of the particles and not their size or number.

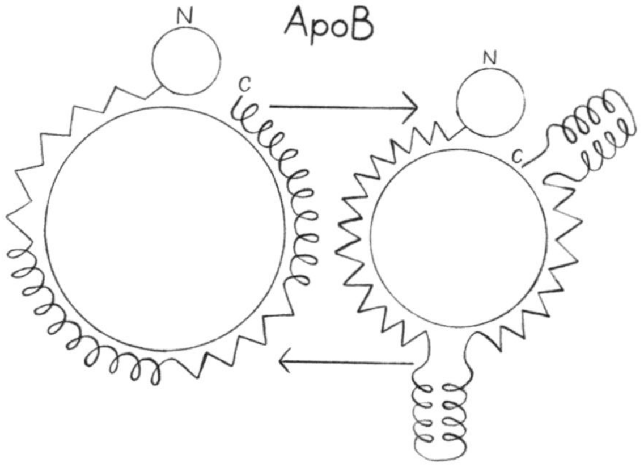

Fig. 2. Apoprotein B100 is a big ringlike flexible molecule holding the whole particle together in its different stages of metabolism and making its binding to LDL-receptor

4. Analytical accuracy of LDL-C in kidney disease and hemodialysis

4.1 Metaanalysis of results achieved with Friedewald equation compared to reference ultracentrifugation method

Our metaanalysis contains data from all available published papers dealing (entirely or as a part of broader study) with analytical accuracy of LDL-C assessment according to the Friedewald equation as compared with the reference UC method in CRI patients. The methodology of the metanalysis is described in our previous paper (Gaško et Sánchez-Meca, 2009). It includes studies from 1990 until the end of year 2010. Four studies were found but two of them were further divided according to the details of the study. The basic data of the studies are summarized in Table 10 and the results of metaanalysis in Fig 3.

Study, Year	Probands	Location	% Weight	Inclusion criteria
Nauck & al 1, 1996	887	Germany	0.0%	healthy (not included)
Nauck & al 2, 1996	136	Germany	23.2%	HD, TG < 4.56 mmol/l
Nauck & al 3, 1996	171	Germany	29.2%	CAPD, TG < 4.56 mmol/l
Pedro-Botet & al, 1996	101	Spain	17.2%	HD, age 20 - 80 years
Bairaktari & al 1, 2001	54	Greece	9.2%	HDs, TG < 2.26 mmol/l
Bairaktari & al 2, 2001	38	Greece	6.5%	HD, TG 2,26 – 4.52 mmol/l
Bairaktari & al, 2004	86	Greece	14.7%	HDs TG < 4.5 mmol/l
	586		100.0%	

Table 10. Studies included in metaanalysis, divided into subgroups according to inclusion criteria.

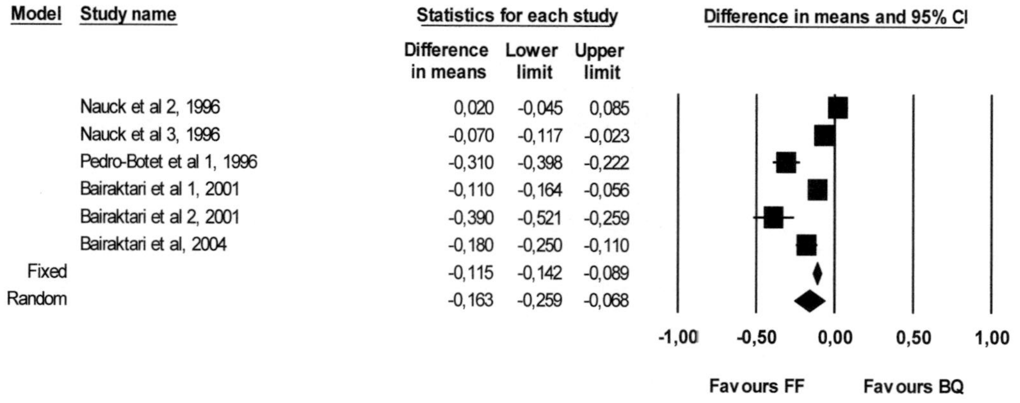

Fig. 3. Difference in means LDL-C with 95% CI in 4 studies included with 6 subgroups of patients with severe nephropathy on different forms of dialysis, with fixed and random effects model summary difference. Forest plot. Units: mmol/l. Patients included 586.

For patients in different dialysis regimes the summary differences of means of LDL-C is 0.234 mmol/l, what presents a bias of -4.9%. The information value of this result is much higher when compared with results on healthy probands od with results of patients with other diseases. We identified 23 publications including 17 213 patients analyzing accuracy of LDL-C assessment on healthy probands or in patients with hyperlipidemia from 1990 until 2009. The summary differences of means in this setting is 0.108 mmol/l and the bias is +2.3%. Furhter 3 papers followed analytical accuracy LDL-C in 350 patients with I and II diabetes mellitus or with hepatopathy. Total difference in means in this group was 0.234 mmol/l, (bias +6.8%; Fig 4).

From these findings it is possible to conclude that calculated concentrations of LDL-C according to the Friedewald equation can differ from the true values by almost 12 % systemic error. For clinical practice this analytical error can have a unwelcome situation because in approximately 7% of patients proper and necessary treatment according to guidelines is not prescribed and in another 5 % superfluous treatment is prescribed. This second group however is not in a danger of non-treated dyslipidemia because but there is problem of pharmacoeconomy.

Model	Study name	Difference in means	Lower limit	Upper limit
	Matas et al 2, 1994	0,370	0,214	0,526
	Matas et al 3, 1994	0,310	0,215	0,405
	Hirany et al 1, 1997	0,180	0,099	0,261
	Hirany et al 2, 1997	0,280	0,234	0,326
	Wägner et al, 2000	0,240	0,197	0,283
	Wägner et al, 2003	0,090	0,038	0,142
Fixed		0,220	0,196	0,245
Random		0,234	0,160	0,309

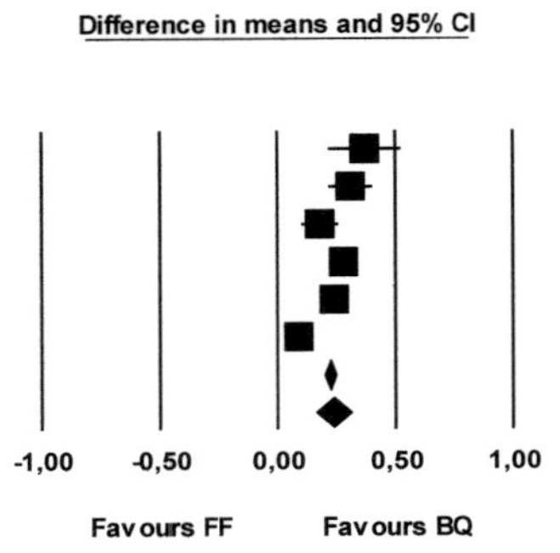

Fig. 4. Difference in means LDL-C with 95% CI in 3 studies included with 6 subgroups of patients with diabetes mellitus or hepatopathy, with fixed and random effects model summary difference. Forest plot. Units: mmol/l. Patients included 350. Figure from Gaško & Sánchez-Meca, 2009, with permision.

4.2 Unreliability of LDL-C assessment in everyday laboratory practice

There is only one method providing a true picture about the composition of the particles ultracentrifugation with subsequent chemical analysis of their composition. This method is the golden standard and the anchor of all methods used in routine clinical practice.

For a couple of years there was only one indirect way to estimate the cholesterol content of LDL particles. Despite modern methods estimating total cholesterol, HDL-cholesterol and triglycerides with a high level of precision and accuracy they have a certain degree of uncertainity and the overall uncertainity is too high to give a reliable picture on LDL-cholesterol even in probands without any confounding factors. In CRI patients the situation is even worse.

Recently clinical chemistry laboratories can use one commercial kits based on 7 different method for direct LDL-C assays. Some laboratories however calculate LDL-C according to the Friedewald formula or use both procedures (e.g. direct assay only in the case of elevated total cholesterol or in patients with otherwise elevated cardiovascular risk). According to

Agrawal et al (2010) in USA in 2009 approximately 2200 laboratories used direct assays but 3300 calculated LDL-C according to Friedewald. In Czech and Slovak republics the ratio was different (159 laboratories on direct assays and only 83 on formula (Gaško et al, 2011).
There is no official recommendation on international level about the methodology of LDL-C estimation. The choice depends solely on the decision of the laboratory and/or the health care provider. Another confounding factor is that the same laboratory can change the actual type of the direct method or use alternatively a direct method or the calculation mostly without any warning towards the clinician.
We realized a multicentric prospective study to compare the results achieved by different direct method compared with the results of Friedewald calculation (Gaško et al, 2011) in 13 laboratories. All of them were controlled also in the frame of an external quality assesment system. All of them diclosed results of the control sera in the appropriate range. Results of the direct assay and the calculation were compared on a set of randomly selected 200 patient samples with a broad range of diseases including CRI. In Fig 5. the average difference between the results of direct (considred in this study as reference) method and the calculated results are shown. The differences are in the range from -8 % ap to + 30 %. Of course the evident limitation of this study is the lack of comparison with the reference ultacentrifugation method. Despite this limitation the results of this simple study combined with the results of metanalysis (4.1.) show an unacceptable degree of uncertainity of LDL-C estimation in individual patients not to mention those who are at special risk.

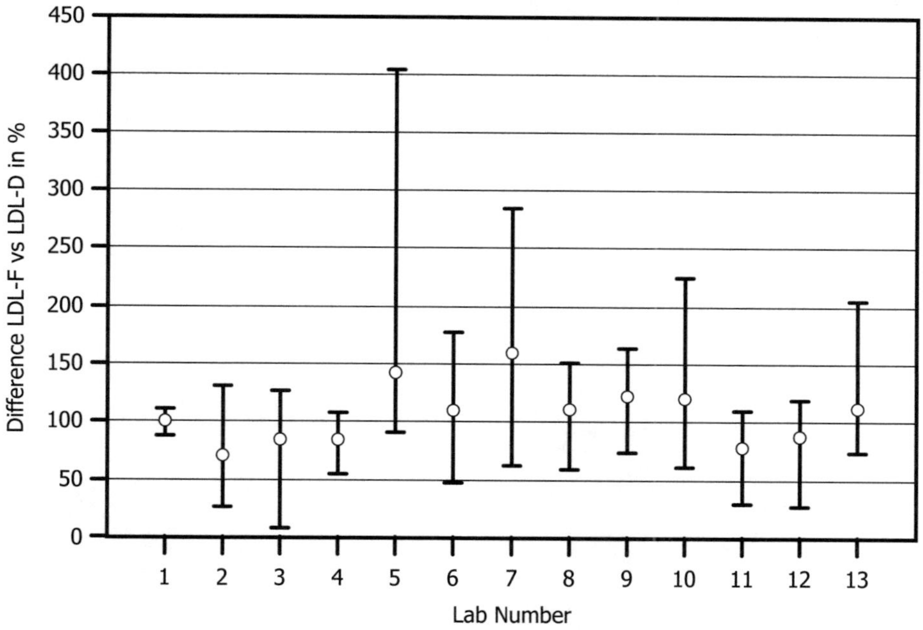

Fig. 5. Average differences (n = 200) in calculated LDL-C compared with results of the direct assay in 13 different laboratories. Value measured by the direct method in each laboratory is considered 100%. Data are shown as median and 2.5 to 97.5 percentiles.

A very interesting question is the situation after kidney transplatation. These patients at the first sight are „cured" but as a matter of fact they are far from being „healthy" beacause of the long-life immunosuppression therapy and of the slightly decreased kidney function in most of them. Balal et al (2010) compared results from 103 renal transplant recipients and the sum of differences between the calculation according to Friedewaldovho and the direct method was - 6,5 % ± 6,6 % (mean ± SD). According to Tsimihodimos et al (2008) after transplantation one very important atherogenic factor disappears - the increased level of Lp(a).

5. Conclusions

5.1 Where we stand today?

From our metaanalysis and the study on the unreliability of LDL-C estimation we conclude that the Friedewald formula seems to be no longer a viable test for appropriate targeted therapy in chronic renal failure and hemodialysis. Direct assays of LDL-C are not absolutely without error but they provide considerably more reliable results as a calculation from three measurements.

Clinicians should be aware that despite our gradually better understanding of the pathobiochemistry, pathobiochemistry and genetic background of atherosclerosis and kidney disease laboratories are not able to provide full explanation about the situation in individual patients. According to McNamara et al (2006) "we are still only scratching the surface, and mich more research and discovery remains to fully understand these critically important particles". As is depicted in Fig. 6 the scientist are looking on the different visible parts of the problem. The situation in clinical chemistry is even more problematic because the currently available methods are showing only the footprints of the real situation, not its essence.

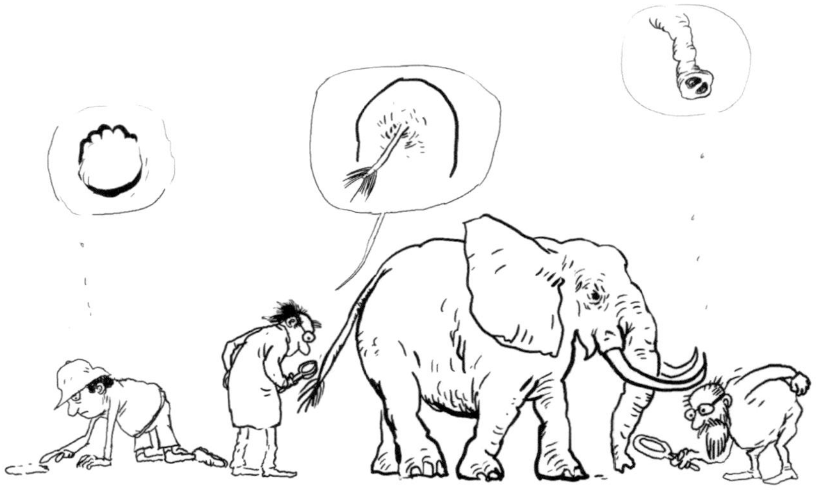

Fig. 6. Scientist looking at miscellaneous aspects of the problem and a clinical chemist trying to gain some information from the footseps.

5.2 Conclusion

In patients with CRI and/or ESRD, HD the pace of atherosclerosis development should be estimated as follows:

Proper clinical and biochemical evaluation of the underlying kidney disease and continuous monitoring of its progression. Special attenttion should be devoted to proteinuria and hypalbuminemia because they directly influence the metabolism of LDL-type particles and their concentration in the blood.

Evaluation of the risk factors not directly associated with the kidney disease (smoking, obesity, diabetes, hypertension, etc.)

Evaluation of lipid parameters - total cholesterol, LDL-cholesterol measured directly, HDL-cholesterol, triglycerides, apoprotein B100, apoporotein AI and Lp(a). The evaluation should not be a mechanistical process but should be based on pathophysiology of atherosclerosis in renal disease and should consider the strengths and weaknesses of the employed methods.

Measurement of other parameters not fully validated yet from analytical point of view and from their clinical usefulness (small dense LDLs, parameters of the oxidative stress and antioxidant systems) is possible for research purposes.

6. List of abbreviations

C	Cholesterol (as LDL-C, HDL-C, nonHDL-C)
CHY	Chylomicron
CKD	Chronic kidney disease
CRI	Chronic renal insufficiency
ESRD	End stage renal disease
HD	Hemodialysis
HDL	High-density lipoprotein
IDL	Intermediate-density lipoprotein
LCAT	Lecithin-cholesterol acyltransferase
LDL	Low-density lipoprotein
TC	Total cholesterol
TG	Triglyceride
TRL	Triglyceride rich particle
VLDL	Very low-density lipoprotein

7. References

Agrawal, M., Spencer, H.J., Fass, F.H. (2010) Method of LDL cholesterol measurement influences classification of LDL cholesterol treatment goals: Clinical research study. *Journal of Investigative Medicine*, Vol.58, No.8, pp. 945-949, ISSN 1081-5589

Attman, P.O., Samuelson, O. & Alaupovic P. (2011) The effect of decreasing renal function on lipoprotein profiles. *Nephrol Dialysis Transplant* doi:10.1093/ndt/gfq762, ISSN 1460 - 2385

Bairaktari, E., Tzallas, C., Kalientzidou, M. & al. (2004) Evaluation of alternative calculation methods for determining low-density lipoprotein cholesterol in hemodialysis patiens. *Clinical Biochemistry*, Vol.37, No.10, pp. 937-940, ISSN 0009-9120

Bairaktari, E., Elisaf, M., Tzallas, Ch. & al. (2001) Evaluation of five methods for determining low-density lipoprotein cholesterol (LDL-C) in hemodialysis patients. *Clinical Biochemistry*, Vol.34, No.8, pp. 593-602, ISSN 0009-9120

Balal, M., Paydas, S., Inal, T. & al. (2010) Validation of the Friedewald formula for the determination of low-density lipoprotein cholesterol in renal transplant recipients. Renal Failure, Vol.32, No. 4, pp. 455-458, ISSN 1525-6049

Basnakian, A.G., Shah, S.V. & Ok, E. (2010) Carbamylated LDL. Advances in Clinical Chemistry, Vol.51, pp. 25-52, ISSN 0065-2423

Batista MC, Welty FK, Diffenderfer MR et al (2004) Apolipoprotein A-I, B-100, and B-48 metabolism in subjects with chronic kidney disease, obesity and the metabolic syndrome. *Metabolism Clin Exp* Vol 53, No, 10, pp. 1255-1261, ISSN 1532 - 8600

Chan, D.T., Dogra, G.K., Irish A.B. et al (2009) Chronic kidney disease delays VLDL-apoB-100 particle catabolism: potential role of apolipoprotein C-III. *J Lipid Res* Vol. 50, pp. 2524-2531, ISSN 1539 - 7262

Danesh, J., Collins, R. & Peto, R. (2000) Lipoprotein(a) and coronary heart disease: Meta-analysis of prospective studies. *Circulation* Vol. 102, pp. 1082-1085, ISSN 0009 - 7322

Felström, B.C., Holdaas, H. & Jardine, A.G. (2003) Why do we need a statin trial hemodialysis patiens? *Kidney International,* Vol. 63, No. S84, pp. S204–S206, ISSN 0085-2538

Foley, R.N., Parfrey, R.S., Sarmak M.J. (1998) Clinical epidemiology of cardiovascular disease in chronic renal disease. *Am J Kidney Dis* Vol. 32, pp. S112-S119, ISSN 0272-6386

Fredrickson, D.S. & Lees, R.S. (1965) A system for phenotyping hyperlipoproteinemias. *Circulation* Vol. 31, pp. 321-327, ISSN 0009-7322

Friedewald, W.T., Levy, R.I., Fredrickson, D.S. (1972) Estimation of the concentration of low-density lipoprotein cholesterol in plasma, without use of the preparative ultracentrifuge. *Clin Chem* Vol. 18, pp. 499–502, ISSN 0009-9147

Fuentes-Arderiu, X., Braga-Fernández, S., Freire-Campo, L. & al. (2009) Comparison of measurement uncertainties in direct plasma low-density lipoprotein cholesterol method of measurement and indirect estimation according to Friedewald equation. *Accreditation and Quality Assurance*, Vol.14, No.2, pp. 179-183, ISSN 1432 0517

Gaško, R. & Sánchez-Meca, J. (2009) LDL cholesterol: A critical assessment of analytical accuracy of Friedewald's formula. Meta-analysis. *Kardiológia/Cardiology,* Vol.18, No.5, pp. 244–255, ISSN 1210-0048

Gaško, R., Rácz, O., Jedličková, B. & al. (2011) Methods for measurement of LDL-cholesterol: a critical assessment of direct measurement versus calculation in the treatment goals by European guidelines (2007), a multicenter study. *Cardiology Letters,* ISSN 1210-0048, accepted

Go, A.S., Chertow, G.M., Fan, D. & al (2004) Chronic kidney disease and the risks of death, cardiovascular events, and hospitalization. N Engl J Med Vol. 351, pp. 1296-1305, ISSN 1533-4406

Ikewaki, K., Schaefer, J.R., Frischmann, M.E. et al (2005) Delayed in vivo catabolism of intermediate-density lipoprotein and low-density lipoprotein in hemodialysis patients as potential cause of premature atherosclerosis. *Arteriosclerosis, Thrombosis & Vasc Biol* Vol 25, pp. 2615-2622, ISSN 1079 - 5642

Karumanchi, S.A. & Thadhani, R. (2010) Kidney complications: Why don´t statins always work? Nature Medicine, Vol.16, pp. 38-40, ISSN 1546-170X

Kwan, B.C.H., Kronenberg, F., Beddhu, S. & Cheing, A.K. (2007) Lipoprotein Metabolism and Lipid Management in Chronic Kidney Disease. *Journal of the American Society of Nephrology,* Vol.18, No.4, pp. 1246-1261, ISSN 1533-3450

Lacquaniti, A., Bolignano, D., Donato, V. & al. (2010) Alterations of lipid metabolism in chronic nephropathies: Mechanisms, diagnosis and treatment. *Kidney&Blood Pressure Research,* Vol.33, pp. 100-110. ISSN 1420-4096

Magnus, P. & Beaglehole, R. (2001) The real contribution of the major risk factors to the coronary factors to the coronary epidemics: time to end the "only 50%" myth. *Arch Intern Med* Vol. 161, pp. 2657-2669, ISSN 1538-3679

McNamara, J.R., Warnick, G.R & Cooper, G.R. (2006) A brief hisstory of lipid and lipoprotein measurements and their contribution to clinical chemistry. *Clin Chim Acta* 369, No 2, pp. 158-167, ISSN 0009-8981

Miller, W.G., Myers, G.L., Sakurabayashi, I. & al. (2010) Seven direct methods for measuring HDL and LDL cholesterol compared with ultracentrifugation. Reference measurement procedures. *Clin Chem* Vol. 56, pp. 1007-1014, ISSN 0065-2423

Nauck, M., Kramer-Guth, A., Bartens, W. & al. (1996) Is the determination of LDL cholesterol according to Friedewald accurate in CAPD and HD patients? *Clinical Nephrology,* Vol.46, No.3, pp. 319-325, ISSN 0301-0430

Olofsson, S.E., Wiklund, O. & Borén, J (2007) Apolipoproteins A-I and B: biosynthesis, role in the development of atherosclerosis and targets for intervention against cardiovascular disease. *Vasc Health Risk Manag* Vol. 3, pp. 491 – 503, ISSN 1178-2048

Pedro-Botet, J., Sentí, M., Rubiés-Prat, J. & al. (1996) When to treat dyslipidaemia of patients with chronic renal failure on haemodialysis ? A need to define specific guidelines. *Nephrology Dialysis Transplantation,* Vol.11, No.2, pp. 308-313, ISSN 1460-2385

Rosenson, R.S., Brewer, H.B., Chapman, M.J. et al (2011) HDL measures, particle heterogeneity, proposed nomenclature, and relation to atherosclerotic cardiovascular events. *Clin Chem* Vol. 57, No 1, pp. 392-410, ISSN ISSN 1530 - 8561

Ritz, E. & Wanner, C. (2008) Lipid abnormalities and cardiovascular risk in renal disease. *J Am Soc Nephrol* Vol 18, pp. 1065-1070, ISSN 1533 - 3450

Saland, J.M. & Ginsberg H.N. (2007) Lipoprotein metabolism in chronic renal insufficiency. *Pediatr Nephrol* Vol 22, pp. 1095-1112, ISSN 1432-198X

SHARP Collaborative Group. (2010) Study of Heart and Renal Protection (SHARP): Randomized trial to assess the effects of lowering low-density lipoprotein cholesterol among 9,438 patients with chronic kidney disease. *American Hearth Journal,* Vol.160, No.5, pp. 785-794, ISSN 1097-6744

Viklický O. (2006) Chronické selhání ledvin a uremický syndrom. *In: Tesař, V. Schück, O. (Eds) Klinická nefrologie. Grada Publishing Praha* pp. 477-511 ISBN 80-247-0503-6

Tsimihodimos, V., Dounousi, E., Siamopoulos, K.C. (2008) Dyslipidemia in chronic kidney disease: An approach to pathogenesis and treatment. *Am J Nephrol* Vol. 28, pp. 958-973, ISSN 1421-9670

Tsimihodimos, V., Mitrogianni Z., Elisaf M. (2011) Dyslipidemia associated with chronic kidney disease. *Open Cardiovasc Med J* Vol. 5, pp. 41-49, ISSN 1874-1924

Vaziri, N.D. (2006) Dyslipidemia of chronic renal failure: the nature, mechanisms, and potential consequences. *Am J Physiol Renal Physiol* Vol. 290, pp. F262-F272, ISSN 1522-1466

Žák, A. (2002) Poruchy metabolismu lipidů a lipoproteinů. *In: Zima T (Ed.) Laboratorní diagnostika. Galén Praha* pp. 125-153 ISBN 80-7262-201-3

20

Hemodialysis Vascular Access Dysfunction

Timmy Lee
Assistant Professor of Medicine
Department of Internal Medicine and Division of Nephrology and Hypertension,
University of Cincinnati and Veterans Affairs Medical Center, Cincinnati, OH;
United States of America

1. Introduction

A successful functioning vascular access is the "lifeline" for a hemodialysis patient. Hemodialysis vascular access dysfunction is a major cause of morbidity and mortality in hemodialysis patients[1-3]. Improving vascular access outcomes remains an ongoing challenge for nephrologists, vascular access surgeons, and interventionists. In arteriovenous fistulas (AVF) and grafts (AVG), the most common cause of this vascular access dysfunction is venous stenosis as a result of neointimal hyperplasia within the peri-anastomotic region (AVF) or at the graft-vein anastomosis (AVG) [4,5]. There have been few effective treatments to-date for venous neointimal hyperplasia in part because of the poor understanding of the pathogenesis of venous neointimal hyperplasia. Central venous catheters (CVC) are prone to frequent thrombosis and infection and the treatment of catheter-related bacteremia (CRB) remains on ongoing debate [6-8]. Therefore, this review will: (1) describe the pathology and pathophysiology of hemodialysis access stenosis in AVFs and AVGs, (2) discuss the pathogenesis of CRB and catheter thrombosis (3) discuss current and future novel therapies for treating venous neointimal hyperplasia, (4) discuss current strategies to treat CRB and catheter thrombosis, and (5) suggest future research areas in the field of hemodialysis vascular access dysfunction.

1.1 Types of hemodialysis access

Successful hemodialysis treatment requires access to the bloodstream to deliver a high enough blood flow to achieve an adequate dialysis dose. There are three primary types of hemodialysis vascular access to achieve this goal: (1) arteriovenous fistula, (2) arteriovenous graft, and (3) tunneled central venous catheter. Each type of access has unique advantages and individual problems.

1.1.1 Arteriovenous fistula

AVFs are the preferred vascular access for hemodialysis patients, because once mature and functional, they require fewer interventions to maintain patency and develop fewer infections compared to AVGs [9-13]. However, AVFs have higher rates of nonmaturation and longer maturation times compared to AVGs, which may lead to prolonged periods of CVC dialysis [9,14,15]. Recent reports from the United States have shown that up to 60% of AVFs never mature adequately to be successfully cannulated for dialysis [16] compared to 20-25 years ago where the nonmaturation rates in AVFs was approximately 10% [12].

1.1.2 Arteriovenous graft

Arteriovenous grafts (made from polytetrafluoroethylene, a synthetic fluoropolymer of tetrafluoroethylene) are advantageous because of short maturation time and relative ease to cannulation compared to AVFs [12,17-19]. Until recently, AVGs were the most common access used in hemodialysis patients in the Unites States [20]. However, the main disadvantages of AVGs are development of recurrent venous stenosis, requiring frequent interventions to maintain patency, and graft infection [19,21-24].

1.1.3 Tunneled central venous catheter

Tunneled central venous catheters have the advantage of immediate use, multiple sites for insertion, and the ability to provide access for hemodialysis for a period of months, permitting time for AVF or AVG maturation, in patients who require immediate hemodialysis [19,25-28]. However, the main disadvantages are the high risks of morbidity and mortality caused by infection [7,29-33], catheter thrombosis [19,34-37], and central venous stenosis [37-39].

2. Epidemiology and clinical significance of hemodialysis vascular access dysfunction

2.1 Epidemiology of hemodialysis vascular access

Due to reduced AVF use and increased AVG (70% in 1993 [40]) and catheter use in the United States from the mid-1980's-1990's, the National Kidney Foundation in 1997, in an effort to improve vascular access outcomes, published the first Kidney Disease Outcome Quality Initiative (K/DOQI) clinical practice guidelines for vascular access to optimize the care of vascular access in hemodialysis patients using evidenced and opinion-based guidelines [41]. Since these initial clinical practice guidelines have been published, we have seen the creation of the Fistula First Breakthrough Initiative (FFBI) [42-45] and two more revised K/DOQI clinical practice guidelines and performance measures for vascular access [19,46], which have clearly impacted and improved hemodialysis vascular access management. The most recent report from the 2009 United States Renal Data System (USRDS) has showed an AVF prevalence of 50% [47], a marked improvement since 2004 (39% AVF prevalence), 2000 (30% AVF prevalence), and 1998 (26% AVF prevalence)[48] in the United States. In contrast, AVF prevalence in Europe and Japan, reported from the Dialysis Outcomes and Practice Patterns Study (DOPPS) has been historically much higher, ranging from 57-91% [20].

While the K/DOQI guidelines and FFBI have clearly played an instrumental role in meeting the initial target goal of 50% AVF prevalence (new goal 66% [19,42]), the prevalence of CVC use continues to remain between 20-30% in the United States [42]. Furthermore, this trend of increased catheter use has also been observed in other countries, such as Spain, France, Belgium, Germany, and Italy [20]. This is likely due to an increase in the number of AVFs that have failed to mature for dialysis use in recent years [14,16].

2.2 Clinical significance and economic implications of hemodialysis vascular access dysfunction

When patients develop vascular access dysfunction, due to an immature AVF or thrombosed AVF or AVG, they are often consigned to CVC use for prolonged periods. Because dialysis with a catheter is associated with increased morbidity and mortality [49-55], CVC use has significant clinical implications such as increased risk of bacteremia which has been reported to occur at a frequency ranging from 2.5 to 5.5 episodes per 1000-catheter days [6,56], increased risk of 1-year mortality [49], and 60-70% higher risk of subsequent AVF failure [32,57]. The cost of treating one CVC-related bacteremia in the United States has been estimated to be as high as $45,000 per episode with an average of $22,000 per bacteremic episode [58].

3. Pathology and pathophysiologic mechanisms of hemodialysis vascular access dysfunction

3.1 Pathology of Hemodialysis Vascular Access Stenosis in AVF and AVG

Venous stenosis that occurs in both AVFs and AVGs is primarily due to neointimal hyperplasia. Venous stenosis in AVGs most frequently arises from the development of aggressive neointimal hyperplasia, characterized by (a) the presence of alpha smooth muscle actin positive cells myofibroblasts, and microvessels within the neointima, (b) an abundance of extracellular matrix components, (c) angiogenesis (neovascularization) within the neointima and adventitia, (d) a macrophage layer lining the perigraft region, and (e) an increased expression of mediators and inflammatory cytokines such as TGF-β, PDGF, and endothelin within the media, neointima and adventitia [59-64].

While the neointimal hyperplasia in AVFs is similar to AVGs in regards to pathogenesis, the venous stenosis that develops in AVFs is highly influenced by the capacity of the vein to vasodilitate and vascular injury from surgical technique [65]. In AVFs the two main etiologies of failure are an initial failure to mature (nonmaturation) and a subsequent (late) venous stenosis [4]. Similar to AVGs, venous neointimal hyperplasia in late AVF stenosis has been shown to be composed primarily of alpha smooth muscle actin positive cells, together with expression of mediators and cytokines such as TGF-β, PDGF, and endothelin within the media and intima of the vein [60,65]. However, recently, the lesion of AVF nonmaturation at 6 weeks after AVF creation has also been described to have significant neointimal hyperplasia [66].

3.2 Pathophysiologic mechanisms of neointimal hyperplasia formation in hemodialysis access dysfunction

The pathogenesis of venous neointimal hyperplasia in AVG stenosis and late AVF stenosis has been well described and is commonly divided into upstream and downstream events[4]. Upstream events are characterized as the initial events and insults that are responsible for endothelial and smooth muscle cell injury, which leads to a cascade of mediators (downstream events) that regulate oxidative stress, endothelial dysfunction, and inflammation (eventually resulting in venous neointimal hyperplasia). Upstream events that are believed to contribute to the pathogenesis of neointimal hyperplasia include [4,62,67-70]: (1) surgical trauma at the time of AV surgery, (2) hemodynamic shear stress at the vein-artery or vein-graft anastomosis, (3) bioincompatability of the AVG, (4) vessel injury due to dialysis needle punctures, (5) uremia resulting in endothelial dysfunction, and (6) repeated angioplasties causing further endothelial injury. Downstream events represent the response to endothelial (vascular) injury from the upstream events, resulting in the migration of smooth muscle cells from the media to the intima and eventually the development of neointimal hyperplasia [65].

The pathogenesis in AVFs that fail to mature (early failure) for dialysis, in contrast to AVG and late AVF failure, remains poorly understood. At a histological level early AVF failure is also characterized by aggressive neointimal hyperplasia in both animal and human models, seen as early as 1 month in animals [63,71] and 3 months in humans [64,66]. The underlying factors

(upstream events) which may contribute to early AVF failure, include [4,72-81]: (1) small diameter sizes in the vein and artery, (2) surgical injury at the time AV fistula placement, (3) previous venipunctures, (4) development of accessory veins after surgery, (5) hemodynamic shear stress at the AV anastomosis, (6) a genetic predisposition to vascular constriction and neointimal hyperplasia, and (7) pre-existing venous neointimal hyperplasia.
The subsequent sections will focus on the downstream events and three main mechanisms responsible for neointimal hyperplasia such as oxidative stress, inflammation, endothelial dysfunction, and alternative origins of neointimal-derived cells.

3.2.1 Oxidative stress

Many of the upstream mechanisms above (particularly hemodynamic shear stress and angioplasty injury) have been documented to result in an increase in the production of free radicals and its downstream products nitrotyrosine and latter (peroxynitrate). The latter is a potent upregulator of the matrix metalloproteinases (MMPs) [82,83]. MMPs are key enzymes that cause breakdown of extracellular matrix proteins such as collagen and elastin which facilitate the migration of vascular smooth muscle cells (VSMCs) in neointimal hyperplasia formation [84]. MMPs, paradoxically, have also been shown to facilitate a beneficial dilatation of the feeding artery (through degradation of the internal elastic laminae) in both rabbit and mouse AVF models [82,85]. Experimental studies of AVGs have demonstrated a differential upregulation of MMP-2 at the graft-vein anastomosis, with early expression (9 days) in the adventitia and a later expression (19 days) within the intima, supporting the concept of cellular migration from the adventitia to the intima [86]. Furthermore, linkages between hemodynamic shear stress and the expression of oxidative stress markers and cytokines have also been described in a porcine model of AVG stenosis [87]. Clinical studies of stenotic and thrombotic AVGs and AVFs have also demonstrated an upregulation of MMPs [88], and have documented the co-localization of oxidative stress markers with inflammatory cytokines such as transforming growth factor-beta (TGF-β), and platelet-derived growth factor (PDGF), within the neointima of both stenotic AVGs and AVFs [60].
Heme-oxygenase-1 (HO-1) is an important enzyme pathway which has been shown to confer protective effects in the vascular endothelium and other organ systems through its anti-inflammatory, antioxidant, or antiproliferative actions and properties [89]. Experimental studies in AVFs have described an increase in both the magnitude of arteriovenous stenosis and the frequency of thrombosis following the creation of AVFs in HO-1 knock out mice (increased baseline oxidative stress) as compared to wild type animals [90]. Furthermore, in the HO-1 knockout mice, there was significant induction of MMP-9 expression in the vein at 1 week compared to wild type mice, suggesting that MMP expression in vascular tissue and its deleterious effects with regard to promoting cellular migration may in part be inhibited by HO-1. Clinical studies have demonstrated a higher frequency of AVF failure in patients with heme-oxygenase-1 (HO-1) gene polymorphisms with long GT repeats (resulting in increased oxidative stress) [73].

3.2.2 Inflammation

ESRD is associated with a chronic inflammatory state, characterized by the elevation of circulating cytokines and chemokines [91]. This inflammation has been proposed to play an important role in the initiation and progression of atherosclerosis in ESRD, but may also play a significant role in vascular access stenosis. Support for this paradigm comes from recent work in which uremic mice developed a 2-3 fold greater magnitude of neointimal hyperplasia at the arteriovenous anastomosis as compared to non-uremic animals in a mouse model of AVF stenosis [92], and a recent study which showed marked upregulation of monocyte chemoattractant protein-1 (MCP-1) in the venous segment of AVF compared to rats deficient in the MCP-1 gene [93].

In clinical studies, possible linkages have described the presence of inflammatory cells (macrophages and lymphocytes), cytokines such as TGF-ß and insulin-like growth factor-1 (IGF-1) and the magnitude of neointimal hyperplasia and venous stenosis within stenotic AVFs [94].

Local bioincompatability to synthetic polytetrafluoroethylene (PTFE) material in AVGs could also result in local inflammation [95]. In vitro studies have demonstrated that conditioned media obtained after the interaction of peripheral blood mononuclear cells (PBMCs) with PTFE graft material resulted in a significant upregulation of smooth muscle cell proliferation as compared to control media [96]. This proliferative response has been shown to be attenuated by tumor necrosis-alpha (TNF-α) inhibitors [96]. Furthermore, the presence of macrophages that line PTFE graft material has been described in both experimental and clinical AVG stenosis with co-expression of inflammatory cytokines such as basic fibroblast growth factor (bFGF) [61,97].

3.2.3 Endothelial dysfunction

An intact and functional endothelium is essential for the vein to properly respond to acute changes in blood flow that occurs after creation of AVFs and AVGs [98]. Nitric oxide (NO) is an important mediator responsible for these transformations [99,100]. The presence of uremia in hemodialysis patients has been shown to exacerbate endothelial dysfunction, possibly through the pathways of inflammation and oxidative stress described above [101,102]. In the specific context of vascular access stenosis, endothelial dysfunction is likely to be responsible for the development of pre-existing venous neointimal hyperplasia [77-81], medial hypertrophy [77,81] and radial artery intima-media thickening [103-105] that is present even before the creation of AVFs in uremic patients. Pre-existing arterial intima-media thickness has been correlated with future AVF dysfunction [103]. Recently, pre-existing venous neointimal hyperplasia has been linked to poor AVF maturation in a small clinical study [77].

Asymmetrical dimethylarginine (ADMA) is an endogenous inhibitor of NO synthase and has been implicated as an important contributor to endothelial dysfunction in ESRD patients [106]. ADMA is not excreted in ESRD patients and its levels have been reported to be two to six times higher in this patient population as compared to non-uremic individuals [107]. In a recent clinical study in AVFs, patients with elevated ADMA levels at the time of percutaneous transluminal angioplasty of an initial AVF stenosis had a significantly increased risk of a recurrent AVF stenosis [108].

3.2.4 Alternative origins of neointimal cells

Although the traditional paradigm for the pathogenesis of neointimal hyperplasia has emphasized the migration of smooth muscle cells from the media to the intima, where they proliferate and contribute to the final volume of neointimal hyperplasia, a number of studies have reported that following coronary angioplasty or saphenous vein bypass grafting there is also a migration of cells (fibroblasts) from the adventitia, through the media, and into the intima, where these cells transform into "myofibroblasts" [109-111]. In dialysis access, a number of recent studies in AVGs have supported the concept of a migration of adventitial cells into the intima where they contribute to final neointimal volume [59,112]. In addition, recent data from several experimental AVF stenosis models have shown that smooth muscle cells in the neointima, may in part, originate from bone-marrow-derived cells that bind to the site of vascular injury and later differentiate into a smooth muscle cell phenotype in the neointima [82,113,114]. From a therapeutic standpoint, it is likely that better information about the true source of neointimal cells will allow for the development of novel therapeutic interventions targeting specific cell types.

3.3 Hemodynamic and vascular remodeling in hemodialysis access dysfunction

A number of experimental studies have shown that turbulent, low flow, low fluid sheer stress are involved in neointimal hyperplasia development [115-119]. High sheer stress has been associated with vascular dilatation through inhibition of smooth muscle cell proliferation and high levels of nitric oxide release, whereas low sheer stress has been associated with smooth muscle cell proliferation and lack of vasodilatation [120-123]. Poor hemodynamic profiles could be a risk factor for neointimal hyperplasia development and poor venous dilatation, and the degree of luminal stenosis is dependent upon both the magnitude of neointimal hyperplasia and the capacity for vasodilatation or vasocontriction. Therefore, a significant amount of neointimal hyperplasia and medial hypertrophy may not result in luminal stenosis in the presence of adequate vasodilatation, while a small amount of neointimal hyperplasia, but with poor vasodilatation, may result in severe venous stenosis [4,124]. Unfortunately, the factors that are responsible for vascular remodeling are unknown, but adventitial angiogenesis and scar formation are hypothesized to play a significant role[125,126]. Thus, the ideal therapy for vascular stenosis would be an intervention that would prevent vascular constriction (adverse remodeling) and neointimal hyperplasia[4]

4. Central venous dialysis catheters

CVC dysfunction and related-infection remains a common cause of morbidity, mortality, and high economic costs in treating chronic hemodialysis patients. This section will provide a brief overview of catheter dysfunction and catheter-related infections.

4.1 Catheter dysfunction

Catheter dysfunction can occur immediately after placement or in a catheter which has been previously functioning without difficulties, and most commonly manifests with low catheter blood flows during dialysis or negative arterial pressures on the dialysis machine [6]. In more severe cases catheter thrombosis is characterized by the inability to aspirate blood from the dialysis port [6]. Catheter dysfunction which occurs immediately after placement is most likely due to placement problems [6].

Installation of a thrombolytic agent for 30 to 60 minutes is a treatment for catheter dysfunction, followed by a second installation if necessary [6]. Recently published studies have reported varied success rate when treating catheter dysfunction with thrombolytics, ranging anywhere between 60-95% [26,28,35,127,128]. When thrombolytic therapy is unsuccessful in providing adequate blood flow and adequate dialysis, despite repeated installations, then catheter exchange needs to be performed. The current K/DOQI guidelines recommends treatment with thrombolytic agents in all catheters with a persistently low blood flow rate (<300 ml/min) [19].

The current standard of care to prevent catheter thrombosis is installation of an anticoagulant in both dialysis ports at the completion of each dialysis session. In the United States, heparin is most commonly used, while in Europe citrate is the more common anticoagulant [6]. The studies to-date have shown similar efficacy when comparing citrate to heparin for prophylaxis of catheter thrombosis, but with fewer complications of systemic bleeding with citrate [129-132]. A recent multicenter, randomized-controlled trial has reported that use of a thrombolytic, tissue plasminogen activator as a locking solution compared to heparin had reduced incidence of catheter dysfunction [34].

4.2 Catheter-related bacteremia

Currently, a precise definition for diagnosis catheter-related bacteremia is lacking. More rigorous definitions require a positive blood culture obtained from the catheter and a peripheral vein with the quantitative colony count being at minimum four-fold higher from the catheter sample [133]. However, recently, the Infectious Disease Society of America has recognized the challenges in obtaining peripheral blood cultures from hemodialysis patients (e.g. priority for preserving veins and difficult cannulations) and has considered a definition of "possible" catheter-related bacteremia as positive blood culture obtained from the catheter in a symptomatic patient [134].

The two main pathways where organisms can gain entry into the blood stream to initiate catheter-related bacteremia are intraluminal and extraluminal [135]. Organisms gain entrance through the bloodstream extraluminally through contact between the skin surface organisms and the external surface of the catheter at the time of catheter placement or following catheter placement before healing of the exit site or endothelialization of the subcutaneous tunnel [7]. Subsequently, the organisms colonize or migrate through the intracutaneous exterior tract of the catheter to the tip, allowing for hematagenous dispersion of the organisms and leading to catheter-related bacteremia [7]. Intraluminal-derived infections results from the transfer of organisms from hand contact with the catheter, leading to contamination of the internal catheter surfaces [7]. Infection from the extraluminal pathway most commonly occurs immediately after catheter insertion, while infections from the intraluminal pathway occurs throughout the life of the catheter [7]. Irrespective of the route of bacterial entry, the bacteria will either adhere to the CVC or become incorporated into a fibrin sheath. Adherence of the bacterial organisms to the CVC initiates a common pathway of biofilm production. A mature biofilm is a self-sustaining colony of microorganism, guarded by an exopolysaccharide matrix, that is stimulated and secreted by the organism and very difficult to eradicate [7,136-140].

Catheter-related bacteremia can result in devastating complications such as endocarditis, osteomyelitis, thrombophlebitis, septic arthritis, spinal epidural abscess, and large atrial thrombi [30,31,141-149]. The majority of isolated organisms from catheter-related bacteremia are gram-positive organisms (52-84%) with *Staph Aureus* responsible for the majority of these organisms [7,30,31,143,150,151]. Gram-negative are isolated in 27-36% of episodes and fungal isolated are relatively uncommon (<10%) [141-143,149,152]. Therefore, it is important to identify catheter-related bacteremia early so treatment can be initiated immediately.

4.2.1 Treatment of catheter-related bacteremia

Initial empiric antibiotic treatment should include broad-spectrum coverage for gram-positive and gram-negative organisms using knowledge of the common organisms and

sensitivity patterns that are grown at the dialysis center. Due to the high prevalence of methicillin-resistant *Staph Aureus* (MRSA), empiric therapy should include coverage for MRSA. When the specific organism and antibiotic sensitivities are identified, it is important to narrow the antibiotic therapy to prevent the development of drug resistant organisms. While the exact duration of antibiotic treatment for catheter-related bacteremia is uncertain, the Infectious Disease society of America recommends a 2 week course of antibiotics [153], while the K/DOQI guidelines recommends a 3 week course of antibiotics [19]. Other therapies, which have been used in conjunction with systemic antibiotics, to treat catheter-related bacteremia are antibiotic catheter locks. A number of studies have shown that antibiotic locks (which may treat the biofilm layer) used in conjunction with systemic antibiotics, in tunneled dialysis catheters, have documented a 70% cure rate [30,145,154-156].
Recent studies have evaluated pharmacologic therapies to prevent catheter-related bacteremia. Routine application of topical antibiotic ointments at the CVC exit such as mupirocin, povidine-iodine, and polysporin triple ointment has been associated with a 73-93% reduction in the risk of catheter-related bacteremia [7,151,157-159]. Prophylactic antibiotic catheter locks have also recently been evaluated. A marked reduction in catheter-related bacteremia has been reported, ranging from 51-99%, with use of a prophylactic antibiotic catheter locking solution [7,160-164]. However, of concern, a recent study has shown emergence of gentamicin-resistant organisms after 6 months when using a gentamicin-heparin prophylactic catheter lock [165].
The above strategies for treatment of catheter-related bacteremia apply to patients who are clinically stable. However, catheter removal, in addition to antibiotic therapy, should be the treatment of choice when patients: (1) are clinically unstable, (2) have persistent fever for 48 hours, (3) have evidence of tunnel infection, or (4) develop metastatic infectious complications [7].

5. Translating science to therapies in hemodialysis vascular access dysfunction: from the bench to bedside

There are currently few if any effective therapies to treat hemodialysis vascular access stenosis and neointimal hyperplasia. However, the knowledge obtained in recent years regarding the pathology and pathogenesis of vascular access access dysfunction has provided a framework for development of therapies that target neointimal hyperplasia and vascular stenosis. The purpose of the next section is to (1) describe current therapies for AVF and AVG stenosis and (2) novel therapies using localized delivery systems for AVF and AVG.

5.1 Systemic therapies

Systemic therapies, such as dipyridamole, angiotensin-converting enzyme inhibitors, aspirin, and fish oil, from small clinical trials and observational studies have been shown to have the potential to block smooth muscle cell proliferation and migration and to prevent thrombosis in AVFs and AVGs [166-170]. Most recently, two large randomized controlled trials, sponsored by the National Institutes of Health, evaluating anti-platelet agents in AVG and AVF to prevent neointimal hyperplasia were published [16,171]. In the AVG study, dipyridamole and aspirin, modestly reduced the risk of stenosis and improved primary unassisted patency [171]. In the AVF study clopidogrel reduced frequency of early thrombosis but did not improve AVF suitability defined as cannulation with two needles, minimum dialysis blood flow of 300ml/min, successful use 8/12 dialysis sessions, and use after 120 days from creation [16]. While these two studies have shown some promising results, the clinical significance of these drugs used as standard treatment for hemodialysis access stenosis remains questionable.

Fish oil has been shown to prevent AVG stenosis and thrombosis in one randomized, controlled trial [172]. Currently, another study evaluating fish oil and AVG stenosis and thrombosis is ongoing [173]. Other systemic agents, though not tested in randomized clinical trials, which have shown potential anti-proliferative effects targeting neointimal hyperplasia in CVD or PVD models, include peroxisome proliferation-activated receptor γ agonist [174-176], sirolimus [177], and imatinib mesylate [176,178,179].

5.2 Radiation therapy

Radiation therapy has been hypothesized to be a potential therapy to treat vascular stenosis due to its antiproliferative effects and potential beneficial effects of vascular remodeling[180-183]. In experimental models, both external beam and endovascular radiation therapy has proven effective to reduce neointimal hyperplasia in AVF and AVG [184,185]. However, in clinical studies, a recent randomized-controlled trial of in AVGs 25 patients showed that 42% of the radiated AVGs achieved the target lesion primary patency end point at 6 months as compared to 0% of the control group ($p = 0.015$), but this did not translate into an improvement in secondary patency at either 6 or 12 months [186].

5.3 Far infrared therapy

Infrared radiation is an invisible electromagnetic wave with a longer wavelength than that of visible light. In experimental models, far infrared therapy has been shown to improve skin blood flow and endothelial function in cardiovascular disease [187-189]. The rationale for far infrared therapy to treat dialysis vascular access stenosis is that the dialysis vascular access in patients are located at a superficial site and improving access flow may improve vascular access performance. In the lone clinical study of far infrared in dialysis access in AVFs, patients who received far infrared therapy had improved access flows and longer unassisted patencies [190].

5.4 Local drug delivery systems for hemodialysis access

The rationale behind local delivery of drugs treat hemodialysis vascular access stenosis is that (1) AVFs and AVGs could be the ideal clinical model for the use of perivascular therapies since these can be easily applied at the time of surgery, (2) perivascular therapies preferentially target the "active" adventitia, (3) studies have demonstrated that lipophilic molecules when placed over the adventitia rapidly diffuse through all the layers of the vessel wall, and (4) small amounts of otherwise toxic drugs can be safely delivered to the site of stenosis using the perivascular approach resulting in high local concentrations with minimal systemic toxicity [4]. The subsequent section will discuss local therapies to treat hemodialysis vascular access stenosis from experimental models and clinical studies.

5.4.1 Drug eluting paclitaxel perivascular wraps

Experimental studies have previously demonstrated the efficacy of paclitaxel eluting wraps in AVG stenosis likely due to anti-proliferative effects [191-193]. In 2007, a large multi-center randomized-controlled study, evaluating the use of paclitaxel-eluting mesh wraps, Vascular

Wrap™, (Angiotech Pharmaceuticals, Inc.; Vancouver, British Columbia, Canada), was initiated to study the effectiveness and safety of this therapy on primary AVG patency compared to a standard AVG. However, this study was recently suspended in 2009 following a data safety monitoring review, due to an imbalance in the incidence of infections in one of the arms (either control or treatment). An alternative approach is the use of sirolimus eluting COLL-R® wraps (Covalon Technologies Ltd: Mississauga, Ontario, Canada). An initial Phase II study demonstrated primary unassisted AVG patency of 75% and 38% at 1 and 2 years respectively with these wraps [194].

5.4.2 Endothelial cell loaded gel foam wraps

The rationale behind the use of these wraps is that the endothelial cell (in addition to lining blood vessels) is also a "bioreactor" which produces a large number of beneficial mediators that reduces thrombosis, inflammation, stenosis, and increases lumen diameter. Initial experimental studies have documented a beneficial effect of endothelial cell loaded gel-foam wraps in porcine models of AV fistula and graft stenosis [195-198]. A recent Phase II study ("V-HEALTH") was able to demonstrate technical feasibility and safety in hemodialysis patients who received a "Vascugel®" wrap loaded with treated human aortic endothelial cells at the time of AVF or AVG placement [97]. A phase III multi-center randomized-controlled study using the Vascugel® (Pervasis Therapeutics, Inc., Cambridge, MA) wraps in human AVGs is currently being designed.

5.4.3 Vascular Endothelial Growth Factor D (VEGF-D) gene therapy

In animal models of angioplasty induced restenosis, the delivery of adenoviral particles encoding for vascular-endothelial growth factor C to the site of vascular injury has been shown to trigger the release of nitric oxide and prostacyclin and reduce neointimal hyperplasia [199]. Preliminary studies on the use of VEGF-D gene therapy (using a packaged adenoviral vector and a biodegradable local delivery device (collar) made of collagen wrapped at the venous anastomosis at the time of surgery), "Trinam®" (Ark Therapeutics; London, UK), in patients receiving AVGs, have been able to document technical feasibility and safety. A phase III study using this technology was initiated in 2009 but terminated in 2010 due to poor enrollment.

5.4.4 Recombinant elastase PRT-201

PRT-201 (Proteon Therapeutics; Waltham, MA) is a recombinant pancreatic elastase topically applied at the outflow vein at the time of surgery access creation which has been shown to result in both arterial and venous dilation and an increase in AVF blood flow in experimental models [200]. The clinical benefit of this approach is the potential ability to enhance AVF maturation (through rapid vascular dilation) and prevent venous stenosis in AVGs. A phase II study using this novel technology is ongoing in the United States evaluating this therapy and whether or not it improves primary patency and cumulative survival in AVG and AVF, as well as safety.

5.5 Endovascular stent therapy

Endovascular vascular therapies (angioplasty or angioplasty with stent placement) remains the only true intervention available to treat vascular stenosis. The main advantage of stent therapy after angioplasty is a reduction in adverse remodeling. In dialysis access, placement of bare metal stents after angioplasty compared to angioplasty [201] alone has been shown to improve primary patency [202,203]. However, bare-metal stents have yielded poor results due to aggressive development of in-stent restenosis. In experimental models of dialysis access in AVGs, drug-eluting stents have shown to reduce neointimal hyperplasia and improve luminal stenosis compared to bare-metal stents [204]. However, there are no clinical studies evaluating drug-eluting stents in dialysis access to date.

Stent grafts (covered stents constructed from the same material of AVGs) have received recent attention as a therapy for prevention of restenosis due to its ability to prevent elastic recoil and inability of the neointimal cells to penetrate the covered barrier. A recently published multicenter, randomized controlled, clinical trial showed stent grafts (Bard Peripheral Vascular, Tempe, AZ), placed after angioplasty, to treat venous stenosis had better primary unassisted patency compared to angioplasty alone [205]. This is the only treatment to date that has shown to be effective to treat vascular access stenosis in a large, randomized, clinical trial.

5.6 Improving hemodynamics

Hemodynamic sheer stresses play a significant role in development of neointimal hyperplasia [87,112,206,207]. Therefore, altering the sheer stress pattern to prevent turbulent, low-flow, and low-sheer stresses could reduce the development of neointimal hyperplasia. Previous clinical data to date to support such an intervention comes from several studies evaluating cuffed AVG grafts ("Venaflo"; Bard Vascular, Tempe Arizona) [208-210]. In a recent randomized control trial evaluating cuffed vs non-cuffed AVG, cuffed AVGs showed better primary patency and cumulative survival [211]. Finally, results from a newly developed anastomotic implant device, "OptiflowTM" (Bioconnect Systems; Ambler, PA), to connect the artery and vein in AVFs and improve hemodynamics by providing a symmetric flow pattern, have shown a primary patency of 83% at 90 days [212]. This primary patency rate was higher compared to other similarly published studies [213].

6. Future perspectives: new frontiers in research

In the last decade our knowledge of vascular access dysfunction has significantly evolved. We now understand that the most common pathologic lesion seen in AVF and AVG dysfunction is aggressive venous neointimal hyperplasia, and biofilms and fibrin sheaths play a major role in CVC infection and dysfunction. In order to advance the field further, we need to further our current understanding of both the clinical and experimental pathways that result in venous neointimal hyperplasia and mechanisms that lead to biofilm and fibrin sheath production in CVCs by using the advanced technologies and tools in cellular and molecular biology, bioengineering, genomics, proteomics, and vascular imaging (ultrasound, computed tomography, and magnetic resonance imaging) [65,124,214]. Finally, small and large animal models of AVF and AVG, which a number of investigators in this field have already developed [61,93,207,215-217], will play an essential role in "translating" our knowledge of pathophysiologic mechanisms in vascular access dysfunction to novel therapies for patients.

7. Conclusion

The magnitude and costs of dialysis access dysfunction is clearly evident, and will only become magnified in the coming years as the prevalent dialysis population continues to increase. Only by launching a "translational" research initiative ("from animal to human") can recent advances in the understanding of the mechanisms of neointimal hyperplasia formation and vascular stenosis and catheter dysfunction be translated to the development of novel effective therapies for patients.

8. References

[1] Collins AJ, Foley RN, Gilbertson DT, Chen SC. The state of chronic kidney disease, ESRD, and morbidity and mortality in the first year of dialysis. Clin J Am Soc Nephrol 2009;4 Suppl 1:S5-11.

[2] Feldman HI, Kobrin S, Wasserstein A. Hemodialysis vascular access morbidity. J Am Soc Nephrol 1996;7:523-35.

[3] Dhingra RK, Young EW, Hulbert-Shearon TE, Leavey SF, Port FK. Type of vascular access and mortality in U.S. hemodialysis patients. Kidney Int 2001;60:1443-51.

[4] Roy-Chaudhury P, Sukhatme VP, Cheung AK. Hemodialysis vascular access dysfunction: a cellular and molecular viewpoint. J Am Soc Nephrol 2006;17:1112-27.

[5] Roy-Chaudhury P, Kelly BS, Melhem M, et al. Vascular access in hemodialysis: issues, management, and emerging concepts. Cardiol Clin 2005;23:249-73.

[6] Allon M. Current management of vascular access. Clin J Am Soc Nephrol 2007;2:786-800.

[7] Lok CE, Mokrzycki MH. Prevention and management of catheter-related infection in hemodialysis patients. Kidney Int 2011;79:587-98.

[8] Moist LM, Trpeski L, Na Y, Lok CE. Increased hemodialysis catheter use in Canada and associated mortality risk: data from the Canadian Organ Replacement Registry 2001-2004. Clin J Am Soc Nephrol 2008;3:1726-32.

[9] Oliver MJ, McCann RL, Indridason OS, Butterly DW, Schwab SJ. Comparison of transposed brachiobasilic fistulas to upper arm grafts and brachiocephalic fistulas. Kidney Int 2001;60:1532-9.

[10] Palder SB, Kirkman RL, Whittemore AD, Hakim RM, Lazarus JM, Tilney NL. Vascular access for hemodialysis. Patency rates and results of revision. Annals of surgery 1985;202:235-9.

[11] Allon M. Current management of vascular access. Clinical journal of the American Society of Nephrology : CJASN 2007;2:786-800.

[12] Allon M, Robbin ML. Increasing arteriovenous fistulas in hemodialysis patients: problems and solutions. Kidney Int 2002;62:1109-24.

[13] Schwab SJ, Harrington JT, Singh A, et al. Vascular access for hemodialysis. Kidney international 1999;55:2078-90.

[14] Lok CE, Allon M, Moist L, Oliver MJ, Shah H, Zimmerman D. Risk equation determining unsuccessful cannulation events and failure to maturation in arteriovenous fistulas (REDUCE FTM I). J Am Soc Nephrol 2006;17:3204-12.

[15] Lee T, Barker J, Allon M. Comparison of survival of upper arm arteriovenous fistulas and grafts after failed forearm fistula. J Am Soc Nephrol 2007;18:1936-41.

[16] Dember LM, Beck GJ, Allon M, et al. Effect of Clopidogrel on Early Failure of Arteriovenous Fistulas for Hemodialysis: A Randomized Controlled Trial. JAMA 2008;299:2164-71.

[17] Raju S. PTFE grafts for hemodialysis access. Techniques for insertion and management of complications. Annals of surgery 1987;206:666-73.

[18] Fan PY, Schwab SJ. Vascular access: concepts for the 1990s. Journal of the American Society of Nephrology : JASN 1992;3:1-11.
[19] Clinical Practice Guidelines for Vascular Access. Am J Kidney Dis 2006;48:S176-S273.
[20] Ethier J, Mendelssohn DC, Elder SJ, et al. Vascular access use and outcomes: an international perspective from the Dialysis Outcomes and Practice Patterns Study. Nephrol Dial Transplant 2008;23:3219-26.
[21] Maya ID, Weatherspoon J, Young CJ, Barker J, Allon M. Increased risk of infection associated with polyurethane dialysis grafts. Semin Dial 2007;20:616-20.
[22] Schwab SJ. Reducing the risk of hemodialysis access. American journal of kidney diseases : the official journal of the National Kidney Foundation 1999;34:362-3.
[23] Akoh JA, Patel N. Infection of hemodialysis arteriovenous grafts. The journal of vascular access 2010;11:155-8.
[24] Schwab SJ, Oliver MJ, Suhocki P, McCann R. Hemodialysis arteriovenous access: detection of stenosis and response to treatment by vascular access blood flow. Kidney Int 2001;59:358-62.
[25] Fan PY. Acute vascular access: new advances. Advances in renal replacement therapy 1994;1:90-8.
[26] Schwab SJ, Buller GL, McCann RL, Bollinger RR, Stickel DL. Prospective evaluation of a Dacron cuffed hemodialysis catheter for prolonged use. American journal of kidney diseases : the official journal of the National Kidney Foundation 1988;11:166-9.
[27] Moss AH, McLaughlin MM, Lempert KD, Holley JL. Use of a silicone catheter with a Dacron cuff for dialysis short-term vascular access. American journal of kidney diseases : the official journal of the National Kidney Foundation 1988;12:492-8.
[28] Moss AH, Vasilakis C, Holley JL, Foulks CJ, Pillai K, McDowell DE. Use of a silicone dual-lumen catheter with a Dacron cuff as a long-term vascular access for hemodialysis patients. American journal of kidney diseases : the official journal of the National Kidney Foundation 1990;16:211-5.
[29] Allon M. Dialysis catheter-related bacteremia: treatment and prophylaxis. Am J Kidney Dis 2004;44:779-91.
[30] Krishnasami Z, Carlton D, Bimbo L, et al. Management of hemodialysis catheter-related bacteremia with an adjunctive antibiotic lock solution. Kidney Int 2002;61:1136-42.
[31] Tanriover B, Carlton D, Saddekni S, et al. Bacteremia associated with tunneled dialysis catheters: comparison of two treatment strategies. Kidney Int 2000;57:2151-5.
[32] Lee T, Barker J, Allon M. Tunneled catheters in hemodialysis patients: reasons and subsequent outcomes. Am J Kidney Dis 2005;46:501-8.
[33] Allon M. Treatment guidelines for dialysis catheter-related bacteremia: an update. Am J Kidney Dis 2009;54:13-7.
[34] Hemmelgarn BR, Moist LM, Lok CE, et al. Prevention of dialysis catheter malfunction with recombinant tissue plasminogen activator. N Engl J Med 2011;364:303-12.
[35] Suhocki PV, Conlon PJ, Jr., Knelson MH, Harland R, Schwab SJ. Silastic cuffed catheters for hemodialysis vascular access: thrombolytic and mechanical correction of malfunction. American journal of kidney diseases : the official journal of the National Kidney Foundation 1996;28:379-86.
[36] Crain MR, Mewissen MW, Ostrowski GJ, Paz-Fumagalli R, Beres RA, Wertz RA. Fibrin sleeve stripping for salvage of failing hemodialysis catheters: technique and initial results. Radiology 1996;198:41-4.

[37] Caruana RJ, Raja RM, Zeit RM, Goldstein SJ, Kramer MS. Thrombotic complications of indwelling central catheters used for chronic hemodialysis. American journal of kidney diseases : the official journal of the National Kidney Foundation 1987;9:497-501.

[38] Maya ID, Saddekni S, Allon M. Treatment of refractory central vein stenosis in hemodialysis patients with stents. Semin Dial 2007;20:78-82.

[39] Schwab SJ, Quarles LD, Middleton JP, Cohan RH, Saeed M, Dennis VW. Hemodialysis-associated subclavian vein stenosis. Kidney international 1988;33:1156-9.

[40] Tokars JI, Miller ER, Alter MJ, Arduino MJ. National surveillance of dialysis-associated diseases in the United States, 1997. Semin Dial 2000;13:75-85.

[41] NKF-DOQI clinical practice guidelines for vascular access. National Kidney Foundation-Dialysis Outcomes Quality Initiative. Am J Kidney Dis 1997;30:S150-91.

[42] Fistula First National Access Improvements Initiative. Available at: http://www.fistulafirst.org/. Accessed January 23, 2011.

[43] Gold JA, Hoffman K. Fistula First: the National Vascular Access Improvement Initiative. Wmj 2006;105:71-3.

[44] Lok CE. Fistula first initiative: advantages and pitfalls. Clin J Am Soc Nephrol 2007;2:1043-53.

[45] Peters VJ, Clemons G, Augustine B. "Fistula First" as a CMS breakthrough initiative: improving vascular access through collaboration. Nephrol Nurs J 2005;32:686-7.

[46] National Kidney Foundation: DOQI Clinical Practice Guidelines for Vascular Access: Update 2000. Am J Kidney Dis 2001;37:S137-S81.

[47] U.S. Renal Data System, USRDS 2009 Annual Data Report: Atlas of CKD and ESRD in the United States, National Institutes of Health, National Institute of Diabetes and Digestive and Kidney Diseases, Bethesda, MD, 2009.

[48] Kinney R. 2005 Annual Report: ESRD Clinical Performance Measures Project. American Journal of Kidney Diseases 2006;48:S1-S105.

[49] Xue JL, Dahl D, Ebben JP, Collins AJ. The association of initial hemodialysis access type with mortality outcomes in elderly Medicare ESRD patients. Am J Kidney Dis 2003;42:1013-9.

[50] Oliver MJ, Rothwell DM, Fung K, Hux JE, Lok CE. Late creation of vascular access for hemodialysis and increased risk of sepsis. J Am Soc Nephrol 2004;15:1936-42.

[51] Allon M, Daugirdas J, Depner TA, Greene T, Ornt D, Schwab SJ. Effect of change in vascular access on patient mortality in hemodialysis patients. Am J Kidney Dis 2006;47:469-77.

[52] Lacson E, Jr., Wang W, Hakim RM, Teng M, Lazarus JM. Associates of mortality and hospitalization in hemodialysis: potentially actionable laboratory variables and vascular access. Am J Kidney Dis 2009;53:79-90.

[53] Foley RN, Chen SC, Collins AJ. Hemodialysis access at initiation in the United States, 2005 to 2007: still "catheter first". Hemodial Int 2009;13:533-42.

[54] Astor BC, Eustace JA, Powe NR, Klag MJ, Fink NE, Coresh J. Type of vascular access and survival among incident hemodialysis patients: the Choices for Healthy Outcomes in Caring for ESRD (CHOICE) Study. J Am Soc Nephrol 2005;16:1449-55.

[55] Bradbury BD, Fissell RB, Albert JM, et al. Predictors of early mortality among incident US hemodialysis patients in the Dialysis Outcomes and Practice Patterns Study (DOPPS). Clin J Am Soc Nephrol 2007;2:89-99.

[56] Allon M. Prophylaxis against dialysis catheter-related bacteremia: a glimmer of hope. Am J Kidney Dis 2008;51:165-8.

[57] Rayner HC, Pisoni RL, Gillespie BW, et al. Creation, cannulation and survival of arteriovenous fistulae: data from the Dialysis Outcomes and Practice Patterns Study. Kidney Int 2003;63:323-30.

[58] Reed SD, Friedman JY, Engemann JJ, et al. Costs and outcomes among hemodialysis-dependent patients with methicillin-resistant or methicillin-susceptible Staphylococcus aureus bacteremia. Infection control and hospital epidemiology : the official journal of the Society of Hospital Epidemiologists of America 2005;26:175-83.

[59] Roy-Chaudhury P, McKee, L., Miller, M., Reaves, A., Armstrong, J., Duncan, H., Munda, R., Kelly, B., Heffelfinger, S. Adventitial fibroblasts contribute to venous neointimal hyperplasia in PTFE grafts [Abstract]. J Am Soc Nephrol 2001;12:301A.

[60] Weiss MF, Scivittaro V, Anderson JM. Oxidative stress and increased expression of growth factors in lesions of failed hemodialysis access. Am J Kidney Dis 2001;37:970-80.

[61] Kelly BS, Heffelfinger SC, Whiting JF, et al. Aggressive venous neointimal hyperplasia in a pig model of arteriovenous graft stenosis. Kidney Int 2002;62:2272-80.

[62] Roy-Chaudhury P, Kelly BS, Miller MA, et al. Venous neointimal hyperplasia in polytetrafluoroethylene dialysis grafts. Kidney Int 2001;59:2325-34.

[63] Wang Y, Krishnamoorthy M, Banerjee R, et al. Venous stenosis in a pig arteriovenous fistula model--anatomy, mechanisms and cellular phenotypes. Nephrol Dial Transplant 2008;23:525-33.

[64] Roy-Chaudhury P, Wang Y, Krishnamoorthy M, et al. Cellular phenotypes in human stenotic lesions from haemodialysis vascular access. Nephrol Dial Transplant 2009;24:2786-91.

[65] Lee T, Roy-Chaudhury P. Advances and new frontiers in the pathophysiology of venous neointimal hyperplasia and dialysis access stenosis. Adv Chronic Kidney Dis 2009;16:329-38.

[66] Roy-Chaudhury P, Arend L, Zhang J, et al. Neointimal hyperplasia in early arteriovenous fistula failure. Am J Kidney Dis 2007;50:782-90.

[67] Ene-Iordache B, Mosconi L, Antiga L, et al. Radial artery remodeling in response to shear stress increase within arteriovenous fistula for hemodialysis access. Endothelium 2003;10:95-102.

[68] Paszkowiak JJ, Dardik A. Arterial wall shear stress: observations from the bench to the bedside. Vascular and endovascular surgery 2003;37:47-57.

[69] Huynh TN, Chacko BK, Teng X, et al. Effects of venous needle turbulence during ex vivo hemodialysis on endothelial morphology and nitric oxide formation. Journal of biomechanics 2007;40:2158-66.

[70] Chang CJ, Ko PJ, Hsu LA, et al. Highly increased cell proliferation activity in the restenotic hemodialysis vascular access after percutaneous transluminal angioplasty: implication in prevention of restenosis. Am J Kidney Dis 2004;43:74-84.

[71] Lin T, Horsfield C, Robson MG. Arteriovenous fistula in the rat tail: a new model of hemodialysis access dysfunction. Kidney Int 2008;74:528-31.

[72] Roy-Chaudhury P, Melhem M, Husted T, Kelly BS. Solutions for hemodialysis vascular access dysfunction: thinking out of the box!! J Vasc Access 2005;6:3-8.

[73] Lin CC, Yang WC, Lin SJ, et al. Length polymorphism in heme oxygenase-1 is associated with arteriovenous fistula patency in hemodialysis patients. Kidney Int 2006;69:165-72.

[74] Heine GH, Ulrich C, Kohler H, Girndt M. Is AV fistula patency associated with angiotensin-converting enzyme (ACE) polymorphism and ACE inhibitor intake? Am J Nephrol 2004;24:461-8.
[75] Heine GH, Ulrich C, Sester U, Sester M, Kohler H, Girndt M. Transforming growth factor beta1 genotype polymorphisms determine AV fistula patency in hemodialysis patients. Kidney Int 2003;64:1101-7.
[76] Girndt M, Heine GH, Ulrich C, Kohler H. Gene polymorphism association studies in dialysis: vascular access. Semin Dial 2007;20:63-7.
[77] Lee T, Chauhan V, Krishnamoorthy M, et al. Severe venous neointimal hyperplasia prior to dialysis access surgery. Nephrology, dialysis, transplantation : official publication of the European Dialysis and Transplant Association - European Renal Association 2011.
[78] Wali MA, Eid RA, Al-Homrany MA. Smooth muscle changes in the cephalic vein of renal failure patients before use as an arteriovenous fistula (AVF). J Smooth Muscle Res 2002;38:75-85.
[79] Wali MA, Eid RA, Dewan M, Al-Homrany MA. Intimal changes in the cephalic vein of renal failure patients before arterio-venous fistula (AVF) construction. J Smooth Muscle Res 2003;39:95-105.
[80] Wali MA, Eid RA, Dewan M, Al-Homrany MA. Pre-existing histopathological changes in the cephalic vein of renal failure patients before arterio-venous fistula (AVF) construction. Ann Thorac Cardiovasc Surg 2006;12:341-8.
[81] Feinfeld DA, Batista R, Mir R, Babich D. Changes in venous histology in chronic hemodialysis patients. Am J Kidney Dis 1999;34:702-5.
[82] Castier Y, Lehoux S, Hu Y, Foteinos G, Tedgui A, Xu Q. Characterization of neointima lesions associated with arteriovenous fistulas in a mouse model. Kidney Int 2006;70:315-20.
[83] Dixon BS. Why don't fistulas mature? Kidney Int 2006;70:1413-22.
[84] Rotmans JI, Velema E, Verhagen HJ, et al. Matrix metalloproteinase inhibition reduces intimal hyperplasia in a porcine arteriovenous-graft model. J Vasc Surg 2004;39:432-9.
[85] Tronc F, Mallat Z, Lehoux S, Wassef M, Esposito B, Tedgui A. Role of matrix metalloproteinases in blood flow-induced arterial enlargement: interaction with NO. Arterioscler Thromb Vasc Biol 2000;20:E120-6.
[86] Misra S, Doherty MG, Woodrum D, et al. Adventitial remodeling with increased matrix metalloproteinase-2 activity in a porcine arteriovenous polytetrafluoroethylene grafts. Kidney Int 2005;68:2890-900.
[87] Misra S, Fu AA, Puggioni A, et al. Increased shear stress with upregulation of VEGF-A and its receptors and MMP-2, MMP-9, and TIMP-1 in venous stenosis of hemodialysis grafts. Am J Physiol Heart Circ Physiol 2008;294:H2219-30.
[88] Misra S, Fu AA, Rajan DK, et al. Expression of hypoxia inducible factor-1 alpha, macrophage migration inhibition factor, matrix metalloproteinase-2 and -9, and their inhibitors in hemodialysis grafts and arteriovenous fistulas. J Vasc Interv Radiol 2008;19:252-9.
[89] Nath KA. Heme oxygenase-1: a provenance for cytoprotective pathways in the kidney and other tissues. Kidney Int 2006;70:432-43.
[90] Juncos JP, Tracz MJ, Croatt AJ, et al. Genetic deficiency of heme oxygenase-1 impairs functionality and form of an arteriovenous fistula in the mouse. Kidney Int 2008;74:47-51.

[91] Sezer S, Ozdemir FN, Arat Z, Turan M, Haberal M. Triad of malnutrition, inflammation, and atherosclerosis in hemodialysis patients. Nephron 2002;91:456-62.

[92] Kokubo T, Ishikawa N, Uchida H, et al. CKD accelerates development of neointimal hyperplasia in arteriovenous fistulas. J Am Soc Nephrol 2009;20:1236-45.

[93] Juncos JP, Grande JP, Kang L, et al. MCP-1 contributes to arteriovenous fistula failure. Journal of the American Society of Nephrology : JASN 2011;22:43-8.

[94] Stracke S, Konner K, Kostlin I, et al. Increased expression of TGF-beta1 and IGF-I in inflammatory stenotic lesions of hemodialysis fistulas. Kidney Int 2002;61:1011-9.

[95] Li L, Terry CM, Shiu Y-TE, Cheung AK. Neointimal hyperplasia associated with synthetic hemodialysis grafts. Kidney Int 2008;74:1247-61.

[96] Mattana J, Effiong C, Kapasi A, Singhal PC. Leukocyte-polytetrafluoroethylene interaction enhances proliferation of vascular smooth muscle cells via tumor necrosis factor-alpha secretion. Kidney Int 1997;52:1478-85.

[97] Conte MS, Nugent HM, Gaccione P, Guleria I, Roy-Chaudhury P, Lawson JH. Multicenter phase I/II trial of the safety of allogeneic endothelial cell implants after the creation of arteriovenous access for hemodialysis use: the V-HEALTH study. J Vasc Surg 2009;50:1359-68 e1.

[98] Shuhaiber JH, Evans AN, Massad MG, Geha AS. Mechanisms and future directions for prevention of vein graft failure in coronary bypass surgery. European journal of cardio-thoracic surgery : official journal of the European Association for Cardio-thoracic Surgery 2002;22:387-96.

[99] Langille BL, O'Donnell F. Reductions in arterial diameter produced by chronic decreases in blood flow are endothelium-dependent. Science 1986;231:405-7.

[100] Ignarro LJ, Buga GM, Wood KS, Byrns RE, Chaudhuri G. Endothelium-derived relaxing factor produced and released from artery and vein is nitric oxide. Proceedings of the National Academy of Sciences of the United States of America 1987;84:9265-9.

[101] Bolton CH, Downs LG, Victory JG, et al. Endothelial dysfunction in chronic renal failure: roles of lipoprotein oxidation and pro-inflammatory cytokines. Nephrol Dial Transplant 2001;16:1189-97.

[102] Ghiadoni L, Cupisti A, Huang Y, et al. Endothelial dysfunction and oxidative stress in chronic renal failure. J Nephrol 2004;17:512-9.

[103] Kim YO, Choi YJ, Kim JI, et al. The impact of intima-media thickness of radial artery on early failure of radiocephalic arteriovenous fistula in hemodialysis patients. J Korean Med Sci 2006;21:284-9.

[104] Kim YO, Song HC, Yoon SA, et al. Preexisting intimal hyperplasia of radial artery is associated with early failure of radiocephalic arteriovenous fistula in hemodialysis patients. Am J Kidney Dis 2003;41:422-8.

[105] Ku YM, Kim YO, Kim JI, et al. Ultrasonographic measurement of intima-media thickness of radial artery in pre-dialysis uraemic patients: comparison with histological examination. Nephrol Dial Transplant 2006;21:715-20.

[106] Zoccali C. Endothelial damage, asymmetric dimethylarginine and cardiovascular risk in end-stage renal disease. Blood Purif 2002;20:469-72.

[107] Cooke JP. Does ADMA cause endothelial dysfunction? Arterioscler Thromb Vasc Biol 2000;20:2032-7.

[108] Wu CC, Wen SC, Yang CW, Pu SY, Tsai KC, Chen JW. Plasma ADMA predicts restenosis of arteriovenous fistula. J Am Soc Nephrol 2009;20:213-22.

[109] Scott NA, Cipolla GD, Ross CE, et al. Identification of a potential role for the adventitia in vascular lesion formation after balloon overstretch injury of porcine coronary arteries. Circulation 1996;93:2178-87.
[110] Shi Y, O'Brien JE, Fard A, Mannion JD, Wang D, Zalewski A. Adventitial myofibroblasts contribute to neointimal formation in injured porcine coronary arteries. Circulation 1996;94:1655-64.
[111] Shi Y, O'Brien JE, Jr., Mannion JD, et al. Remodeling of autologous saphenous vein grafts. The role of perivascular myofibroblasts. Circulation 1997;95:2684-93.
[112] Li L, Terry CM, Blumenthal DK, et al. Cellular and morphological changes during neointimal hyperplasia development in a porcine arteriovenous graft model. Nephrol Dial Transplant 2007;22:3139-46.
[113] Caplice NM, Wang S, Tracz M, et al. Neoangiogenesis and the presence of progenitor cells in the venous limb of an arteriovenous fistula in the rat. Am J Physiol Renal Physiol 2007;293:F470-5.
[114] Diao Y, Guthrie S, Xia SL, et al. Long-term engraftment of bone marrow-derived cells in the intimal hyperplasia lesion of autologous vein grafts. Am J Pathol 2008;172:839-48.
[115] Haruguchi H, Teraoka S. Intimal hyperplasia and hemodynamic factors in arterial bypass and arteriovenous grafts: a review. Journal of artificial organs : the official journal of the Japanese Society for Artificial Organs 2003;6:227-35.
[116] Sivanesan S, How TV, Black RA, Bakran A. Flow patterns in the radiocephalic arteriovenous fistula: an in vitro study. Journal of biomechanics 1999;32:915-25.
[117] Krishnamoorthy MK, Banerjee RK, Wang Y, et al. Hemodynamic wall shear stress profiles influence the magnitude and pattern of stenosis in a pig AV fistula. Kidney Int 2008;74:1410-9.
[118] Paszkowiak JJ, Dardik A. Arterial wall shear stress: observations from the bench to the bedside. Vasc Endovascular Surg 2003;37:47-57.
[119] Corpataux JM, Haesler E, Silacci P, Ris HB, Hayoz D. Low-pressure environment and remodelling of the forearm vein in Brescia-Cimino haemodialysis access. Nephrol Dial Transplant 2002;17:1057-62.
[120] Mondy JS, Lindner V, Miyashiro JK, Berk BC, Dean RH, Geary RL. Platelet-derived growth factor ligand and receptor expression in response to altered blood flow in vivo. Circulation research 1997;81:320-7.
[121] Sterpetti AV, Cucina A, Santoro L, Cardillo B, Cavallaro A. Modulation of arterial smooth muscle cell growth by haemodynamic forces. Eur J Vasc Surg 1992;6:16-20.
[122] Kraiss LW, Geary RL, Mattsson EJ, Vergel S, Au YP, Clowes AW. Acute reductions in blood flow and shear stress induce platelet-derived growth factor-A expression in baboon prosthetic grafts. Circulation research 1996;79:45-53.
[123] Ueba H, Kawakami M, Yaginuma T. Shear stress as an inhibitor of vascular smooth muscle cell proliferation. Role of transforming growth factor-beta 1 and tissue-type plasminogen activator. Arteriosclerosis, thrombosis, and vascular biology 1997;17:1512-6.
[124] Roy-Chaudhury P, Lee TC. Vascular stenosis: biology and interventions. Curr Opin Nephrol Hypertens 2007;16:516-22.
[125] O'Brien JE, Jr., Shi Y, Fard A, Bauer T, Zalewski A, Mannion JD. Wound healing around and within saphenous vein bypass grafts. The Journal of thoracic and cardiovascular surgery 1997;114:38-45.

[126] Kwon HM, Sangiorgi G, Ritman EL, et al. Enhanced coronary vasa vasorum neovascularization in experimental hypercholesterolemia. J Clin Invest 1998;101:1551-6.
[127] Daeihagh P, Jordan J, Chen J, Rocco M. Efficacy of tissue plasminogen activator administration on patency of hemodialysis access catheters. American journal of kidney diseases : the official journal of the National Kidney Foundation 2000;36:75-9.
[128] Lund GB, Trerotola SO, Scheel PF, Jr., et al. Outcome of tunneled hemodialysis catheters placed by radiologists. Radiology 1996;198:467-72.
[129] Grudzinski L, Quinan P, Kwok S, Pierratos A. Sodium citrate 4% locking solution for central venous dialysis catheters--an effective, more cost-efficient alternative to heparin. Nephrology, dialysis, transplantation : official publication of the European Dialysis and Transplant Association - European Renal Association 2007;22:471-6.
[130] Lok CE, Appleton D, Bhola C, Khoo B, Richardson RM. Trisodium citrate 4%--an alternative to heparin capping of haemodialysis catheters. Nephrology, dialysis, transplantation : official publication of the European Dialysis and Transplant Association - European Renal Association 2007;22:477-83.
[131] Dogra GK, Herson H, Hutchison B, et al. Prevention of tunneled hemodialysis catheter-related infections using catheter-restricted filling with gentamicin and citrate: a randomized controlled study. J Am Soc Nephrol 2002;13:2133-9.
[132] Weijmer MC, van den Dorpel MA, Van de Ven PJ, et al. Randomized, clinical trial comparison of trisodium citrate 30% and heparin as catheter-locking solution in hemodialysis patients. Journal of the American Society of Nephrology : JASN 2005;16:2769-77.
[133] Mermel LA, Farr BM, Sherertz RJ, et al. Guidelines for the management of intravascular catheter-related infections. Clinical infectious diseases : an official publication of the Infectious Diseases Society of America 2001;32:1249-72.
[134] Mermel LA, Allon M, Bouza E, et al. Clinical practice guidelines for the diagnosis and management of intravascular catheter-related infection: 2009 Update by the Infectious Diseases Society of America. Clinical infectious diseases : an official publication of the Infectious Diseases Society of America 2009;49:1-45.
[135] Cheesbrough JS, Finch RG, Burden RP. A prospective study of the mechanisms of infection associated with hemodialysis catheters. The Journal of infectious diseases 1986;154:579-89.
[136] Costerton JW. In response to: In vivo efficacy of silver-coated (Sil-zone) infection-resistant polyester fabric against a biofilm-producing bacteria, Staphylococcus epidermidis. J Heart Valve Disease; 1998;7:524-530. J Heart Valve Dis 1999;8:346-8.
[137] Costerton JW. Introduction to biofilm. Int J Antimicrob Agents 1999;11:217-21; discussion 37-9.
[138] Costerton JW, Stewart PS, Greenberg EP. Bacterial biofilms: a common cause of persistent infections. Science 1999;284:1318-22.
[139] Donlan RM, Costerton JW. Biofilms: survival mechanisms of clinically relevant microorganisms. Clin Microbiol Rev 2002;15:167-93.
[140] Hoyle BD, Alcantara J, Costerton JW. Pseudomonas aeruginosa biofilm as a diffusion barrier to piperacillin. Antimicrobial agents and chemotherapy 1992;36:2054-6.
[141] Mokrzycki MH, Zhang M, Cohen H, Golestaneh L, Laut JM, Rosenberg SO. Tunnelled haemodialysis catheter bacteraemia: risk factors for bacteraemia recurrence, infectious complications and mortality. Nephrology, dialysis, transplantation :

official publication of the European Dialysis and Transplant Association - European Renal Association 2006;21:1024-31.

[142] Beathard GA. Management of bacteremia associated with tunneled-cuffed hemodialysis catheters. Journal of the American Society of Nephrology : JASN 1999;10:1045-9.

[143] Marr KA, Sexton DJ, Conlon PJ, Corey GR, Schwab SJ, Kirkland KB. Catheter-related bacteremia and outcome of attempted catheter salvage in patients undergoing hemodialysis. Annals of internal medicine 1997;127:275-80.

[144] Negulescu O, Coco M, Croll J, Mokrzycki MH. Large atrial thrombus formation associated with tunneled cuffed hemodialysis catheters. Clinical nephrology 2003;59:40-6.

[145] Poole CV, Carlton D, Bimbo L, Allon M. Treatment of catheter-related bacteraemia with an antibiotic lock protocol: effect of bacterial pathogen. Nephrol Dial Transplant 2004;19:1237-44.

[146] Kovalik EC, Raymond JR, Albers FJ, et al. A clustering of epidural abscesses in chronic hemodialysis patients: risks of salvaging access catheters in cases of infection. Journal of the American Society of Nephrology : JASN 1996;7:2264-7.

[147] Ghani MK, Boccalandro F, Denktas AE, Barasch E. Right atrial thrombus formation associated with central venous catheters utilization in hemodialysis patients. Intensive Care Med 2003;29:1829-32.

[148] Obrador GT, Levenson DJ. Spinal epidural abscess in hemodialysis patients: report of three cases and review of the literature. American journal of kidney diseases : the official journal of the National Kidney Foundation 1996;27:75-83.

[149] Hemmelgarn BR, Moist LM, Lok CE, et al. Prevention of dialysis catheter malfunction with recombinant tissue plasminogen activator. The New England journal of medicine 2011;364:303-12.

[150] Saad TF. Bacteremia associated with tunneled, cuffed hemodialysis catheters. American journal of kidney diseases : the official journal of the National Kidney Foundation 1999;34:1114-24.

[151] Lok CE, Stanley KE, Hux JE, Richardson R, Tobe SW, Conly J. Hemodialysis infection prevention with polysporin ointment. J Am Soc Nephrol 2003;14:169-79.

[152] Zhang J, Melhem M, Kassing W, et al. In vitro paclitaxel and radiation effects on the cell types responsible for vascular stenosis: a preliminary analysis. Blood Purif 2007;25:155-60.

[153] Mermel LA, Farr BM, Sherertz RJ, et al. Guidelines for the management of intravascular catheter-related infections. Clin Infect Dis 2001;32:1249-72.

[154] Capdevila JA, Segarra A, Planes AM, et al. Successful treatment of haemodialysis catheter-related sepsis without catheter removal. Nephrology, dialysis, transplantation : official publication of the European Dialysis and Transplant Association - European Renal Association 1993;8:231-4.

[155] Fernandez-Hidalgo N, Almirante B, Calleja R, et al. Antibiotic-lock therapy for long-term intravascular catheter-related bacteraemia: results of an open, non-comparative study. J Antimicrob Chemother 2006;57:1172-80.

[156] Vardhan A, Davies J, Daryanani I, Crowe A, McClelland P. Treatment of haemodialysis catheter-related infections. Nephrology, dialysis, transplantation : official publication of the European Dialysis and Transplant Association - European Renal Association 2002;17:1149-50.

[157] Levin A, Mason AJ, Jindal KK, Fong IW, Goldstein MB. Prevention of hemodialysis subclavian vein catheter infections by topical povidone-iodine. Kidney international 1991;40:934-8.
[158] Sesso R, Barbosa D, Leme IL, et al. Staphylococcus aureus prophylaxis in hemodialysis patients using central venous catheter: effect of mupirocin ointment. Journal of the American Society of Nephrology : JASN 1998;9:1085-92.
[159] Johnson LB, Jose J, Yousif F, Pawlak J, Saravolatz LD. Prevalence of colonization with community-associated methicillin-resistant Staphylococcus aureus among end-stage renal disease patients and healthcare workers. Infection control and hospital epidemiology : the official journal of the Society of Hospital Epidemiologists of America 2009;30:4-8.
[160] James MT, Conley J, Tonelli M, Manns BJ, MacRae J, Hemmelgarn BR. Meta-analysis: antibiotics for prophylaxis against hemodialysis catheter-related infections. Annals of internal medicine 2008;148:596-605.
[161] Yahav D, Rozen-Zvi B, Gafter-Gvili A, Leibovici L, Gafter U, Paul M. Antimicrobial lock solutions for the prevention of infections associated with intravascular catheters in patients undergoing hemodialysis: systematic review and meta-analysis of randomized, controlled trials. Clinical infectious diseases : an official publication of the Infectious Diseases Society of America 2008;47:83-93.
[162] Jaffer Y, Selby NM, Taal MW, Fluck RJ, McIntyre CW. A meta-analysis of hemodialysis catheter locking solutions in the prevention of catheter-related infection. American journal of kidney diseases : the official journal of the National Kidney Foundation 2008;51:233-41.
[163] Snaterse M, Ruger W, Scholte Op Reimer WJ, Lucas C. Antibiotic-based catheter lock solutions for prevention of catheter-related bloodstream infection: a systematic review of randomised controlled trials. The Journal of hospital infection 2010;75:1-11.
[164] Pervez A, Ahmed M, Ram S, et al. Antibiotic lock technique for prevention of cuffed tunnel catheter associated bacteremia. The journal of vascular access 2002;3:108-13.
[165] Landry DL, Braden GL, Gobeille SL, Haessler SD, Vaidya CK, Sweet SJ. Emergence of gentamicin-resistant bacteremia in hemodialysis patients receiving gentamicin lock catheter prophylaxis. Clinical journal of the American Society of Nephrology : CJASN 2010;5:1799-804.
[166] Diskin CJ, Stokes TJ, Jr., Pennell AT. Pharmacologic intervention to prevent hemodialysis vascular access thrombosis. Nephron 1993;64:1-26.
[167] Sreedhara R, Himmelfarb J, Lazarus JM, Hakim RM. Anti-platelet therapy in graft thrombosis: results of a prospective, randomized, double-blind study. Kidney Int 1994;45:1477-83.
[168] Schmitz PG, McCloud LK, Reikes ST, Leonard CL, Gellens ME. Prophylaxis of hemodialysis graft thrombosis with fish oil: double-blind, randomized, prospective trial. Journal of the American Society of Nephrology : JASN 2002;13:184-90.
[169] Gradzki R, Dhingra RK, Port FK, Roys E, Weitzel WF, Messana JM. Use of ACE inhibitors is associated with prolonged survival of arteriovenous grafts. American journal of kidney diseases : the official journal of the National Kidney Foundation 2001;38:1240-4.
[170] Saran R, Dykstra DM, Wolfe RA, Gillespie B, Held PJ, Young EW. Association between vascular access failure and the use of specific drugs: the Dialysis Outcomes and Practice Patterns Study (DOPPS). Am J Kidney Dis 2002;40:1255-63.

[171] Dixon BS, Beck GJ, Vazquez MA, et al. Effect of dipyridamole plus aspirin on hemodialysis graft patency. N Engl J Med 2009;360:2191-201.
[172] Schmitz PG, McCloud LK, Reikes ST, Leonard CL, Gellens ME. Prophylaxis of hemodialysis graft thrombosis with fish oil: double-blind, randomized, prospective trial. J Am Soc Nephrol 2002;13:184-90.
[173] Lok CE, Allon M, Donnelly S, et al. Design of the fish oil inhibition of stenosis in hemodialysis grafts (FISH) study. Clin Trials 2007;4:357-67.
[174] Murthy SN, Obregon DF, Chattergoon NN, et al. Rosiglitazone reduces serum homocysteine levels, smooth muscle proliferation, and intimal hyperplasia in Sprague-Dawley rats fed a high methionine diet. Metabolism 2005;54:645-52.
[175] Takagi T, Yamamuro A, Tamita K, Katayama M, Morioka S. Thiazolidinedione treatment attenuates diffuse neointimal hyperplasia in restenotic lesions after coronary stent implantation in type 2 diabetic patients: an intravascular ultrasound study. J Cardiol 2005;45:139-47.
[176] Davies MG, Owens EL, Mason DP, et al. Effect of platelet-derived growth factor receptor-alpha and -beta blockade on flow-induced neointimal formation in endothelialized baboon vascular grafts. Circ Res 2000;86:779-86.
[177] Hausleiter J, Kastrati A, Mehilli J, et al. Randomized, double-blind, placebo-controlled trial of oral sirolimus for restenosis prevention in patients with in-stent restenosis: the Oral Sirolimus to Inhibit Recurrent In-stent Stenosis (OSIRIS) trial. Circulation 2004;110:790-5.
[178] Rutherford C, Martin W, Salame M, Carrier M, Anggard E, Ferns G. Substantial inhibition of neo-intimal response to balloon injury in the rat carotid artery using a combination of antibodies to platelet-derived growth factor-BB and basic fibroblast growth factor. Atherosclerosis 1997;130:45-51.
[179] Leppanen O, Rutanen J, Hiltunen MO, et al. Oral imatinib mesylate (STI571/gleevec) improves the efficacy of local intravascular vascular endothelial growth factor-C gene transfer in reducing neointimal growth in hypercholesterolemic rabbits. Circulation 2004;109:1140-6.
[180] Fareh J, Martel R, Kermani P, Leclerc G. Cellular effects of beta-particle delivery on vascular smooth muscle cells and endothelial cells: a dose-response study. Circulation 1999;99:1477-84.
[181] Rubin P, Williams JP, Riggs PN, et al. Cellular and molecular mechanisms of radiation inhibition of restenosis. Part I: role of the macrophage and platelet-derived growth factor. International journal of radiation oncology, biology, physics 1998;40:929-41.
[182] Sabate M, Serruys PW, van der Giessen WJ, et al. Geometric vascular remodeling after balloon angioplasty and beta-radiation therapy: A three-dimensional intravascular ultrasound study. Circulation 1999;100:1182-8.
[183] Mayberg MR, Luo Z, London S, Gajdusek C, Rasey JS. Radiation inhibition of intimal hyperplasia after arterial injury. Radiat Res 1995;142:212-20.
[184] Kelly BS, Narayana A, Heffelfinger SC, et al. External beam radiation attenuates venous neointimal hyperplasia in a pig model of arteriovenous polytetrafluoroethylene (PTFE) graft stenosis. International journal of radiation oncology, biology, physics 2002;54:263-9.
[185] Sun S, Beitler JJ, Ohki T, et al. Inhibitory effect of brachytherapy on intimal hyperplasia in arteriovenous fistula. The Journal of surgical research 2003;115:200-8.

[186] Misra S, Bonan R, Pflederer T, Roy-Chaudhury P. BRAVO I: A pilot study of vascular brachytherapy in polytetrafluoroethylene dialysis access grafts. Kidney Int 2006;70:2006-13.

[187] Yu SY, Chiu JH, Yang SD, Hsu YC, Lui WY, Wu CW. Biological effect of far-infrared therapy on increasing skin microcirculation in rats. Photodermatology, Photoimmunology & Photomedicine 2006;22:78-86.

[188] Akasaki Y, Miyata M, Eto H, et al. Repeated thermal therapy up-regulates endothelial nitric oxide synthase and augments angiogenesis in a mouse model of hindlimb ischemia. Circulation journal : official journal of the Japanese Circulation Society 2006;70:463-70.

[189] Ikeda Y, Biro S, Kamogawa Y, et al. Repeated thermal therapy upregulates arterial endothelial nitric oxide synthase expression in Syrian golden hamsters. Jpn Circ J 2001;65:434-8.

[190] Lin CC, Chang CF, Lai MY, Chen TW, Lee PC, Yang WC. Far-infrared therapy: a novel treatment to improve access blood flow and unassisted patency of arteriovenous fistula in hemodialysis patients. J Am Soc Nephrol 2007;18:985-92.

[191] Kelly B, Melhem M, Zhang J, et al. Perivascular paclitaxel wraps block arteriovenous graft stenosis in a pig model. Nephrol Dial Transplant 2006;21:2425-31.

[192] Melhem M, Kelly B, Zhang J, et al. Development of a local perivascular paclitaxel delivery system for hemodialysis vascular access dysfunction: polymer preparation and in vitro activity. Blood Purif 2006;24:289-98.

[193] Masaki T, Rathi R, Zentner G, et al. Inhibition of neointimal hyperplasia in vascular grafts by sustained perivascular delivery of paclitaxel. Kidney international 2004;66:2061-9.

[194] Paulson WD, Kipshidze N, Kipiani K, et al. Safety and Efficacy of Locally Eluted Sirolimus for Prolonging AV Graft Patency (PTFE Graft Plus Coll-R) First in Man Experience. Journal of the American Society of Nephrology 2008:252A.

[195] Nugent HM, Edelman ER. Endothelial implants provide long-term control of vascular repair in a porcine model of arterial injury. J Surg Res 2001;99:228-34.

[196] Nugent HM, Groothuis A, Seifert P, et al. Perivascular endothelial implants inhibit intimal hyperplasia in a model of arteriovenous fistulae: a safety and efficacy study in the pig. J Vasc Res 2002;39:524-33.

[197] Nugent HM, Rogers C, Edelman ER. Endothelial implants inhibit intimal hyperplasia after porcine angioplasty. Circ Res 1999;84:384-91.

[198] Nugent HM, Sjin RT, White D, et al. Adventitial endothelial implants reduce matrix metalloproteinase-2 expression and increase luminal diameter in porcine arteriovenous grafts. J Vasc Surg 2007;46:548-56.

[199] Hiltunen MO, Laitinen M, Turunen MP, et al. Intravascular adenovirus-mediated VEGF-C gene transfer reduces neointima formation in balloon-denuded rabbit aorta. Circulation 2000;102:2262-8.

[200] Burke SK, LaRochelle A, Mendenhall HV. Local Application of Recombinant Human Type I Pancreatic Elastase (PRT-201) to an Arteriovenous Fistula (AVF) Increase AVF Blood Flow in a Rabbit Model. Journal of the American Society of Nephrology 2008:252A.

[201] Haskal ZJ, Trerotola S, Dolmatch B, et al. Stent graft versus balloon angioplasty for failing dialysis-access grafts. The New England journal of medicine 2010;362:494-503.

[202] Maya ID, Allon M. Outcomes of thrombosed arteriovenous grafts: comparison of stents vs angioplasty. Kidney Int 2006;69:934-7.
[203] Chan MR, Bedi S, Sanchez RJ, et al. Stent placement versus angioplasty improves patency of arteriovenous grafts and blood flow of arteriovenous fistulae. Clin J Am Soc Nephrol 2008;3:699-705.
[204] Rotmans JI, Pattynama PM, Verhagen HJ, et al. Sirolimus-eluting stents to abolish intimal hyperplasia and improve flow in porcine arteriovenous grafts: a 4-week follow-up study. Circulation 2005;111:1537-42.
[205] Haskal ZJ, Trerotola S, Dolmatch B, et al. Stent graft versus balloon angioplasty for failing dialysis-access grafts. N Engl J Med 2010;362:494-503.
[206] Krishnamoorthy MK, Banerjee RK, Wang Y, et al. Hemodynamic wall shear stress profiles influence the magnitude and pattern of stenosis in a pig AV fistula. Kidney Int 2008.
[207] Misra S, Woodrum DA, Homburger J, et al. Assessment of Wall Shear Stress Changes in Arteries and Veins of Arteriovenous Polytetrafluoroethylene Grafts Using Magnetic Resonance Imaging. Cardiovasc Intervent Radiol 2006.
[208] Nyberg SL, Hughes CB, Valenzuela YM, et al. Preliminary experience with a cuffed ePTFE graft for hemodialysis vascular access. Asaio J 2001;47:333-7.
[209] Tsoulfas G, Hertl M, Ko DS, et al. Long-term outcome of a cuffed expanded PTFE graft for hemodialysis vascular access. World journal of surgery 2008;32:1827-31.
[210] Sorom AJ, Hughes CB, McCarthy JT, et al. Prospective, randomized evaluation of a cuffed expanded polytetrafluoroethylene graft for hemodialysis vascular access. Surgery 2002;132:135-40.
[211] Ko PJ, Liu YH, Hung YN, Hsieh HC. Patency rates of cuffed and noncuffed extended polytetrafluoroethylene grafts in dialysis access: a prospective, randomized study. World journal of surgery 2009;33:846-51.
[212] Roy-Chaudhury P, Wang Y, Krishnamoorthy M, Dakin A. Optiflow: A Novel Anastomotic Conduit for Reducing AV Fistula Dysfunction. J Am Soc Nephrol 2008;19:253A.
[213] Falk A. Maintenance and salvage of arteriovenous fistulas. J Vasc Interv Radiol 2006;17:807-13.
[214] Yevzlin AS, Chan MR, Becker YT, Roy-Chaudhury P, Lee T, Becker BN. "Venopathy" at work: recasting neointimal hyperplasia in a new light. Transl Res 2010;156:216-25.
[215] Misra S, Fu AA, Anderson JL, et al. The rat femoral arteriovenous fistula model: increased expression of matrix metalloproteinase-2 and -9 at the venous stenosis. J Vasc Interv Radiol 2008;19:587-94.
[216] Croatt AJ, Grande JP, Hernandez MC, Ackerman AW, Katusic ZS, Nath KA. Characterization of a model of an arteriovenous fistula in the rat: the effect of L-NAME. Am J Pathol 2010;176:2530-41.
[217] Croatt AJ, Juncos JP, Hernandez MC, et al. Upregulation of Inflammation-Related Genes and Neointima Formation in Arteriovenous Fistula (AVF) Model in the Rat (Abstract). J Am Soc Nephrol 2008;19:252A.

21

Nontraditional Anti - Infectious Agents in Hemodialysis

Martin Sedlacek
Dartmouth Hitchcock Medical Center, One Medical Center Drive
Lebanon

1. Introduction

The distinction between antibiotic and non antibiotic medications is in fact quite arbitrary as drugs against bacteria can have unpredictable side effects in man and drugs developed for use in humans can affect microbes. It would be extremely surprising if it was otherwise, as eukaryotes and prokaryotes are related by evolution and share conserved molecular mechanisms. Many antibiotic and non antibiotic medications have closely related chemistries and share the same historic roots.

For example, both antimicrobial activity and an affinity for brain tissue of the phenothiazine compound methylene blue were described by Paul Ehrlich in the 19th century. Early uses of phenothiazines included treatment of urinary tract infection and postoperative analgesia. As a positive effect on psychotic patients was discovered, phenothiazines became with the development of chlorpromazine an important tool in psychiatry (Williams, 1995). With the discovery of penicillin the antimicrobial activities of phenothiazines and other earlier compounds fell into the background, but with the emergent problem of antibiotic resistance in more recent years there was new interest. Phenothiazines have activity against multidrug resistant *Staphylococcus aureus* and *Enterococcus faecalis*, presumably through the inhibition of bacterial efflux pumps (Kristiansen J.E. et al., 2007).

As a routine, antibiotic medications are tested for their effects on the eukaryotic host as these constitute potential side effects. While the ideal antibiotic would have no side effects at all, the discovery of unexpected side effects has lead to important drug developments. For instance, the clinical observation of a hypoglycemic effect of sulfonamide antibiotics led to the development of sulfonylureas for the treatment of diabetes. Likewise the observation that Sulfanilamide causes hens to lay eggs without shells because of alkaline diuresis led to the development of acetazolamide and ultimately the thiazide diuretics. The initial observation derived from the similarity between the sulfonamide ion and the bicarbonate ion. The antiviral amantadine was found to be useful in the treatment of Parkinson's disease and motility agents to treat gastroparesis are derived from the observation of the bothersome gastrointestinal side effects of erythromycin. As described below, even Lipitor, the "best selling drug in the world" with $11 Billion of annual sales according to Forbes magazine, was developed from a compound initially discovered as an antibiotic originating from a fungal broth.

On the other hand side, the efforts to look into the unintended effects on microbes of non antibiotic medications have been less systematic. Non antibiotic medications can affect

microbes in various ways: Compounds may have direct anti microbial effects in vitro, similar to traditional antibiotics. However, to be clinically useful the drug level to achieve minimum inhibitory concentration has to be within a range that is achievable and tolerable in humans. Compounds can exert an antimicrobial effect by inhibition of bacterial pumps. A well known example is the potentiation of antibiotic treatment against *Helicobacter pylori* through omeprazole. Many psychotropic medications including the phenothiazines fall into this category. Aspirin appears to modulate the expression of genes that are important for Staphylococcal virulence and the statins appear to have immune modulatory effects. Both medications are discussed in more detail below.
This chapter deals with the anti microbial effects of medications that are not traditionally regarded as antibiotics with regards to dialysis.

2. A combination of unfortunate events: infection in dialysis

The current epidemic of obesity and, as a complication, diabetic nephropathy associated to type 2 diabetes mellitus has fueled the spectacular growth of hemodialysis into an industry that is dominated by a handful of large companies. Infection is a leading cause of morbidity and mortality in dialysis patients and the annual mortality rate caused by sepsis is several hundred folds higher in patients with end stage renal disease than in the general population (Laupland et al., 2004). The incidence of bacteremia has increased in hemodialysis patients over the years, mainly because of increased rates of serious *Staphylococcus aureus* infection in this population (Foley at al., 2004). *S. aureus* has its name from a gold coloured caroten virulence factor called staphyloxanthin which allows the bacteria to survive oxidative bursts of neutrophils (Liu G.Y. & Nizet V., 2009). *S.aureus* produces a battery of surface proteins, enzymes and toxins which enable the bacteria to both persist in intracellular locations and in biofilms for long periods of time, and to rapidly disseminate in the host in an opportunistic fashion which makes it one of the most dangerous and pathogenic bacteria in humans.
The use of dialysis catheters is a major risk factor for developing *S.aureus* infection because of disruption of the normal skin barrier, thus forming a gateway for bacterial entry into the blood stream (Vandecasteele S.J. et al., 2009). Despite Kidney Disease Outcomes Quality Initiative clinical practice guidelines recommending the use of auto logos arterio-venous fistulae as dialysis access and other efforts, the overall prevalence of hemodialysis catheter use has been increasing, approaching 30% in the United States (Rayner et al., 2004). Humans are the main natural reservoir for *S.aureus* which can colonize skin, gastrointestinal and urogenital tracts. The most frequent site of colonization is the anterior nose and longitudinal studies have shown that there are three types of *S.aureus* nasal carriage in healthy adults: fifty percent are persistent non carriers, thirty percent are intermittent carriers and twenty percent are persistent carriers (VandenBergh et al., 1999). Hands are the main vector of transmission and in the majority of cases the same strain that is found in the bloodstream is also found on the hands and in the nose (von Eiff C. et al., 2001). It follows that rigorous hand washing is extremely important to prevent infection in the dialysis units as it is elsewhere in the medical setting. The majority of *S.aureus* infections has its source in the endogenous reservoir in the nose of the same person and can thus be considered an "autoinfection" (Boelart et al., 1995 as quoted in Vandecasteele et al., 2009). Consistent with this view is that in prospective studies the interval between catheter placement and staphylococcemia can be very short, with 23% of episodes occurring less than one week after catheter insertion (Little M.A. et al., 2001). *S.aureus* bacteremia is associated frequently with

metastatic infection such as endocarditis, osteoarticular infection, septic pulmonary embolism and epidural abscess and carries a mortality that is higher than with other pathogens. While the original observation by Fleming that led to the discovery of penicillin involved the accidental overgrowth of an *S.aureus* culture with fungus, staphylococcal resistance to penicillin has since become very frequent both in community and hospital acquired infections. A recent study in the US found that methicillin resistant *S.aureus* accounted for 65% of isolates from the nose in hospitalized dialysis patients (Johnson L.B. et al., 2009). As with methicillin sensive *S.aureus*, colonization seems to precede clinical infection. A scheme of three times a week nasal mupirocin ointment can decrease nasal carriage but is cumbersome, the rate of recurrence is high and rapid development of resistance has been observed (Vandecasteele et al., 2009).

3. Salicylic acid

Salicylic acid, the active ingredient of willow bark, is one of the oldest medicines still in use, in the buffered form of aspirin. The beneficial effect on fever, pain and inflammation were already described by Hippocrates. Fallen out of favour because of other non steroidal anti inflammatory drugs with more favorable side effects profiles aspirin has made a spectacular come back fifty years ago as the antiplatelet effects of aspirin were discovered. Since then aspirin has found widespread therapeutic use in the treatment of cardiovascular disease. Chronic treatment with Aspirin may prevent colorectal cancer, presumably by inhibition of cyclooxygenase 2 (COX-2) which is expressed in large amounts in adenocarcinoma (Ruder E.H. et al., 2011). Salicylic acid is ubiquitous in plants as a phytohormone. It is part of the innate immune system of plants, involved in local resistance to pathogens and in systemic acquired resistance (SAR), where a pathogenic attack one part of a plant induces resistance in other parts. Depending on the amount of fruit and vegetables in the diet humans have detectable serum levels of salicylic acid. It has been hypothesized that diet derived salicylic acid could in part account for the observed link between diet and colorectal cancer (Paterson J.R.& Lawrence J.R., 2001) and this might possibly apply to the relation between diet and cardiovascular disease as well. Salicylic acid is used as a food preservative and an antiseptic in toothpaste. Aspirin is thus not only one of the oldest but also one of the most versatile and successful drugs known.

3.1 Laboratory evidence for an anti staphylococcal effect of salicylic acid

Early studies in the rabbit endocarditis model showed that platelets provide a nidus for bacteria and that aspirin can decrease vegetation size (Pujadas et al., 1988). The observation was made that aspirin can reduce not only the weight of vegetations in a rabbit model of *S.aureus* endocarditis but also bacterial density although neither aspirin nor salicylic acid have known antibacterial effects at the low concentrations employed (Nicolau D.P. et al., 1993). This benefit was seen if aspirin was given together with antibiotics but also if aspirin was provided prior to the infectious challenge with which endocarditis was induced (Nicolau D.P. et al., 1995). Even more puzzling in this study was that vegetation weight and bacterial density were higher if higher doses of aspirin were administered while the optimum beneficial effect was seen at a lower dose, suggesting that serum levels may be very important. Subsequently this observation has been called the "Goldilocks effect" in which too little and too much aspirin may cause paradoxically diminished effects on outcome parameters in the infectious endocarditis model (Eisen et al., 2008). The beneficial

effects of aspirin in the rabbit model of endocarditis have been recapitulated with salicylic acid, its major biometabolite (Kupferwasser et al., 1999). As salicylic acid has no anti-platelet properties, this indicates that platelet independent mechanisms are likely to have a more significant role in the action of aspirin on *S.aureus* endocarditis that the platelet dependant effects. Further experimental work in vivo in animal models of infectious *S.aureus* endocarditis showed that aspirin reduced a multitude of measurable parameters of the severity of the infection and metastasis such as vegetation weight and the bacterial density in vegetations and the number of renal emboli and these effects were dose dependant, more pronounced at lower rather than higher doses (Kupferwasser et al., 1999). In vitro studies showed that salicylic acid inhibits the expression of two key virulence genes in *S. aureus* that are involved in endovascular pathogenesis: alpha-toxin [hla] and fibronectin-binding adhesion [fnbA], through activation of genetic pathways involving the major stress response operon, sigma factor B (Kupferwasser et al., 2003). These aspirin mediated effects on sigma factor B were observed at serum concentrations that are achieved by usual clinical dosages of aspirin in humans (Kupferwasser et al., 2003). On the other hand side, it has been shown that the presence of salicylic acid decreases expression of capsular polysaccharides. It has been hypothesized that the loss of these capsular virulence factors could lead to an increased capacity of *S.aureus* to invade epithelial cells and that chronic treatment with aspirin could potentially lead to more persistent or recurrent infection (Alvarez C.P. et al., 2010).
In conclusion a significant body of in vitro and in vivo evidence indicates that aspirin may have the potential to be useful in the treatment of *S.aureus* infection by down modulating key regulator and structural genes resulting in the abrogation of virulent phenotypes but it has to be noted that important questions remain.

3.2 Clinical evidence for a beneficial effect of aspirin in *S.aureus* endocarditis

The earliest clinical observations of a potential salutatory role of aspirin come from the study of bacterial endocarditis. In a small retrospective study a decreased rate of embolic events was found in patients with native valve endocarditis who were on long term aspirin treatment (11% versus 47%), although the number of patients treated with aspirin was too small to be conclusive (Schunemann S. et al., 1997). A small preliminary prospective observational study conducted in 9 patients found adjunctive treatment of established endocarditis with aspirin beneficial (Taha et al., 1992).
Subsequently, a Canadian prospective multicenter study in 115 patients with endocarditis showed no benefit of the adjunctive treatment with a 325mg dose of aspirin (Chan et al., 2003). Despite its prospective design this study was criticized as patients on chronic aspirin treatment were excluded from this study although the greatest benefit might be expected in this population. Moreover, Aspirin was added only after an average of 35 days after onset of symptoms. Only 14 patients (25%) in the Aspirin treatment group had *Staphylococcus aureus* endocarditis while the majority had streptococcal endocarditis. As the putative mechanism of action of aspirin involves the inhibition of *S.aureus* virulence factors, the benefit of aspirin is likely greatest if it is used before infection occurs. The benefit of aspirin is also very likely to be limited to *S.aureus* as the mechanism seems to be specific to this pathogen. The same authors presented a post hoc analysis of their data in 2008, comparing 84 patients who had been excluded from their previous study because of long term aspirin treatment with 54 patients in the placebo arm and again found no significant clinical differences in the outcome between both groups (Chan et al., 2008). Only 29% of patients, 16 and 24 patients

respectively, in both arms had *S.aureus* endocarditis and thus the same concern that the study was underpowered to detect a difference was voiced for this study as well (Eisen D.P. & Bayer A.S., 2008).

A retrospective single center cohort study of 600 patients with infectious endocarditis, who were treated over a 18 year period at the Mayo Clinic, found that the odds of suffering symptomatic embolic events was decreased by 64% in patients who were treated with antiplatelet agents for at least 6 months prior to the diagnosis: Aspirin was the antiplatelet agent in 98% of cases and an 81mg daily dose was used in the majority of patients (Anavekar et al., 2007).

Eisen et al. used the International Collaboration on Endocarditis –Prospective Cohort Study (ICE-PCS) database to assess the influence of aspirin usage at the time of diagnosis on the outcome of definitive *S.aureus* endocarditis. A cohort of 670 patients had both information on prior aspirin use and *S.aureus* endocarditis. Aspirin use at the time of diagnosis in 132 patients was a predictor for a decreased risk of acute valve surgery, independent of methicillin resistance status. A statistically significant decrease in embolic events in aspirin users was found in a univariate analysis that became a trend in multivariate analysis. A comparison of groups with and without aspirin use among patients with Streptococcal endocarditis was made and no association of aspirin with improved outcomes was found (Eisen et al., 2009).

Thus the data on aspirin use in *S.aureus* endocarditis suggests that aspirin likely does alter the course of illness. The non dependence of the effect on methicillin resistance status and the absence of an observed effect of aspirin on other pathogens are consistent with the proposed specific mechanism of aspirin on staphylococcal virulence factors. It is also noteworthy that Staphylococcal endocarditis is rather difficult to study in adequate numbers as the population incidence is fortunately low.

3.3 Aspirin and *S.aureus* nasal carriage

Karabay et al. investigated the prevalence of *S.aureus* nasal carriage in an outpatient cardiology clinic. Of a total of 346 patients 199 were chronic aspirin user while 147 patients were not. The prevalence of *S.aureus* nasal carriage was 5% on patient treated chronically with aspirin versus 16% in those that did not take aspirin. Only aspirin was found to be associated with a decreased rate of nasal carriage in a multivariate analysis (Karabay et al., 2006). These findings are of obvious significance to hemodialysis patients as nasal colonization is considered the initiating event that leads to catheter associated staphylococcal bacteremia. If confirmed, aspirin could decrease nasal carriage at a fraction of the cost and effort of mupirocin ointment. Given the fact that aspirin is a very old drug the findings of Karabay et al. have another potential significance: If a clinical effect of aspirin on *S.aureus* can still be detected after decades of over-the-counter use it would be unlikely that *S.aureus* would develop resistance to this effect in the future. It is clear that the important findings of Karabay et al. merit further investigation both in hemodialysis and in the general population.

3.4 A potential beneficial effect of aspirin in hemodialysis patients

Patient undergoing hemodialysis treatments suffer staphylococcal infections with increased frequency because of a high prevalence of tunneled or non tunneled dialysis catheters. The hemodialysis setting is thus well suited to study the potential beneficial clinical anti staphylococcal effects of aspirin.

We conducted a single center retrospective study in 872 patients with tunneled catheters who dialyzed over a ten year time period from 1995 to 2005. During this time period our patients had 1853 tunneled dialysis catheters placed and accumulated more than 476 patient-catheter-years and had 4722 blood cultures performed. Temporary dialysis catheters were excluded because of the high variability in the circumstances of placement of temporay catheters and also greater difficulty in tracking them retrospectively. The overall incidence of bacteremia was 7.2 episodes per 100 patient-catheter-months and the incidence of *S.aureus* bacteremia was 2.1 episodes per 100 patient-catheter-months. The incidence of *S.aureus* endocarditis was 0.16 episodes per 100 patient-catheter-months. These numbers are within the range reported in the literature. Blood cultures were obtained at the discretion of the treating physician if infection was suspected. Tunneled catheters that were a suspected source of infection were usually removed and negative cultures were required before insertion of a new tunneled catheter. All tunneled catheters were placed and removed by the same interventional radiology service. Suspected infection was the principal reason for tunneled catheter removal (19%), followed by poor catheter blood flow (14%) and presence of a mature permanent vascular access (14%). Infection rates were compared by Poisson regression analysis. In this study catheter associated bacteremia was defined as one or more positive blood cultures in a patient with a tunneled catheter. In retrospect it was impossible to exclude other sources of infection and contamination and for this reason all positive blood culture results that were obtained in the presence of a tunneled catheter were included without discrimination. Blood cultures that were obtained after a tunneled catheter was removed were excluded per definition. Our institution is a tertiary care medical center that offered hemodialysis in two outpatient units, serving a population of about 400,000 people. Because of location in a rural area, limited availability of hemodialysis and other geographical factors limiting access to other institutions the long term follow up of patients was excellent. A proprietary medical record system integrated electronic inpatient and outpatient records with procedure notes and laboratory, radiological and microbiological test result and was ideally suited for a large retrospective study. As a result the fate of only 8 catheters (<0.5%) was unaccounted for.

The number of episodes and rates of catheter associated bacteria is shown in Table 1 which includes repeated episodes and polymicrobial infections with more than one bacterial isolate. As expected, Gram positive bacteria accounted for the majority of bacteremic episodes. When all bacteremic episodes were considered together, there was no difference between patients treated with aspirin or not. In fact, the only pathogen with a lower rate of catheter-associated bacteremia in patients treated with aspirin was *S.aureus* which caused only half as many episodes in the aspirin group compared to patients not treated with aspirin (0.17 versus 0.34 events/patient-catheter-years, $p=0.003$). In addition to blood cultures 369 catheter tip cultures were performed in the same time interval, albeit in a less systematic fashion. Of these 53 catheter tip cultures grew *S.aureus*. In such a case treatment is usually recommended because *S.aureus* bacteremia is considered more likely than contamination (Peacock et al., 1998). If these tip cultures were added to bona fide blood cultures in the analysis, the difference was statistically more significant: 83 instances (0.36 events per patient-catheter-year) of *S.aureus* in the non aspirin treated group versus 45 (0.18 event per patient-catheter-year) in the aspirin treated group ($p=0.001$).

Moreover, if we excluded repeated events in the same patient from our data and considered only first episodes of *S.aureus* bacteremia, the difference looked between the two groups looked even more impressive: 28 first episodes of *S.aureus* bacteremia in patients treated with aspirin (0.23 events per patient-catheter year) versus more than double, 64 first episodes of *S.aureus* bacteremia (0.57 events per patient catheter year) in patient not treated with aspirin (p<0.001).

We explored the association between aspirin dose and rates of catheter associated *S.aureus* and *MRSA* bacteremia in table 2. There was a dose effect as only a 325mg dose of Aspirin, but not an 81mg dose (common formulations in the United States), was associated with a decreased rate of *Staphylococcus aureus* infection compared to patients not treated with aspirin. Importantly there was a significantly lower rates of *Methicillin resistant Staphylococcus aureus* bacteremia (*MRSA*) in patients treated with 325mg of aspirin a day.

	No Aspirin		**Aspirin**		***P***
	978 Catheters/227.4 Patient-Catheter-Years		**875 Catheters/ 249.3 Patient-Catheter-Years**		
	No.	**Rate (/patient-catheter-y)**	**No.**	**Rate (/patient-catheter-y)**	
All positive	232	1.02	207	0.83	0.30
Gram-positive					
Coagulase-negative *Staphylococcus*	96	0.42	93	0.37	0.85
S aureus	77	0.34	43	0.17	0.003*
MRSA	19	0.08	11	0.04	0.16
Enterococcus species	21	0.09	30	0.12	0.18
Corynebacterium species	7	0.03	6	0.02	0.82
Streptococcus species	4	0.02	7	0.03	0.34
Bacillus species	4	0.02	4	0.02	0.97
Gram-negative					
Enterobacter species	20	0.09	21	0.09	0.81
Pseudomonas species	11	0.05	13	0.05	0.64
Serratia species	12	0.05	9	0.04	0.55
Klebsiella species	9	0.04	10	0.04	0.77
Escherichia coli	7	0.03	4	0.02	0.39
Acinetobacter species	4	0.02	4	0.02	0.97
Bacteroides species	3	0.01	3	0.01	0.78

Note: Multiple bacterial isolates and repeated episodes were included in this table. Fungal isolates and bacterial species found fewer than 5 times during the 10-year study period were omitted.
*Significant difference by Poisson regression.

Table 1. Number of Episodes and Rates of Catheter-Associated Bacteremia in a 10-Year Period from 1995 to 2005
Reprinted from Sedlacek et al.: "Aspirin Treatment Is Associated With a Significantly Decreased Risk of Staphylococcus aureus bacteremia in Hemodialysis Patients With Tunneled Catheters", Am J Kidney Dis Vol49, pp401-408 with permission from Elsevier

	No Aspirin		81 mg Aspirin		325 mg Aspirin	
	978 Catheters/227.4 Patient-Catheter-Years		367 Catheters/116.2 Patient-Catheter-Years		508 Catheters/133.1 Patient-Catheter-Years	
	No.	Rate (/patient-catheter-y)	No.	Rate (/patient-catheter-y)	No.	Rate (/patient-catheter-y)
S aureus	77	0.34	26	0.22	17	0.13
No Aspirin vs 81 mg Aspirin		*P* = 0.26				
No Aspirin vs 325 mg Aspirin		*P* < 0.001*				
MRSA	19	0.08	10	0.09	1	0.01
No Aspirin vs 81 mg Aspirin		*P* = 0.62				
No Aspirin vs 325 mg Aspirin		*P* = 0.001*				

Table 2. Association between Aspirin Dose and Rates of Catether-Associated *S aureus* and MRSA Bacteremia
Reprinted from Sedlacek et al.: "Aspirin Treatment Is Associated With a Significantly Decreased Risk of Staphylococcus aureus bacteremia in Hemodialysis Patients With Tunneled Catheters", Am J Kidney Dis Vol49, pp401-408 with permission from Elsevier

We used Cox proportional hazard analysis to study risk factors for developing a first episode of *S.aureus* bacteremia. Table 3 shows the patient characteristics and distribution of covariates that were used for this analysis. Patient treated with aspirin were on average 10 years older and had a higher prevalence of coronary artery disease, peripheral vascular disease, history of stroke, hypertension and diabetes mellitus than patients not treated with aspirin.
Table 4 shows the result of the Cox proportional hazard analysis. Aspirin decreased the odds of developing a first episode of *S.aureus* bacteremia by 54% (with a confidence interval of 72% to 24%, p=0.002). No other cardiovascular medication and neither clopidogrel nor Warfarin had a similar effect. Also, no beneficial effect of statins on the odds of *S.aureus* bacteremia was observed in this study. On the opposite side, the presence of diabetes mellitus increased the risk of developing a first episode of catheter associated *S.aureus* bacteremia, as was previous recognized (Breen et al. 1995). COPD decreased the odds of a first episode *S.aureus* bacteremia in this study. A potential explanation for this observation could be more frequent antibiotic use in this condition which might reduce nasal carriage. A greater incidence of *S.aureus* bacteremia was reported in patients with cardiovascular disease (K/DOQI, 2005) but the opposite, lower numbers of *S.aureus* bacteremia was observed in this sicker patient population which may be taken as a sign of the potential clinical importance of the anti staphylococcal effects of aspirin. Similar results were obtained when multiple logistic regression analysis was used instead of Cox analysis.
Data on metastatic infection (endocarditis, osteomyelitis, septic arthritis) was analyzed as well. There were significantly less events in patients treated with aspirin compared with events in patients not treated with aspirin (3 versus 11 events, p=0.04).
A Kaplan-Meier plot of cumulative catheter failure associated with *S.aureus* bacteremia is shown in Figure 1. Grouping by aspirin treatment resulted in two divergent graphs with catheter failure caused by *S.aureus* infection significantly more frequent in the non aspirin group (p<0.001). The two graphs diverge very early which is consistent with the clinical observation that almost a quarter of *S.aureus* infection occur very early within a week after catheter insertion (Little M.A. et al., 2001). Figure 1 also illustrates another measure of the beneficial anti staphylococcal effect of aspirin: delayed onset of infection.

	No Aspirin (454 patients)	Aspirin (418 patients)	P
Age (y)	59 ± 19*	68 ± 13*	<0.0001
Time on dialysis (d)	362 ± 810	346 ± 542	0.73
Catheter no.	1.8 ± 1.8	1.9 ± 1.7	0.70
Female sex	194 (42)	186 (44)	0.54
Tobacco use	205 (45)*	225 (54)*	0.01
Diabetes mellitus	170 (38)*	236 (56)*	<0.0001
Hypertension	333 (74)*	364 (87)*	<0.0001
COPD	92 (20)*	117 (28)*	0.009
Coronary artery disease	159 (35)*	309 (79)*	<0.0001
Peripheral vascular disease	113 (25)*	200 (48)*	<0.0001
Stroke	66 (15)*	99 (24)*	0.007
Arthritis	141 (31)*	164 (39)*	0.01
Cancer	102 (23)	80 (19)	0.24
Previous transplant	50 (11)*	14 (3)*	<0.0001
Clopidogrel	12 (3)*	40 (10)*	<0.0001
Warfarin	61 (14)	60 (14)	0.77
Statin	69 (15)*	172 (41)*	<0.0001
B-Blocker	248 (55)*	315 (75)*	<0.0001
ACE inhibitor/ARB	136 (30)*	187 (45)*	<0.0001
Calcium channel blocker	216 (48)	216 (52)	0.28
Aspirin	0	418	<0.0001

Note: Values expressed as mean ± SD or number (percent).
Abbreviations: ACE, angiotensin-converting enzyme; ARB, angiotensin receptor blocker.
*Statistically significant difference between aspirin-treated and non–aspirin-treated groups by means of Fisher exact test or unpaired Student *t*-test, as appropriate.

Table 3. Patient Characteristic and Distribution of Covariates for the Cox Proportional Hazard Analysis
Reprinted from Sedlacek et al.: "Aspirin Treatment Is Associated With a Significantly Decreased Risk of Staphylococcus aureus bacteremia in Hemodialysis Patients With Tunneled Catheters", Am J Kidney Dis Vol49, pp401-408 with permission from Elsevier

A second study that addressed the anti staphylococcal effects of aspirin in hemodialysis patients was published in abstract form (Sedlacek et al., 2008). We performed a historical cohort study of the United States Renal Data System (USRDS) Dialysis Morbidity and Mortality Study (DMMS) Wave II data, linking medication data to mortality data from the core files. The updated USRDS Wave II data comprise 4024 patients, 16% of which were treated with Aspirin at study start date and 2776 of whom died. 54 of 2262 deaths (2.39%) in patients not treated with aspirin were attributed to septicemia due to vascular access either as primary or secondary cause, while there were only 4 of 510 deaths (0.78%) in patients treated with aspirin that were attributed to this cause (p<0.02, 2-tailed Fisher's Exact Test). Although anti platelet agents and other cardiovascular medications are underused in dialysis patients, we still find a strong negative association between aspirin treatment and death from septicemia due to vascular access in USRDS data. These results provide a confirmation of a clinical anti-staphylococcal effect of aspirin in hemodialysis patient that is independent from the data pool used in our first study.

	Relative Risk (95% CI)	*P*
Age (y)	1.0 (1.0-1.0)	0.99
Time on dialysis (d)	1.0 (1.0-1.001)	0.88
Catheter no.	0.95 (0.83-1.09)	0.45
Female sex	1.19 (0.76-1.86)	0.45
Tobacco use	0.78 (0.49-1.24)	0.30
Diabetes mellitus	1.65 (1.02-2.67)	0.04*
Hypertension	1.36 (0.74-2.51)	0.33
COPD	0.49 (0.24-0.97)	0.04*
Coronary artery disease	0.80 (0.48-1.34)	0.40
Peripheral vascular disease	1.01 (0.62-1.65)	0.97
Stroke	1.11 (0.63-1.96)	0.72
Arthritis	1.22 (0.78-1.92)	0.39
Cancer	1.04 (0.59-1.83)	0.89
Previous transplant	1.19 (0.55-2.55)	0.66
Clopidogrel	1.06 (0.40-2.83)	0.91
Warfarin	1.79 (1.03-3.10)	0.04*
Statin	1.08 (0.63-1.85)	0.79
B-Blocker	1.13 (0.70-1.83)	0.62
ACE inhibitor/ARB	0.79 (0.50-1.25)	0.31
Calcium channel blocker	0.73 (0.46-1.15)	0.17
Aspirin	0.46 (0.28-0.76)	0.002*

Abbreviations: ACE, angiotensin-converting enzyme; ARB, angiotensin receptor blocker.
*Statistical significance in Cox proportional hazard model.

Table 4. Risk of First *S aureus* Bacteremia Episode in 872 Dialysis Patients with a Tunneled Catheter by using Cox Proportional Hazard Analysis
Reprinted from Sedlacek et al.: "Aspirin Treatment Is Associated With a Significantly Decreased Risk of Staphylococcus aureus bacteremia in Hemodialysis Patients With Tunneled Catheters", Am J Kidney Dis Vol49, pp401-408 with permission from Elsevier

3.5 Concerns about aspirin use in hemodialysis patients

The abuse of non steroidal inflammatory drugs is a well described risk factor for upper gastrointestinal bleeding. The concern has been raised that the use of aspirin in dialysis patients could be harmful by causing bleeding (Chan et al., 2003 and 2008). As noted in a recent metanalysis the available data is conflicting for a variety of reasons such as selection bias, insufficient length of follow up and concomitant treatment with proton pump inhibitors (Hiremath et al., 2009). In the study of Chan et al a trend towards a higher incidence of bleeding was observed which did not reach statistical significance as both the initial study as well as the subsequent post hoc analysis was underpowered to either

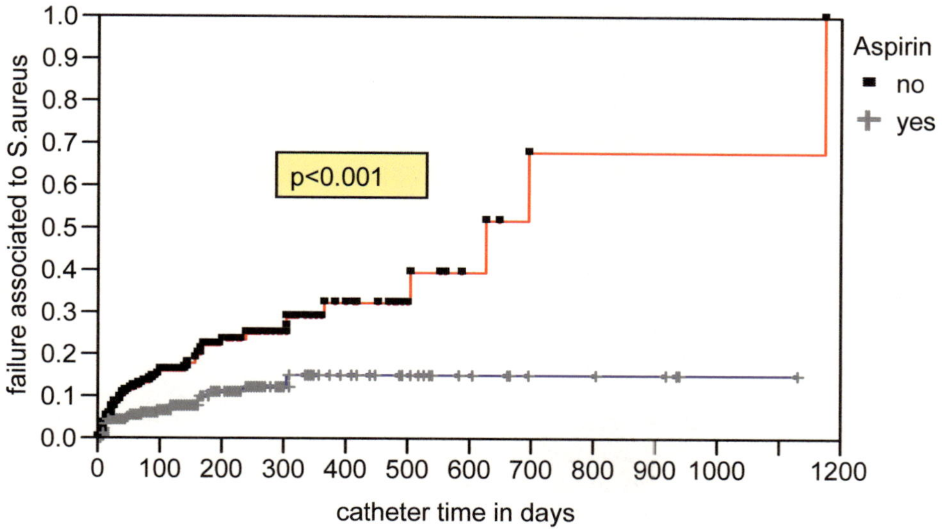

patients at risk:

ASA	417	142	66	35	25	16	9	6	5
no ASA	452	118	61	37	22	11	6	3	2

Fig. 1. Cumulative plot of tunneled catheter failure associated with *S aureus* bacteremia. The failure plot was obtained using the Kaplan-Meier method. Tics represent censoring of catheter removal unrelated to *S aureus* bacteremia. Log-rank test was used to calculate *P*. Reprinted from Sedlacek et al.: "Aspirin Treatment Is Associated With a Significantly Decreased Risk of Staphylococcus aureus bacteremia in Hemodialysis Patients With Tunneled Catheters", Am J Kidney Dis Vol49, pp401-408 with permission from Elsevier

support or refute this hypothesis. In our own study no increased risk of bleeding was observed (unpublished data, Sedlacek et al., 2008). A study on aspirin use in 28320 patients from the Dialysis Outcomes and Practice Patterns Study I and II found neither a decreased cardiovascular risk nor an increase in the gastrointestinal bleeding with the use of aspirin (Ethier J et al., 2007). (Of note, no data on infectious complications was included in this manuscript which why it was not discussed in the above sections.)

While there is no unequivocal proof that aspirin increases the risk of upper gastrointestinal bleeding in dialysis patients, it must not be forgotten that upper gastrointestinal bleeding is a well documented part of the uremic syndrome and that anticoagulation is routinely used during the hemodialysis procedure. It would thus seem reasonable to adopt a similar approach to high risk dialysis patients as has been recommended in high risk cardiac patients who would benefit from aspirin. Patients can be screened and treated for *H.pylorii* and proton pump inhibitors may be considered. Lastly it has to be noted that upper gastrointestinal bleeding is more amenable to treatment and represents a lesser risk to a high risk dialysis patient than for example cardiac stent occlusion.

4. Statins

Statins are cholesterol reducing medications that similarly to aspirin have become a cornerstone in the prevention and treatment of cardiovascular disease. The antimicrobial effects of statins have been known for a long time. In fact, statins were discovered by searching for compounds that would inhibit HMG-CoA reductase in microbes that require sterols or other isoprenoids, which are part of bacterial cytoskeleton, for growth. The first statins were described as antibiotics secreted by Penicillium species. The first statin compound, mevastatin, is derived from a culture of *Pythium ultimum* and *Penicillium citrinum* and under the name compactin the same compound was isolated from a culture of *Penicillium brevicompactum* (Endo et al., 1976). A mevastatin analog currently in use, lovastatin, was isolated from a culture of *Aspergillus terreus*. (Endo A., 1992). The antimicrobial effects of statins were rediscovered at a later time and it was noted that the minimum inhibitory concentration of simvastatin for *S.aureus* was much higher than the serum levels that can be achieved during routine treatment at recommended doses (Jerwood S. & Cohen J., 2008). Direct antimicrobial effects with potential clinical relevance have been postulated for HIV, CMV, HCV, Salmonella and yeast (Gupta et al., 2007) but are perhaps less relevant for dialysis catheter associated infection. Newer laboratory evidence shows that the interferon response to viral infection of the innate immune immune system is coupled to the mevalonate-isoprenoid arm of the sterol pathway. These findings may explain the observation that the CMV and HCV viruses are sensitive to statin administration and that treatment with interferon decreases plasma cholesterol levels similar to treatment with statins (Blanc M et al., 2011).

Several observational studies in patients with severe bacterial infections have reported improved survival in patients treated with statins (Bjoerkheim-Bergman et al., 2010). These beneficial effects appear to be greater than what might be expected with lipid lowering alone and are attributed to pleiotropic effects of statins. Such effects involve improving endothelial function, decreasing oxidative stress and inflammation and inhibiting the thrombogenic response (Liao J.K. & Laufs U., 2005).

The hypothesis that treatment with statins could have an influence on the rate of septic events in dialysis patients was investigated by Gupta et al in 2007. The authors used data from a prospective study to investigate choices and outcomes of dialysis care, which enrolled 1041 patients from 1995 to 1998, the majority of which dialyzed in units associated with Dialysis Clinic Inc in Nashville TN. These patient data were linked to United States Renal Data System administrative data which included hospitalizations and data from other treatment settings, including outpatient and skilled nursing facilities. Primary outcome were sepsis events but "only episodes in which the primary event was sepsis were included (…) to avoid including cases in which infection was acquired as a secondary phenomenon" (Correction by the same authors in JAMA Vol 299 P 765). The correction to their method section published later by the authors raises the possibility that their data analysis could come to a different conclusion if all episodes of sepsis were considered, not only the events that were considered"primary". The authors found that 143 patients (14%) received statin treatment compared with 898 patients (86%) who were not. Among all 1041 patients there were a total of 303 events of primary sepsis during a mean follow up of 3.4 years. The crude incidence rate of sepsis events was 63% lower in patients treated with statins compared with the control group (41 events per 1000 patient-years compared with 110 events per 1000 patient years) The authors found that the odds ratio for a primary septic event in statin users was 0.38 (95% CI 0.21-0.67) with adjustments for demographics, dialysis modality, comorbidities and laboratory values. In a propensity-matched subcohort analysis statin use was even more protective with an odds ratio of 0.24 (CI 0.11-0.49) (Gupta et al., 2007). In

contrast to the results of this study no difference in the rate of death from fatal infection with the use of atorvastatin was found in the 4D study (Wanner et al., 2005).
An interesting question that is raised by the study by Gupta et al. is whether the observed benefit could be due to concomitant treatment with aspirin (Gupta et al., 2007). Both statins and aspirin are used for the treatment of coronary artery disease and a head to head comparison would be instructive. Our aspirin study did not find a beneficial effect of statins on the risk of septic events (Sedlacek et al., 2007) and the study by Gupta et al. did not control for aspirin use.
It has to be noted that the relation between lipid parameters and mortality in dialysis patients is complex, confounded by the fact that elevated serum cholesterol levels are paradoxically protective in this population, probably because they are a marker for the absence of malnutrition and inflammation. In practical terms it is advised to use low doses of statins to reduce side effects and to avoid the concomittant administration of other drugs metabolized by the cytochrome P-450 system such as cyclosporine, azole antifungals and fibrates (Olyaei et al., 2011).

5. Effects of other drugs used on dialysis

Several other drugs that are frequently used on dialysis have known interactions with microbes. Heparin is used frequently to block dialysis catheters when not in use to preserve their patency. Unfortunately, heparin has been found to promote growth of bacterial biofilm in dialysis catheters (Shanks et al., 2005). Citrate has been used as an alternative to heparin to block catheters and was found to have inhibitory effects on biofilms at elevated concentration. Reminiscent of the "Goldilocks effect" observed with aspirin, citrate stimulates biofilm formation at sub inhibitory concentrations, an effect which might have clinical relevance at catheter tips (Shanks et al., 2006). EDTA also has an inhibitory effect on biofilm. The mechanism for both EDTA and citrate is thought to be through chelation of divalent ions essential to the extracellular matrix structure of biofilm (Percival et al., 2005).
Diltiazem, Amlodipine and the angiotension converting enzyme inhibitor Zofenopril have modest in vitro antimicrobial activity against S.aureus. Most of these effects are bacteriostatic and occur at higher drug concentrations in vitro than the therapeutic concentrations that are usually achieved during therapy in vivo. It has to be noted however, that drug concentration can vary considerably throughout different organs and body compartments. In the case of Amiloride it has been determined that urine concentrations achieved in patients are not sufficient to replicate the antibacterial effects that are observed in vivo (Cederlund et al., 1993). The relevance of these observations probably concerns more microbial purity testing of drugs during the fabrication process rather than clinical effects.
Emla cream, a mixture of lidocaine, prilocaine and preservatives, which is used for topical anesthesia at the site of dialysis fistula puncture, has no effect on microbial growth (Kruszewska et al., 2010). Other drugs relevant to ESRD that have been tested and were found to be devoid of antimicrobial effects are the loop diuretics furosemide and bumetanide.
The antihistaminic drug diphenhydramine has been reported to be synergistic with the penicillins (Kristiansen, 1992) and amiloride reportedly enhances uptake of tobramycin in pseudomonas aeruginosa (Cederlund et al., 1993).

6. Last but not least: Honey

Honey has been used for the treatment of wounds since ancient times and its medicinal use is sanctioned by the Bible, Torah and Koran (Namias N., 2003). Johnson et al. conducted a prospective trial of topical honey versus topical Mupirocin ointment for the prevention of dialysis catheter associated infection. In a two year study period the authors enrolled 101 patients with tunneled dialysis catheters in their hospital based dialysis unit. Honey was applied three times a week to the dialysis catheter exit site in 51 patients while mupirocin ointment was used in 50 patients. No exit site infections were observed in either group and no difference in the rate of catheter associated bacteremia could be demonstrated. The cost of the Australian grown medicinal honey that the authors used was equivalent to mupirocin. As the authors noted, it is interesting that at the time of the study about 2% of staphylococcal isolates in their hospital were resistant to mupirocin while no bacterial resistance to honey has yet been reported despite millennia of being around (Johnson D.W. et al., 2005).

7. Conclusion

In summary, a couple of observational studies have shown that both aspirin and statins might have significant salutatory effects on infectious complications in hemodialysis patients. Of note, aspirin does not have growth inhibitory or bactericidal activity at pharmacologically relevant concentrations and thus may be less likely to promote bacterial resistance as traditional antimicrobials do (Eisen et al., 2009). The same might apply for statins as well (Jerwood & Cohen, 2008). However, retrospective and observational studies are prone to multiple sources of bias that are unquantifiable and of indeterminate direction. Thus, randomized prospective trials are needed to further investigate this exciting new approach to the prevention of infectious complications in dialysis patients.

8. References

Alvarez, L.P.; Barbagelata, M.S.; Gordiola M.; Cheung A.L.; Sordelli D.O.& Buzzola F.R. (2010). Salicylic acid diminishes staphylococcus aureus capsular polysaccharide Type 5 expression. *Infection Immunology,* Vol.78, (2010), pp. 1339-1344

Anavekar, N.S.; Tleyjeh, M.; Anavekar, N.S.; Mirzoyev, Z.; Steckeleberg, J.M.; Haddad, L.; Khandaker, M.H.; Wilson, W.R.; Chandrasekaran, K.& Baddour, L.M. (2007). Impact of prior antiplatelet therapy on risk of embolism in infectious endocarditis. *Clinical Infectious Disease,* Vol. 44, (2007), pp.1180-1186

Bjoerkhem-Bergman, L.; Bergman, P.; Andersson, J. & Lindh, J. (2010). Statin treatment and mortality in bacterial infections - a systematic review and meta-analysis. *PlosONE,* Vol5, No5, (2010), e10702

Blanc, M.; Hsieh, W.Y.; Robertson, K.A.; Watterson, S.; Shui, G.; Lacaze, P.; Khondoker, M.; Dickinson, P.; Sing, G.; Rodrigues-Martin, S.; Phelan, P.; Forster, T.; Strobl, B.; Mueller, M.; Riemersma, R.; Osborne, T.; Wenk, M.R.; Angulo, A. & Ghazal, P. (2011). Host Defense against viral infection involves interferon mediated down-regulation of sterol biosynthesis. Plos *Biology,* Vol 9,(2011) e1000598

Boelaert, J.R.; Van Landuyt, H.W.; De Baere, Y.A; Deruyter, M.M.; Daneels, R.F.; Schurgers, M.L.; Matthys, E.G.& Gordts,B.Z. (1950). Staphylococcus aureus infections in haemodialysis patients: pathophysiology and use of nasal mupirocin for prevention. *Journal of Chemotherapay,* Vol.7, Suppl. 3, (1950), pp.43-53

Breen, J.D. & Karchmer, A.W. (1995). Staphylococcus aureus infections in diabetic patients. *Infectious Disease Clinic of North America,* Vol.9, (1995), pp. 11-24

Cederlund H., Mardh P.A. (1993). Review: Antibacterial activities of non-antibiotic drugs. *Journal of Antimicrobial Chemotherapy* Vol. 32, (1993) pp.355-365

Chan, KL., Dumesnil, J.G., Cujec, B., Sanfilippo, A., Jue, J., Turek, M., Robinson, T., & Moher, D.(2003). A randomized trial of aspirin on the risk of embolic events in patients with infective endocarditis. *Journal of the American College of Cardiology,* Vol. 42, No 5, (2003), pp.775-780

Chan, K.L.; Tam, J.; Dumesnil, J.G.; Cujec, B.; Sanfilippo, A.J.; Jue, J,; Turek, M.; Robinson, T.& Williams, K. (2008). Effect of long-term aspirin use on embolic events in infective endocarditis. *Clinical Infectious Disease,* Vol46, (2008), pp. 37-41

Endo, A.; Kuroda, M. & Tsujita, Y. (1976). ML-236A, ML-236B and ML-236C, new inhibitors of cholesterogenesis produced by Penicillium citrinium. *Journal of Antibiotics,* Vol29. (1976) pp. 1346-1348

Endo, A. (2004) The origin of the statins. *Artherosclerosis Supplemen,t* Vol.5, (2004), pp. 67-80

Eisen, D.; Corey,G.,;McBryde,E.; Flowler, V.; Miro, J.; Cabell, C.; Street, A.; Goulart Paiva, M.; Ionac, A.; Tan, R.; Tribouilloy, C.; Pachirat, O.; Braun Jones, S.; Chipina, N.; Naber, C.; Pan, A.; Ravasio, V.; Gattringer, R.; Chu, V. &Bayer, A. (2009). Reduced valve replacement surgery and complication rate in Staphylococcus aureus endocarditis patients receiving acetyl-salicylic acid. *Journal of Infection,* Vol.58, No.5,(2009), pp.332-338

Eisen, D.P. & Bayer, A.S. (2008). Aspirin use in infective endocarditis. *Clinical Infectious Disease,* Vol. 46, (2008), pp. 1481-1482

Ethier, J.; Bragg-Gesham, J.L.; Piera, L.; Akizawa, T.; Asano, Y.; Mason, N.; Gillespie, B.W.& Young, E.W. (2007). Aspirin prescription and outcomes in hemodialysis patients: the dialysis outcomes and practice patterns study (DOPPS). *American Journal of Kidney Diease,* Vol.50, (2007), pp.602-611

Foley, R.N.; Guo, H.; Snyder, J.J.; Gilbertson, D.T. & Collins, A.J. (2004). Septicemia in the United States dialysis population, 1991 to 1999. *Journal of the American Society of Nephrology,* Vol. 15, (2004), pp. 1038-1045

Gupta, R.; Plantinga, L.; Fink, N.; Melamed, M., Coresh, J., Fox, C., Levin, N. & Powe,N. (2007). Statin use and hospitalization for sepsis in patients with chronic kidney disease. *Journal of the American Medical Association,* Vol. 297, No.13, (2007), pp. 1455-1464

Gupta, R.; Plantinga, L.; Fink, N.; Melamed, M.; Coresh, J.; Fox, C.; Levin, N. & Powe,N. (2008). Corrections. *Journal of the American Medical Association,* Vol. 299, No.7, (2008), p.765

Hiremath, S.; Holdren, R.M.; Fergusson, D. & Zimmerman, D.L. (2009). Antiplatelet medications in hemodialysis patients: a systematic review of bleeding rates. *Clinical Journal of the American Society of Nephrology,* Vol.4, (2009), pp1347-1355

Jerwood, S. & Cohen, J. (2008). Unexpected antimicrobial effects of statins. *Journal of Antimicrobial Chemotherapy,* Vol.61, No.2, (2008), pp.362-364

Johnson, D.W.; van Eps, C.; Mudge, D.W.; Wiggins, D.W.; Armstrong, K.; Hawley, C.M.; Campbell, S.B.; Isbel, N.M.; Nimmo, G.R. & Gibbs, H. (2005). Randomized controlled trial of topical exit-site application of honey (Medihoney) for the prevention of catheter-associated infections in hemodialysis patients. *Journal of the American Society of Nephrology*, Vol. 16, (2005), pp. 1456-1462

Karabay, O.; Arinc, H.; Gundu, Z.; Tamer, A.; Ozhan, H. & Uyan, C. (2006). A new effect of acetylsalicylic acid? Significantly lower prevalence of nasal carriage of staphylococcal aureus among patients receiving orally administered acetylsalicylic acid. *Infection Control Hospital Epidemiology*, Vol 27, (2006),pp. 317-319

National Kidney foundation: K/DOQI Clinical Practice guidelines for cardiovascular diease in dialysis patients. (2005) *American Journal of Kidney Diseases*, Vol. 45, Suppl.3, (2005), pp. S1-S153

Kristinasen, J.E. (1992). The antimicrobial activity of non-antibiotics. Report from a congress on the antimicrobial effect of drugs other than antibiotics on bacteria, viruses, protozoa and other organisms. *APMIS* Suppl.30, Vol.100, (1992), pp.7-14

Kristiansen, J.E.; Hendricks, O.; Delvin, T.; Butterworth, T.S.; Aagaard, L.; Christensen, J.B.; Flores, V.C. & Keyzer, H. (2007). Reversal of resistance in microorganisms by help of non-antibiotics. *Journal of Antimicrobial Chemotherapy*, Vol.59, (2007), pp 1271-1279

Kruszewska, H.; Zareba, T. & Tyski, S. (2010). Examination of antimicrobial activity of selected non-antibiotic products. *Acta Poloniae Pharmaceutica Drug Research*, Vol.67 No.6, (2010), pp.733-736

Kupferwasser, L.I.; Yeaman, M.R. & Shapiro, S.R. (1999). Acetylsalicylic acid reduces vegetation, bacterial density, hematogenous bacterial dissemination and frequency of embolic events in experimental staphylococcus aureus endocarditis through antiplatelet and antibacterial effects. *Circulation*, Vol.99, (1999),pp. 2791-2797

Kupferwasser, L., Yeaman,M.R., Nast, C., Kupferwasser,D.; Xiong,Y., Palma, M., Cheung,A., & Bayer, A. (2003). Salicylic acid attenuates virulence in endovascular infections by targeting global regulatory pathways in staphylococcus aureus. Journal of *Clinical Investigation*, Vol.122, No.2, (2003),pp. 222-233

Laupland, K.B.;Gregson ,D.B.; Zygun, D.A.; Doig, C.J,.; Mortis, G. & Church, D.L. (2004). Severe blood stream infections: a population based assessment. *Critical Care Medicine*, Vol. 32, (2004), pp. 992-997

Liao, J.K. & Laufs, U. (2005) Pleiotropic effects of statins. *Annual Review of Pharmacology and Toxicology*, Vol.45, (2005), pp. 89-118

Little, M.A.; O'Riordan, A.; Lucey, B. et al. (2001). A prospective study of complications associated with cuffed tunneled haemodialysis catheters. *Nephrology Dialysis Transplantation*, Vol 16,(2001), pp. 2194-2200

Liu, G.Y. & Nizrt, V. (2009). Colour me bad: microbial pigments as virulence factors. *Trends in Microbiology*, Vol. 17, (2009), pp. 406-413

Namias, N. (2003) Honey in the management of infections. *Surgical Infection*, Vol.4, (2003), pp. 219-226

Nicolau, D.P.; Freeman, C.D.; Nightingale, C.H.; Quintiliani, R.; Coe, C.J.; Maderazo, E.G. & Cooper, B.W. (1993). Reduction of bacterial titers by low-dose aspirin in experimental aortic valve endocarditis. *Infection and Immunity*, Vol.61, (1993), pp. 1593-1595

Nicolau, D.P.; Marangos, M.N.; Nightingale, C.H. & Quintiliani, R. (1995). Influence of Aspirin on development and treatment of experimental Staphylococcus aureus endocarditis. *Antimicrobial Agents and Chemotherapy*, Vol.39, (1995), pp. 1748-1751

Olyaei, A.; Greer, E.; Delos Santos, R. & Rueda, J. (2011) The efficacy and safety of 3-hydroxy-3-methylglutaryl-CoA esterase inhibitors in chronic kidney disease, dialysis and transplant patients. *Clinical Journal of the American Society of Nephrology*, Vol6, (2011), pp. 664-678

Paterson, J.R. & Lawrence, J.R. (2001), Salicylic acid: a link between aspirin, diet and the prevention of colorectal cancer. *Quarterly Journal of Medicine*, Vol. 94, (2001), pp. 445-448

Peacock, S.J.; Eddleston, M.; Emptage, A.; King, A. & Crook, D.W. (1998) Positive intravenous line tip cultures as predictors of bacteremia. *Journal of Hospital Infection*, Vol. 40, (1998), pp. 35-38

Percival, S.L.; Kite, P.; Eastwood, K.; Murga, R.; Carr, J.; Arduino, M.J. & Donlan, R.M. (2005). Tertrasodium EDTA as a novel central venous catheter lock solution against biofilm. *Infection Control Hospital Epidemiology* Vol. 26 (2005), pp.511-514

Pujadas, R.E.; Escriva, F.; Jane, J.; Argimon, J.; Fava, P. & Calera, M.C. (1988). Effect of various doses of aspirin on the development of aseptic thrombotic aortic endocarditis experimentally induced in the rabbit. *Revista Espanola de Cardiologia*, Vol. 41,(1988), pp 31-34

Rayner, H.C.; Besarab, A.; Brown, W.; Disney, A.; Saito, A. & Pisoni, R.L. (2004). Vascular access results from the Dialysis Outcomes and Practice Patterns Study (DOPPS): performance against kidney disease outcomes quality initiative (K/DOQI) clinical practice guidelines. *American Journal of Kidney Disease*, Vol. 44, Suppl.2, (2004), pp. S22-S26

Ruder, E.H.; Layemo, A.O.; Graubard, B.I.; Hollenbeck, A.R.; Schatzkin, A & Cross, A.J. (2011). Non steroidal anti-inflammatory drugs and colorectal cancer risk in a large prospective cohort. *American Journal of Gastroenterology*, (2011), (e-published before print)

Sedlacek, M.; Gemery, J.; Cheung, A.; Bayer, A. & Remillard, B. (2007). Aspirin Treatment is associated with a significantly decreased risk of Staphylococcus aureus bacteremia in Hemodialysis patients with tunneled catheters. *American Journal of Kidney Diseases*, Vol. 49, No.3, (2007), pp. 401-408

Sedlacek, M.; Kaneko, T.; Schoolwerth, A. & Remillard, B.(2008) Septicemia due to vascular access is a rare cause of death in dialysis patients treated with aspirin. *Journal of the American Society of Nephrology*, Vol.19, (2007), abstract F-PO1586

Schunemann, S.; Werner, G.S.; Schulz, R.; Bitsch, A.; Prange, H.W. & Kreutzer, H. (1997). Embolische Komplikationen bei bacterieller Endokarditis. *Zeitschrift fuer Kardiologie*, Vol.86,(1997), pp1017-1025

Shanks, R.M.Q.; Donegan, N.P.; Graber, M.L.; Buckingham, S.E.; Zegans, M.; Cheung, A.L. & O'Toole, G.A. (2005). Heparin stimulates staphylococcus aureus biofilm formation. *Infection and Immunity*, Vol. 73, No 8, (2005), pp. 4596-4606

Shanks, R.M.Q.; Sargent, J.L.; Martinez, R.M.; Graber, M.L. & O'Toole, G.A. (2006). Catheter lock solutions influence staphylococcal biofilm formation on abiotic surfaces. *Nephrology Dialysis Transplantation*, Vol. 21, (2006), pp. 2247-2255

Taha, T.H.; Durrant, S.S.; Mazeika, P.K.; Nihoyannopoulos,P. & Oakley, C.M. (1992). Aspirin to prevent growth of vegetations and cerebral emboli in infective endocarditis. *Journal of Internal Medicine,* Vol. 231, (1992), pp. 543-546

Vandecasteele, S.J.; Boelaert , J.R. & De Vriese, A.S. (2009). Staphylococcus aureus infections in hemodialysis: what a nephrologist should know. *Clinical Journal of the American Society of Nephrology,* Vol.4, (2009), Pp. 1388-1400

VanderBergh, M.F.; Yzerman, E.P.; van Belkum, A.; Boelens, H.A;, Sijmons, M. & Verbrugh, H.A (1999). Follow up of Staphylococcus aureus nasal carriage after eight years: redefining the persistent carrier state. *Journal of Clinical Microbiology,* Vol 37, (1999), pp .3133-3140

Von Eiff, C.; Becker, K.; Machka, K.; Stammer, H. & Peters, G. (2001). Nasal carriage as a source of staphylococcus aureus bacteremia. *New England Journal of Medicine,* Vol. 344, (2001), pp11-16

Williams J.D. (1995). The Garrod lecture: Selective toxicity and concordant pharmacodynamics of antibiotics and other drugs. *Journal of Antimicrobial Chemotherapy,* Vol35, (1995), pp.721-737

Wanner, C.; Kanne, V. & Marz, W. (2005). Atorvastatin in patients with type 2 diabetes mellitus undergoing hemodialysis. *New England Journal of Medicine,* Vol. 353, (2005), pp 238-248

22

Sleep in Patients with ESRD Undergoing Hemodialysis

Mukadder Mollaoğlu
Cumhuriyet University
Turkey

1. Introduction

Sleep has been identified as an essential human need; this is partly because of the metabolic activities that occur while the individual is sleeping. Normal sleep is divided into non–rapid eye movement (NREM) and rapid eye movement (REM) sleep. NREM sleep comprises 75% to 80% of total sleep time (TST), and is characterized by relatively quiescent brain activity and decreased metabolic rate (Carskadon & Dement, 2000). NREM sleep consists of four stages (S1-S4), with each stage leading to a progressively deeper sleep. REM sleep follows slow wave sleep (SWS), or deep sleep, and increases over the night, comprising 20% to 25% of TST. REM sleep is characterized by an activated EEG pattern, muscle atonia, and episodic bursts of rapid eye movements. Normal sleep provides a period of physiologic and mental rest. During sleep, sympathetic tone decreases and parasympathetic tone increases, leading to a reduction in heart rate, arterial blood pressure, and cardiac output (Rosenthal, 1998). Deep sleep is theorized to be necessary for physiologic restoration. REM sleep is associated with dreaming, and is essential for maintaining emotional and cognitive well-being (Redline et al., 2004).
Waking and consciousness depend on the activity, of neurons in the ascending reticular activating system of the brainstem. These neurons project into the thalamus, hypothalamus and basal forebrain and eventually send projections to the cortex. There are particular neurotransmitters, such as the catecholamines, acetylcholine, histamine, glutamate and aspartate, that are localized within the reticular formation and have important roles in cortical activation and arousal (Jones, 1989). Sleep-promoting neurotransmitters include gamma aminobutyric acid (GABA), adenosine, and melatonin. Specific stages of sleep are regulated by the turning "on" and "off" of various neurons. REM "on" cells use GABA, acetylcholine, and glutamine, whereas REM "off" cells use norepinephrine and serotonin." REM On cells" are cholinergic cells in the lateral pontine and medial medullary reticular areas that innervate the thalamus, hippocampus and hypothalamus. These cells discharge at high rates during REM and show little or no activity during NREM."REM Off cells" are noradrenergic and serotonergic cells found in the locus coeruleus and raphe. These are cells which are slow or silent during REM sleep. Affecting levels of norepinephirne or serotonin can have an effect on REM sleep (Hoyt, 2005).
Sleep regulation is a balance between a homeostatic sleep need and an intrinsic body clock, or circadian pacemaker. Located in the suprachiasmic nucleus, the circadian pacemaker determines the onset and termination of sleep, and is partially regulated by environmental

cues such as light and ambient temperature (Rosenthal, 1998). Melatonin, a physiologic sleep promoter, is inhibited by ambient light, and its circulation is decreased during daylight hours. The adrenal secretion of cortisol, which is associated with wakefulness, follows a circadian pattern. Regulated by the hypothalamic-pituitary axis, cortisol levels peak in the early morning hours in preparation for the increased metabolic demands during wakefulness (Mahowald, & Schenk, 1989).

Some medical illnesses, such as congestive heart failure (CHF), diabetes mellitus, chronic obstructive pulmonary disease and renal disease, can directly impair sleep physiology, leading to a cyclical interaction (Ballard, 2005). End-stage renal disease (ESRD) is one of these diseases. Approximately 50% of patients with chronic end-stage renal disease undergoing hemodialysis (HD) have insomnia and other sleep disorders (Hanly, 2007). Patients often complain of restless leg syndrome (RLS), periodic limb movement disorder (PLMD), bone pain, nausea, and pruritus (Merlino et al., 2006). The etiology of sleep disorders appears to be related to metabolic derangements associated with ESRD or from coexisting diabetes mellitus (Ballard, 2005).

2. Sleep problems in hemodialysis patients

Sleep complaints and sleep disorders are common in patients with end-stage renal disease. Although variable, their prevalence has been reported to be higher when compared to the general population (Merlino et al., 2006). The experiences of sleep alteration in ESRD patients have been studied. Interestingly, 80% of hemodialysis patients suffer from sleep abnormalities and the prevalence is higher than that in the general population (Gul et al., 2006). Holley et al. (1992) surveyed 70 dialysis patients, and reported sleep disturbance experienced mainly included trouble falling asleep (67%), nighttime waking (80%), early morning waking (72%), restless legs (83%), and jerking legs (28%). However, Walker et al. (1995) found daytime sleepiness was the most commonly reported problem (66.7%) followed by restless legs syndrome (57.4%). Generally, the most prominent sleep disorders among hemodialysis patients are sleep apnea syndrome, restless leg syndrome, periodic limb movement disorders, and insomnia (De Santo et al., 2005; Holley et al., 1992; Sabry et al., 2010).

2.1 Sleep apnea syndrome

The prevalence of sleep apnea syndrome in hemodialysis patients is at least 10 times higher (Kraus & Hamburger, 1997) than those values reported in the general population (Young et al., 1993). In another recent investigation, an apnea/hypopnea index higher than 5 was found in 31% of the (young) non-diabetic HD patients studied (Rodriquez et al, 2005).

Sleep apnea syndrome (SAS) is a major clinical disturbance defined as an intermittent interruption of air flow at the level of nose and mouth during sleep. These abnormalities cause frequent decreases in O_2 saturation and awakenings. Episodes of apnea are considered clinically significant if they persist for more than 10 s; however, apnea episodes may last up to 2 min. SAS is the clinical consequence of frequent (at least 10 events per hour) episodes of apnea during sleep (Tatomir et al., 2007). There are three major types of sleep apnea: obstructive sleep apnea (OSA), the central type (CSA), and the mixed type, which includes features of both obstructive and central apnea. OSA is characterized by obstruction of the air flow determined by the occlusion of the oropharyngeal tract (Zoccali et al., 2001).

OSA occurs when the patient no longer has airflow but there is respiratory effort. CSA is determined by the transient abolition of nerve conduction to the respiratory muscles. Central apnea is defined when the patient has both cessation of airflow and the lack of respiratory effort followed by spontaneous resumption of breathing. Mixed apnea is the combination of central and obstructive apneas. All of these conditions can cause arterial oxygen desaturation and they may even be present in the same person (Tatomir et al., 2007; Zoccali et al., 2001). Researchers have speculated that the chronic metabolic acidosis suffered by patients with hemodialysis causes these sleep disorders; as the body attempts to correct the acidosis, the patient exhales more carbon dioxide and the hypocapnia that results may be inadequate to fuel respiration (Kimmel, 1989). Another theory is that these patients frequently have peripheral neuropathy, either from the ESRD or diabetes mellitus, and if the neuropathy affects the nerves innervating the upper airway, then SAS will occur (Fletcher, 1993). There is also evidence that SAS is associated with increased morbidity, and mortality, as the patient with ESRD who suffers with SAS is looking at a future with probable pulmonary hypertension and right heart failure, as well as a shortened lifespan (Fletcher, 1993; Parker, 1997). While, there are no ready answers for the causes of these sleep disorders seen in patients with ESRD undergoing HD, it is crucial that the health care provider be aware of the syndrome.

The awareness of SAS as a potent cardiovascular risk factor in ESRD undergoing HD has generated new enthusiasm in examining novel therapeutic strategies to modify sleep apnea in the patient population. To date, conservative non-pharmacological treatments (e.g. weight loss and avoidance of potentiating medications) have yielded limited success. Nasal continuous positive airway pressure therapy remains a mainstay of treatment of SAS in the non-ESRD population. Continuous positive airway pressure involves a mask fitting over the nose or mouth in which positive pressure is administered to the airway keeping the upper airway patent during sleep. In the general population, the treatment of sleep apnea with continuous positive airway pressure improves quality of life (D'Ambrosio et al.,1999), vigilance, cognition, sexual performance, and normalizes nocturnal blood pressure profile (Faccenda et al., 2001). In the HD population, continuous positive airway pressure was used in a small study of eight patients with some improvement in nocturnal oxygenation, and five of six patients reporting improved daytime alertness (Pressman, 1993). Finally, given the contribution of uremia in the pathogenesis of SAS in ESRD, attempts in optimizing uremia control in the forms of nocturnal hemodialysis (NHD) and renal transplantation have shown early clinical success (Auckley et al, 1999;Hanly & Pierratos, 2001). It is tempting to speculate that similar to those with refractory hypertension, the treatment of sleep apnea in the HD population would improve their quality of life, augment rehabilitation, and perhaps impact on the poor survival of patients.

2.2 Restless Legs Syndrome

Restless Legs Syndrome (RLS) is a neurological movement disorder that is common, under-diagnosed, under-treated, and has a poorly understood etiology (Patrick,2007). Restless legs syndrome (RLS) is a sensorimotor movement disorder characterized by the irresistible need to move associated with feelings of discomfort and parasthesias (International Restless Legs Syndrome Study Group, 2003). The incidence of idiopathic RLS (iRLS) varies between 5-15% in the general population (Nicholas et al., 2003). In the HD population, the prevalence of secondary RLS may be greater, reported to be between 6-62% (Takaki et al., 2003;Unruh et al.,2004) with some geographic variability (Kavanagh et al., 2004). With employment of standardized criteria by IRLSSG, this decreased to 12–48% (Siddiqui et al.,2005; Takaki et al, 2003;Unruh et al., 2004). RLS is observed more commonly in women than men, more commonly with increasing age and with co-morbid diabetes. Other potential correlates of RLS include lower socio-economic status, worse somatic and mental health and diabetes (Berger et al., 2004; Siddiqui et al.,2005). A high correlation between RLS and PLMS has also been noted (Allen et al. 2003, Liao et al.,2008).

The pathophysiology of RLS in uremia remains unknown however, several theories have been proposed. Potential risk factors include anemia, iron deficiency, dialysis vintage, calcium/phosphate imbalance, and peripheral and central nervous system abnormalities(Berger et al., 2004;Unruh et al.,2004).

Evidence for a possible relationship of iron deficiency to RLS in this patient population has been explained by the universal occurrence of anemia, which is commonly acquired in patients with end-stage renal disease due to inadequate production of erythropoietin (Gigli et al.,2004). Anemia in ESRD is associated with several co-morbid conditions, including congestive heart failure, stroke, cognitive dysfunction, left ventricular hypertrophy,and worsening iron deficiency due to loss from hemodialysis (Allen,2004; Gigli et al.,2004) Ferritin levels under 100 ng/mL reflect depletion of iron stores and complicate the treatment of anemia in patients on dialysis (Easom, 2006; Patrick ,2007)

Multiple causes of secondary RLS including iron deficiency anemia, diabetes mellitus, Parkinsons disease, pregnancy, rheumatic disease, venous insufficiency and less commonly in association with peripheral neuropathies, vitamin deficiencies, lumbosacral radiculopathy, spinal stenosis, excess caffeine intake, administration of some tricyclic antidepressants, hypoglycemia and hypothyroidism (Nichols et al.,2003; Siddiqui et al.,2005;Unruh et al.,2004).

The revised IRLSSG criteria (Allen et al. 2003) for RLS included four essential diagnostic criteria additional supportive features. The criteria include unpleasant and uncomfortable sensations associated with an urge to move the limbs with symptoms worsened by rest, relieved by activity and typically worse toward the evening. Positive family history, initial therapeutic response to L-dopa or a dopamine-receptor agonist are supportive evidence. At least 85% of patients with RLS may also have concomitant periodic limb movements (PLMS) though this may be the result of other disorders such as obstructive sleep apnea.

Treatment of ESRD-associated anemia with erythropoietin has been shown to decrease arousal due to PLMS and produce trends toward higher sleep quality (Benz et al 2000). As will be reviewed later, intravenous (I.V.) iron in ESRD patients has been shown to be highly effective in causing remission of RLS symptoms (Sloand et al., 2004).

Given that alterations of the dopaminergic pathways may contribute to the development of RLS in ESRD, pharmacological treatment of RLS with Levodopa (L-DOPA) has been studied and was shown to improve sleep and reduce nocturnal limb movements in three prospective trials (Sandyk et al.1987; Trenkwalder et al., 1995; Walker, 1996). Recently, treatment with pergolide, a dopamine agonist was also examined in a double-blind placebo-controlled crossover study in ESRD patients (Pieta et al., 1998). In contrast to the use of L-DOPA, pergolide resulted in decreased symptoms without objective improvements in nocturnal limb movement or sleep architecture. Limited beneficial data regarding the use of other dopamine agonists have also been reported (Miranda et AL., 2004; Pellecchia et al., 2004). Folate is also involved in the production of dopamine in the CNS. Folate, as 5-methyltetrahydrofolate, increases production of CNS tetrahydrobiopterin, a cofactor in tyrosine hydroxylase production significant reduction in RLS symptoms and decreased leg movements during sleep (p=0.018). With the exception of this one trial, there is only limited information from case reports of significant symptom reduction in pediatric RLS using dopaminergic agents (Konofal et al.,2005)

2.3 Periodic Limb Movement Disorder

Periodic limb movement disorder (PLMD) is a condition characterized by periodic episodes of repetitive and highly stereotyped limb movements that occur either during sleep (PLMS) or in wakefulness (PLMW) (Walker et al., 1995). This syndrome is more often seen in the patient with ESRD than in the general population (Pressman et al., 1995). The presence of PLMS is responsible for sleep problems in up to 72% of patients with ESRD (Benz et al., 2000) and the presence of PLMS is a more accurate predictor of mortality than coexisting diseases, serum albumin, or urea reduction ratio (Winkelman et al., 1996). A high correlation between RLS and PLMS has also been noted (Allen et al. 2003).

Treatments with high-dose iron dextran and normalization of hematocrit with recombinant human erythropoietin have been demonstrated to improve RLPLMD in ESRD patients (Benz et al, 1999; Sloand et al., 2004). Alterations in dopamine and opioid synthesis may also play a role in the high prevalence of RLS and PLMD in uremia; however, data are limited. Indirect evidence stems from the notion that treatment with dopamine agonists, dopamine precursors in ESRD patients may improve RLS and PLMD symptoms (Sandyk et al.1987; Trenkwalder et al., 1995; Walker, 1996).

2.4 Insomnia

Insomnia is defined as a disorder of difficulty initiating sleep (DIS), difficulty maintaining sleep (DMS), and/or early morning awakening (EMA). Insomnia is commonly defined as the subjective sensation of short, unsatisfying sleep, despite the ability to sleep (Sabbatini et al., 2002). It may be secondary either to trouble falling asleep and/or to night-time waking, which must be persistently present (i.e. three to four times a week for several weeks) (Leger et al.,2002). The prevalence estimates of insomnia vary because of differences in definition, diagnosis, population characteristics, and research methodologies. Insomnia is a common sleep problem, however, and its prevalence in the general population ranges from 4% to 64% (Terzano et al., 2004; Chesson et al., 2000). The prevalence of insomnia is substantially greater in dialysis patients and has been reported to range from 45% to 59% (İliescu et al., 2003; İliescu et al., 2004; Sabbatini et al., 2002).

Insomnia is characterized by one or more of the following symptoms: difficulty falling asleep ("sleep onset insomnia"), difficulty staying asleep ("sleep maintenance insomnia"), early awakening or poor sleep quality ("non-restorative sleep") (Ohayon et al., 2002; Meyer, 1998). Insomnia is primarily a clinical diagnosis and it is most frequently diagnosed from data obtained from the history and from sleep diaries. PSG is not indicated in the initial evaluation of insomnia but may be necessary in chronic treatment-resistant cases and in patients in whom specific sleep disorders (SASRLSPLMS) are suspected (Bonner et al., 2008).

Insomnia may be caused by a variety of reasons, with the most frequent causes listed by researchers as: restless legs syndrome (RLS), periodic leg movements during sleep (PLMS), sleep apnea syndrome (SAS) and depression (Kimmel, 1989; Parker, 1997; Welch & Austin, 2001). The prevalence of insomnia due to RLS in dialysis patients ranges from 57% to 83% (Holley et al., 1992; Sabbatini et al., 2002; Walker et al., 1995). Elderly patients, those with longer dialysis durations, dialysis shift, and those with high levels of parathyroid hormone (PTH) or diabetes mellitus are at higher risk of insomnia; however, the dialysis type and biochemical parameters are not important determinants of insomnia (Han et al., 2002; Sabbatini et al., 2002).

Most studies assessing the effectiveness of different treatment modalities in insomniacs address short-term treatment of insomnia (Montgomery &Dennis., 2004; Morgan et al., 2003; Smith et al., 2002). Extra care and caution has to be exercised when treating insomnia in patients with renal impairment. Most hypnotics should be administered in appropriately reduced doses and interactions with the numerous medications used in the different HD populations should be considered carefully when prescribing a hypnotic to patients with renal failure (Novak et al., 2006). Surprisingly there is an almost complete lack of pharmacologic studies in renal patients suffering from insomnia. In a small randomized study using the PSQI Sabbatini et al. (2003). suggested that zaleplon improved sleep efficacy in maintenance hemodialysis patients.

Nonpharmacologic interventions include sleep hygiene measures relaxation therapy and biofeedback stimulus control therapy sleep restriction and cognitive behavioral therapy (Montgomery &Dennis., 2004; Morgan et al., 2003). These interventions have been shown to be beneficial in the long-term management of patients with chronic hypnotic use. Cognitive behavioral therapy for insomnia in the routine general practice setting improved sleep quality reduced hypnotic drug use and improved health-related quality of life at a favorable cost in chronic insomniacs.

3. Related factors with sleep problems in hemodialysis patients

A multitude of causes including anemia, blood urea levels, plasma creatinine levels, parathyroid hormone (PTH) concentrations, increased blood pressure, quality of life, and illness intrusiveness may contribute to sleep disturbances in patients on maintenance hemodialysis (Hanly et al., 2003; Iliescu et al., 2004; Sabbatini et al.,2003). Furthermore, there is a positive correlation between sleep disturbances and increased morbidity and mortality related to cardiovascular disease and infectious complications, the 2 major causes of death in hemodialysis patients (De Santo et al., 2005). Sleep disorders in hemodialysis patients is a multifactorial complaint, stemming from Uremic toxins and dialysis procedure, other medical problems, psychiatric or psychosocial background.

3.1 Uremic toxins

Several studies in the past 30 years have shown that uremic patients are at great risk for disordered sleep. A study by Millman et al. (1985) noticed a slight but significant relationship between sleep apnea syndrome and azotemia. In a recent prospective study of incident HD patients followed-up for 1 year, higher dialysis efficiency was associated with fewer sleep disturbances (Unruh et al., 2006). These latter data are further supported by the results of Hanly et al. (2001), who studied patients on conventional hemodialysis (4 h three times a week) who then switched to nocturnal (intensive) dialysis (8 h for 6 or 7 days/week). A spectacular correction of sleep apnea was recorded in this small-scale study (Hanly et al., 2001). Finally, the impact of uremic toxins is highlighted by the fact that sleep disorders are more frequent and more severe in dialyzed patients compared with subjects with pre-dialysis CKD (Merlino et al., 2006).

3.2 Interdialytic weight gain and hypertension

Excessive interdialytic weight gain has been associated with poor compliance and high blood pressure (Rahman et al., 2000). While the mechanism of the association between interdialytic weight gain and sleep problems is unclear, we speculate that large interdialytic weight gains result in expanded intravascular volume, which has been associated with upper airway obstruction (Chiu et al., 2006).

The length of sleep during the night before a hemodialysis session after a long interdialytic interval (3 days, the "weekend interval") is significantly shorter compared to the usual sleep length following a short interdialytic interval. This led to some speculation regarding the possible effect of interdialytic weight gain (IWG) on sleep (Bertini et al., 1999). Furthermore, patients with uncontrolled pre-dialysis systolic pressure (usually a sign of hypervolemia in these patients) experience clinically overt insomnia more frequently (De Santo et al., 2001); in patients with chronic diseases, systolic hypertension appears to be a cause of sleep disturbances (Katz & McHorney 1998; Sabbatini et al., 2002; Thase, 2005).

3.3 Dialysis shift

The dialysis shift has several effects on patients with ESRD. Morning-shift HD patients experience more insomnia (Sabbatini et al., 2002), but also have longer survival times (Bliwise., 2001) than patients on other dialysis shifts. In according to another study (Merlino et al., 2006), for patients undergoing HD in the morning shift, the risk of subclinical insomnia is up to 18 times higher than for those who have their dialysis session in the afternoon. However, morning-shift HD patients have higher intradialytic sleepiness, which is associated with more decreased body temperature during HD, than patients on other dialysis shifts (Parker et al., 2003).

3.4 Dialysis vintage

The longer the dialysis vintage, the more significant is the prevalence of sleep quality disorders (Veiga et al., 1997). In a study by De Santo et al., (2005), patients with subclinical or clinical sleep disorders had double the dialysis vintage of those without sleep complaints; in patients with a medium dialytic age of 75 months, the prevalence of sleep disorders is close to 80%. These data are not surprising, taking into account the accumulation of comorbidites, including peripheral neuropathy and CVD, whilst on dialysis on long-term. In a polysomnographic study by Tatomir et al.,(2007) in patients hemodialyzed for more than 10 years, all patients has disturbed sleep with frequent awakening and reduced sleep efficiency. One-half of these patients had sleep-related breathing disorders, i.e. sleep apnea syndrome.

3.5 Restless legs syndrome

Restless legs syndrome (RLS) usually becomes apparent during resting and may significantly interfere with sleep. An association between RLS and insomnia in patients on maintenance hemodialysis has been suggested already by a few papers (Musci et al., 2005; Sabbatini et al., 2002; Walker et al., 1995). Moreover, RLS is associated with a low quality of sleep and lower quality of life.

3.6 Other medical factors

Other medical factors include the pain and discomfort caused by illnesses such as arthritis, cardiovascular disease, chronic obstructive pulmonary disease (COPD), cerebrovascular disease, neurological disorders, asthma, headaches, and more. The prognosis of patients with chronic uremia is influenced by the presence of comorbidities, mainly by cardiovascular disease (CVD), which causes roughly 50% of deaths (Covic et al., 2006). A study by Mucsi et al. (2004), demonstrated that comorbidities are independent predictors of sleep disturbances in patients on maintenance dialysis. According to another study, the average Charlson Comorbidity Index (CCI) in patients without sleep disorders was 4.10, while scores in patients with subclinical and clinically overt sleep disorders were 6.10 and 6.81, respectively (De Santo et al.,2005). This highly significant association in the Italian HD population was maintained regardless of age. To conclude so far, any in-depth research on the quality of sleep in renal patients must consider the magnitude of comorbidities.

3.7 Age

Sleep difficulties are closely correlated with older age in patients with chronic uremia (Iliescu et al., 2003). Yoshioka et al.(1993) found that advanced age and long-term dialysis therapy directly affected patients experiencing sleep problems. The disorders are similar to those described in the general population, where the prevalence and severity of sleep disorders are also associated with old age. Each decade of age increases the risk of insomnia by 239%, and the risk of overt clinical insomnia by 51% (De Santo et al., 2005). Mollaoğlu (2004) reported a negative correlation between age and sleep quality, with sleep quality decreasing with advanced age in their study of 105 HD patients. In addition, community-based studies have shown that sleep quality could be deteriorated in elderly patients due to increased frequency of physical diseases, multiple drug use, primary sleep disturbances, or lifestyle modifications (Brandenberger et al., 2003; Kamel & Gammack 2006).

3.8 Depression

The psychiatric condition most commonly causing sleep disorders is depression that may affect up to 50% of this patient population (Covic et al., 2006). The relationship between depression and sleep disorders is well known both in the general population and in patients undergoing hemodialysis (İliescu et al.,2003). Depression can be a cause, as well as a result, of insomnia. Dialysis patients with a Pittsburg Quality Index Sleep score of >5 (patients with a "difficult sleep") have a prevalence of overt depression of 20%, while among ESRD patients reporting a normal sleep, the prevalence of depression is almost nil (İliescu et al.,2003).

3.9 Medications and other substances

Medications and other substances which may cause insomnia include beta-blockers, bronchodilators, corticosteroids, CNS stimulants, Tagamet, cardiovascular drugs, neurological drugs, alcohol, caffeine and nicotine (Merlino et al., 2006; Rosenthal, 1998; Unruh et al., 2006). Most prescribed as well as over-the-counter medications produce side effects which are either sedating or stimulating. Drugs which cause daytime sleepiness include analgesics, benzodiazepines and antihistamines (Rosenthal, 1998; Unruh et al., 2006). According to recent investigations, the use of hypnotic medication in dialysis patients is rather modest: 8–10% (De Santo et al., 2005; De Santo et al., 2001). In a large study, the reported use of sleep-inducing medication was even lower—3.6% (Merlino et al., 2006). However, dialysis patients with severe sleep disorders use specific medication more frequently (24%) (De Santo et al., 2005). Improved hemodialysis techniques, socio-economical disparities in the studied populations, and reluctance by nephrologists to prescribe psychotropic medication may explain these disparities. However, we must be aware that chronic auto-administration of hypnotic medication may be more frequent in

ESRD patients compared to the general population. Moreover, according to recent data from the CHOICE incident dialysis population, use of benziodiazepines is associated with altered sleep quality during the first year of dialysis. Although this study was unable to distinguish between cause and effect, more effective dialysis and cognitive behavioral therapy have been suggested in patients with sleep disorders in need of sleep-inducing medication (Unruh et al., 2006). Moreover, many antidepressants actually cause paradoxical restlessness, therefore systematic administration of these drugs should be subjected to close clinical follow-up, which should be easy to accomplish in hemodialysis patients.

Alcohol is widely used as a sleep aid. Although it does shorten sleep latency, it also causes sleep fragmentation, decreased REM, REM rebound and early morning awakenings. The use of alcohol combined with hypnotics may exacerbate sleep difficulties even more (Rosenthal, 1998). Alcohol and (particularly) tobacco abuse is highly associated with increased prevalence of sleep disorders in ESRD (Merlino et al., 2006). Caffeine and other stimulants such as nicotine have been shown to increase sleep latency and sleep fragmentation, and to decrease total sleep time (Rosenthal, 1998). Current smoking is also related with decreases in sleep quality during the first year of dialysis therapy in incident patients (Unruh et al., 2006). Caffeine intake appears to have no significant impact on insomnia in ESRD (Sabbatini et al., 2002).

4. Sleep quality and evaluation of sleep in hemodialysis patients

Sleep quality is an important clinical construct for two major reasons. First, complaints about sleep quality are common; epidemiological surveys indicate that 15-35 % of the adult population complain of frequent sleep quality disturbance, such as difficulty falling asleep or difficulty maintaining sleep. Second, poor sleep quality can be an important symptom of many sleep and medical disorders (Buysse et al., 1989).

Sleep quality" is sometimes used to refer to a collection of sleep measures including total sleep time (TST), sleep onset latency (SOL), degree of fragmentation, total wake time, sleep efficiency, and sometimes sleep disruptive events such as spontaneous arousals or apnea. The widely employed Pittsburgh Sleep Quality Index (PSQI), for example, provides a measure of global sleep quality based on a respondent's retrospective appraisal (past month) of an array of sleep measures, including sleep latency, sleep duration, habitual sleep efficiency, sleep disturbances, use of sleeping medication, and daytime dysfunction (Krystal & Edinger, 2008). Sleep quality is also sometimes inferred from a collection of objective indices taken from polysomnography (PSG). PSG is the most valid and accurate way to assess sleep. Measures derived from PSG include: (a) total sleep time, (b) sleep efficiency (ratio of time spent asleep/time in bed), (c) sleep latency (time to fall asleep after lights out), (d) amount of wake time during sleep periods (waking after sleep onset, WASO), (e) number of awakenings, and (f) amount of each sleep stage (Landis al., 2002).

Among these objective indices are measures such as sleep onset latency, total sleep time, wake time after sleep onset, sleep efficiency, and number of awakenings that correspond to like measures taken from various available self-report instruments (e.g., sleep diaries, PSQI, etc.) (Buysse et al., 2006). However, PSG also provides a number of measures that reflect the architecture of sleep such as the percentage or temporal amounts of stage 1 sleep, stage 2 sleep, slow wave sleep or rapid eye movement (REM) sleep. Despite having no self-report analogues, these latter measures also have been employed by some as indices of sleep quality (Krystal & Edinger, 2008).

Most of the recent studies on quality of sleep use different questionnaires assessing various aspects of sleep. The Pittsburgh Sleep Quality Index, the Epworth Sleepiness Scale, and the Berlin Questionnaire are most frequently applied. Results derived from these questionnaires are limited by the subjective perception/sincerity of the patients, and thus are an imperfect substitute for more objective research methods on sleep in patients with chronic uremia (Chen et al, 2006; Iliescu et al., 2003; Mollaoglu & Mollaoglu, 2009; Sabbatini et al., 2003).

Researchers have documented that ESRD patients reported significantly poorer subjective quality of sleep in comparison to the general population (Holley et al., 1992; Parker, 2005). The reported prevalence of 'poor sleep', including sleep-wake complaints, sleep-disordered breathing and excessive sleepiness, in dialysis patients is in the range of 45–80% (Afshar et al., 2011; Parker, 1996; Walker et al., 1995; Wei et al., 2011). In a another study It was examined the quality of sleep in 89 subjects with ESRD on haemodialysis using the PSQI and found a prevalence of 'poor sleep' (global PSQI>5) of 71% (Iliescu et al., 2003). Also, decreased quality of sleep is common in dialysis patients and is associated with decreased health-related quality of life (Iliescu et al., 2003; Williams et al., 2002).

The complex evaluation of sleep in patients with renal disease may be accomplished only by means of polysomnography. Polysomnography includes the comprehensive evaluation of the patient during sleep by electroencephalography, electrooculography, myography, quantification of respiratory efforts (by plethysmography), pulseoxymetry and noninvasive evaluation of CO2 blood level, and heart rate measuring (Tatomir et al., 2007). Parker et al. (2003) examined by polysomnography 16 patients with HD and 8 patients with pre-dialysis CKD. Dialysis patients, in comparison with non-dialyzed CKD subjects, have a shorter sleep time. The REM phase is also shortened, time until falling asleep is longer, and respiratory events are more frequent. The sleep latency period was double in renal patients without dialysis compared to those with dialysis. Moreover, the prevalence and severity of periodical limb movement is higher in dialysis patients, as well as the number of short-term awakening periods (Parker et al., 2003). The authors suggest that sleep disturbances may have a different etiology in dialyzed patients compared to pre-dialysis CKD subjects. Functional and psychological factors may play a more prominent role in the pre-dialysis group, whereas intrinsic sleep disruption (arousals, apneas and limb movements) secondary to intermittent daytime HD sessions may play a more prominent role in patients with chronic uremia. Taken as a whole, renal patients experience a significant reduction in sleep length and efficiency compared to the general population (Parker et al., 2005).

The studies have shown poor the quality of sleep in HD patients to be associated with female sex, older age, caffeine intake, recombinant erythropoietin therapy, pain, cardiovascular disease, physical functioning, larger body mass index (BMI), exercise, dialysis adequacy, parathyroid hormone, serum creatinine and quality of life (QOL) (Benz et al., 1999; Sabatini et al., 2002; Walker et al., 1995). Hanly et al. (2003) examined daytime sleepiness with multiple sleep latency tests in 24 haemodialysis patients and found strong correlation between sleep latency and BUN. In addition, psychological problems do represent crucial factors in influencing the quality of sleep in hemodialysis patients, as emphasized by all the previous studies in prevalent patients with renal disease, with depression playing a prominent role, followed by anxiety, sexual problems, financial strains, and isolation (İliescu et al., 2003; İliescu et al., 2004; Markou et al.,2006; Novak et al.,2006).

Considering the strict linkage between some of these factors affecting sleep and hemodialysis, it is tempting to speculate that treating sleep problems, while improving the overall quality of life, might positively affect hemodialysis. In addition, with this point of

view, psychological, behavioural and pharmacologic interventions that promote sleep will represent a more than promising area for future research in hemodialysis patients.
The above studies results show that the sleep characteristics of hemodialysis patients need to be routinely evaluated. In addition to medical treatment to eliminate the sleep problems of hemodialysis patients and increase their sleep quality, the implementation of sleep hygiene interventions that can play a part in the regularity of patients' sleep could also be beneficial. These interventions would include an environment with a comfortable room temperature and ventilation, minimal noise, a comfortable bed, and proper lighting. These interventions should apply to each patient's personal routines (Mollaoglu & Mollaoglu, 2009).

5. Management of sleep problems in hemodialysis patients

Proper management of sleep problems in ESRD patients requires in the first instance a proper identification of sleep abnormalities (extensively discussed above). Although significant research has been done to characterize sleep abnormalities in hemodialysis patients (Holey et al., 1992; De Santo et al., 2005; Merlino et al., 2006), little has been published regarding proper treatment. In the absence of guidelines, nephrologists rely largely on some published data and on opinion-based medicine. Sleep problems lower quality of life and contribute to physical and mental health problems. Sleep disorders and lack of sleep are an under treated threat to the public health. Sleep professionals have recognized the behavioral components of sleep disorders for decades, yet most patients never get a proper diagnosis and treatment (Mollaoglu & Mollaoğlu, 2009).
Periodic clinical assessment of sleep complaints should become routine for dialysis staff. Early identification of sleep problems and interventions to improve sleep quality is essential, because sleep disturbance that persists for a long period of time could decrease general health and functioning (Sabbatini et al., 2003; Tatomir et al., 2007). Increasing evidence supports the effectiveness of both pharmacologic and nonpharmacologic therapies for sleep problems (Edinger et al., 2001; Montgomery & Dennis, 2004; Smith et al., 2002). Pharmacologic therapy are discussed in the sleep disorders section.
The most effective nonpharmacologic interventions tested to date include all or most of the following components: *sleep hygiene instruction, sleep restriction, stimulus control, relaxation training, and cognitive modification* (Edinger et al., 2001; Montgomery & Dennis, 2004).

5.1 Sleep hygiene

Sleep hygiene involves basic education on how the sleep environment, caffeine, alcohol, nicotine, food and exercise affect sleep (Smith et al., 2002). Sleep Hygiene is an educational approach designed to teach insomnia patients as well as the population at large how to maintain healthy behavioral habits which promote better sleep. It is important to understand that successful treatment is only possible if the patient complies with suggestions to improve sleep hygiene (*Edinger et al., 2001).* Below are summarized tips for sleep hygiene

Sleep hygiene tips

- Sleep only when sleepy. If you can't fall asleep within 20 min get up and do something boring until you feel sleepy,
- Don't take nap sunless your doctor advises so.

- Regular sleep-wake schedule is important. Get up and go to bed the same time every day even on weekends.
- Regular exercise improves sleep but most people should refrain from exercise at least 4 hr before bedtime.
- Develop sleep rituals (listening to musicetc.). It is important to give your body cues that it is time to slow down and sleep.
- Only use your bed for sleeping and intimacy. Refrain from using your bed to watch TV or work.
- Stay away from caffeine-containing beverages foods and medications nicotine and alcohol at least 4–6 hr before bedtime.
- Have a light snack before bed with a glass of milk which contains sleep-promoting tryptophan.
- Take a hot bath 90 min before bedtime. A hot bath will raise your body temperature but it is the drop in body temperature that may leave you feeling sleepy.
- Make sure your bed and bedroom are quiet and comfortable. Use appropriate curtains ear plugs or a white noise machine if necessary. A cooler room is recommended. Use a humidifier if the air is too dry.

These suggestions often combine several methods and may sound trivial. Compliance with such advice is still relatively poor however as it frequently requires changes in persistent "bad" habits which are ingrained (Morin et al., 1999). Building a regular sleep schedule and creating an appropriate sleeping environment as well as regular physical activity are very important in combating insomnia or insomnia-like presentations in RLS/PLMD (Montgomery & Dennis, 2004).

In terms of sleep hygiene for RLS/PLMD, there are a two main points that bear highlighting. First, the avoidance of alcohol, caffeine and nicotine may be underscored because of their potential contribution to RLS symptoms and/or PLMs. Second, other sleep hygiene practices may or may not have any utility for patients with RLS. Particularly when sleep hygiene is provided to patients as a handout or pamphlet, there is no indication that this helps promote sleep in any patient group. (Martin, 2000; Pigeon &Yurcheshen, 2009).

5.2 Relaxation and biofeedback techniques

Relaxation and biofeedback techniques for treating insomnia are based on the assumption that insomnia patients are overly aroused and anxious, and this interferes with their ability to initiate and/or maintain sleep (Lacks, 1993). Relaxation techniques are designed simply to teach patients to relax, and thus improve their ability to sleep. Of several relaxation methods, none has been shown to be more efficacious than the others. Progressive muscle relaxation, autogenic training and electromyographic biofeedback seek to reduce somatic arousal (e.g., muscle tension), whereas attention-focusing procedures such as imagery training and meditation are intended to lower presleep cognitive arousal (e.g., intrusive thoughts, racing mind) (Spielman et al., 1987).

In general, biofeedback training is an effective treatment for some insomnia patients, and is as effective as other non-pharmacologic interventions (Morin et al., 1999). If patients can train themselves to relax before sleep or at night after an awakening, they are more capable or falling asleep and staying asleep. It is believed that the beneficial effects of these methods extend beyond the sleep problems in that they facilitate better coping skills in general (Martin, 2000).

Structured exercise programs may also improve symptoms of insomnia (Montgomery & Dennis., 2004). Despite the promise of CBT the relative efficacy of these various nonpharmacologic approaches has not been well established. Data also suggest that CBTin contrast to medications may have a lasting effect beyond the termination of treatment. The extent to which the concomitant use of nonpharmacologic therapy augments the performance of pharmacologic treatments needs to be established in further studies (Novak et al., 2006).

5.3 Stimulus-control therapy

Stimulus-control therapy is a behavioral approach based on the premise that some sleep disturbances are behaviorally conditioned, so that the patient associates the bedroom environment with arousal. The main objective of stimulus control therapy is to reassociate the bed and bedroom with the rapid onset of sleep.

Below are summarized instructions for stimulus-control therapy (Martin, 2000).

Instructions for Stimulus-Control Therapy

- Patient goes to bed only when sleepy.
- If not asleep within about 10 minutes, patient gets out of bed, and does not return to bed until sleepy.
- When patient returns to bed, if not asleep within 15 minutes, gets out of bed.
- Pattern is repeated until patient can fall asleep within a few minutes.
- Must get up at the same time each morning (even if only slept 2 hours).
- Bed is used only for sleeping (not for watching television, reading exciting books, etc).
- All naps during the day must be avoided.

This method focuses primarily on shortening sleep onset, however, in the case of sleep maintenance insomnia, the instructions may be followed when the patient awakens and cannot fall back to sleep during the night. The patient should avoid lying awake in bed as much as possible and only go to bed when sleepy. No stimulating or distracting activities (e.g. reading exciting books or articles, watching television, looking at a clock) should be available. Although the patient cannot control sleep onset, wake up time should be fixed, so that a regular sleep/wake schedule will develop. Pro hibiting daytime naps is important to take advantage of the sleep deficit accumulated since the sleep period on the previous night, which in itself can shorten sleep onset. As with all psychological therapies, compliance is enhanced when the instructions and their rationales are explained to the patient.

Stimulus control therapy has been shown to be effective in shortening sleep latency compared with placebo intervention in insomnia patients (Lacks, Bertelson, Gans & Kunkel, 1996). Clinical trials have documented the efficacy of stimulus control therapy for both sleep onset and sleep-maintenance insomnia (Espie et al., 1989; Lacks et al., 1993)

5.4 Sleep restriction therapy

Sleep restriction therapy, is based on the observation that many insomnia patients spend an excessive amount of time in bed in futile attempts to achieve more sleep (Spielman, Saskin, & Thorpy, 1987).. Sleep restriction therapy consists of curtailing the amount of time spent in bed to increase the percentage of time spent asleep. This improves the patient's sleep efficiency (time asleep/time in bed). For example, a person who reports staying in bed for eight hours but sleeping an average of five hours per night would initially be told to decrease the time spent in bed to five hours. The allowable time in bed per night is increased 15 to 30 minutes as sleep efficiency improves. Adjustments are made over a period of weeks until an optimal sleep duration is achieved. Typically, it is best to alter the bedtime and to keep the rising time constant in order to maintain a regular sleep-wake rhythm. By creating a mild state of sleep deprivation, this therapy promotes more rapid sleep onset and more efficient sleep (Hauri, 2000). To minimize daytime sleepiness, time in bed should not be reduced to less than five hours per night. Sleep restriction therapy is modified in older adults by allowing a short afternoon nap.

Lichstein and Reidel (1994) concluded that sleep restriction therapy is actually the preferred technique for insomnia in older patients. In a later study they combined sleep restriction with sleep education for older insomnia patients, comparing a self-help technique (a guiding video) with therapist guidance (Riedel et al., 1995). While the self-help technique alone showed improvement on some sleep variables, therapist guidance was superior in that it improved sleep latency, wake time after sleep onset and sleep satisfaction.

Implementation of this technique requires a high level of motivation and compliance on the patient's part, and close follow up by the clinician. Below are listed the rules for sleep restriction therapy.

Instructions for Sleep Restriction Therapy

- Patient is only allowed to stay in bed for the amount of time they think they sleep each night, plus 15 minutes. For example, if patient reports sleeping only 5.75 hours, they are allowed to stayin bed for 6 hours.
- Patient must get up at the same time each day. If normal waking time is 6:30, patient is allowed to go to bed at 12:30.
- Napping is not allowed.
- When sleep efficiency has reached 85%, the patient can go to bed 15 minutes earlier.
- This procedure is repeated until the patient can sleep for the desired amount of time.

5.5 Weight loss

Upper-body obesity is a risk factor for OSA, and it is well documented that weight loss has a notable ameliorative impact on the occurrence of OSA (Ancoli-Israel et al., 1996; Smith et al., 1985). Since OSA results from closure of the airway, excess fatty tissue in theneck area may be a contributing factor. This supports the notion that weight plays a significant role in the presence and severity of sleep disordered breathing although no conclusive treatment trials have been published at this time.

5.6 Light therapy

The most influential treatment for circadian rhythm disturbances is increased exposure to bright light. This form of therapy, which directly targets the circadian system, is much preferred over hypnotics and other sedative medications. Since light is the most important synchronizer in our circadian system, increasing bright light exposure during certain times of the day can shift circadian rhythm phase and increase its amplitude. Specifically, bright light exposure in the evening causes a phase delay, while morning bright light exposure causes a phase advance in circadian rhythms, including rhythms of melatonin, core body temperature and sleepiness (Martin et al., 2000).

5.7 Cognitive-behavioral therapies

Many behavioral sleep medicine interventions are based on cognitive-behavioral therapies (CBT). The focus is on systematically introducing behavioral changes that have been proven to improve sleep. This could include changes in sleep schedule and changes in the contingencies and reinforcers that promote sleep. The cognitive approach focuses on looking internally to examine, manage, or modify sleep interfering thoughts and beliefs that can interfere with sleep. Cognitive behavioral therapy for insomnia in the routine general practice setting improved sleep quality reduced hypnotic drug use and improved health-related quality of life at a favorable cost in chronic insomniacs. Randomized controlled trials (RCTs) report somewhat conflicting results on the effectiveness of CBT in patients with insomnia but one systematic review including six RCTs (282 people) found that group or individual cognitive behavioral therapy (including sleep hygiene stimulus control sleep restriction muscle relaxation and sleep education) significantly improved PSQI scores compared with no treatment immediately after treatment and at 3 months (*Montgomery &Dennis, 2004)*. Furthermore another meta-analysis involving 2102 patients in 59 trials found that sleep restriction and stimulus control therapies were more effective than relaxation techniques when used alone (*Edinger & Sampson., 2003)*.

6. Conclusion

Considering that the most frequent sleep complaints, such as insomnia, OSAS and RLS, are related to a significant negative impact on functional health status in uraemic patients, the nephrologists should improve their recognition and treatment of these conditions to restore the quality of life of their patients. A good sleep history and, when indicated, a sleep recording, will help the clinician to make an accurate diagnosis and thus identify the best treatment. Nonpharmacologic methods such as behavioral techniques and cognitive therapyas well as pharmacologic approaches and combinations of these methods should be used for the treatment of sleep problems in hemodialysis patients.

7. References

Afshar, R., Emany, A. Saremi, A., Shavandi, N., & Sanavi, S. (2011). Effects of intradialytic aerobic training on sleep quality in hemodialysis patients. *Iranian Journal of Kidney Diseases,* Vol. 5, No. 2, Apr, pp. 119-23.

Allen, R. (2004). Dopamine and iron in the pathophysiology of restless legs syndrome (RLS). *Sleep Med,* Vol. 5, pp. 385-391.

Allen, R.P., Picchietti, D., Hening, W.A., Trenkwalder, C., Walters, A.S., & Montplaisi, J. (2003). Restless legs syndrome: Diagnostic criteria, special considerations, and epidemiology. A report from the restless legs syndrome diagnosis and epidemiology workshop at the National Institute of Health. *Sleep Med,* pp. 101–119

Ancoli-Israel, S., Kripke, D. F., Klauber, M. R., Fell, R., Stepnowsky, C., Estline, E., Khazeni, N. & Chinn, A.(1996). Morbidity, mortality and sleep disordered breathing in community dwelling elderly. *Sleep,* Vol. 19, pp. 277–282.

Auckley, D.H., Schmidt-Nowara, W., & Brown, L.K. (1999). Reversal of sleep apnea hypopnea syndrome in end-stage renal disease after kidney transplantation. *Am J Kidney Dis,* Vol. 34, pp. 739–744.

Ballard, R. D. (2005). Sleep and medical disorders. *Prim Care,* Vol. 35, pp. 511–533.

Benz, R.L., Pressman, M.R., Hovick, E.T. , & Peterson, D. D. (1999). A preliminary study of the effects of anemia with recombinant human erythropoietin therapy on sleep,

sleep disorders, and daytime sleepiness in hemodialysis patients (the SLEEPO study). *Am J Kidney Dis,* Vol. 34, pp. 1089–1095

Benz,R.L., Pressman, M.R., Hovik, E.H., & Peterson, D.D. (2000). Potential novel predictors of mortality in end-stage renal disease patients with sleep disorders. *American Journal of Kidney Disease,* Vol. 35, No. 6, pp. 1052-1060.

Berger, K., Luedemann, J., Trenkwalder, C., John, U. & Kessler, C. (2004). Sex and the risk of restless legs syndrome in the general population. *Arch Intern Med,* Vol. 164, pp. 196–202.

Bertini, M., Lucidi F, & De Santo RM (1999). Effeti dell' emodialisi sulla qualita del sonno, In: *Qualita della vita, etica ed economia in Nefrologia,* Bertini M, Di Iorio BR (eds). pp 79–90 Editoriale Bios, Cosenza.

Bliwise, D.L., Kutner, N.G, Zhang, R., & Parker, K.P. (2001). Survival by time of day of hemodialysis in an elderly cohort. *JAMA,* Vol. 286, pp.2690–4

Bonner, A., Wellard, S., & Caltabiano, M. (2008). Levels of fatigue in people with ESRD living in far North Queensland. *J Clin Nurs,* Vol. 17, No. 1, pp. 90-98.

Brandenberger, G., Viola, A.U., Ehrhart, J., Charloux, A., Geny, B. Piquard, F. & Simon C. (2003). Age-related changes in cardiac autonomic control during sleep. *J Sleep Res,* Vol. 12, No. 3, pp. 173–180.

Buysee, D.J., Reynolds, C.F., Monk, T.H., Berman, S.R., & Kupfer, D.J. (1989). The Pittsburgh Sleep Quality Index: A new ınstrument for psychiatric practice and research. *Psychiatry Research,* Vol. 28, pp. 93-213.

Buysse, D.J., Ancoli-Israel, S., Edinger, J.D., Lichstein, K.L., & Morin, C.M. (2006). Recommendations for a standard research assessment of insomnia. *Sleep,* Vol. 29, No. 9, pp. 1155–73.

Carskadon, M. A. and W. C. Dement (2000). Normal human sleep, In: *Principles and Practice of Sleep Medicine,* Kryger, M. H., Roth, T., Dementi, W. C., (editors), pp.15-16, W.B.Saunders,978-1416066453, Philadelphia.

Chen, W.C., Lim, P.S., Wu, W.C., Chiu, H.C., Chen, C.H., Kuo, H.Y., Tsai, T.W., Chien, P.I., Su, Y.J., Su, Y.L., Hung, S.H., & Woods, H.F. (2006). Sleep behavior disorders in a large cohort of chinese (Taiwanese) patients maintained by long-term hemodialysis. *Am J Kidney Dis.,* Vol.33 2, No. 48, pp. 277-284.

Chesson, A. J., Hartse, K., & Anderson, W.M. (2006). Practice parameters for evaluation of chronic insomnia. An American Academy of sleep medicine report. *Sleep,* Vol. 29, No. 11, pp. 1415-1419.

Chiu K-L, Ryan CM, Shiota S, Ruttanaumpawan P, Arzt M, Haight JS, Chan CT, Floras JS & Bradley TD (2006). Fluid shift by lower body positive pressure increases pharyngeal resistance in healthysubjects. *Am J Resp Crit Care Med,* Vol. 174, pp.1378–1383.

Covic, A., Gusbeth-Tatomir, P., & Goldsmith, D.J. (2006). The epidemics of cardiovascular disease in elderly patients with chronic kidney disease—two facets of the same problem. *Int Urol Nephrol,* Vol. 38, pp. 371–379.

D'Ambrosio, C., Bowman, T., & Mohsenin, V. (1999). Quality of life in patients with obstructive sleep apnea: effect of nasal continuous positive airway pressure - a prospective study. *Chest,* Vol. 115, pp. 123–129.

De Santo, R.M., Lucidi , F., Violani C, & Bertini, M. (2001). Insomnia is associated with systolic hypertension in uremic patients on hemodialysis. *Int J Artif Organs*, Vol. 24, pp. 853–862

De Santo, R.M., Lucidi, F., Violani, C., & Di Iorio, B.R. (2005). Sleep disorders in hemodialyzed patients—the role of comorbidities. *Int J Artif Organs*, Vol. 28, pp. 557–565.

Easom, A. (2006). The challenges of using serum ferritin to guide I.V. iron treatment practices in patients on hemodialysis with anemia. *Nephrol Nurs J*, Vol. 33, pp. 543-551.

Edinger, J.D., & Sampson, W.S. (2003). A primary care "friendly" cognitive behavioral insomnia therapy. *Sleep*, Vol. 26, pp. 177–182.

Edinger, J.D., Wohlgemuth, W.K., Radtke, R.A., Marsh, G.R., & Quillian, R.E. (2001). Cognitive behavioral therapy for treatment of chronic primary insomnia: a randomized controlled trial. *JAMA*, Vol. 285, pp. 1856–1864.

Espie, C.A., Lindsay, W.R., Brooks, D.N., Hood, E.M., & Turvey, T.A. (1989). Controlled comparative investigation of psychological treatments for chronic sleep-onset insomnia. *Behav Res Ther*, Vol. 27, pp. 79-88.

Faccenda, J.F., Mackay, T.W., Boon, N.A., & Douglas, N.J. (2001). Randomized placebo-controlled trial of continuous positive airway pressure on blood pressure in the sleep apnea–hypopnea syndrome. *Am J Respir Crit Care Med*, Vol. 163, pp. 344–348.

Fletcher, E.C. (1993). Obstructive sleep apnea and the kidney. *Journal of the American Society of Nephrology*, Vol. 4, No. 5, pp. 1111-1121.

Gigli, G.L., Adorati, M., Dolso, P., Piani, A., Brotini, S., & Budai, R. (2004). Restless legs syndrome in end-stage renal disease. *Sleep Med*, Vol. 5, pp. 309–315.

Gul, A., Aoun, N., & Trayner, E.M. (2006). Why do patients sleep on dialysis? *Semin Dial*, Vol. 19, No. 2, pp. 52-157.

Han, S.Y., Yoon, J.W., Jo, S.K., Shin, J.H., Shin, C., Lee, J.B., Cha, D.R., Cho, W.Y., Pyo, H.J.,Kim, H.K., Lee, K.B., Kim, H., Kim,. K.W., Kim, Y.S., Lee, J.H., Park, S.E., Kim, C.S., Wea, K.S., Oh, K.S.,Chung, T.S., & Suh, S.Y. (2002). Insomnia in diabetic hemodialysis patients. Prevalence and risk factors by a multicenter study. *Nephron*, Vol. 92, No. 1, pp. 127- 32.

Hanly, P.J., & Pierratos, A. (2001). Improvement of sleep apnea in patients with chronic renal failure who undergo nocturnal hemodialysis. *N Engl J Med*, Vol. 344, pp. 102–107.

Hanly, P.J., Gabor, J.Y., Chan, C., & Pierratos, A. (2003). Daytime sleepiness in patients with CRF: impact of nocturnal hemodialysis. *Am J Kidney Dis*, Vol. 41, pp. 403-410.

Hauri, P. J. (2000). The many faces of insomnia. In D. I. Mostofsky & D. H. Barlow (Eds.), The management of stress and anxiety in medical disorders (pp. 143-159). Needham Heights, MA: Allyn & Bacon.

Holley, J.L., Nespor, S., & Rault, R. (1992). A comparison of reported sleep disorders in patients on chronic dialysis and continuous peritoneal dialysis. *American Journal of Kidney Disease*, Vol. 14, No. 2, pp. 156–161.

Hoyt, B.D. (2005). Sleep in patients with neurologic and psychiatric disorders. *Prim Care*. Vol. 32, pp. 535–548.

Iliescu, E.A., Yeates, K.E., & Holland, D.C. (2004). Quality of sleep in patients with chronic kidney disease. *Nephrol Dial Transplant*, Vol. 19, pp. 95–99.

Iliescu, E.A., Coo, H., McMurray, M.H., Meers, C.L., Quinn, M.M., Singer, M.A., & Hopman, W.H.l. (2003). Quality of sleep and health-related quality of life in haemodialysis patients. *Nephrol Dial Transplant*, Vol. 18, No. 1, pp. 126–132.

International Restless Legs Syndrome Study Group (IRLSSG) (2003). Validation of the international restless legs syndrome study group rating scale for restless legs syndrome. *Sleep Med*, Vol. 4, pp. 121–132.

Jones, B.E., (1989). Basic mechanisms of sleep-wake states, In: *Principles and Practice of Sleep Medicine*, Kryger, M. H., Roth, T., Dementi, W. C., (editors), pp.121-140, W.B. Saunders , 978-1416066453, Philadelphia.

Kamel, N.S., & Gammack, J.K. (2006). Insomnia in the elderly: cause, approach, and treatment. *Am J Med*, Vol. 119, No. 6, pp. 463–469.

Katz, D.A., & McHorney, C.A. (1998). Clinical correlates of insomnia in patients with chronic illness. *Arch Intern Med*, Vol. 158, pp. 1099–1107.

Kavanagh, D., & Siddiqui, S. (2004). Restless legs syndrome in patients on dialysis. *Amer J Kidney Dis*, Vol. 43, No. 5, May, pp.763–771.

Kimmel, P.L. (1989). Sleep disorders in chronic renal disease. *Journal of Nephrology*, Vol. 1, pp. 59-65.

Konofal, E., Arnulf, I., Lecendreux, M., & Mouren, M.C. (2005). Ropinirole in a child with attention-deficit hyperactivity disorder and restless legs syndrome. *Pediatr Neurol*, Vol. 32, pp. 350-351.

Kraus, M.A., & Hamburger, R.J. (1997). Sleep apnea in renal failure. *Adv Perit Dial* Vol. 13, pp. 88–92.

Krystal, A.D.& Edinger, J.D. (2008). Measuring sleep quality. *Sleep Medicine*, Vol. 9, Suppl. 1, pp: 10–17.

Lacks, P, Morin, CM. (1993). Recent advances in the assessment and treatment of insomnia. *J Consult Clin Psychol*. Vol.60, pp.586.

Lacks, P., Bertelson, A.D., Sugerman, J., & Kunkel, J. (1996). The treatment of sleep maintenance insomnia with stimulus-control techniques. *Behav Res Ther*, Vol. 21, pp. 291-295.

Landis, C.A., Lentz, M.J., Tsuji, J., Buchwald, D., & Shaver J.L. (2004). Pain, psychological variables, sleep quality, and natural killer cell activity in midlife women with and without fibromyalgia, *Brain, Behavior, and Immunity*, Vol. 13, pp. 304–313.

Leger, D., Guilleminault, C., Dreyfus, J.P., Delahaye, C., & Paillard, M. (2000). Prevalence of insomnia in a survey of 12,778 adults in France. *J Sleep Res*, Vol. 9, pp. 35–42.

Liao, W.C., Ming-Jang Chiu, M.J., & Landis,C.A., (2008). A Warm Footbath before Bedtime and Sleep in Older Taiwanese with Sleep Disturbance. *Res Nurs Health*. Vol. 31, No. 5, pp. 514–528.

Lichstein, K. L. & Reidel, B. W. (1994). Behavioral assessment and treatment of insomnia: a review with anemphasis on clinical application. *Behavior Therapy*, Vol. 25, pp. 659–688.

Mahowald, M.W. and Schenk, C.H.(1989). "REM sleep behavior disorder" In: *Principles and Practice of Sleep Medicine*, Kryger, M. H., Roth, T., Dementi, W. C., (editors), pp.389-401, W.B. Saunders , 978-1416066453, Philadelphia.

Markou, N., Kanakaki, M., Myrianthefs, M., Hadjiyanakos, D., Vlassopoulos, D., Damianos, A., Siamopoulos, K., Vasiliou, M., & Konstantopoulos, S. (2006). Sleep-disordered breathing in nondialyzed patients with chronic renal failure. *Lung,* Vol. 184, pp. 43–49.

Martin, J. (2000). Assessment and treatment of sleep disturbances in older adults *Clinical Psychology Review,* Vol. 20, No. 6, pp. 783–805.

Merlino, G., Piani, A., Dolso, P.1, Adorati, M., Cancelli, I., Valentel, M., & Gigli, G.L. (2006). Sleep disorders in patients with end-stage renal disease undergoing dialysis therapy. *Nephrol Dial Transplant,* Vol. 21, pp. 184–190.

Meyer, T.J (1998). Evaluation and management of insomnia. *Hosp Pract (Minneap),* Vol. 33, No. 12, pp. 75-8, 83-6.

Millman, R.P., Kimmel, P.L., Shore, E.T., & Wasserstein, A.G. (1985). Sleep apnea in hemodialysis patients: the lack of testosterone effect on its pathogenesis. *Nephron,* Vol. 40, pp.407–410.

Miranda, M., Kagi, M., Fabres, L., Aguilers, L., Alvo, M., Elgueta, L., Erazo, S., & Venegas, P. (2004). Pramipexole for the treatment of uremic restless legs in patients undergoing hemodialysis. *Neurology,* Vol. 62, pp. 831–832.

Mollaoğlu, M. (2004). Depression and Health Related Quality of Life in Hemodialysis Patients. *Dialysis Transplant,* Vol 33, pp. 544-555

Mollaoğlu, M., & Mollaoğlu, M. (2009). Sleep Quality in Hemodialysis Patients. *Neurology Psychiatry &Brain Research,* Vol.15, pp.179-184.

Montgomery, P., & Dennis, J. (2004). A systematic review of non-pharmacological therapies for sleep problems in later life. *Sleep Med Rev,* Vol. 8, pp. 47–62.

Morgan, K., Dixon, S., Mathers, N., Thompson, J., & Tomeny, M (2003). Psychological treatment for insomnia in the management of long-term hypnotic drug use: a pragmatic randomised controlled trial. *Br J Gen Pract,* Vol. 53, pp. 923–928.

Morin, C.M., Colecchi, C., Stone, J., Sood, R., & Brink, D. (1999). Behavioral and pharmacological therapies for late-life insomnia: a randomized controlled trial. *JAMA,* Vol. 281, pp. 991–999.

Mucsi, I., Molnar, M.Z., Ambrus, C., Szeifert, L., Kovacs, A.Z., Zoller, R., Barotfi, S., Remport, A., & Novak, M. (2005). Restless legs syndrome, insomnia and quality of life in patients on maintenance dialysis. *Nephrol Dial Transplant,* Vol. 20, pp. 571–577

Mucsi, I., Molnar, M.Z., Rethelyi, J., Vamos, E., Csepanyi, C., Tompa, C., Barotfi, S., Marton, A., & Novak, M. (2004). Sleep disorders and illness intrusiveness in patients on chronic dialysis. *Nephrol Dial Transplant,* Vol. 19, pp. 1815–1822.

Nichols, D.A., Allen, R..P, Grauke, J.H., Brown,. J.B., Rice, M.L., Hyde, P.R., Dement, W.C., Kushida, C.A. (2003). Restless legs syndrome symptoms in primary care: a prevalence study. *Arch Intern Med,* Vol. 163, pp. 2323–2329.

Novak, M., Shapiro, C.M., Mendelssohn, D., & Mucsi, I. (2006). Diagnosis and management of insomnia in dialysis patients. Semin. Dial., Vol.19, pp.25–31.

Ohayon, M.M. (2002). Epidemiology of insomnia: what we know and what we still need to learn. *Sleep Med Rev* Vol. 6, No. 2. pp. 97-111.

Parker, K.P. (1997). Sleep and dialysis: A research-based review of the literature. *ANNA Journal,* Vol. 24, No. 6, pp. 626-641.

Parker, K.P., Bliwise, D.L., Bailey, J.L., & Rye, D.B. (2005). Polysomnographic measures of nocturnal sleep in patients on chronic, intermittent daytime haemodialysis vs those with chronic kidney disease. *Nephrol Dial Transplant,* Vol. 20, pp.1422–1428.

Parker, K.P., Kutner, N.G., Bliwise, D.L., Bailey, J.L., & Rye, D.B. (2003). Nocturnal sleep, daytime sleepiness, and quality of life in stable patients on hemodialysis. *Health Qual Life Outcomes,* Vol. 1, pp. 68.

Patrick, L. (2007). Restless Legs Syndrome: Pathophysiology and the Role of Iron and Folate. *Alternative Medicine Review,* Vol. 12, No. 2, pp. 101-112.

Pellecchia, M.T., Vitale, C., Sabatini, M., Longo, K., Amboni, M., Bonavita, V., & Barone, P. (2004). Ropinirole as a treatment of restless legs syndrome in patients on chronic hemodialysis: an open randomized crossover trial versus levodopa sustained release. *Clin Neuropharmacol,* Vol. 27, pp. 178–181.

Pieta, J., Millar, T., Zacharias, J., Fine, A., Kryger, M. (1998). Effect of pergolide on restless legs and leg movements in sleep in uremic patients. *Sleep,* Vol. 21, pp. 617–622.

Pigeon, W.R., & Yurcheshen, M. (2009). Behavioral Sleep Medicine Interventions for Restless Legs Syndrome and Periodic Limb Movement Disorder. *Sleep Med Clin,* Vol. 1, No. 4, December, pp. 487–494.

Pressman, M.R. Benz,.R.L., & Peterson, D.D. (1995). Periodic leg movements in sleep index(PLMSI) predicts mortality in end stage renal disease patients. *Sleep Research,* Vol. 24, pp. 416.

Rahman, M., Fu,P., Sehgal,A., & Smith, M.(2000). Interdialytic weight gain, compliance with dialysis regimen, and age are independent predictors of blood pressure in hemodialysis patients. *American Journal of Kidney Diseases,* Vol. 35, pp. 257-265

Redline, S., Kirchner, H.L., Quan, S.F., Gottlieb, D.J., Kapur, V., & Newman, A. (2004). The effects of age, sex, ethnicity, and sleep-disordered breathing on sleep architecture. *Arch Intern Med,* Vol. 164, pp. 406–418.

Riedel, B. W., Lichstein, K. L. & Dwyer, W. O. (1995). Sleep compression and sleep education for older insomniacs: Self-help versus therapist guidance. *Psychology and Aging,* Vol. 10, pp. 54–63.

Rodrigues, C.J.O., Marson, O., Tufic, S., Kohlmann, O., Guimar, S.M., Togeiro, P., Ribeiro, A.B., & Tavares, A. (2005). Relationship among end-stage renal disease, hypertension, and sleep apnea in nondiabetic dialysis patients. *Am J Hypertens,* Vol. 18, pp. 152–157.

Rosenthal, M.S. (1998). Physiology and Neurochemistry of Sleep. *American Journal of Pharmaceutical Education,* Vol. 62, pp. 204-208.

Sabbatini, M., Crispo, A., Pisani, A., Cesaro, A., Mirenghi, F., Cianciaruso, B., & Federico, S. (2003). Zaleplon improves sleep quality in maintenance hemodialysis patients. *Nephron Clin Pract,* Vol. 94, pp. 99–103.

Sabbatini, M., Minale, B., Crispo, A. Pisani, A., Ragosta, A., Esposito, R., Cesaro, A., Cianciaruso, B., & Andreucci, V.E. (2002). Insomnia in maintenance hemodialysis patients. *Nephrol Dial Transplant,* Vol. 17, pp. 852–856.

Sabry, A.A., Abo-Zenah, H., Wafa, E., Mahmoud, K., El-Dahshan, K., Hassan, A., Abbas, T.M., Saleh, A.M., & Okasha, K.. (2010). Sleep disorders in hemodialysis patients. *Saudi J Kidney Dis Transpl,* Vol. 21, pp. 300-305.

Sandyk, R., Bernick, C., Lee, S.M., Stern, L.Z., Lacono, R.P., & Bamford, C.R. (1987). L-dopa in uremic patients with the restless legs syndrome. *Int J Neurosci,* Vol. 35, pp. 233–235.

Siddiqui, S., & Kavanagh, D. (2005). Risk factors for restless legs syndrome in dialysis patients. *Nephro Clin Pract,* Vol. 101, pp. 155–60.

Sloand, J.A., Shelly, M.A., Feigin, A., Bernstein, P., & Monk, R.D. (2004). A double blind,placebo-controlled trial of intravenous iron dextran therapy in patients with ESRD and restless legs syndrome. *Am J Kidney Dis,* Vol. 43, pp. 663-670.

Smith, M.T., Perlis, M.L. Park, A., Smith, M.S., Pennington, J., Giles, D.E., & Buysse , D.J. (2002). Comparative meta-analysis of pharmacotherapy and behavior therapy for persistent insomnia. *Am J Psychiatry,* Vol. 159, pp. 5–11.

Smith, P.L., Gold, A.R., Meyers, D.A., Haponik, E.F., & Bleecker, E.R. (1985). Weight loss in mildly to moderately obese patients with obstructive sleep apnea. *Ann Intern Med,* Vol. 103, pp. 850-855.

Spielman, A.J., Saskin, P., & Thorpy, M.J. (1987). Treatment of chronic insomnia by restriction of time in bed. *Sleep,* Vol. 10, pp. 45-56.

Takaki, J., Nishi, T., Nangaku, M., Shimoyama, H., Inada, T., Matsuyama, N., Kumano, H., & Kuboki, T. (2003). Clinical and psychological aspects of restless legs syndrome in uremic patients on hemodialysis. *Am J Kidney Dis,* Vol. 41, pp. 833–839.

Tatomir, P., Seic, D.B. A., Buga, C., & Covic, A. (2007). Sleep disorders: a systematic review of an emerging major clinical issue in renal patients. *Int Urol Nephrol,* Vol.. 39, pp. 1217–1226

Terzano, M.G., Parrino, L., Cirignotta, F., Ferini-Strambi, L., Gigli, G., Rudelli, G., Sommacal, S., Studio Morfeo Committee (2004. Studio Morfeo: insomnia in primary care, a survey conducted on the Italian population. *Sleep Med,* Vol. 5, No. 1, pp. 67-75.

Thase, M.E. (2005). Correlates and consequences of chronic insomnia. *Gen Hosp Psychiatry,* Vol. 27, pp. 100–112.

Trenkwalder, C., Stiasny, K., Pollmacher, T., Wetter, T., Schwarz, J., Kohnen, R., & Kazenwadel, J. (1995). L-dopa therapy of uremic and idiopathic restless legs syndrome: a double-blind, crossover trial. *Sleep,* Vol. 18, pp. 681–688.

Unruh, M.L, Levey, A.S., D'Ambrosio, C. Fink, N.E., Powe, N., & Myer, B.K. (2004). Restless legs symptoms among incident dialysis patients: Association with Lower Quality of Liver and Shorter Survival (CHOICE). *Amer J Kidney Dis,* Vol. 43, No. 5, May, pp. 900–909.

Unruh, M.L., Sanders, M.H., Redline, S., Piraino, B.M., Umans, J.G., Hammond, T.C., Sharief, I., Punjabi, M., & Newman, B. (2006). Sleep apnea in patients on conventional thrice-weekly hemodialysis: comparison with matched controls from the sleep heart health study. *J Am Soc Nephrol,* Vol. 17, pp. 3503–3509

Veiga, J., Gonçalves, N., Gomes, F., Santos, N., Baptista, A., Paiva, T. (1997).Sleep disturbances in end-stage renal disease patients on hemodialysis. *Dial Transplant,* No.26, pp.380-384

Walker, S., Fine, A., & Kryger, M.H., (1995). Sleep complaints are common in a dialysis unit. *American Journal of Kidney Disease,* Vol. 5, No. 26, pp. 751–756.

Walker, S.L., Fine, A., & Kryger, M.H. (1996). L-DOPA/carbidopa for nocturnal movement disorders in uremia. *Sleep,* Vol. 19, pp. 214–218.

Wei, C.Y., Chung, T.C., Wu, S.C., Chung, C.F., & Wu, W.F. (2011). The Subjective sleep quality and heart rate variability in hemodialysis patients. *Ren Fail.* Vol. 5, No. 26, pp. 109-117.

Welch, J.L. & Austin, J.K. (2001). Stressors, coping and depression in haemodialysis patients. *Journal of Advanced Nursing,* Vol. 33, No. 2, pp. 200-207.

Williams, S.W., Tell, G.S., Zheng, B., Shumaker, S., Rocco, M.V., & Sevick, M.A. (2002). Correlates of sleep behavior among hemodialysis patients. *Am J Nephrol*, Vol. 22, pp. 18–28.

Winkelman, J.W., Chertow, G.M., & Lazarus, J.M. (1996). Restless legs syndrome in end-stage renal disease. *American Journal of Kidney Diseases,* Vol. 28, No. 3, pp. 372-378.

Yoshioka, M., Ishii ,T., & Fukunishi, I. (1993). Sleep disturbance of end-stage renal disease. *Jpn J Psychiatry Neurol.*, Vol. 47, pp.847-851.

Young , T., Palta, M., Dempsey, J., Skatrud, J., Weber, S., & Badr, S. (1993). The occurrence of sleep-disordered breathing among middle-aged adults. *N Engl J Med* Vol. 328, pp. 1230–1235.

Zoccali, C., Mallamaci, F., & Tripepi, G. (2001). Sleep Apnea in Renal Patients. *J Am Soc Nephrol*, Vol. 12, pp. 2854–2859.

23

The Importance of Exercise Programs in Haemodialysis Patients

Susanne Heiwe[1], Andrej Ekholm[2] and Ingela Fehrman-Ekholm[3,4]
[1]*Dept of Physiotherapy, Karolinska Institutet, Dept of Medicine & Dept of Clinical Sciences,*
[2]*Karolinska Institutet*
[3]*Dept of Renal Medicine, Karolinska University Hospital,*
[4]*Stockholm and Transplantation Centre, Sahlgrenska Academy, Göteborg,*
Sweden

1. Introduction

The lifestyle today is new. We sit with our computers, televisions etc. Usually, we do not carry heavy things. We gain weight and loose muscle strength. Through history the life has included moments with physical efforts. The body has not changed. It still needs physical training and efforts. The person who is untrained gets quickly tired. Therefore it is important to make the efforts regularly. The capacity of the heart to transport oxygen increases and the energy increases with physical training. The muscle condition is important. The mitochondria in the muscles cells may increase with 30-40 % after one month of exercise. With more mitochondria more fat is consumed and less carbohydrate is needed. Consequently, less lactic acid is formed and the blood does not change the pH towards acidosis as easily.

Thus, modern people need exercise. You need not to go to a gym or run every day. It is more about having an active life. Take the cycle or walk to the job or to the shop, take the stairs instead of escalator or elevator. The exercise is a part of the natural common life and the body is a tool which needs to be used. It could be enough with 30 minutes of activity to reach physical efforts the heart rate has to increase, maybe to 120 beats/minute. This could be a dilemma for many patients since they have decreased maximal capacity and interacting medication. The training program has to be individualized but the goal is to improve the capacity. If success the daily normal activities feel easier and the patients get more improved trust and comfort. Physical activities mean also better control and less fear of having fall accidents. With a feeling of control there are fewer obstacles.

Thus exercise and effort are important to all of us which are true for many people with different diseases. For patients with cardiac diseases, hypertension, diabetes mellitus there are often exercise programs but for patients with different stages of chronic kidney disease, CKD, there is no obvious exercise treatment program. However, more and more evidence exists that exercises are important for these patients. The dialysis treatment hours have increased more and more to increase KT/V, the dialysis dose, but this also means less time for activities like exercise, work, family life and spear time. How could we help these patients?

Hence, this chapter is chosen with the intention to provide the reader with information concerning exercise capacity and level of physical activity in adults with chronic kidney disease. It also has the aim to make health-care providers within renal medicine aware of exercise training as an evidence-based intervention to improve health and well-being in adults with CKD. Despite the fact that exercise training is easy, cost effective and preventive, exercise training has not been implemented into clinical practice. We hope that this chapter will stimulate to action and provide some knowledge about these patients and their problems in order to understand why exercise training should be included in the standard care for adults with CKD. The chapter also contains general information about exercise and expected effects in healthy individuals.

2. What is a training program for grown-up people?

It is important to consider the training models, methodology, and expected changes that happen at regular physical activity in general. We consider different measures to describe the activities.

- *Frequency* - That means how often we do the training. A daily dosage of effort like taking walks, taking stair-cases is basic.
- *Intensity* - This is how the levels of efforts are. A common used definition is RM that is repetition maximum. One RM is the weight or load you are able to lift once but not twice. It has been shown that 60-70% of 1 RM could be enough for the starter to give an increase of muscle strength. For the well-trained it is necessary with almost 70-84% for the increase of muscle mass and strength (Kramer et al 1997).
- *Duration* - It is the length of the exercise period at a time. A 30 minute period of physical exercise is nowadays a common, recommended duration. A simple and common instrument is the pedometer, which could quantify the number of steps and calculate the calories, the walking distance one could obtain during a period.

Concerning intensity this could be varied by adding different muscle groups. The level of effort and the muscle groups involved are important for the results. If you add walking with sticks, the shoulder and arm muscles become involved and increase the results. In these moments also the important coordination becomes involved.
The general effects of training are many. Below are some aspects and findings.

Muscles

Skeletal muscle is not a simple homogenous group of fibers. Type I fibers are characterized by slow speed of contraction, low activity of myosin ATPase and are well suited for prolonged aerobic exercise. Type II fibers have the ability to generate energy for quick and forceful contractions. At training there is an increase in both muscle fibre size and muscle number, the largest effect being increase of muscle size. The number of mitochondria and the small vessels in the muscles increase. Interestingly, even very old people could increase the strength. In an interesting study it was shown that 90-year old persons living at a nursing home could double the muscle strength, increase the quadriceps muscular volume with 10 % as well as increase the daily function after 8 weeks of bodybuilding (Fiatarone et al 1990).

Cardiosvascular system

The cardiac output will increase. The normal pulse will be reduced. The small arteries will dilate which contribute to decreasing blood pressure. The blood circulation to the heart and muscles will increase and both the blood volume and the haemoglobin level will increase.

Many patients with CKD have hypertension. In dialysis the hypertension is most linked to salt and water over load. After kidney transplantation the immunosuppressive drugs CNI (calcineurin inhibitors such as tacrolimus and ciclosporin) and corticosteroids contribute to hypertension. In transplants patients with CAN (chronic allograft nephropathy) ischemia in the kidneys aggravate the situation and give severe hypertension with often therapy resistant blood pressure.

The basis of treatment in hypertension is life style changes, exercise, stop smoking habits and decrease of the sodium chloride in the diet. These are basic advice applicable also to the CKD patients. Many patients have treatment with diuretics to decrease salt and water. Beta-blockers protect the heart from stress and lower the pulse rate, sometimes hamper maximal training efforts. Calcium blockers are frequently used, cause relaxation of the muscles and vasodilatation.

ACE-inhibitors block the angiotensin system and are often well tolerated. It could however be important to be aware of the fact that severe dehydration could be dangerous due to risk of high serum potassium and loss of blood pressure which is a severe condition. This information is important to give to the patient in case of any situation with loss of water like gastrointestinal acute diseases.

Regular physical activity lowers the blood pressure but the blood pressure increases during exercise, mostly the systolic blood pressure. With a stress ECG the individual patient could get information about the level of blood pressure and ECG changes during efforts. There are recommended levels not to exceed.

Nerve system

Regular physical activity affects the nerves. The coordination, the balance and the ability to react becomes better. Most of the persons who do regular exercise have better sleep, less depressions and more self-esteem.

Hormone system

The exercise increases the insulin sensitivity in the skeletal muscle and decreases the insulin in the blood. This means less adiposities and a more healthy profile of the lipids with increased HDL-cholesterol and decreased triglycerides. For body builders the growth hormone may increase. Also testosterone levels have been found to increase and androgen receptors which increase the effect of testosterone (Kraemer et al 2005). Added testosterone has a much stronger effect, both increasing the muscle mass and adding new cells. However, this substance is classified as doping preparation. Cortisol is a catabolic substance and could be increased at stress caused by some exercises and exercisers. However, cortisol is a life-necessary substance. Catecholamine (noradrenalin and adrenalin) are also produced in the moments of stress, fight and flight response. There is probably an anabolic effect on the skeletal muscles which has been shown in certain animal studies. That is why these preparations are on the doping list. Insulin-like growth factor (IGF-1) could also be produced locally in the muscle but the systemic effect is unclear.

3. Physical fitness and physical functioning and self-evaluation in patients with CKD

The physical fitness and physical functioning (= the ability and capacity to perform activities of daily living) is severely reduced in adults with CKD (Kettner-Melsheimer et al 1987;

Kouidi et al 1998; Heiwe et al 2003; Johansen et al 2003; Heiwe et al 2005). It is declining from 70% of the expected norm in a pre-uremic phase to 50% of the expected norm when starting dialysis therapy (Painter et al 1986; Kettner-Melsheimer et al 1987; Brodin et al 2001). However, also ageing decreases muscle mass. The median age at dialysis start in Sweden is 66 years. The muscle mass in 70-year old person is 25% lower compared with 25-year old persons (Klitgaard et al 1990).

Patients with a renal transplant have a lower physical fitness of approximately 70-80% of the age-matched controls (Painter et al 1986). Here, the corticosteroids, still a basic immunosuppressive treatment, contribute to muscular atrophy. Thus, the physical fitness in adults with CKD is reduced and affects the capacity of the patients to perform activities in everyday life and occupational tasks.

Physical functioning in patients with CKD is affected by several factors like consequences of CKD in it-self, the original disease process that brought about the patient's kidney disease and the treatment of CKD which may have further detrimental effects (Marlowe et al 2001). The main factors causing reduced physical fitness are anaemia (Clyne et al 1987; McMahon et al 1999) and muscular weakness (Bohannon et al 1994; Johansen et al 2003). This results in fatigue and increasing inactivity, which in turn reduces physical fitness even further and increases impairments in physical functioning (Bohannon et al 1994; Nielens et al 2001; Johansen et al 2003).

Today, anaemia is successfully corrected by erythropoietin treatment and results in an improved, but not normalised, physical fitness (McMahon et al 1999). When analysing muscle biopsies it has been shown that adults with CKD have muscular histopathological abnormalities already in the pre-uremic phase (Heiwe et al 2005). The causes of muscular weakness in patients with CKD have, however, not been fully elucidated. Muscle atrophy, a neuropathic process and myopathy are potential causes of the muscular weakness. It is suggested that myopathy is due to abnormal energy metabolism (Thompson et al 1993), secondary hyperparathyreoidism (Ritz et al 1980), malnutrition (Guarnieri et al 1983), prolonged physical inactivity (Jones et al 1990) and to uraemia itself (Sakkas et al 2003).

It is important that the consultant renal physiotherapist, renal nurse, renal dietician and renal physician have an understanding of limitations in physical fitness and physical functioning that adults with CKD are expected to face and how various unique issues may alter the treatment approach. All training methods have to start with cautions and feed-back to the patients.

It has been shown that adults with CKD experience limitations in their daily life due to insufficient physical fitness. In a previous study (Heiwe et al 2003) it was shown that adult with CKD experience fatigue both mental and physical fatigue. This results in a reduced physical fitness and reduced physical functioning in terms of impact on performance and endurance. The experienced fatigue appeared frequently and varied in strength.

The informants described having a more or less always-present mental fatigue, which was experienced as something that they really had to fight to overcome. Feeling listless and paralysed by fatigue was a common trait of this group of descriptions. The feeling of physical fatigue appeared as soon as they started performing a physical activity and could vary in extent from day to day. They experienced muscular weakness and rapid onset of tiredness. Pagels et al (2006) have shown that when asked to rate the level of physical activity 40% of the adults being in a pre-uremic phase had a low activity and 11% were mostly sitting or lying down. Thus, the daily basic walks became an effort.

Many adults with CKD experience difficulties in walking if the ground is not level, as in the case of stairs or steps, uphill slopes, etc. In such conditions, they experience physical resistance very quickly. Many elderly with CKD also have difficulties in performing everyday chores, such as managing their personal hygiene, making their bed, hanging up laundry, vacuum-cleaning, lifting things, rising from a squatting position, cleaning, etc. They also experience difficulty in performing a physical activity over a prolonged period of time, for instance, hanging up laundry, without having to pause several times, which they have not had to do prior to the disease. Most of the patients also have difficulties in performing physical activities at the same pace as they did prior to the CKD.

Adults with CKD may also experience temporal stress since they cannot do as much as they would have liked to. They need more time to perform various activities, partly due to "internal demands", like the need for physical rest and partly due to their experiences of external demands as a result of all the medical appointments and other appointments. All these factors may have a negative impact on the patients' level of activity and participation as well as their social life (Heiwe et al 2003). It seems urgent to do something for these patients.

Rehabilitation has a positive effect on physical fatigue and improves both 'endurance' and physical 'performance', which, in turn, could reduce the need for more time to be able to perform everyday chores or other physical activities. It would then be possible for the patients to find more time for their own activities, increasing their physical activity level. It is important to make clear to patients that just by putting time and effort into physical exercise or activity they can improve several aspects of their experience of fatigue, reduced physical fitness and temporal stress. It is, though, important that appointments for physical exercise training are co-ordinated, as far as possible, with the patients' other medical appointments. This would give the patients more time to perform their own physical activities.

It is also important that physiotherapists consider patients' views when reflecting upon and interpreting how they can support and strengthen patients in their effort to be able to perform physical activities as well as social activities that are of importance to them.

Adults with CKD are subjected to multiple physiological and psychological stressors. Welch et al (1999) have for instance showed that the most common treatment-related stressors in patients with haemodialysis are fluid limitations, the length of dialysis and vacation limitations. When adults with CKD rank the stressors that they are subjected to, it is limitation of physical activity which is the number one stressor (Lok et al 1996). Therefore, it is important to include questions concerning physical activity when meeting these patients.

Coping has been proposed as an important mediating factor with regard to adaptation to illness. Coping refers to 'an individual's efforts to master demands that are appraised (or perceived) as exceeding or taxing his or her resources. It is a process that may consist of behaviours and intra-psychic responses designed to overcome, reduce or tolerate these demands (Lazarus et al 1984). There are many ways in which coping responses can be grouped, but the two general categories of coping strategies are problem-solving efforts and strategies aimed at the regulation of emotions (Lazarus et al 1984). Problem-focused coping refers to efforts to improve the troubled person-environment relationship by changing things, for instance by seeking information about what to do. Emotional-focused (or palliative) coping refers to thoughts or actions whose goal is to relieve the emotional impact of stress (for example, bodily or psychological disturbances). Although both sets of strategies are brought to bear on most stressful events, problem-solving efforts are especially useful for managing controllable stressors, and emotional-regulation efforts are well suited to managing the impact of uncontrollable stressors.

It has been shown that in order to cope with the limited physical fitness three coping activities are used: 1) avoiding physical activities, 2) adjusting pace and 3) scheduling. The strategies were problem-focused, and patients used active-, avoidant- and social-support coping strategies. When coping with limited physical fitness, adults with CKD tend to use coping strategies that have a positive short-term outcome. These strategies are, however, also associated with negative long-term outcomes. The individual is placed in an evil circle where the physical functioning decreases as the experience of mental and physical fatigue increases (Heiwe et al 2004). It is therefore important that renal physicians and renal nurses identify these patients and refer them to a renal physiotherapist at an early stage, so that they can get information and help with physical exercise training. This could contribute to the patients' own resources which can then be used to improve the level of participation and also to improve some parts of the patient's social life.

All people employ different combinations of problem-focused and emotion-focused methods to cope with stress. The conditions determining our coping methods in specific situations are complex and at present largely unknown, but they are likely to depend on the conditions being faced, the options available to us and our personality. An issue often emerging in discussions about coping is whether some coping processes are more effective than others. For instance, whether avoidant responses to stressful events are more adaptive or whether more confrontational coping methods are superior. However, coping processes have both positive and negative consequences for an individual. A behaviour that might be effective from, say, the physiological perspective might have devastating consequences for the psychological or sociological domains. Moreover, what is an optimal response in one situation at a particular point in time may be damaging in some other situation or at a different point in time. Most people appear to use a variety of coping strategies to deal with a stressor. Successful coping may depend more on a match of different coping strategies to the features of the stressful event than on the relative efficacy of one coping strategy over another. Therefore, when meeting a patient with CKD and evaluating his or her coping and adaptation, the health-care provider must take into account diverse levels of analysis (physiological, psychological, sociological), short versus long-term consequences and the specific nature of the situation in question.

4. Evidence based effects of exercise training in patients with CKD

There is scientific evidence showing that if adults with CKD do not exercise only having a certain level of physical activity in their daily living:

- The muscle mass and physical fitness will continue to decrease (Painter et al 1986; Kettner-Melsheimer et al 1987; Bohannon et al 1994; Brodin et al 2001; Heiwe et al 2001; Sakkas et al 2003; Heiwe et al 2005; McIntyre et al 2006; Zamojska et al 2006)
- The patient's possibility to maintain, for him or her, a satisfyingly active and social life will be reduced = reduced health-related quality of life (Brodin et al 2001; Fukuhara et al 2003; Heiwe et al 2003; Heiwe et al 2004)

- An already high cardiovascular risk factor and co-morbidity burden (Yao et al 2004; Venkataraman et al 2005) will increase even more due to the severely reduced level of physical activity

Published articles concerning effects of physical exercise on patients with CKD started to appear in the 1980s. Since then, interest in effects of physical exercise has increased in renal medicine, and today there are numerous published articles showing positive effects of exercise training. Data from previously and recently published studies have shown that exercise training in adults with CKD can affect the following factors:

- Muscular hypotrophy, -strength, -endurance & physical functioning (Kouidi et al 1998; Mercer et al 2002; Painter et al 2002; DePaul et al 2002; Sakkas et al 2003; Heiwe et al 2005; McIntyre et al 2006; Heiwe & Jacobson 2011)
- The structure and number of capillaries and mitochondria (Kouidi et al 1998; Sakkas et al 2003, Cheema et al 2010)
- Glucose metabolism (Goldberg et al 1983)
- Aerobic capacity (Painter et al 1986; Painter et al 2002; DePaul et al 2002)
- Blood pressure (Goldberg et al 1983; Pechter et al 2003)
- Cardiac performance (i.e. augmentation of cardiac vagal activity, decrease of vulnerability to arrhythmias) and improvement of coronary risk profiles (Venkataraman et al 2005)
- Depression, performance of pleasant activities in daily living and health-related quality of life (Suh et al 2002; Molsted et al 2004; van Vilsteren et al 2005)
- Circulating cytokines (Cheema BS et al 2010)
- Nutritional parameters and energy expenditure using SWA, SenseWear™ Armband (Cupusti A el al 2011)

A review article, based on 29 trials on this issue, shows that exercise training in dialysis patients improves arterial compliance, cardiac autonomic control and left ventricular systolic function. Moreover, exercise diminishes oxidative stress, blood pressure and inflammation. As shown in Table 1, significant effects of exercise and training were found.

It is interesting to notice that haemoglobin levels, s-albumin, PCR (protein catabolic rate) and KT/V increase. This tells us that less erythropoietin is needed, which means that training is cost-effective. The patients have better protein intake. They probably eat more to get energy. The recommended protein intake at training in general is 1.6-1.7 g/kg. The recommendations for uremic patients in dialysis are a protein intake above 1.3 g/kg body weight.

Also, the decrease in CRP is an interesting finding. CRP is connected to residual renal function (Pecoits-Filho et al 2003). The low inflammatory process in the dialysis patients becomes thus better after 6 months of repeated cycle training and this might be an adequate prescription! Actually, today the physiotherapists give prescriptions on physical activities like the doctors do on medication. The difficulties could be the compliance or adherence of the patient to the physical program suggested but the same problem exists with the prescribed drugs.

Here is a prescription or suggestions to patients with CKD. To obtain improvements it is, however, important that the exercise program has an adequate intensity, frequency and duration. Examples and type of exercises are given (Table 2).

prescription	duration	variable	% change	significance
Cycle ergometer, walking, jogging	8-9 months	HDL cholesterol Hemoglobin Plasma insulin fasting Plasma glucose	+23% +29% -40% -6.3%	< 0.05 < 0.05 <0.01 <0.01
Cycle ergometer 3 times/week	12 weeks	Max workload	Increase	< 0.05
Aerobic strength training 90 min 3 times per week	6 months	VO2 peak Peak blood lactate Isometric strength Type muscle fibre area I Type muscle fibre area II	Increase Decrease Increase Increase	< 0.05 < 0.05 < 0.05 < 0.05
Cycle ergometer 30 min 3 times per week	6 months	Albumin CRP PCR KT/V	Increase Decrease Increase Increase	< 0.024 < 0.046 < 0.001 < 0.026
Treadmill walking or cycle ergometer	3 months	Arterial stiffness Pulse pressure Systolic blood pressure	Decrease Decrease Decrease	0.01 <0.05 <0.05

Table 1. 29 studies and effects of physical activity in dialysis patients on metabolic and nutritional parameters. (Cheema BS, Sing MA 2005).

Activity	Example	Intensity	Duration	Frequency
Muscular Sustained training	Sequential exercise Individual program with weight cuffs as resistance	50 % 1RM	Maximal number of correctly performed repetitions. Corresponding to self-rated total exertion 13-15 according to Borg's RPE-scale	3 times/w
Functional training (including walking-, balance- and coordination-training)	Walking, eg on treadmill or balance carpet. Standing on balance plate Knee bow Stairs Standing up from knee bow		Maximal walking and number of correctly performed repetitions. Corresponding to self-rated total exertion 13-15 according to Borg's RPE-scale	3 times/w
Isometric strength	Sequence training Individual training with weight cuffs or other things as resistance	80% 1RM	1 set á 8-10 reps	3 times/w

Borg´s RPE scale = Borg rating of perceived exertion. It was constructed in the 60-ties by Gunnar Borg, professor in perception and psychophysics in Stockholm. The scale indicates different degrees of effort from 6 to 20. The rated RPE shows a linear relation to workload and heart pulse frequency. It is used within rehabilitation and training (Borg 1970).
VO2 peak: This is the oxygen uptake which reflects the maximal performance of the individual. This has to be measured before start of programme and this helps to adjust the programme for each individual.
Reps = repetitions, **RM** repetition maximum see page 2

Table 2. Prescription on physical activities in patients with CKD and explanations

5. Details and aim of physical training

- Get the patient informed about the importance of physical training in CKD both in dialysis and after kidney transplantation.
- To make the patient independent in the daily life and to keep/increase the quality of life.
- Diminish the risk of cardiovascular disease, osteoporosis and loss of muscle mass. Increase/maintain muscular strength and endurance, balance as well as the sub maximal oxygen uptake.
- Minimize the risk of fall accident.
- Minimize depression.

Dynamic muscular endurance	• Maximal number of muscle contractions with a strain corresponding to 50 % of 1RM and at fixed frequency. • Standing heel-rise test. • Sit-to-stand-to-sit
Static muscular endurance	• Maximal number of seconds the patient is able to maintain an isometric muscle contraction, for example knee extension, with loading corresponding to 50% of 1RM. • Unilateral isotonic shoulder flexion, bilateral isometric shoulder abduction
Functional capacity	• 6-minutes walking test with patient's experienced leg fatigue, breathlessness and possible cardiac pain is rated by the patient according to Borg's CR-10 scale and the total effort according to Borg's RPE-scale before and after the test performed • Walking 30 meters in self-selected normal rate and maximal rate • Timed "Up & Go" • Stand on one leg Functional reach • Stairs
Muscular strength	• One repetition maximum (1RM) • GRIPPIT(grip strength), Jamar hand dynamometer: correlating to muscular mass • Isometric leg strength.
Self-rated physical level of activity	• Disability Rating Index (DRI). Activity rating according to Grimby Frändin
Physical capacity	• Standardized, symptom limited ergometer cycling with patient's experienced leg fatigue, breathlessness and possible cardiac pain is rated by the patient according to Borgs CR-10 scale and the total effort according to Borg's RPE-scale.
Quality of life	• SF-36

Notes: **General about CKD 4-5**

- For patients with secondary kidney diseases it is important to consider the original disease at assessment of physical capacity, general advice and follow-up. For patients with diabetes mellitus for instance it is important to consider the present foot status and the insulin regimen.

- Patients with polycystic kidney disease should avoid contact sports like karate since hard hits against the kidneys may cause bleeding and pain. There is also a higher risk of hernia of the abdominal wall in this disease. Patients with kidney transplants should also avoid contact sports like ice-hockey and land-hockey due to risk of tackling moments.
- Patients with CKD 4 and 5 suffer more easily from tendinitis. Treatment with chinolones means increased risk of tendinitis. Because of this it is important with heating and cool-down to be prolonged. Also the training of mobility and agility should be prolonged and the training intensity and duration increase smoothly.

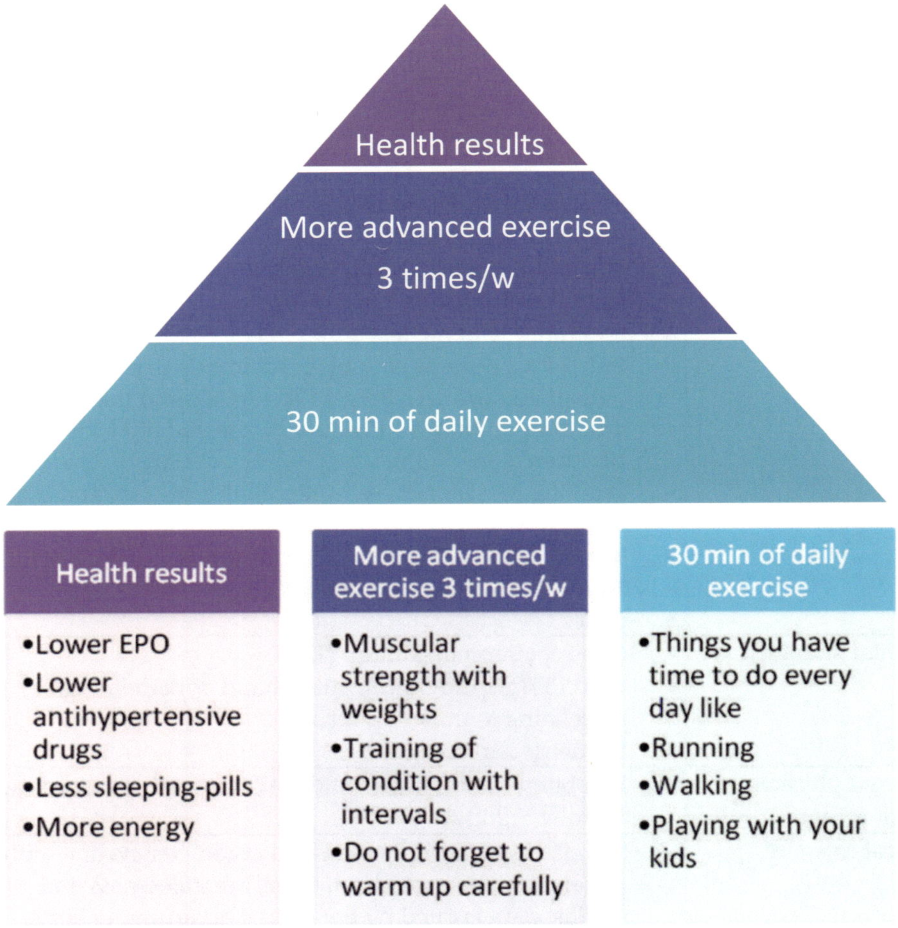

Fig. 1. The amount of training and training effects in CKD patients in a schematic form

Concerning haemodialysis patients:

- When is the physical training to be performed? It is the medical condition of the patient and the desire of the patient which decide the optimal timing for the training. The most optimal training effect is obtained with the physical activity on dialysis free days. If this is a problem for the patient, for instance far distance to travel, confinement to the hospital etc, the training may be performed before the dialysis treatment or during the first two hours in dialysis. It is not recommended to do the exercise after dialysis treatment since the patients are dehydrated and there is great risk of hypotensive episodes. Since the patients often have lack of time, it is important to coordinate the different treatments within the team.

- The amount of fluid, sodium, potassium and blood pressure is constantly variable in a dialysis patient. As a physical therapist it is important to consider these factors in planning the training schedule and in every training opportunity. Consider the restriction of water in individual patients! However, in jogging and running all need water. The simplest method is to instruct the patient to weigh himself/herself before and after the running episodes.
- The signs of exercise-induced hyponatremia should be recognized by everyone handling dialysis patients. These are symptoms of cerebral over hydration: nausea, malaise when sodium is below 125-130 mmol/L. If plasma sodium falls below 115 to 120 mmol/L there are adding symptoms with headache, lethargy, seizures, and coma. This is a risk identified in marathon runners (Ayes et al 2000).
- Avoid circular pressure in the arm with arteriovenous (AV)-fistula/graft. The blood pressure should not be measured in that arm because of risk to strangle and destroy the important blood flow to the access.
- Before surgery of AV-fistula/graft it is important to perform endurance training of the muscles in the forearm and the hand. This may increase the size of the vena cephalica which is valuable. During a short period after the surgery the patient should not use watches, bracelets or carry heavy bags which may hamper the blood flow in the important AV access. Training the arm with squeezing a soft ball could be important to increase the blood flow in the vein. This makes the AV-fistula more strong and useful. Shoulder and elbow move ability should be alerted and the arm/hand could be used for easier house and family work. Depending on the surgeon's prescription and the status of the patient it may be valuable to start strength training after 3-4 weeks to maintain muscular fitness.
- Patients with central dialysis catheters (CDK) on the neck or frontal thorax may start training of muscle and motility. If the sutures cause pain or prevent movements in the neck/shoulder, the physician is consulted for possible adjustment. Considering the risk of infection the patient with CDK is not allowed to exercise in a pool.

6. Nutrition and exercise

Nutrition is a most important issue in CKD patients. Before start of dialysis many patients have protein restricted diet. This has to be changed as soon as dialysis treatment is initiated. The protein intake has instead to be increased. Both the dialysis process and the physical activities need proteins and amino acids. We usually calculate the PCR = protein catabolic rate every month in the dialysis patients based on urea determinations before and after dialysis session and urea before the next dialysis. The patients could get feedback on their protein intake and add protein supplements if needed.
Carbohydrates are important to refill the glycogen stores in the liver and the muscles. The more glycogen, the more energy is available for the exercise. It is considered that 5-7 g/kg/day on training days are needed. If we eat too much more fat is stored instead.

Fats are needed, in the first hand, the essential fatty acids. But any fat to get the important energy balance is important.

Fruit and vegetables are recommended to sportsmen and sportswomen. However, due to risk of hyperpotassemia and high water content in fruits, caution is needed for patients in dialysis. The patients should have lists from dieticians to find the most proper fruits.

Vitamins are needed. Especially C-vitamins since they are removed at hemodialysis or hemofiltration (Fehrman-Ekholm et al 2008). D-vitamins are needed for the skeleton and in treatment of secondary hyperparathyroidism. Iron is necessary in anemia treatment and today most patients have intravenous iron supply at dialysis sessions.

General recommendation is to eat often and to eat after the exercise to fill up the glycogen stores again.

In co work with other team members the physical therapist works to motivate the patient to continue exercises for the rest of life. Regular check-ups by physiotherapist with knowledge of renal medicine and transplant medicine are of greatest importance to maintain maximal physical performance whatever CKD treatment the patient has. We also know that there are several national guidelines that include exercise training and physical activity as part of the treatment for problems that are common in patients with CKD, i.e. high blood pressure, hyperlipidemia and cardiovascular diseases. Within renal care and -medicine we spend a lot of time trying to find ways to optimise the outcome of the care that is given to our patients. But there is already an easy, low-tech intervention that has multiple advantages for these patients' health and well-being, but which hasn't been implemented as a part of the standard care for patients with CKD: Exercise training and physical activity in daily living! Another question is if aerobic exercise and strength training starting early in renal disease could play an important role in prevention or progression of CKD (Moinuddin et al 2008).

7. Conclusion

- The physical fitness is severely reduced among adults with haemodialysis treatment
- Physical exercise programs should be initiated with gentle start and preferably non-dialysis days or before dialysis treatment
- Exercise training including various programs improves aerobic capacity, muscular strength and endurance, physical functioning, physical- and psychological well-being if the program is regular and monitored
- Exercise training has positive effects on the cardiovascular risk profile, oxidative stress and inflammation
- Exercise training improves protein intake (PCR), dialysis effects (KT/V), haemoglobin and the endothelial function which are important treatment parameters in hemodialysis patients.

We need to encourage our patients with CKD to get more physically active and to start exercising. We need to refer them to physiotherapists with special knowledge in renal medicine that can give them adequate, individually adapted exercise recommendations.

8. References

Ayus JC, Varon J, Arieff AI. Hyponatremia, cerebral edema, and noncardiogenic pulmonary edema in marathon runners. Ann Intern Med 2000; 132:711

Bohannon RW, Hull D, Palmeri D. Muscle strength impairments and gait performance deficits in kidney transplantation candidates. Am J Kidney Dis. 1994 Sep;24(3):480-5.

Borg G. Perceived exertion as an indicator of somatic stress. Scandinavian J Rehabilitation Medicine 1970;2:92.

Brodin E, Ljungman S, Hedberg M, Sunnerhagen KS. Physical activity, muscle performance and quality of life in patients treated with chronic peritoneal dialysis. Scandinavian journal of urology and nephrology. 2001 Feb;35(1):71-8.

Cheema BS, Abas H, Smith B, O'Sullivan AJ, Chan M, Patwardhan A, Kelly J, Gillin A, Pang G, Lloyd B, Berger K, Baune BT, Fiatarone Singh MA. Investigation of skeletal muscle quantity and quality in end-stage renal disease. Nephrology (Carlton). 2010 Jun;15(4):454-63.

Cheema BS and Singh MA. Exercise of training in patients receiving maintenance hemodialysis: a systematic review of clinical trials. Am J Nephrol 2005; 25: 352-364.

Cheema BS, Abas H, Smith B, O'Sullivan AJ, Chan M, Patwardhan A, Kelly J, Gillin A, Pang G, Lloyd B, Berger K, Baune BT, Fiatarone Singh MA. Effects of resistance training during hemodialysis on circulating cytokines: a randomised controlled trial. Eur J Appl Physiol 2010 Dec (Epub ahead of print).

Clyne N, Jogestrand T, Lins LE, Pehrsson SK, Ekelund LG. Factors limiting physical working capacity in predialytic uraemic patients. Acta medica Scandinavica. 1987;222(2):183-90.

Cupisti A, Capitanini A, Betti G, D´Allesasandro C and Barsotti G. Assessment of habitual physical activity and energy expenditure in dialysis patients and relationships to nutritional parameters. Clin Nephrology 2011; 75:218-25.

DePaul V, Moreland J, Eager T, Clase CM. The effectiveness of aerobic and muscle strength training in patients receiving hemodialysis and EPO: a randomized controlled trial. Am J Kidney Dis. 2002 Dec; 40(6):1219-29.

Fehrman-Ekholm I, Lotsander A, Logan K, Dunge D, Odar-Cederlöf I and Kallner A. Concentrations of vitamin C, vitamin B12 and folic acid in patients treated with hemodialysis and on-line hemodiafiltration or hemofiltration. Scand J Urology and Nephrology 42: 74-80, 2008.

Fiatarone M, Marks E, Ryan N, Meredith C, Lipsitz L et al. High intensity strength training in nonagenarians. Effects on skeletal muscle. JAMA 1990; 263; 3029-34.

Fukuhara S, Lopes AA, Bragg-Gresham JL, Kurokawa K, Mapes DL, Akizawa T, et al. Health-related quality of life among dialysis patients on three continents: the Dialysis Outcomes and Practice Patterns Study. Kidney Int. 2003 Nov;64(5):1903-10.

Goldberg AP, Geltman EM, Hagberg JM, Gavin JR, 3rd, Delmez JA, Carney RM, et al. Therapeutic benefits of exercise training for hemodialysis patients. Kidney International. 1983 Dec; 16: 303-9.

Guarnieri G, Toigo G, Situlin R, Faccini L, Coli U, Landini S, et al. Muscle biopsy studies in chronically uremic patients: evidence for malnutrition. Kidney international. 1983 Dec;16: 187-93.

Heiwe S & Jacobson H S. Effects of regular exercise training in adults with chronic kidney disease – a Cochrane Collaboration meta-analysis. In publication 2011.

Heiwe S, Abrandt-Dahlgren M. Living with chronic renal failure: coping with physical activities of daily living. Advances in Physiotherapy. 2004;6:147-57.

Heiwe S, Clyne N, Dahlgren MA. Living with chronic renal failure: patients' experiences of their physical and functional capacity. Physiother Res Int. 2003;8(4):167-77.

Heiwe S, Clyne N, Tollback A, Borg K. Effects of regular resistance training on muscle histopathology and morphometry in elderly patients with chronic kidney disease. American journal of physical medicine & rehabilitation / Association of Academic Physiatrists. 2005 Nov; 84(11):865-74.

Johansen KL, Shubert T, Doyle J, Soher B, Sakkas GK, Kent-Braun JA. Muscle atrophy in patients receiving hemodialysis: effects on muscle strength, muscle quality, and physical function. Kidney Int. 2003 Jan;63(1):291-7.

Jones D, Round J. Skeletal muscle in health and disease. Manchester: University Press 1990.

Kettner-Melsheimer A, Weiss M, Huber W. Physical work capacity in chronic renal disease. The International journal of artificial organs. 1987 Jan;10(1):23-30.

Klitgaard H, Mantoni M, Schiaffino S, Ausoni S, Gorza et al. Function, morphology and protein expression of ageing skeletal muscle: a cross-sectional study of elderly men with different training backgrounds. Acta Physiol Scand 1990; 140:41-54.

Kouidi E, Albani M, Natsis K, Megalopoulos A, Gigis P, Guiba-Tziampiri O, et al. The effects of exercise training on muscle atrophy in haemodialysis patients. Nephrol Dial Transplant. 1998 Mar;13(3):685-99.

Kraemer WJ, Ratamess NA. Hormonal responses and adaptations to restistance exercise and training. Sports Med 2005;35; 339-61.

Kramer J, Stone M, O´bryant H et al. Effects of single vs multiple sets of weight training: impact of volume, intensity, and variation. J Strength Cond Res 1997;11: 143-147.

Lazarus R, Folkman S. Stress, Appraisal, and Coping. New York: Springer 1984.

Lok P. Stressors, coping mechanisms and quality of life among dialysis patients in Australia. Journal of advanced nursing. 1996 May;23(5):873-81.

Marlowe E. Rehabilitation concerns in the treatment of patients with chronic renal failure. American journal of physical medicine & rehabilitation / Association of Academic Physiatrists. 2001 Oct;80(10):762-4.

McIntyre CW, Selby NM, Sigrist M, Pearce LE, Mercer TH, Naish PF. Patients receiving maintenance dialysis have more severe functionally significant skeletal muscle wasting than patients with dialysis-independent chronic kidney disease. Nephrol Dial Transplant. 2006 Aug;21(8):2210-6.

McMahon LP, McKenna MJ, Sangkabutra T, Mason K, Sostaric S, Skinner SL, et al. Physical performance and associated electrolyte changes after haemoglobin normalization: a comparative study in haemodialysis patients. Nephrol Dial Transplant. 1999 May;14(5):1182-7.

Moinuddin I, Leehey DJ. A comparison of aerobic exercise and resistance training in patients with and without chronic kidney disease. Adv Chronic Kidney Dis 2008; 15: 83-89

Molsted S, Eidemak I, Sorensen HT, Kristensen JH. Five months of physical exercise in hemodialysis patients: effects on aerobic capacity, physical function and self-rated health. Nephron Clin Pract. 2004; 96(3): 76-81.

Nielens H, Lejeune TM, Lalaoui A, Squifflet JP, Pirson Y, Goffin E. Increase of physical activity level after successful renal transplantation: a 5 year follow-up study. Nephrol Dial Transplant. 2001 Jan;16(1):134-40.

Nilsen T, Hermann M, Eriksen CS, Dagfinrud et al. Grip force and pinch grip in adult population: Reference values and factors associated with grip force. Scand J Occup Ther 2011 Feb 28 (Epub ahead of print).

Pagels A, Heiwe S, Hylander B. Nutritional status and handgrip strength in pre-dialysis patients. Journal of Renal Care. 2006;XXXII:151-55.

Painter P, Messer-Rehak D, Hanson P, Zimmerman SW, Glass NR. Exercise capacity in hemodialysis, CAPD, and renal transplant patients. Nephron. 1986;42(1):47-51.

Painter PL, Hector L, Ray K, Lynes L, Dibble S, Paul SM, et al. A randomized trial of exercise training after renal transplantation. Transplantation. 2002 Jul 15;74(1):42-8.

Pechter U, Ots M, Mesikepp S, Zilmer K, Kullissaar T, Vihalemm T, et al. Beneficial effects of water-based exercise in patients with chronic kidney disease. International journal of rehabilitation research Internationale Zeitschrift fur Rehabilitationsforschung. 2003 Jun;26(2):153-6.

Pecoits-Filho R, Heimburger O, Barany P, Suliman M, Fehrman-Ekholm I, Lindholm B and Stenvinkel P. Associations between circulating inflammatory markers and residual renal function in CRF patients. American Journal of Kidney Diseases. 2003 Vol 41, 6: 1212-1218.

Ritz E, Boland R, Kreusser W. Effects of vitamin D and parathyroid hormone on muscle: potential role in uremic myopathy. The American journal of clinical nutrition. 1980 Jul 33(7):1522-9.

Sakkas GK, Ball D, Mercer TH, Sargeant AJ, Tolfrey K, Naish PF. Atrophy of non-locomotor muscle in patients with end-stage renal failure. Nephrol Dial Transplant. 2003 Oct;18(10):2074-81.

Sakkas GK, Sargeant AJ, Mercer TH, Ball D, Koufaki P, Karatzaferi C, et al. Changes in muscle morphology in dialysis patients after 6 months of aerobic exercise training. Nephrol Dial Transplant. 2003 Sep;18(9):1854-61.

Sonn U, Frändin K, Grimby G. Instrumental activities of dailys living related to impairments and functional limitations in 70-year-olds and changes between 70 and 76 years of age. Scand J Rehabil Med 1995;27: 119-28.

Thompson CH, Kemp GJ, Taylor DJ, Ledingham JG, Radda GK, Rajagopalan B. Effect of chronic uraemia on skeletal muscle metabolism in man. Nephrol Dial Transplant. 1993;8(3):218-22.

van Vilsteren MC, de Greef MH, Huisman RM. The effects of a low-to-moderate intensity pre-conditioning exercise programme linked with exercise counselling for sedentary haemodialysis patients in The Netherlands: results of a randomized clinical trial. Nephrol Dial Transplant. 2005 Jan;20(1):141-6.

Venkataraman R, Sanderson B, Bittner V. Outcomes in patients with chronic kidney disease undergoing cardiac rehabilitation. American heart journal. 2005 Dec;150(6):1140-6.

Welch JL, Austin JK. Factors associated with treatment-related stressors in hemodialysis patients. ANNA journal / American Nephrology Nurses' Association. 1999 Jun;26(3):318-25; discussion 26.

Yao Q, Pecoits-Filho R, Lindholm B, Stenvinkel P. Traditional and non-traditional risk factors as contributors to atherosclerotic cardiovascular disease in end-stage renal disease. Scandinavian Journal of urology and nephrology. 2004;38(5):405-16.

Zamojska S, Szklarek M, Niewodniczy M, Nowicki M. Correlates of habitual physical activity in chronic haemodialysis patients. Nephrol Dial Transplant. 2006 May;21(5):1323-7.